LIBRARY
HOLY CROSS JUNIOR COLLEGE
NOTRE DAME, INDIANA

D1258408

Building

the

Health Bridge

Selections from the Works of
Fred L. Soper, M.D.

In a world that is haunted by fear and torn by hate, public health can be one of the rallying points of unity. It can be one more bridge across the political and ideological gulfs that divide mankind. Health is something that all nations desire, and no nation by the process of gaining it takes it away from another. There is not a limited supply of health for which nations must compete. Rather, every nation by promoting its own health adds to the better health of other nations, just as by assisting in the public health efforts of other nations it protects itself.

Raymond B. Fosdick, 1945

BUILDING

THE

HEALTH BRIDGE

Selections from the Works of
FRED L. SOPER, M.D.

Edited by
J. AUSTIN KERR, M.D.

Indiana University Press
Bloomington   London

LIBRARY
HOLY CROSS JUNIOR COLLEGE
NOTRE DAME, INDIANA

614.4
S712b

Copyright © 1970 by Indiana University Press
All rights reserved

*No part of this book may be reproduced or utilized in any
form or by any means, electronic or mechanical, including
photocopying and recording, or by any information storage
and retrieval system, without permission in writing from
the publisher. The Association of American University
Presses Resolution on Permissions constitutes the only exception to this prohibition.*

Published in Canada by Fitzhenry & Whiteside Limited,
Don Mills, Ontario

Library of Congress Catalog Card Number: 78-77804
Standard Book Number: 253-31295-7
Manufactured in the United States of America

Contents

*The asterisks indicate that excerpts only of the paper have been included.
†The numbers in parentheses are those assigned to the papers in the Bibliography.

Foreword

An alternative subtitle of this volume of "Selections from the Works of Fred L. Soper" might well be "Reports and Discussions on the Eradication of Infectious Diseases in Various Parts of the World, 1924–1967" by Fred Lowe Soper and his associates and collaborators. Most of the biological, demographic, and scientific investigations and the practical field work were carried out by Dr. Soper while he was a staff member of the Rockefeller Foundation's International Health Division.

The book is composed of reproductions of selected publications on the subject of eradication and related problems. During the period of the indicated 43 years Dr. Soper published 123 "papers." Of these, 45 were selected for inclusion in this volume—some in full; some short transcriptions of remarks made at medical, scientific, or administrative meetings; some long enough to be considered monographs. Overcoming difficulties and the hardships of campaigning against diseases, and making new knowledge available by discoveries, Dr. Soper conducted effective enterprises of epidemiology and public health. He did this in small villages and in great cities, in counties and states, in islands and continents, in hemispheres of the earth, and in areas of global dimensions. In all his writings, such as those included in this volume, is heard the authentic voice of an original, forceful, courageous, and indomitable man—a scientist, philosopher, administrator, strategist, and humanitarian.

The proposal for the publication of selections from the papers of Dr. Fred L. Soper came from the Indiana University Press in a letter written February 22, 1967. This letter explained that the Indiana University Press "has been planning a small series of books in which are collected the papers, essays, and reviews of eminent American scientists in the fields of medicine and public health," and that the Press would hope that Dr. Soper as a creative scientist in the field of epidemiology would consider preparing such a volume. After due consideration, and because he had in his possession, as a result of his habitually thorough "bookkeeping," a practically complete set of his publications, Dr. Soper accepted the invitation of the Indiana University Press and agreed to furnish the material for this book.

Fortunately, Dr. Soper secured as Editor, to assist him in the preparation of this volume, his close friend and collaborator in disease eradication, J. Austin Kerr, M.D., formerly a member of the staff of the International Health Division of The Rockefeller Foundation. Dr. Kerr met Dr. Soper first in Northeast Brazil in January 1928, in connection with the control of yellow fever. During the next 41 years, to October 1968 (and to continue thereafter in another phase of joint literary work), Dr. Soper and Dr. Kerr were associated from time to time and in one way or another in work on yellow fever and malaria in Brazil, Central America, Colombia, and Mexico, with excursions in Paraguay and to places of concern to the Pan American Health Organization (PAHO) and the World Health Organization (WHO). They had common interests in the attempts to eradicate malaria vectors in Sardinia and Egypt. From 1947 to 1951 Dr. Kerr was concerned with studies of influenza and of arboviruses at laboratories of the International Health Division (IHD) at New York and in Berkeley, California. Both men were prominently engaged at various times in investigations of insecticides, particularly DDT, for species eradication of *Aëdes aegypti* in yellow fever, and for the attack on various anopheline mosquito vectors of malaria. Dr. Kerr has contributed to this volume in an important degree. In intimate association with Dr. Soper at the National Library of Medicine, he assisted in making the Selections and in editing them. He is the author of the Introduction, which is not only a comprehensive summary and analysis of each paper included in this volume but is also a detailed and deeply interesting biography of Dr. Soper. To Dr. Soper, Dr. Kerr, and Mrs. Minnis N. Coe is due appreciation for the compilation of Dr. Soper's bibliography.

The Selections are presented in twelve parts under titles that indicate their content in general terms. These titles, gathered in the table of contents, form the material for a rapid survey of the whole volume. They appear to be in order in a time series, but they could not be so consecutively arranged. As publications in one field were sometimes delayed, and as activities of various kinds intermingled irregularly with the issuance of papers and reports, editorial compromises had to be made between chronology and subject matter. On the whole, however, the progression from observations to philosophical ideas and public health administration moves in a logical course which is clearly charted in Dr. Kerr's introduction. A recapitulation with brief commentary follows.

Dr. Soper's first assignment under the International Health Board of the Rockefeller Foundation was to work on ancylostomiasis in a period when the control of hookworm disease was a major program of the Foundation. In this undertaking, he spent approximately six years in the field, from 1920 to 1927, in administrative work and investigations, first in Northeast and South Brazil and later in Paraguay.

He found that the most important factors which influence the choice of an anthelmintic for field work are efficiency, toxicity, and ease of administration. Oil of chenopodium and carbon tetrachloride, separately or in mixture, were used effectively, but the long-term reduction of infestation depended upon the introduction and use of the sanitary privy.

In a cognate investigation in the newly developed science of comparative helminthology, Dr. Soper added information on the ethnological significance of the ratios of *Ancylostoma duodenale* and *Necator americanus* found in the Lengua Indians living in the Gran Chaco Paraguayo. He was prompted to this study by Dr. S. T. Darling, who had stated in 1920: "The races of mankind, living in tropical and subtropical regions, are infested with one or more species of hookworms. In the migrations of these peoples the immigrants have carried their peculiar species of hookworms into regions occupied by people having a different worm-species-content, and by an examination of the intestinal worms of a people, the geographical and ethnic origin of their hosts can, within certain limits, be divined." The correlation of Dr. Soper's *Ancylostoma/Necator* ratio of 13:1 among the Lengua Indians in Paraguay with the distribution of hookworms by races and geographical areas indicated that "the original Amerind race origi-nated in Asia or Indonesia, north of latitude 20° N" and that migrations to America were either through the Pacific or via Bering Strait. This paper is full of interesting history and folklore in addition to observations on tech-nical helminthology. It has a distinctly Darwinian flavor.

The extinction or extirpation of certain species of mosquitoes for the control of yellow fever and malaria, with a view to eventual eradication of these diseases, in accordance with the extensive programs of The Rocke-feller Foundation, as visualized by Mr. Wickliffe Rose and others, has been the driving motivation of Dr. Soper's greatest efforts and the chief setting of his monumental accomplishments during the years 1927 to 1947. These efforts and their results are described and discussed with relation to *Aëdes aegypti* and yellow fever in Parts II, III, IV, V, VI, and VIII; with relation to *Anopheles gambiae* in malaria in Northeast Brazil and Egypt and *Anopheles labranchiae* in malaria in Italy and Sardinia in Parts VII, VIII, and XI. The Selections from Dr. Soper's papers reproduced in these parts are full of detailed descriptions of the public health campaigns waged by him in collaboration with entomological, epidemiological, and demograph-ical experts of various nationalities, thousands of assistant workmen, with cooperative financial and administrative (and even legislative) support by foundations and governments. The work was unremitting. The latest knowledge of insecticidal preparations was applied. Developed were new phases of epidemiological investigations, made possible by the introduction of serological surveys for protective antibodies in yellow fever and by the examination of tens of thousands of specimens of liver tissue obtained by viscerotomy for the postmortem removal of pieces of liver from persons dying of an acute febrile illness—an indispensable method for the discovery of cases of yellow fever. A potent and safe vaccine against yellow fever was developed, tested, and widely used.

As for results, Dr. Soper has been able to write about malaria as "a disap-pearing disease," because it has been eradicated in large areas in the Americas, Europe, and Asia. Attesting to this possibility was the rapid disappearance of malaria following the suppression of the person-to-person transmission of this disease by the eradication of *Anopheles gambiae* in Brazil in 1940 and in Egypt in 1945—brilliant feats which convinced even the most ardent believers in the immortality of species that this modern species had been eradicated in these countries like the dodos and dinosaurs of the past. But species eradication of vectors of malaria is not generally feasible; what is needed is species eradication of the plasmodia of malaria. It was the discovery of the long-lasting residual properties of DDT and other insecticides when used inside human habitations that made it possible to plan the interruption of malaria transmission and thereby its eventual eradication without eradicating the anopheline vectors.

Yellow fever is a different story. Urban yellow fever, transmitted by *Aëdes aegypti,* has been eradicated in Brazil and the Americas by eradicating the mosquito vector. *Aëdes aegypti,* however, has not yet been eradicated from the United States and hence remains a threat here as it does in India. For complete elimination of this species in all the Americas, the cooperation and effort of the United States is needed.

The discovery of jungle yellow fever (1932–1935), basically a disease of monkeys transmitted by forest mosquitoes, as a source of virus for the reinfection of cities infested with aegypti, made it obvious that yellow fever could not be eradicated from the world. With regard to this, Dr. Soper wrote in 1960: "The yellow fever eradication program is the most magnificent failure in public health history," because yellow fever persisted in the forest animals of Africa and South America, in an environment and under conditions in which neither the virus nor its vector could be reached by the arm of extermination.

Descriptions of principles and methods of control of louse-borne epidemic typhus fever, and of yaws, tuberculosis, and smallpox, are presented in Parts IX, and XII. From the delineation of problems of eradication in these diseases a general principle emerges to the effect that in each eradication situation there are numerous distinctive elements. The problems of each situation must be studied and understood and appropriate procedures applied for control, prevention, and eradication. It is confidently expected that smallpox will be eradicated within a few years.

Among the principles of eradication of disease on a continental or global scale the mechanisms for cooperation of individuals and agencies are shown to be of cardinal importance for mounting a concerted attack. A number of imperatives for such collaboration and coordination are described and discussed in Part X which deals with international health administration. For this discourse Dr. Soper has drawn on his experiences with the World Health Organization and the Pan American Sanitary Bureau, of which latter he was Director. The ten positions in public health organizations occupied by Dr. Soper from 1920 to 1968 are listed at the end of the Introduction. They bear witness to the validity of his discussions and advice on health administration.

Dr. Soper's essay, "The Philosophy of Eradication," in Part VIII contains selections from papers written in 1942, 1952, 1960, and 1965 (actually written in 1959). In these papers both a personality and a point of view unfold. They are the expressions of both development and maturity. He points out that the eradication concept as applied to communicable diseases and disease vectors means permanent nonrecurrence in the absence of all preventive measures, unless reintroduction occurs. He points out further that the conception of eradication had to await the recognition of the specificity of communicable diseases and the demonstration of means of prevention. Local and national eradication of communicable diseases of animals began in the last decades of the nineteenth century. This was accomplished by the ruthless slaughter of infected animals and herds and by strict quarantine of "eradicated" areas. As human beings could not be slaughtered in the veterinary manner, nor could strict embargoes on the movement of persons from one area to another be enforced, the eradication of communicable diseases of man had to await the development of effective nonlethal preventive measures and the creation of an international mechanism for the coordination of national and regional campaigns in a global effort.

According to the records, the period between the late 1920s and early 1930s was this century's low point in acceptance of the eradication concept. Failures caused loss of faith in the concept. Control took the place of eradication. But the situation has changed since then. In Selection 33 Dr. Soper notes a number of events which have spurred the rehabilitation of the eradication concept. Dr. Soper, in paper *106* of the Bibliography has listed "ten milestones on the way back," substantially as follows:

1. The eradication of the Mediterranean fruit fly from Florida, 1930–1931.

2. The observation in 1933 that the *Aëdes aegypti* mosquito, the vector of urban yellow fever, could be eradicated.

3. The eradication, in 1940, of *Anopheles gambiae* from Brazil—Africa's worst malaria vector, which had invaded Brazil in 1930.

4. The eradication of *Anopheles gambiae* from Egypt, 1944–1945.

5. The introduction of DDT in World War II, and the development of malaria eradication programs in Italy, Venezuela, British Guiana, and the United States.

6. The Pan American Sanitary Bureau's program, beginning in 1947, for the eradication of *Aëdes aegypti* from the Western Hemisphere for the elimination of the threat of urban yellow fever.

7. The action of the XIIIth Pan American Sanitary Conference (1950) approving programs for the eradication of yaws, smallpox, and malaria.

8. The Pan American Sanitary Conference's (1954) reinforcement of the malaria eradication program, with a budget for its proper administration.

9. The approval, in 1955, of malaria eradication as a global interest of UNICEF and the World Health Organization.

10. The widespread acceptance of the concept of eradication in malaria campaigns in the principal malarious countries of the world, outside of Africa, south of the Sahara.

Reviewing the past and estimating the future, Dr. Soper has written that "eradication is neither easy nor cheap; it is most difficult and expensive, requiring a type of coverage and careful administration not dreamed of in most public health programs. In disease control programs the public health officer may protect as many individuals as possible with available funds, generally in the most accessible section of the population for which he is responsible. Eradication, on the other hand, represents a complete change in philosophy and a recognition of the equal rights of all citizens to protection from infection, no matter where they live. Eradication, by its very nature, is public health with a conscience. The public health control officer can sleep tranquilly, salving his conscience with the thought that most of his responsibility has been discharged—that he did not have enough money to do any more. The eradicator knows that his success is not measured by what has been accomplished but, rather, is the extent of his failure indicated by what remains to be done. He must stamp out the last embers of infection in his jurisdiction. His slogan must be: ANY IS TOO MANY."

Stanhope Bayne-Jones, M.D.
Brigadier General, USAR, Retired
Consultant in Medical Research to
The Surgeon General, United States Army

Washington, D.C.
April 1969

Introduction

The type and scope of the varied activities of Dr. Soper during his long career in public health are indicated by the titles of the twelve parts comprising this book. He is perhaps best known for his enunciation and support of the policy of disease eradication. This activity derived from the successes in the eradication of two widely different mosquito species in Brazil. But the organization, financing, and administration of an eradication operation is such a difficult and complex task that one needs to consider how the process developed.

An eradicationist has to be a judicious perfectionist; so a look at Dr. Soper's tendencies is in order, starting with his university training. He entered the Universty of Kansas of 1910, three months before his seventeenth birthday, and decided after his second year there that he would study medicine. He received his A.B. degree in June 1914, after which he interrupted his studies for a year to earn the money he needed to attend medical school. His early bent toward research is revealed by his decision to obtain a Master of Science degree in embryology in the Anatomy Department of the medical school. The content of his master's thesis is not included herein but is summarized in paper *4* of the Bibliography.

The experience gained in obtaining his Master of Science degree under an inspiring teacher, George E. Coghill, provided him with a sound background in the scientific method. This background was to be very important in his later work.

Fred Lowe Soper was born on December 13, 1893, the third of eight children of Socrates John and Mary Ann Soper. All the children were born and grew up in Hutchinson, Kansas, at a time when life in the prairie country of central Kansas was still strongly influenced by the spirit of the frontier.

To earn the money needed to pay for his education, young Mr. Soper sold books and stereoscopic slides during summer vacations and also throughout two school years. Twenty years later, when Dr. Soper recounted some of his youthful adventures in various parts of the Prairie States, he often ended by saying that the experience he gained in meeting people while selling stereoscopes had been invaluable in his professional career.

The boy was father to the man in regard to salesmanship—for Dr. Soper devoted much effort to "selling" the public health projects in which he eventually became involved. The sales to The Rockefeller Foundation, to governments, and to international organizations involved the funding to initiate new pioneering projects and to support ongoing ones. Sales to his peers in the investigation and control of a number of important diseases involved the preparation of many of the published papers included herein. It was evident to his associates that Dr. Soper enjoyed selling and that he was good at it.

The material presented in this book shows that Dr. Soper possessed the three talents needed for success in pioneering public health projects. First, he had the competence needed to carry out meticulous laboratory research himself and the wisdom to support his colleagues who were doing such research. Second, he rapidly developed the entrée and prestige required to obtain the government funds, in amounts that were relatively large for the time and place, needed for the support of the programs he was heading. Third, he had the vision and energy to inspire his colleagues and staff to perfect the organization needed to make good use of the newly discovered facts and the newly devised techniques.

We may now return to biographical data. After completing the first two years of medicine at the University of Kansas Medical School at Lawrence, Kansas, young Soper transferred to Rush Medical College, which was then the medical school of the University of Chicago, graduating in 1918. His final years in medicine were somewhat irregular because of the demand for doctors created by World War I; he spent the year of 1919 as an interne at the Cook County Hospital in Chicago.

On January 2, 1920, immediately after finishing his internship and marrying Miss Juliet Snider at Fort Scott, Kansas, Dr. Soper reported for duty with the International Health Board of The Rockefeller Foundation. After all of three weeks of intensive training in parasitology at the recently established School of Hygiene and Public Health of Johns Hopkins University, Dr. Soper sailed for Brazil, accompanied by Mrs. Soper. Dr. Soper was assigned to work on hookworm disease, first in Northeast Brazil and later in South Brazil. This was in the era when hookworm control was a major Foundation activity, directly beneficial for its effect on hookworm disease and indirectly useful in creating popular interest in public health and in promoting the development of permanent official agencies for the control of preventable diseases.

Part I. Hookworm Infestation: Investigation, Control, and
          Ethnological Implications

After his first tour of duty in Brazil, Dr. Soper spent one academic year at the Johns Hopkins School of Hygiene, receiving the Certificate in Public Health in 1923. This degree was a precursor to the present Master of Public Health. In 1925 he received the degree of Doctor of Public Health from Hopkins in absentia.

Dr. Soper's second tour of duty was in Paraguay, where he organized and directed the cooperative hookworm control program, jointly financed by

the Government of Paraguay and the International Health Board, which
continued for five years.

Seven papers resulted from Dr. Soper's six years of hookworm work,
1920–1927. One of these (6, in the Bibliography), not included here, dealt
with the pioneering use of marginal punch cards for the analysis of hookworm survey data. This paper is more than a description of some gadgetry;
it foreshadows Dr. Soper's later insistence on the need for efficient "bookkeeping" on the results of the public health work that was being carried
out. This concept was of prime importance in the administration of the
Aëdes aegypti control operations in later years.

Part I comprises three Selections: 1 and 2 deal with the investigation and
control of hookworm disease, and 3 deals with the ethnological significance
of the hookworm parasites of the Lengua Indians in the Paraguayan Chaco.
These papers grew out of research projects that Dr. Soper carried out along
with his administrative duties as chief of nationwide hookworm programs.

In 1927, at the age of 33, Dr. Soper was transferred to Rio de Janeiro as
Representative of the International Health Division of the Foundation,
responsible for supervising its programs in Argentina, Brazil, and Paraguay. This supervision did not at first include the technical aspects of the
program for the "eradication" of yellow fever. This program, believed to
be in its terminal stages, was directed by an experienced yellow fever
worker of the Foundation's staff.

The other programs included hookworm control, malaria control, nursing education, public health nursing services, medical education, and
county health programs. The selection and training of public health workers through fellowships was an important activity.

Part II. Vector Eradication in the Prevention of Aëdes aegypti-
Transmitted Yellow Fever in the Americas:
Worldwide Implications

All Dr. Soper's papers published in the years 1924–1928 dealt with
hookworm disease, and none of his later papers did. In Parts II through
XII the selection of papers has required much compromise between chronology and subject matter. Part II contains papers published between 1934
and 1966, and Part V, the largest of all the parts, covers 1932 to 1964.

The chronological order of presentation is a bit unfortunate in Part II
because Dr. Soper's first contact with Aëdes aegypti and with yellow fever
had occurred in 1920 but is not recounted until 1963, in Selection 9. My
own first contact with the disease in Brazil occurred in 1926, during my
first tour of duty with the Foundation. The difference between the operating methods of the Foundation-supported aegypti-control program of that
day and of the highly efficient Cooperative Yellow Fever Service of 1937 is

not fully or adequately documented in any of Dr. Soper's published papers.

One of the yellow fever experts of the Foundation who was working in Brazil in the early days told Dr. Soper that he believed in having his men get out and work and not spend their time writing reports. The utter and complete contrast between this orientation and Dr. Soper's concept of making the inspectors' reports as certifiable as a bank balance is evident. It was my good fortune to have been able to observe both concepts in operation. Needless to say, it required the efficient execution of the latter concept to eradicate aegypti.

In June 1930 Dr. Soper was placed in full charge of The Rockefeller Foundation's cooperative yellow fever control activities in Brazil, which were being conducted only in North Brazil. Because of the importance of yellow fever in Brazil at that time almost all of the Foundation's other activities in Brazil had been terminated.

In December 1930 the Cooperative Yellow Fever Service was made responsible for the yellow fever program in all of Brazil except the city of Rio de Janeiro, then the national capital. The responsibilities of the cooperative service became nationwide on January 1, 1932 when the operations in Rio de Janeiro were entrusted to it. The wave of jungle yellow fever discussed in Part V obliged the national service to extend its operations to the southernmost states of Brazil; it absorbed the yellow fever service of the State of São Paulo in 1938.

The very incomplete and inaccurate epidemiological picture of yellow fever as it was known in 1920 is contrasted in Selection 4 with the much more accurate picture that had been established by 1933. Although jungle yellow fever had been identified in 1932, its epidemiology was still far from clear in 1933.

The methods that led to the eradication of aegypti in a number of Brazilian cities as early as 1933—long before the advent of DDT—are summarized in Selection 5.

The eradication of aegypti requires the discovery and the elimination or treatment of all the breeding places of the species. Vitally important was the discovery of hidden residual breeding places, after the initial reduction of aegypti infestation had been accomplished.

"Adult capture," or the search for adult aegypti that were resting inside houses, was the procedure that proved to be of crucial importance in the discovery of the residual breeding places. This procedure provided a cross-check on the results of the search for aegypti larvae. The distribution of the captured aegypti adults usually made it possible to pinpoint the location of the hidden breeding place, such as an abandoned cistern, within a radius of 25 yards.

When I first heard of this procedure in Nigeria in 1931 I thought it was a crazy idea, as did most of the colleagues who were working in Brazil. But

Dr. Soper pointed out that the method gave an independent check on the presence or absence of aegypti in an area, and before long the value of the method became evident to all.

A short excerpt from a 137-page book describing the organization of the nationwide service in Brazil that had eradicated aegypti from many of the previously infested areas in the country comprises Selection 6. This service was, in the main, a creation of Dr. Soper, who provided the leadership for the large staff of Brazilian and American professionals, working under difficult conditions but effectively motivated by the cumulative success of the operations. The effort was a cooperative one in several respects: first, between The Rockefeller Foundation and the Government of Brazil; second, among the subordinate employees who responded loyally to efficient direction; and, third, to the help given by yellow fever itself. This cryptic remark is made merely to emphasize the fact that the whole of Brazil was markedly yellow fever conscious. Both the people and the doctors knew the way it could kill when the classical triad of symptoms developed: jaundice, hemorrhage, and anuria.

Dr. Soper's first proposal for the extension of aegypti eradication from the nationwide program in Brazil to the entire Western Hemisphere was made in 1942, (Selection 7). This was followed by Selection 8, written in 1947, when Dr. Soper was the newly elected Director of the Pan American Sanitary Bureau. The Bureau had just been made responsible for coordinating the hemisphere-wide aegypti-eradication campaign.

Dr. Soper recounts in Selection 9 some of his personal contacts with aegypti, beginning in 1920. Maps showing the differences in the known distribution of yellow fever in 1900 compared with 1963 in the Americas and in Africa are included in Selection 11. These show the effect of the eradication of aegypti from large areas in the Americas, counterbalanced by the recognition and diagnosis of jungle yellow fever. The fact that aegypti is a hazard not only in the Americas, but in the rest of the tropics as well, is pointed out in Selection 10, which contains two maps: one shows in detail the status of the aegypti eradication campaign in the Americas; the other gives the distribution of the reported cases of dengue fever—transmitted by aegypti—during the extensive epidemic of that disease that occurred in the Caribbean area in 1962–1965.

Selection 12 considers the dynamics and density of aegypti and shows the distribution of the aegypti-infested areas in the Americas as of December 1965.

Part III. Viscerotomy: The Routine Postmortem Removal of Liver
          Tissue from Persons Dying of an Acute Febrile Illness

This section documents the development of a new diagnostic procedure that was to have far-reaching effects in the clarification of the epidemiology of yellow fever. With rare exceptions epidemiologists had overlooked the fact that the histopathological lesions of yellow fever in the liver are upward of 99 per cent pathognomonic when studied by adequately trained pathologists. In 1928 it was still possible for a well-known yellow fever worker to go so far as to insist that the epidemiological findings in an isolated fatal case of yellow fever were more important diagnostically than the histopathological diagnosis on the liver.

Henrique da Rocha-Lima, a Brazilian pathologist of great competence who worked for years at the Tropical Diseases Institute in Hamburg, Germany, published a classical description of these lesions in 1912. His findings were published in a monograph in German and were documented by a superbly executed colored lithograph. (It was exciting to find the monograph, with its colored lithograph perfectly preserved, in the stacks of the National Library of Medicine, Bethesda, Maryland, during the preparation of this book.)

Unfortunately, Rocha-Lima's paper made little impression in Brazil, possibly because it was published in an era (1908–1928) during which yellow fever was quiescent in Rio de Janeiro. Diagnosed cases of the disease continued to occur during these two decades in many places in North Brazil, however.

In 1928, when Rio de Janeiro was hit by the epidemic of classical yellow fever, Prof. Rocha-Lima had just returned to São Paulo, Brazil, because he suffered severely from hay fever in Hamburg. In Rio de Janeiro there were several experienced pathologists in the Oswaldo Cruz Institute and in the national health department who soon confirmed the accuracy of Rocha-Lima's published description of the microscopic lesions in the liver tissues of fatal cases.

Thus an accepted diagnostic procedure was available by which to determine when and where people were dying of yellow fever. But the problem was to obtain the specimens of human livers upon which to make the diagnoses and to do so in a vast inland rural area with a very low ratio of doctors to population.

The fact that doctors could do a partial autopsy, removing only a small piece of liver, was not a satisfactory solution, because of the very restricted distribution of practicing doctors and the difficulty of getting them to do autopsies. The availability of health service physicians was even more restricted, but such personnel did obtain much useful information by doing complete or partial autopsies on cases that were brought to their attention.

The solution lay in devising some technique by which laymen could obtain the necessary liver specimens from persons who died of a febrile illness lasting ten days or less in the thousands of communities where there was no medical attention, and to do this regardless of whether or not they had received medical attention. The first requisite was a simple, safe instrument with which to obtain the liver specimen from the people who died. This necessity mothered the invention of the "viscerotome," as explained in Selection 13.

Enabling legislation was obtained for the routine collection of the liver specimens, and the channels for the shipment of the specimens from the point of origin to the Yellow Fever Laboratory in Salvador, Bahia State, were developed. The laboratory had been established in 1928 by The Rockefeller Foundation to carry out research with the newly isolated virus of yellow fever. In addition to its research activities, the laboratory performed the routine tests that were needed in the yellow fever operations, including the examination of viscerotomy specimens.

A succinct description of the histopathological lesions of yellow fever in the human liver is given in Selection 14. Viscerotomy was applied irrespective of any diagnosis that a doctor may have made; the perfected operations of the "viscerotomy service" as they were carried out in Brazil in 1937 are described in Selection 15. By that date aegypti-transmitted yellow fever had been eliminated and the importance of jungle yellow fever demonstrated.

This segment of Dr. Soper's work comprised the recognition of the value of a previously neglected histopathological phenomenon and the establishment of the administrative machinery needed to exploit its usefulness. The result, within five years, was the clarification of the epidemiology of yellow fever. Three clearly different types emerged: aegypti-transmitted urban, aegypti-transmitted rural, and jungle (of which the aegypti was not the vector).

The ability of the yellow fever service to determine when and where people were actually dying from the disease immediately placed upon the service the responsibility for preventing such deaths. The efficient fulfillment of the responsibility thus imposed was a continuing stimulus to the morale of the service personnel of all ranks and levels.

Part IV. Serological Studies of Human Yellow Fever in South America

The results of serological studies during a period in which the techniques of the serological tests were being developed are presented in Selections 16 and 17. This pioneering work provided part of the basis for the very extensive studies reported in Selection 18 the results of which contributed much to the elucidation of the epidemiology of the three types of yellow fever.

It was indeed fortunate that the original technique of the mouse protection test was highly specific, but not very sensitive, for if it had been more sensitive we now know that there would have been much confusion from cross-reactions with the antibodies of related arbovirus infections. It may be noted that the procedures described in the titles as protection tests have for many years been designated, more accurately, neutralization tests.

Part V. The Discovery of Jungle Yellow Fever and Studies
         of Its Epidemiology

The longest part in this book is Part V, partially because of the excite-
ment that the steadily unfolding aspects of the problem held for those of us
who participated in its study—for the discovery of a new disease was essentially what was involved. In his position as Representative in South America of the International Health Division of The Rockefeller Foundation,
Dr. Soper was favorably situated to serve as the coordinator of the studies
of jungle yellow fever in all the affected countries of South America.

Later, when Dr. Soper became the Director of the Pan American Sanitary
Bureau, he arranged for its staff to participate in studies of the 1948–1958
epidemic that spread from Panama to southern Mexico.

By great good fortune two diagnostic techniques had been perfected
prior to the discovery of jungle yellow fever: viscerotomy and the neutralization test in mice. Clinical observation and the isolation of yellow fever
virus in laboratory animals supplemented the two new diagnostic procedures and established the jungle disease as yellow fever.

Unfortunately, effective vaccination for the protection of the population
exposed to infection with the jungle virus had to wait almost five years for
the perfection of the 17D vaccine against yellow fever.

Selection 19 describes the study of a rural epidemic of fully confirmed
yellow fever in 1932 in an area without *Aëdes aegypti,* situated in a mountainous area north of Rio de Janeiro known as the Valley of Canaan (in
translation). The title describes only what was observed, and the clear
association of yellow fever with the forest was not evident during this first
episode. The fact that the aegypti mosquito was absent from the valley
itself and was well on its way to being eradicated from the coastal cities
and towns of Espírito Santo State greatly simplified the epidemiological
study.

By November 1934, when Dr. Soper delivered Selection 20 at the Pan
American Sanitary Conference in Buenos Aires, yellow fever without
aegypti had been confirmed by histopathological diagnosis in Mato Grosso
State in the center of South America, in Brazilian Amazonia, and in the
Amazonian lowlands of Bolivia. In Colombia it had been found in the
southwesternmost fringe of the Orinoco River basin and in the Valley of
the Magdalena River.

The name "jungle yellow fever" was first proposed in Selection 21, which
Dr. Soper read in Bogotá, Colombia. He presented additional viscerotomy
evidence of the presence of jungle yellow fever in the Magdalena River
Valley in that country, where serological evidence of the disease had previously been found. He also used the term "rural yellow fever" to describe
the yellow fever that had been widespread in Northeast Brazil, where

aegypti had been found breeding in four fifths of the houses of the rural population.

A summary of the epidemiology of jungle yellow fever in South America as it was known in October 1935 appears in Selection 22. This was followed by Selection 23, which is a summary for the Royal Society of Tropical Medicine and Hygiene in London of the yellow fever situation—jungle, rural, and urban—as it existed in South America in late 1938.

Those were very exciting days for the yellow fever workers in South America. The first large epidemic wave of jungle yellow fever was spreading widely in Brazil, having come down from Goiás and Mato Grosso through Minas Gerais and São Paulo to the coast around the city of Rio de Janeiro. Aegypti had been eradicated from the city and environs, so there was no possibility of the "urbanization" of yellow fever, even though some cases did come into the city. The newly available 17D vaccine was being widely used in the rural areas.

Subsequent developments with jungle yellow fever in Brazil and Panama are described in Part VIII, Selection 31. In Selection 24 of this part, the history is reviewed of the epidemic wave that crossed the Panama Canal in 1949 and spread north through Central America. This epidemic, or epizootic, wave was characterized by spectacular mortality of howler monkeys in the forest; in places the forest reeked with the stench of dead monkeys. It finally died out in southern Mexico when it reached areas in which conditions were unfavorable for its continued spread.

Part VI. Yellow Fever Vaccines and Field Studies of Vaccination

One of the more satisfying aspects of the yellow fever program of The Rockefeller Foundation was the success of its decade-long search for an effective, safe, and cheap vaccine against the disease. The Foundation staff in South America, under the leadership of Dr. Soper, played a major role in the field testing of the various vaccination procedures that became available, culminating with 17D vaccine.

The three vaccination procedures that were used before 17D virus became available are described and discussed in Selection 25, as are the first field experiments with 17D. The organization of the mass-vaccination campaign of the rural population at risk to jungle yellow fever is described in Selection 26, and the results of limited serological studies to determine the results are presented.

The three serious complications that occurred following the use of 17D vaccine prepared in the Rio de Janeiro Laboratory are discussed in Selection 27. These were the failure to immunize due to loss of antigenicity of the virus used; the sporadic occurrence of postvaccination hepatitis, attributable to the human serum used in the preparation of the vaccine; and, finally, the occurrence of postvaccination encephalitis associated with the strain of seed virus that was used to replace the one that had been contaminated with hepatitis virus.

Since 1941, when the present technique of primary and secondary "seed lots" was instituted, 17D has proved to be one of the best vaccines ever invented, on the basis of its high degree of efficacy and the low incidence of adverse reactions following its use, combined with moderate cost.

Part VII. The Eradication of *Anopheles gambiae* from Brazil and Egypt

The eradication from Brazil of *Anopheles gambiae,* the phenomenally efficient vector of malaria that had been introduced from West Africa, was favored, in retrospect, by a combination of several unusual factors. First there was the ecological vulnerability of gambiae during the dry season when its breeding places were limited almost exclusively to shallow, sunlit pools in the beds of the rivers and creeks. This made it relatively easy to find and to apply Paris green to all the potential breeding places of gambiae during six months of the year. However, the attack measures were successful even during the typical rainy season of 1940—January to June— when the number of potential breeding places for gambiae was maximal.

The species had been able to survive from 1930 until 1938 in the State of Rio Grande do Norte and had greatly extended its range to the northwest while so doing. There is no doubt that gambiae was in the Americas to stay unless its spread could be halted in Brazil in 1939.

The professional staff that formed the nucleus of the Malaria Service of the Northeast (MSNE), which was responsible for the eradication of gambiae from Northeast Brazil, under the leadership of Fred Soper and Bruce Wilson, had been transferred from the Brazilian Yellow Fever Service, where they had become thoroughly imbued with the Philosophy of Eradication. Nobody on the staff, including Drs. Soper and Wilson, was a malariologist, but they were eradicationists.

The Malaria Service of the Northeast was established by Presidential decree signed on January 11, 1939. From the first it was established as a temporary service to operate wherever *Anopheles gambiae* might be found in Brazil. At its peak of activity, the MSNE had some 4000 employees, and after the eradication of gambiae had been confirmed the Service was completely phased out. Flexibility in transferring staff from the Yellow Fever Service to the MSNE and then back from the MSNE to the YFS was most important in creating an efficient field organization and also in easing the shock of unemployment when the task of the MSNE was finished.

Other factors of importance were the recognition not only by the health authorities of Brazil, but also by its President, Getulio Vargas, that there was a grave emergency. Dr. Soper had established his reputation as an efficient and dynamic administrator, and the local people were well known for their efficient hard work when capably directed.

In January 1939 the MSNE took over the personnel and equipment and supplies of the previously established "Obras Contra A Malaria," the personnel of which then numbered about 700 and included doctors and engineers. Rapid expansion of the field operations was begun, and there were difficulties at first. These were best characterized by the comment of a famous American malariologist-consultant who said that he did not quite see how a shade-loving service could get the best of a sun-loving mosquito.

The MSNE operated for three and one-half years, continuing its surveillance operations for almost two years after the last gambiae was found. Long excerpts from the book describing the eradication operations comprise Selection 28.

Scarcely had the eradication of *Anopheles gambiae* from Brazil been verified in mid-1942 than the occurrence of a devastating epidemic of malaria, transmitted by gambiae, was reported in Upper Egypt, that is, the part of the country lying south of Cairo. Dr. Soper arrived in Egypt, quite fortuitously, in January 1943 as a member of the United States of America Typhus Commission. His advice was sought by the Egyptian Government, and after visiting the affected area he recommended measures almost identical with those that had been successful in Brazil. His suggestion that The Rockefeller Foundation be invited to collaborate in the eradication of gambiae in Egypt was not acted upon until after a second disastrous epidemic of malaria killed thousands of people in the same portion of Upper Egypt that had been desolated in 1942. In February 1944 King Farouk visited Luxor, which was in the affected area, and following that visit the invitation to the Foundation was issued. Dr. Soper was in Italy at the time, and in May 1944 he returned to Egypt and concluded the agreement under which the Foundation cooperated with government in the eradication of gambiae from Egypt. Foundation personnel directed the service, all the expense of which was borne by the Egyptian Government.

The title of Selection 29 is a bit misleading, in that Paris green will not apply itself once a week to all the potential breeding places of *Anopheles gambiae*. Such application requires an organization. Following Dr. Soper's visits in 1943, the Egyptian health authorities had established the area-wide eradication service adapted from the Brazilian organization but based primarily on the use of oil as the larvicide. Results were not satisfactory, as shown by the widespread epidemic of fatal malaria that occurred in the fall of 1943. But the basic organization was invaluable after a Rockefeller Foundation staff member was appointed Director of the Gambiae Eradication Service on July 15, 1944. Three additional Foundation staff members were eventually assigned to the project. The larvicide was changed from oil to Paris green as quickly as possible, and gambiae did not survive the winter of 1944–1945, the last individual having been collected on February 19, 1945. Although the winters in Egypt are much colder than in Northeast Brazil, gambiae had survived the two previous winters.

Once again the vulnerability of gambiae to attack with Paris green was its undoing when this insecticide was properly applied during an adequate length of time.

The brief excerpt, Selection 29, is Dr. Soper's only published statement regarding his vitally important contribution to the gambiae problem in Egypt during 1943–1946, when he was the senior Rockefeller Foundation staff member in the Mediterranean area.

An interesting activity of Dr. Soper that is not covered by any published paper is his participation in the planning of the attempt to eradicate *Anopheles labranchiae* from the island of Sardinia, Italy.

Conversations in 1944 and 1945 with Mr. S. M. Keeny, Chief of the United Nations Relief and Rehabilitation Administration (UNRRA) Mission to Italy, and with Prof. Alberto Missiroli, a famous Italian malariologist, led to the creation of a quasi-governmental regional entity in Sardinia that was made responsible for the eradication of labranchiae, the species of anopheles that was responsible for the notorious malaria on the island. The entity was called ERLAAS (Ente Regionale per la Lotta Anti-Anofelica in Sardegna). There was to be an island-wide attack on both the adults and larvae of the mosquito. Major costs would be defrayed with counterpart lire derived from the sale to the Italian Government of commodities furnished by UNRRA, and Rockefeller Foundation staff would direct the program.

The ERLAAS was established by Royal Decree signed on April 12, 1946, and field operations began in the winter of 1946–1947 with the residual spraying with DDT of all the human habitations on the island, except those in the cities. Comprehensive antilarval work was carried out in the spring and summer of 1947 in the southern part of the island and in the entire island in the following summer seasons.

It proved impossible to eradicate *A. labranchiae,* but vivax and falciparum malaria were eradicated. Quartan malaria, in truly negligible amount, lingered on for many years, owing to the ability of the quartan parasite to produce relapses for a long time after a primary attack of the disease.

Part VIII. The Philosophy of Eradication

As previously mentioned, the arrangement of the parts of this book is a compromise between chronology and subject matter. Thus it is that the first Selection (30) in this part, dealing with the Philosophy of Eradication, was published in 1942, the second (31) was published in 1952, the third (32) was published in 1960, and the fourth (33) was read in 1959 but not published until 1965. In the meantime, Dr. Soper had moved from Brazil to the Mediterranean and finally to Washington, D.C., and had been the Director of the Pan American Sanitary Bureau for 12 years. That position, from which he retired in 1959, afforded him many opportunities for the application of the philosophy.

To Dr. Soper the term "mosquito eradication" means the complete extermination of the species under consideration. This concept is not to be confused with the mosquito reduction that is so widely referred to as eradication, and this is true in regard to many other insect vectors and even of pest insects that are not known to be involved in the transmission of any disease. Thus eradication is an "all-or-none" phenomenon; either you eradicate or you do not, and you do this in a geographical area of significant size.

Dr. Soper's first formal presentation of the eradication concept is Selection 30, written jointly with D. Bruce Wilson, his alter ego for species eradication. The concept developed out of the success in eradicating *Aëdes aegypti*—after the discovery of jungle yellow fever made it obvious that the disease could not be eradicated. This was followed by the success in eradicating *Anopheles gambiae,* which became evident in 1941, and which convinced the senior officers of The Rockefeller Foundation of the validity of the eradication concept. The summary of the article contains the suggestion that eradication may be feasible for aegypti and gambiae in other countries, and even for some other species under certain conditions. Some of these subsequent events have been discussed in earlier parts.

Several diseases that can be said to have elephantine memories are discussed in Selection 31. More accurately, the natural history of the various diseases contains hazards that we tend to forget in normal times but which can bring disaster if preventive measures are neglected or are impossible to carry out, as in wartime. One of these is louse-borne typhus, regarding the control of which a Rockefeller Foundation team under Dr. Soper made important contributions during World War II (see Part IX).

After describing the advantages of eradication over control, Dr. Soper mentions the newly created international agencies: Pan American and World Health Organizations. He points out in Selection 31 that these international organizations can furnish uniform technical orientation to national health services with no loss of sovereignty by any nation, and can thus provide new opportunities for implementing the philosophy of eradication. In subsequent parts, the manner in which these possibilities have been carried out are described.

At a congress of veterinary medicine, Dr. Soper discussed (Selection 32) the philosophy of eradication in relation to diseases of domestic animals and to the zoonoses—diseases of lower animals that are transmissible to man.

When Dr. Soper retired as Director of the Pan American Sanitary Bureau in 1959, after 12 years of pioneering work, the staff of the Bureau sub-scribed funds sufficient to defray the expenses of a series of lectures to be known as the Fred L. Soper Lectures. Each of the five lectures was given at a different school of public health in the Americas—Brazil, Canada, Chile, Mexico, and the United States. The first lecture was given in Octo-ber 1959 by Dr. Soper himself at the Johns Hopkins School of Hygiene and Public Health, from which he had received the degree of Doctor of Public Health in 1925.

This lecture (Selection 33) was not published until 1965; it contains a history of the development of the Philosophy of Eradication. The concept had been in limbo for many years but was due for revival because of the availability of improved technology involving new drugs and new insecti-cides.

The duplication in this paper of some material that is presented in Parts II and VII, as well as X, is explained by the difference in the viewpoint from which the material is presented. Here the information is basically conceptual or philosophical; elsewhere the emphasis is on the technologi-cal and administrative aspects.

Part IX. The Control of Epidemic (Louse-Borne) Typhus Fever by Insecticide Powders

After nearly 23 years of duty in South America, Dr. Soper left Rio de Janeiro in late 1942. After his return to the United States, he was appointed a civilian member of the newly created United States of America Typhus Commission (USATC). When the advance unit of the USATC, of which he was a member, reached Cairo, it was learned that typhus was epidemic in Egypt. It was decided that the Commission would not proceed to Iran as planned, but would establish its field laboratory in Cairo.

Early in 1943, the Director of the International Health Division of The Rockefeller Foundation, Dr. Wilbur A. Sawyer, remarked in my presence that he expected that Dr. Soper's very "peculiar" talents would be useful in studies of louse-borne typhus fever. The Foundation had been engaged for some months in studies of insecticide powders in the United States.

With great foresight, the Typhus Commission was organized in 1942 to investigate and control the rickettsial diseases, one of which, epidemic typhus, had always been one of the major scourges of war in Europe.

Dr. Soper worked as a member of the Typhus Commission in Cairo from January to June 1943. Except for time spent visiting the gambiae-infested area in Upper Egypt and in entertaining a febrile disease that was almost certainly typhus fever, he was in charge of studies on the use of louse pow-der for killing lice and preventing typhus. During this period, it was demonstrated that two applications of MYL powder (pyrethrum plus a synergist) with a 14-day interval between treatments would reduce the louse infestation of the treated individual to a low level. It was also shown that with proper organization large numbers of persons could be deloused at dusting stations in spite of the time consumed in removing the clothing of each individual for dusting. Furthermore, in a village where typhus was epidemic, the spread of the disease was radically checked following insecticidal delousing of the population.

These studies with the Typhus Commission in Egypt convinced Dr. Soper that the louse burden of a population could be drastically reduced with louse powders and that typhus outbreaks could be aborted.

In June 1943 Dr. Soper became the head of the Rockefeller Foundation Health Commission's Typhus Team with headquarters in Algiers. The team included another physician, a medical entomologist, and a bacteriologist, and equipment for laboratory studies of typhus was on hand. However, the preliminary experience with louse powder in Egypt led Dr. Soper to suggest concentrating the efforts of the team on the chemical attack on the body louse, and this was agreed to by the other members of the team. Extensive confirmatory studies on MYL powder were made and pioneering studies were done with DDT, the then-new miracle chemical which fortunately became available to the team for testing in July 1943. Especially important was the demonstration in August 1943 that effective chemical delousing of infested populations did not require the removal of clothing. The application of insecticide by mechanical dusters was found to be very effective and surprisingly easy.

The effect of MYL powder on the louse population of civilian and military prisoners and of rural populations in Algeria is reported in Selection 34. (The use of louse powder in the control of typhus fever could not be studied because the disease was not reported in Algeria during the six months the team remained there.) Studies of louse-infested prisoners demonstrated that DDT was a very effective and long-lasting chemical for delousing individuals and keeping them free of infestation.

By early October these studies had progressed to a point where it was obvious that epidemic typhus could be dominated with louse powders applied en masse to infested populations without the removal of clothing. This method received its first full-scale test in the typhus epidemic of Naples in 1943–1944.

The outbreak of typhus in Naples in 1943–1944 and its control with louse powders is described in Selection 35. The Foundation's Typhus Team worked in the prevention of typhus as part of the Allied Control Commission in Italy from December 8, 1943, until July 31, 1945. During the intervention of the United States of America Typhus Commission in the Naples typhus control program from January 3 to February 20, 1944, the Rockefeller Foundation team continued to be responsible for the mass-delousing program.

The rapid success of the Naples campaign in early 1944 led to the widespread use of DDT powder for the control of typhus in western Europe in 1944–1945; there was no serious epidemic of typhus following World War II similar to that which occurred after World War I.

Part X. International Health Administration

This part deals with a field of Dr. Soper's activities that is in marked contrast to that described in Part IX, in that purely administrative tasks supplanted the meticulous field research that had been followed by the creation of an organization to make use of the newly acquired data.

The Charter of the United Nations (December 1945) provided for the creation of associated specialized agencies. Steps to create the World Health Organization (WHO) were taken early in 1946, and it was officially established in 1948. The Constitution of WHO provides for its operation through regional organizations throughout the world.

This development stimulated the creation of the Pan American Health Organization (PAHO) in 1947, to continue the program of the Pan American Sanitary Bureau (PASB) and also to serve as the Regional Organization of WHO throughout the Americas. The preexisting PASB, with activities previously limited to programs among the American republics, became the operating agency of PAHO.

Dr. Soper was elected Director of the PASB early in 1947, at the time when the PAHO was being created. By formal agreement with the WHO in 1949, the PAHO also became the Regional Office for the Americas of the WHO.

The Pan American Health Organization is funded by separate contributions from the countries of the Americas, but the programs of the two organizations are very closely coordinated.

The governing body of the WHO is the World Health Assembly (WHA), which meets once a year for three weeks. Dr. Soper attended the First Assembly in Geneva as an observer from the PASB.

The excerpts from the Official Records of the WHO (Selection 36) deal with Dr. Soper's promotion of the immediate establishment of the Regional Organizations of the WHO.

Dr. Soper's first quadrennial review (Selection 37) as Director of PASB to its supreme Governing Body, the Pan American Sanitary Conference, contains an account of PAHO's relations with the Organization of American States and with WHO and gives a summary of the diverse activities of PASB during the first four years of expanding activity.

The last quadrennial review (Selection 38) that Dr. Soper submitted to the Pan American Sanitary Conference during his 12-year tenure of office is an exposition of the continuously expanding field of international health and the growth of the program, particularly as related to the prevention of communicable diseases.

Comparison of the first and last quadrennial reports reveals the change in nature and the great expansion of international health work in the Americas in the intervening years. An important development in 1958, the last year of Dr. Soper's tenure but not covered by the 1954–1957 quadrennial report, is the extensive use of live oral poliomyelitis vaccine. Late in 1957 the Pan American Sanitary Bureau became involved in pilot studies of poliomyelitis vaccination in Minneapolis. Beginning in May 1958, PASB sponsored and participated in the vaccination of more than 150,000 children in Colombia; in September of the same year, more than 50,000 children were similarly vaccinated in Nicaragua. In each country vaccination was initiated in the face of an active outbreak of paralytic poliomyelitis.

These field trials of oral vaccine were important because of the reluctance of other responsible authorities to sponsor similar field trials. When Dr. Soper reported the Colombian experience to the Eleventh World Health Assembly (1958), the World Health Organization dissociated itself from the program, emphasizing that it was an independent activity of PAHO. (A summary of the discussion at the Assembly is to be found in paper F in the Addendum to the Bibliography, but it is not included herein.)

Discussion of Dr. Soper's contributions to international health administration would not be complete without mention of his activities in his last three positions listed at the end of this Introduction.

In 1959–1960, Dr. Soper served as a Consultant to the International Cooperation Administration (ICA), the quondam name of the agency that administers the foreign aid program of the United States. His work dealt mainly with assistance the agency was giving to the global malaria eradication campaign, then in its heyday.

In 1960–1962, Dr. Soper, for the first time in his long career, accepted a position in the Far East. He was named Director of the Pakistan-SEATO Cholera Research Laboratory at Dacca, East Pakistan, in the heartland of Asiatic cholera, which had been established to carry out comprehensive studies of cholera in a highly endemic area. Dr. Soper's task was to free the laboratory of local bureaucratic procedures and to establish it as a viable international entity which could carry out long-term coordinated field and laboratory investigations. Dr. Soper's experience as representative of The Rockefeller Foundation in developing long-term field and laboratory studies of yellow fever in the countries of South America was not applicable to work with cholera in Asia. Instead he turned to his more recent experience in the modern era of international health organizations. The Institute of Nutrition of Central America and Panama (INCAP) is the pioneering model of a regional entity organized, under the aegis of the Pan American Health Organization, to permit Panama and the countries of Central America to collaborate freely in the study and solution of their common problems in nutrition. Modifying somewhat the INCAP structure, an acceptable formula was found by which the Cholera Research Laboratory was established as an international agency administered by a small international governing body. The original participating countries were Pakistan, the United Kingdom, and the United States.

Since 1962 Dr. Soper has served as a Special Consultant, Office of International Health, Public Health Service. In this position he has been able to follow the progress and the vicissitudes of the continental campaign for the eradication of *Aëdes aegypti* in the Americas and to participate in discussions of the role of this mosquito as the vector of hemorrhagic dengue in Asia.

Part XI. The Eradication of Malaria: Local, Continental, Global

The importance of Dr. Soper's contributions to the eradication of malaria makes it proper to devote a separate section to that subject.

The story starts in Natal Province, South Africa, in 1935, where Dr. Soper saw malaria control based on weekly space spraying of native homes with pyrethrum to kill infected mosquitoes.

The story continues in Algiers, in the summer of 1943, when Dr. Soper noted that intoxicated house flies kept on falling for many weeks into the soup from the ceiling of the dining room of the billet of the Typhus Team after a single spraying of a solution of DDT in kerosene. He reasoned that if DDT residues would continue to kill mosquitoes day and night for a long period, it would be much more effective in the prevention of malaria than the periodic killing of mosquitoes with pyrethrum. And, much more important, it should be sufficiently economical to justify its use to control rural malaria.

The story continues the following year in Italy. As the typhus epidemic in Naples waned dramatically in the early weeks of 1944, the Rockefeller Foundation Health Commission was invited, while continuing to work on typhus, to undertake the study of how to use DDT most effectively in the prevention of malaria among the Allied troops in Italy.

The invitation was accepted, and a Malaria Control Demonstration Unit of the Allied Control Commission was created to carry out the projected studies. In addition to collaborating in testing the airplane spraying of DDT as a larvicide, a study of the effect of DDT applied to the interior surfaces of human habitations was planned. The study at Castel Volturno, near Naples, began in the spring of 1944; it is believed to be the first practical field test of DDT as a residual wall spray for community-wide malaria control. This study continued in 1945; it was supplemented that year by an extensive and most valuable study in the Tiber Delta area near Rome. The observation by Prof. Alberto Missiroli that malaria transmission had been completely interrupted in this area, where he had studied malaria for many years, led him to plan for and eventually to execute the eradication of malaria in Italy. The results of the studies on residual DDT in Italy are set forth in Selection 39.

These and similar results obtained in other countries by other workers in the following years made it apparent that the new antimalaria measure was so highly effective that one could dream of eradicating malaria, not only from local areas but even from an entire continent, specifically the Americas. The rationale of this program as set out in Selection 40 comprises the progress from a series of isolated nationwide programs to a coordinated continental one.

In the same year, 1950, the XIIIth Pan American Sanitary Conference called upon the Pan American Sanitary Bureau, of which Dr. Soper was the Director, "to provide for greatest intensification and coordination of antimalaria work in the Hemisphere . . . with a view to achieving the eradication of malaria from the Western Hemisphere."

Little came of this mandate, and in 1954 the XIVth Pan American Sanitary Conference reiterated its instructions and made funds immediately available for a planning office for malaria eradication. The regional malaria eradication campaign in the Americas can be said to date from this action.

Immediately after his retirement as Director of the Pan American Sanitary Bureau in 1959, Dr. Soper made a trip to the Far East and observed the operations of a number of national malaria-eradication programs, which he reported in Selection 41. The global malaria-eradication campaign had been approved in 1955 by the Eighth World Health Assembly, and the campaign was in full swing in most of the malarious countries of the world except Communist China and the countries of tropical Africa. The results were generally encouraging, but the serious difficulties that existed in verifying that malaria incidence had, in fact, been reduced to very low levels had not yet been recognized.

The problem of the resistance of anopheles mosquitoes to DDT had been recognized and dire consequences were feared. Subsequent events have revealed that the phenomenon was of relatively slight overall importance. And it had not been generally recognized that the striking successes with DDT had been obtained where the malaria was transmitted by anopheline vectors that rested on the inside walls of human habitations. By and large, these were the only vector species that were amenable to successful attack by the residual spraying of DDT in human habitations.

Nevertheless, the overall decline in the incidence of malaria in the population of the huge areas under attack was heartening, and the optimistic forecasts are entirely understandable.

Selection 42 deals with the relationship of the "public health infrastructure" of a country to its national malaria eradication program. To those who maintain that the former is a prerequisite for a successful outcome of the latter, Dr. Soper points out that malaria—and other diseases as well—have been eradicated in several countries that did not have the widespread network of rural health units that comprise a true public health infrastructure.

Part XII. Disease Eradication: Yaws, Tuberculosis, Smallpox

The pioneer yaws eradication campaign in Haiti, which began in 1950, is described in Selection 43. The eradication method was the single injection treatment with penicillin of all cases and their immediate contacts—an entirely different modus operandi from the methods used for eradicating malaria. The incidence of the disease was high in Haiti, and in spite of many difficulties the program progressed well until a very low incidence was reached. Thereafter, a variety of administrative difficulties made it impossible to find and cure the last few infectious cases; lately there has been a considerable percentage increase in the incidence to levels that would be tolerated in a control operation but are not acceptable in an eradication campaign. Although eradication has not been achieved, the results of this program have been well worthwhile.

The essentials for eradication of tuberculosis in the United States are discussed in Selection 44; it contains a number of concepts that were provocative and refreshing to those responsible for the present antituberculosis work in the United States. These efforts are so highly fragmented in the health departments of our states, counties, and municipalities that the concept of a "national" eradication entity is logical.

The eradication of smallpox is discussed in Selection 45; the campaign is based on the use of vaccine to produce herd immunity against a disease that is acute and self-limited. This eradication procedure is very different from those used with malaria and yaws.

The feasibility of the global campaign is attested by the successful results of numerous national and regional smallpox eradication programs in many different parts of the world. These data fully justify the conclusion that the only thing that prevents the eradication of the disease from the world is the failure to immunize an adequate percentage of the people in the countries that still have smallpox. These countries are all developing countries, and great difficulties are known to exist in the distribution of the vaccine and in its actual administration. Nevertheless, the campaign appears to be based on sound data that are adequate in amount, and the expected results justify the low per capita cost when the total cost is apportioned to the population of the entire world, not merely to the people in the countries involved.

A final consideration is that epidemic smallpox is easy to diagnose, and an outbreak in most countries would be cause for great alarm and for the immediate vaccination of the population at risk. Vitally important is the fact that surveillance and maintenance measures would be relatively inexpensive and simple to provide.

During his half century of work in public health, Dr. Soper has held the ten positions listed below; they provide a vignette of his varied career:

Staff Member of the International Health Board (Division) of The Rockefeller Foundation, 1920–1950 (Associate Director, 1945–1950).

Representative in South America (Rio de Janeiro Office) of the International Health Division of The Rockefeller Foundation, 1927–1942.

Member of the Rockefeller Foundation Health Commission, 1942–1946.

Representative of the International Health Division of The Rockefeller Foundation for Africa and Middle East, 1946.

Director of the Pan American Sanitary Bureau (Pan American Health Organization,) 1947–1959.

Regional Director for the Americas of the World Health Organization, 1949–1959.

Director Emeritus of the Pan American Sanitary Bureau, 1959–.

Consultant to the International Cooperation Administration of the United States, 1959–1960.

Director, Pakistan-SEATO Cholera Research Laboratory, 1960–1962.

Special Consultant, Office of International Health, Public Health Service. 1962–.

Dr. Soper has been decorated by seven countries: Cuba (1940), Brazil (1942 and 1966), the United States of America (1944), Egypt (1947), Colombia (1959), the Dominican Republic (1960), and Venezuela (1960); he has been honored with eight awards or medals: Lasker Award (1946), Theobald Smith Gold Medal (1949), Kansas University Distinguished Service Citation (1949), Pan American Health Organization Gold Medal (1959), Pan American Medical Society Gold Medal (1962), Samuel J. Crumbine Medal (1964), Sedgwick Memorial Medal (1966), and the Léon Bernard Foundation Medal and Prize (1967); and he has received two honorary degrees: Doctor of Science from Jefferson Medical College (1955) and Doctor Honoris Causa from the University of Brazil (1963).

Washington, D.C.
April 1969

Building
the
Health Bridge

Selections from the Works of
Fred L. Soper, M.D.

Part I | Hookworm Infestation: Investigation, Control, and Ethnological Implications

Selection 1 | Factors Which Should Determine
the Selection of an Anthelmintic
in a Geographical Area*

The most important factors which influence the choice of an anthelmintic for field work are efficiency, toxicity, ease of administration, and cost of the standardized drug. Special local conditions which may affect one or more of these factors are the degree and character of the local hookworm infestation; the degree of infestation with other parasites, especially *Ascaris;* the alcoholic habits of the people; the distribution of population; the presence of malaria; and the character and aim of the local campaign. *Ancylostoma* is notoriously more resistant to chenopodium and thymol than is *Necator.* The same has been reported for carbon tetrachloride. Fatal cases of intoxication have been reported in children harboring *Ascaris* and treated with carbon tetrachloride. Carbon tetrachloride has been found to be toxic for alcoholics. Where the population is widely scattered the necessity of dividing the dose and administering a delayed purge may easily double or treble the cost of administration. A local campaign based on the dispensary plan may be able to use a method of treatment which would not be suitable for house-to-house campaigns. If the end sought is a rapid reduction of soil pollution, an anthelmintic with selective action against females might be chosen in preference to one with selective action against males. The presence of malaria is probably of importance only if beta-naphthol is the anthelmintic under consideration, when the toxicity may be enhanced.

Work in recent years has practically reduced the choice of an anthelmintic for field work to oil of chenopodium, carbon tetrachloride, or a combination of these.

The writer in January 1924 faced the problem of selection of an anthelmintic for field work in an area where, with a high known rate of infestation, the degree and character of hookworm infestation was unknown; where the *Ascaris* rate (percentage of population infested) was calculated at 5 per cent; where alcohol is widely and freely used; where the popula-

* This report is based on experimental and field work carried out as a part of the campaign against hookworm disease in Paraguay, conducted with the financial cooperation of the International Health Board and the Republic of Paraguay. Dr. Soper was a staff member of the International Health Board of The Rockefeller Foundation.

This article was first published (*5 in the Bibliography*) in the *American Journal of Hygiene 5:* 408–453, 1925. (About 35 pages of the original text have been omitted, including 17 tables and 10 figures.)

3

tion is largely rural; and where the program of the local campaign called for the treatment of all families in their homes. After reviewing the then-available published reports of the use of carbon tetrachloride and oil of chenopodium, a 3:1 mixture of these drugs in adult dosage of 2.4 cc, with delayed purge of magnesium sulfate after 2 hours, was adopted as the standard treatment for hookworm disease in the Campaña Sanitaria of the Republic of Paraguay. This standard treatment has since been altered to a 2:1 mixture of carbon tetrachloride and oil of chenopodium in an adult dose of 2.4 cc, with simultaneous purge of magnesium sulfate in concentrated solution. This report is based on the carefully controlled experiments which led to this change of treatment for Paraguayan conditions.

Several tests of anthelmintic efficiency have been proposed, based on worm counts and microscopical examinations; but by far the most important measure of efficiency for field work, where the objective is the maximum reduction of human infestation and soil pollution in the minimum time, is the average percentage of all hookworms present removed by first treatment, as determined by subsequent "test treatment" of 3 cc of oil of chenopodium. Many recent workers have taken the percentage of "cures," as determined by microscopic reexamination, as a measure of equal value, and others consider it the only valid measure of efficiency.

Total anthelmintic efficiency will depend upon individual efficiencies for male and female *Necator* and male and female *Ancylostoma* and the incidence of each of these forms in the total worm population. As noted above, *Ancylostoma* is more resistant to anthelmintics than is *Necator*. Females of both species are more resistant than are males of the same species to the action of chenopodium. On the contrary, the female *Necator* is less resistant than the male is to carbon tetrachloride. Sawyer failed to find such selectivity for this drug with *Ancylostoma*. In the use of maximum doses, the study of individual species and sex selectivity is relatively unimportant, as such selectivity tends to disappear as the dose of anthelmintic is increased. But where it is desired to employ the minimum dose for effective results, a careful study should be made of such selective action of the drugs employed, as well as the species character of the worm population.

Although it is interesting and important to know the percentage efficiency of subsequent treatments with the same anthelmintic, the first treatment efficiency rate is the important factor to be considered in the choice of anthelmintic for field work today. With the development of more effective methods of treatment, the so-called "mass treatment" method has been widely adopted, and second and subsequent treatments, always more difficult to administer than first treatments, have rapidly diminished. The International Health Board, in cooperation with various governmental agencies, administered during the year 1923 717,191 first treatments and but 269,806, or 37.6 per cent, second treatments. The importance of first-treatment efficiency is clear.

However, it must be remembered that the character as well as the degree of infestation may be altered by previous treatments with anthelmintics of species and sex selectivity, and probably with all anthelmintics, through removal on first treatment of immature and nonresistant individuals. Smillie found that "worms resistant to first treatment are resistant to the second also" (using a mixture of carbon tetrachloride and oil of chenopodium). It has recently been suggested that the *Necator/Ancylostoma* ratio of a geographical area may be altered through campaigns of selective medication. Thus it may be found advantageous to use a different anthelmintic for follow-up campaigns from that used in the preliminary campaign.

Polyparasitism, especially where *Ascaris lumbricoides* is the offending organism, is an important problem in field work. The expulsion of *Ascaris* in quantity is a visual demonstration of anthelmintic efficiency of great popular appeal and not to be ignored. Lambert attributes fatalities in children treated with carbon tetrachloride to *Ascaris* intoxication and reports that no cases have occurred after combining an ascaricide with this anthelmintic.

Extensive use of an anthelmintic in field work has proved a more delicate test of toxicity for the human host than has the study of controlled groups, which of necessity are small. Lambert treated over 40,000 cases before encountering a fatal case of intoxication with carbon tetrachloride. A wider margin of safety must be allowed for field work than for private or hospital practice.

Oil of chenopodium is particularly toxic for children under 9 years of age and should not be administered to severe heart and kidney cases or to menstruating or pregnant women. Well-nourished individuals seem to resist intoxication better than do undernourished ones. A high carbohydrate diet protects against intoxication with oil of chenopodium *in human subjects*. A similar protective influence against liver destruction is exerted by the administration of a high carbohydrate diet to dogs for several days preceding the administration of carbon tetrachloride. Fats and alcohol when given with carbon tetrachloride greatly increase its toxicity for dogs.

Hall, taking advantage of the work of Macht and Finesilver, who demonstrated that the simultaneous administration of a concentrated solution of magnesium sulfate with many drugs causes a reduction in the amount of such drugs absorbed into the blood from the intestine, administered simultaneously carbon tetrachloride and magnesium sulfate to dogs without any apparent reduction in the anthelmintic action of this drug. Lambert adopted this method for field work and reports decreased toxicity with no decrease in anthelmintic efficiency. Soper showed by worm counts that the simultaneous administration of a concentrated solution of magnesium sulfate with a mixture of carbon tetrachloride and oil of chenopodium caused no reduction in efficiency but a marked delay in the time of expulsion of worms.

The simultaneous administration of the purge should not only reduce the toxicity of the anthelmintic but should markedly increase the number of treatments which can be given by a force in the field.

Any attempt to establish systematic therapeutic measures for hookworm disease must be based on drugs of known standard anthelmintic action and toxicity. Carbon tetrachloride is a simple chemical product, easily purified and relatively cheap. Oil of chenopodium, purchased by the International Health Board, is now being sent to the field with a statement of the ascaridol content of the particular lot shipped. That purchased during 1925 ranged from 68.5 to 78.7 per cent ascaridol.

Scope of the Study

The object of the experiments on which the present report is based was the determination of the optimum safe dose and method of administration of carbon tetrachloride, oil of chenopodium, or a combination of carbon tetrachloride and oil of chenopodium, for field work in the Republic of Paraguay. It is hoped that the presentation of the original data and the analysis of the efficiency rates are such that the findings may be of value in any geographical area *where the character and degree of hookworm infestation is known.*

This report is limited to the following points:

1. Degree and character of Paraguayan helminthological infestation.

2. Comparison of experimental species and sex efficiencies, as influenced by choice of anthelmintic, dosage, and method of administration.

3. Comparison of Willis' flotation, Stoll's egg-count, and Darling's worm-count methods as measures of anthelmintic efficiency.

4. Discussion of toxicity in controlled groups and in field campaign.

The *Necator/Ancylostoma* ratio is much lower than was anticipated. In Puerto Rico, where the ethnic stocks are Spanish, Negro, and Amerind, no *Ancylostoma duodenale* occurs, and in Brazil, among natives of Portuguese, Negro, and Indian descent, the *Necator/Ancylostoma* ratio is more than five times as great. The ethnic stocks of Paraguay are Spanish and Amerind. The occasional traces of Negro descent noted in the population are said to have had their origin in the Brazilian occupation following the Paraguayan War, as there was never any important importation of Negro slaves.

Local authorities claim that hookworm disease did not exist in Paraguay before the Brazilian occupation. If it be true that hookworm disease in Paraguay is entirely due to postwar infestation, the only possible explanation of present findings is that Paraguayan conditions are so much more favorable to the spread of *Ancylostoma duodenale* than to the dissemination of *Necator americanus* that the *Necator/Ancylostoma* ratio has been greatly altered since the supposed original infection 60 years ago.

That hookworm disease was not entirely absent from Paraguay in early colonial days is indicated by the occurrence of the word "pyseboí" in the Guarani (Indian)-Spanish dictionary prepared by Antonio Ruiz de Montoya, a Jesuit priest, and published in 1639 A.D., 104 years after the founding of Asunción by the Spaniards. Montoya translates "py-seboí" as "itching or irritation of the feet," and the word is currently used today to designate "ground itch." Strangely enough, the analysis of the compound word "py-seboí" ("py"—foot, "seboí"—worm) suggests that the aborigines had an inkling of biological facts not established by helminthologists until some centuries later.

The probable explanation of the character of hookworm infestation encountered today is that there has existed in Paraguay an infestation with *Ancylostoma* since early Spanish colonial days, and that on this has been superimposed a Brazilian infestation, largely of *Necator*.

Although the *Necator* problem is of the greatest importance in Paraguay, there is a sufficiently high *Ancylostoma* infestation to justify its consideration in the selection of the anthelmintic for field work.

Summary and Conclusions

1. Four hundred and nineteen cases were treated with carbon tetrachloride, oil of chenopodium, or a combination. Efficiency rates of such treatments were calculated for species and sex on the basis of percentage removed by first treatment, as tested by the administration of 3 cc of oil of chenopodium.

2. The average hookworm infestation among Paraguayan soldiers and prisoners is high; among boys and girls of the asylum a much lower degree of infestation exists. Seven per cent of 82,856 hookworms classified were *Ancylostoma duodenale*. The present ratio between *Ancylostoma* and *Necator* is probably due to three factors: early introduction of *Ancylostoma* by Spanish colonists, the absence of Negro slaves, and the occupation of Paraguay by the Brazilian army with its known heavy *Necator* infestation, following the Paraguayan war.

3. *Ascaris* infestation in Paraguay is relatively low (11.7 per cent), being but one fourth that of *Trichuris* (43.4 per cent). No judgment of the relative value of the anthelmintics used as ascaricides can be made from the present study. The efficiency of all combinations used is low for *Trichuris*.

4. Correction of total efficiency rates for distribution of worm population by species and sex of each group failed to cause more than a 2.5 per cent difference in such rate of any group. Correction of species efficiency rates for equal sex distribution caused no appreciable difference in *Necator* rates, where the number of worms was relatively large; a maximum change of 3.3 per cent occurred in certain groups in *Ancylostoma* rates where the number of worms was small.

5. Oil of chenopodium and carbon tetrachloride both possess a species and sex selective action on *Necator* and *Ancylostoma*. Both are more active against *Necator* than against *Ancylostoma*. Oil of chenopodium is more efficient for males than for females; carbon tetrachloride is more efficient for females than for males. The decreasing order of resistance is as follows:

Oil of chenopodium	Carbon tetrachloride	2:1 combination
Female *Ancylostoma*	Male *Ancyclostoma*	Female *Ancylostoma*
Male *Ancyclostoma*	Female *Ancylostoma*	Male *Ancyclostoma*
Female *Necator*	Male *Necator*	Male *Necator*
Male *Necator*	Female *Necator*	Female *Necator*

6. The species selectivity of both oil of chenopodium and carbon tetrachloride is greater than the sex selectivity. The selectivity of oil of chenopodium for males is more marked with *Ancylostoma* than with *Necator,* whereas the selectivity of carbon tetrachloride for females is more marked with *Necator* than with *Ancylostoma*. A 3:1 mixture of carbon tetrachloride and oil of chenopodium has slightly less oil of chenopodium than is necessary, in the dosages used, to overcome the female selectivity of carbon tetrachloride in *Necator,* but somewhat more than is required for the same purpose with *Ancylostoma*.

7. Simultaneous administration of concentrated magnesium sulfate with combinations of carbon tetrachloride and oil of chenopodium, such as used in this study, delays the expulsion of worms but does not impair the ultimate anthelmintic result. The larger the dose of carbon tetrachloride administered with simultaneous purge, the larger is the percentage of worms expelled in the first 24 hours. Oil of chenopodium gives a delayed expulsion in comparison with carbon tetrachloride.

8. One and a half cubic centimeters of a 2:1 mixture of carbon tetrachloride in undivided dose and with simultaneous purge of magnesium sulfate in concentrated solution gave very high efficiency for *Necator*. This dosage should be sufficient for treating lightly infested areas where *Ancylostoma* does not occur. Areas with heavy infestation of *Necator* should never require a larger adult dose than 2.5 cc of this combination.

9. The best results were obtained for *Ancylostoma* with 2.8 cc of a 9:5 mixture of carbon tetrachloride and oil of chenopodium (1.8 cc carbon

tetrachloride and 1.0 cc oil of chenopodium). From a study of the efficiency curve a dosage of 3.5 cc of a 2:1 combination would be required to give the same efficiency for *Ancylostoma* as is secured for *Necator* with 2.4 cc. This dosage is probably above the limit of safety for field work but should be applicable to controlled institutional groups. Further controlled groups are required to determine the proper combination and dosage of carbon tetrachloride and oil of chenopodium for maximum efficiency for *Ancylostoma* within limits safe for wide application in the field.

10. The Willis flotation method is not a safe criterion of efficiency of anthelmintic action.

11. The Stoll egg-count method gave the same percentage total reduction in hookworm infestation in 150 cases following trial treatment, as did the more laborious worm-count method.

12. The worm-count method was shown to be superior to the Willis and Stoll methods as a means of diagnosis of the presence of hookworm. The method is *indispensable for the determination of the degree and character of infestation* and the study of *sex and species selectivity of anthelmintics.*

13. No serious toxic symptoms were noted in 419 cases of this series. The maximum doses administered were 3 cc of oil of chenopodium; 2.4 cc carbon tetrachloride; and 2.8 cc of a 9:5 mixture of carbon tetrachloride and oil of chenopodium.

14. Five serious (two fatal) cases (four alcoholics and one child with heavy *Ascaris* infestation) have been encountered in 36,000 treatments with an adult dose of 2.4 cc of 3:1 and 2:1 combinations of carbon tetrachloride and oil of chenopodium.

15. Pregnant women may be treated with moderate doses of carbon tetrachloride without danger.

Selection 2 | Comparison of Stoll and Lane Egg-Count Methods for the Estimation of Hookworm Infestation*

Following the publication of Stoll's original work on a dilution method for estimating the number of hookworm eggs contained in 1 gram of feces, high hopes were entertained by many that an easy, reliable method of estimating the degree of group hookworm infestation had been developed. Further work by Stoll and by others of the Cort group seemed to confirm these hopes.

Lane, however, not only attacked Stoll for having ignored antecedent work of his in estimating the egg content of feces but also published data to show the unreliability of the Stoll method. After comparing a number of control methods, among them a *modified* Stoll technique he concluded: "The individual count obtained by this technique (*Lane's modification of the Stoll method*) has given no guide to the true ovum content of the feces. It has proved *most definitely the least reliable method* of control yet advocated."

Davis, working in a lightly infested area, and making Stoll counts on a 1-day's stool, per case, and calculating the *EPDP* ♀ and *EPGP* ♀ from worm counts, made under *field conditions,* came to the conclusion "that a combination of direct smears and the Willis brine flotation method gives sufficiently reliable data for routine inspection and treatment campaigns." That is, he failed to find the Stoll method of real value in the field.

Following the publication by Maplestone of results showing a lack of correlation between egg counts as made by the Stoll salt "concentration" and culture methods, Dr. G. K. Strode suggested to the writer in September 1924 a comparative study of the Stoll and Lane techniques. The present paper gives the results of such a comparative study, based on work done at Asunción, Paraguay, between June 1 and November 1, 1925; a later

* This report is based on experimental work carried out as part of the cooperative program against hookworm disease in the Republic of Paraguay, financed by the International Health Board and the National Department of Health of the Republic of Paraguay. Dr. Soper was a staff member of the International Health Board of The Rockefeller Foundation.

This article was first published (7) in the *American Journal of Hygiene 6* (*Suppl.*): 62-102, 1926. (About 37 pages of the original text have been omitted, including 16 tables and 17 figures.)

paper will present the correlation of these results with the degree of infestation, as disclosed by the worm-count method.

SUMMARY AND CONCLUSIONS

1. Between-spin stirring of the contents of the Lane tube is necessary to secure complete egg counts.

2. The Lane count must be "pushed to finality" to be of value as a measure of the number of eggs present; this requires so much time that the method is not practical for field surveys.

3. The Lane "pour-off" removes objectionable *substances from certain stools,* thus increasing the visibility of the eggs.

4. There is a limit to the effective concentration of hookworm eggs by the Lane method.

5. The Stoll suspension does not secure an even distribution of eggs; the frequency distribution of repeated counts on two tubes indicates that variations in count follow the normal curve of random sampling and tend to be compensatory. In lightly infested cases the *actual error in the estimated number* of female worms present should be small, whereas in heavily infested cases, the *percentage error in the estimated number* of female worms should be small.

6. The Stoll method is greatly inferior to the Lane method as a measure of the *rate of infestation* in groups containing lightly infested individuals.

7. From the data of this study, it is believed that average Stoll counts are as reliable as average Lane counts for estimating the *average degree of infestation* of groups containing *lightly infested individuals* and are probably superior for the same purpose in groups containing *heavily infested individuals.* The comparative value of the two methods will depend to a certain extent on the percentage of stools of the type mentioned in 3 and the degree of infestation.

8. Egg-per-gram values are less variable than are daily stool weights, but egg-per-gram counts cannot be blindly accepted as measures of hookworm infestation in individual cases.

Selection 3 | The Report of a Nearly Pure
Ancylostoma duodenale Infestation
in Native South American Indians
and a Discussion of Its
Ethnological Significance*

Few contributions of the late Dr. S. T. Darling are of more fundamental interest than those touching the ethnological significance of various *Ancylostoma/Necator* ratios found in different parts of the world. What proved to be a posthumous publication of his was concerned with some of the possibilities inherent in comparative helminthology in the solution of certain ethnological problems. Earlier he had stated a principle as applicable to comparative hookworm infestations:

> The races of mankind, living in tropical and subtropical regions, are infested with one or more species of hookworms. In the migrations of these peoples the immigrants have carried their peculiar species of hookworms into regions occupied by people having a different worm-species-content, and by an examination of the intestinal worms of a people, the geographical and ethnic origin of their hosts can, within certain limits, be divined. I refer particularly to migrations within 35° N. and 30° S. latitudes, for when migrations are made into colder climates the hookworm infection is ultimately lost through inability of the embryos to persist during the phase of their life cycle spent in the soil.

Following the reported finding of *Ancylostoma duodenale* in appreciable numbers in Paraguay, Darling requested the writer to secure data regarding the species distribution of hookworms among Indians living in the more remote parts of that country, where they would not easily become infected with *Necator americanus* from Negroes. In this paper data will be presented on the species infestation of the Lengua Indians living in the Gran Chaco Paraguayo, and attention will be called to the possible bearing of such data on the question of the origin of the Amerind race. Darling would have relished these data as another block in his world map mosaic of hookworm distribution and as an added bit of evidence in support of his theory.

* This paper is a contribution from the Department of Medical Zoology of the School of Hygiene and Public Health of the Johns Hopkins University, the data having been gathered in Paraguay under the auspices of the International Health Board of The Rockefeller Foundation, of which Dr. Soper was a staff member.

This article was first published *(9)* in the *American Journal of Hygiene 7:* 174–184, 1927.

In considering data of any kind from Paraguay, one must take account of the peculiar division of that country into two widely differing regions by the Paraguay river. That region lying on the left bank is a rolling, well-watered, agricultural, grazing, and forest district, about the size of the state of Missouri, which has supported a population of hundreds of thousands for many centuries. The original population consisted of Guarani Indians, a part of that great Tupi-Guarani stock which roamed from the Caribbean Sea to the Rio de la Plata, east of the Paraguay River. This Guarani stock has in great measure persisted and amalgamated with the Spanish, thus forming the Paraguayan race of today.

The contacts of this part of Paraguay with the outside world have been constant since the early part of the sixteenth century except for a period of about 20 years at the beginning of the nineteenth century, when, at the will of her first dictator, Paraguay became a hermit nation. From 1865 to 1870 the Triple Alliance waged a war, almost of extermination, against Paraguay. During and after this war many thousands of Brazilian troops, with a known heavy infestation of *Necator americanus,* were in the country and undoubtedly made their contribution to the hookworm picture of the survivors. The great apparent increase in hookworm disease in Paraguay following this war was so marked that local authorities attributed its existence to the presence of Brazilian troops, although from etymological considerations the existence of hookworms in Paraguay since early colonial times seems established. Classification of hookworms from Paraguay east of the Paraguay River shows a *Ancylostoma/Necator* ratio of 1:14.

That part of Paraguay lying on the right bank of the Paraguay River and known as the Gran Chaco Paraguayo is an area of unknown extent and without definite boundaries to the north and west. Of geologically recent formation, the Chaco is thought to have been the bottom of an inland sea; low-lying and flat, it suffers from both floods and droughts. Quite close to the surface is found an impermeable layer of gumbo which prevents the absorption of the rainfall; thus the rain which falls first floods the country and then drains off or evaporates rapidly. Wells sunk through this impermeable layer usually give water too salty for use. Rivers one sees on maps of this region are wide swamps during wet seasons and but dry water courses during periods of drought.

The Chaco, then, at least that part visited by the writer, is ill adapted to agriculture or to the support of a moderately dense aboriginal population depending on hunting and fishing; it has attracted neither the strong Guarani Indians nor the modern Paraguayans to take possession of it in force, and one can encounter today within a few days' ride of the Paraguay River Indian tribes whose contact with the outside world has been very limited.

The making of complete worm counts on aborigines is not easily accom-

plished, and the success of the work here reported is due to the full cooperation of all the members of the Anglican Mission at Makthlawaia, where
they have had a station since 1908, although their work in this region dates
back to 1889.

Makthlawaia, 25 or 30 leagues due west of Concepcion, is situated on
a small island lying in the center of a circular lagoon; its population consists of a few white mission workers and about 200 Indians, mostly of the
Lengua tribe, living under very primitive conditions. Some gardening
is attempted, but the principal occupation is cattle raising; some 2000 or
3000 head of cattle are to be found in the herds belonging to the Indians.

The Lengua is not considered a pure tribal type but rather a fusion of
types. The Lenguas are reputed to have come to the Chaco from the west
and to have furnished the ruling dynasties for several of the older tribes,
for example, Sugines, Tozles, and others. The Sanapaná, Carotuguis, Can-
aguatsan, Conamesma, and some others are probably derived from the
original Lenguas.

Careful worm counts were made on complete 48-hour stools of 71 Indians at Makthlawaia following treatment with either 3 cc of oil of chenopodium or with 3.5 cc of a 2:1 mixture of carbon tetrachloride and oil of
chenopodium with graduations of 1/18 dose per year of age for children.
The group treated included 8 women, 17 boys, 21 girls, and 25 men, 5 of
whom were nonresidents of the village and came from the region lying
west of Makthlawaia. The data from these nonresident cases will be
presented separately. The boys and girls studied ranged in age from 1 to 17
years; the 1-year-old child treated proved negative and has been eliminated
in the presentation of data.

Of 70 infected cases 41, or 59 per cent, harbored *Necator americanus*
and 70, or 100 per cent, harbored *Ancylostoma duodenale*. Of a total of
3217 hookworms recovered, 228, or 7 per cent, were *Necator*; 2989, or 93
per cent, were *Ancylostoma*. Table 1 shows the distribution of hookworm
infection by species in the various groups treated. All individuals examined
were infested with *Enterobius vermicularis*; no *Ascaris lumbricoides* or
Trichuris trichiura were found.

Table 1

Group	No. in Group	Percentage with *Necator*	Percentage of *Necator*	Average no. of *Necator*	Average no. of *Ancylostoma*
Men	20	85.0	10.8	7.5	62.6
Women	8	87.5	4.4	3.4	73.7
Boys	17	52.9	4.0	1.4	32.6
Girls	20	40.0	4.5	1.3	27.6
Nonresidents	5	20.0	2.4	0.2	8.0

In considering the data from Paraguay, the author wishes to call attention to the fact that the dosage of anthelmintic used was sufficient to guarantee a high percentage (probably over 95 per cent) of the number of hookworms harbored being expelled; further that *A. duodenale* is known to be remarkably more resistant to medication than is *Necator* and fails to be revealed in proper percentages in worm counts unless powerful doses have been administered. (This difference in resistance may help to explain the failure to report the existence of *Ancylostoma* in some regions where the Amerind race has fused with the white or Negro races.) The data from the Chaco are comparable with those reported for eastern Paraguay, since the same anthelmintics, the same technique, and the same assistant were employed.

None of the cases treated in the Chaco had ever received treatment for hookworm disease, which precludes the possibility of previous medication having altered the *Ancylostoma/Necator* ratio.

In Table 1, the *Ancylostoma/Necator* ratio is lower for men than for women and that for both boys and girls is approximately the same as for the women. This is interpreted to indicate that the village infestation is predominantly *Ancylostoma* and that *Necator* is a newcomer, being brought in by the men, who make occasional trips to the river for supplies for the mission, and who have had during the past 2 years some contact with Paraguayan soldiers from east of the river, known to carry a heavy hookworm infestation with a low *Ancylostoma/Necator* ratio. That a pure *A. duodenale* infestation has been introduced into the Chaco in modern times is not probable, considering the difficulty with which *Necator* is becoming established, even with much greater contact with outside sources of infection than has ever occurred in the past.

It is not surprising to find that the men carry a lighter infestation than do the women, since much of the time they are working away from the village.

The percentage of each group infected with *Necator* seems to depend on the degree of total infestation of the group rather than on the degree of *Necator* infestation in the group; data based on percentage of group infested with a given species of hookworm do not give the same impression of relative importance of the two species in the group as do data based on the *Ancylostoma/Necator* ratio of the whole group. Hill and Earle found 25 per cent of one group of 64 cases in Puerto Rico infected with *Ancylostoma,* but only 1 per cent of all hookworms present were of this species; in the present study 59 per cent of the cases harbored *Necator,* although 93 per cent of the hookworms found were *Ancylostoma.*

Smillie examined 34 Indians of the Terenos tribe, probably of the Tupi-Guarani race, living near Miranda, Matto Grosso, Brazil, close to the Paraguay River and found an *Ancylostoma/Necator* ratio of 1:57. This ratio was enough higher than that found among native Brazilians, 1:94, to suggest that the infestation had not been entirely derived from contact with Brazilians. Smillie describes these Indians as "pure-blooded semi-civilized Indians with no contact with whites or blacks although in the past there has been some communication with both Brazilians and Paraguayans," and later makes the significant statement, "They have had little contact with the whites though they fought in the Paraguayan War." This will explain the presence of *Necator americanus,* and from the present *Ancylostoma/ Necator* ratio it seems probable, without referring to historical records, that they spent the 7 years of that war with the Brazilian rather than the Paraguayan troops.

Soper has reported finding an *Ancylostoma/Necator* ratio of 1:14 in Paraguay, east of the Paraguay River, and has explained this ratio as representing a heavy *Necator* infestation, derived partially from Negro slaves, but more largely from Brazilian troops, superimposed on a light *Ancylostoma* infestation present since early colonial days. The data in Table 2 summarize the available information regarding species distribution of hookworm in native Brazilians, Brazilian Indians, native Paraguayans, and Chaco Indians. The *Ancylostoma/Necator* ratio in these groups is progressively larger as one goes from zones of greater to zones of lesser contact with Negroes.

The use of comparative parasitology in the study of species origins, of zoogeography, and of genetic relationships is relatively recent. It has been used, however, in helping solve many complex problems in a wide variety of fields. Von Ihering, working with helminths, used the distribution of entoparasites to help explain the genetic relationships of their hosts. Zschokke concluded from the relative importance of marine and freshwater entozoa in certain species of salmon that the original home of these species

Table 2

Group	Location	No. of cases	Aver-age Ancylo-stoma per case	Aver-age Necator per case	Ancylo-stoma/ Necator ratio	Percent-age of cases with Ancylo-stoma	Percent-age of cases with Necator
Brazilians	São Paulo	112	0.4	52	1:194	10	?
Terenos Indians	Matto Grosso	34	1.7	87	1:57	62	?
Paraguayans	East of River Paraguay	419	13.4	184	1:14	78	98
Lengua Indians	Chaco Para-guayo	70	42.7	3.3	13:1	100	59

was marine, although spawning now occurs in fresh water. Zschokke again used the same method in explaining the distribution of certain cestodes of the marsupial mammals. Johnston, working with trematodes of Australian frogs, called attention to the tendency of helminths to occur in faunal groups and stated the principle "that the helminths found parasitic in any particular class of host in a definite zoo-geographical region, find their nearest relatives not in that region in which themselves occur, but in the same class of host living in other zoo-geographical regions." Later Johnston extended his observations to include trematodes of mammals and birds and cestodes of marsupials, birds, and amphibia.

Kellogg, by a study, first of bird hosts and later of mammals, showed that certain ectoparasites, although less completely isolated from the effects of changing environment than are entoparasites, show much less tendency to be modified than do their hosts and hence may be used to indicate relationships between certain groups of birds or animals having common ancestry.

Metcalf called attention to the importance of studies on *Opalina* parasites of frogs in determining the geographical distribution and former migrations of *Anura* and shows that to explain the existing relationships, it is necessary to assume that there was previously a continental land connection between Australia and southern South America. The principle on which these conclusions are based is thus stated: "Having once met the conditions of parasitism and having undergone the initial modification to adapt them to the conditions of the new environment, some of their species are rather prone to persist without much further change, living as they do in a secluded, protected and remarkably uniform habitat."

Following a detailed description of present racial and geographical distributions of the two common species of hookworm, Darling pointed out the possibility of either *Necator americanus* or *Ancylostoma duodenale* or both having been introduced into the American continent from Asia, Indonesia, or Polynesia by voyagers or storm-tossed fishermen. He stated that migrations to America may have come (1) from Asia by way of Bering Strait, in which case, unless the temperature of that region in times past was warmer than it now is, hookworm infection would not be expected to persist; (2) from Asia or Indonesia by way of the Pacific, in which case either or both *A. duodenale* and *N. americanus* might persist; or (3) from Polynesia by way of the Pacific, in which case only *N. americanus* would be found. Darling concludes that

If certain tribes in America are found to be infected with *A. duodenale* as well as *Necator* this will suggest their having come to this continent via the sea from those countries in Asia where *A. duodenale* and *N. americanus* are found to be infecting the natives, i.e., Japan and China. . . . A careful hookworm survey of

existing Indian tribes may disclose the presence of more than one primitive
stock. . . .

It is interesting to note that since the above was written, Hill and Earle
have reported finding *A. duodenale* in Puerto Rico, previously believed to
have a pure *Necator* infestation, and Warren and Carr have found an
appreciable infestation with *Ancylostoma* among native Mexicans where
the ethnic stocks are white and Amerind.

As stated above, the data from the Chaco are interpreted to indicate that
A. duodenale came to this region with the Indian tribes, whereas *Necator*
is only now being introduced from outside contacts; this would, according
to Darling's theory, indicate that the original Amerind stock originated in
Asia or Indonesia, north of latitude 20°N and migrated to America via the
Pacific. Had migration been limited to Bering Strait, it must have occurred
when the temperature of that region was more favorable to hookworm
larvae than it now is, or it must have occurred from a region which was
favorable to hookworm in Asia to a favorable zone in America in less than
the maximum life span of the hookworm.

Hrdlička, from ethnological data, considers all the Amerinds to be of
Mongoloid origin and believes that a triple invasion occurred via Bering
Strait. Further helminthological studies on other isolated regions of the
Americas may reveal whether all immigrants carried the same species of
worms or not and whether all invasions were by the same route.

It is, of course, possible that both *A. duodenale* and *Necator* came to
America together and that adverse conditions of soil, climate, or mode of
life have blotted out *Necator* in certain districts or in certain tribes. All too
little is known about the comparative life histories of *A. duodenale* and
Necator. However, Smillie stated: "We were able to prove readily that
the factors of age, sex, soil, type of work and mode of life, though they
greatly affect total infection with hookworms, do not affect the relative
prevalence of *Ancylostoma* and *Necator*." Darling believed that there is no
difference between the adaptability of *Ancylostoma* and *Necator* to temperate, subtropical, and tropical climates. Nevertheless, although it is true
that under certain conditions the two species develop equally well, there
is some evidence to suggest that under adverse conditions one species may
survive and the other perish. Sawyer et al. reported finding an institutional
infestation, predominantly *A. duodenale,* in a hospital lying outside the
hookworm belt and drawing most of its patients from districts where
Necator is the predominating species. Svensson found that there is a difference between the optimum developmental temperatures of *Necator* and
Ancylostoma larvae and that larvae of *A. duodenale* live twice as long as
do larvae of *Necator* at icebox temperature.

The finding of a nearly pure infestation of *Ancylostoma duodenale* among the Indians of the Chaco must be explained in one of two ways:

1. That the *Necator* element of a mixed *Ancylostoma* and *Necator* infestation has succumbed to conditions not sufficiently adverse to eliminate *A. duodenale*. If the mixed infection was of Asiatic origin, such adverse conditions may have been encountered en route to the Chaco or may exist in the Chaco; if it was of Paraguayan origin, that is, from east of the Paraguay River, such adverse conditions must exist in the Chaco.

2. That the *Ancylostoma* infestation antedates that of *Necator,* in which case it must have come with the race from Asia or have been introduced by the early Spanish conquistadores. In the light of local conditions and the past history of the Chaco, it seems most reasonable to believe that the *Ancylostoma* infestation of the Lengua Indians existed before the advent of the Spanish and that the *Necator* now present represents a very recent importation from east of the Paraguay River. Studies must be made in other regions before the possibility of an original mixed infestation of the Amerind stock with *Necator* can be ruled out.

SUMMARY

1. Seventy Lengua Indians living under semicivilized conditions in the Paraguayan Chaco were found to have an *Ancylostoma/Necator* ratio of 13:1; this is by far the highest ratio reported for any group on the American continent.

2. The correlation of this finding with the species distribution of hookworms by races and geographical areas indicates that the Amerind race originated in Asia or Indonesia, north of latitude 20°N; that migrations to America were either through the Pacific or via Bering Strait; if by the latter route, special conditions (either climatic or of rapidity of migration) must have obtained at the time of migration.

3. Further studies on various isolated tribes in other parts of the Americas should be made; such studies may be expected to throw more light on the origin and migrations of the American Indian.

Part II | Vector Eradication in the Prevention of *Aëdes aegypti*–Transmitted Yellow Fever in the Americas: Worldwide Implications

Selection 4 | Some Notes on the Epidemiology of Yellow Fever in Brazil*

The extent to which present beliefs regarding the epidemiology of yellow fever differ from those of 10 or 15 years ago is not generally appreciated outside the small group of workers actively engaged in the control and study of this disease.

My first contact with the problem of yellow fever control came in the year 1920, when, shortly after attending what was probably the last lecture on yellow fever delivered by General Gorgas, I visited Pernambuco and saw at first hand the work of the Comissão de Febre Amarela of the National Department of Health.

[Dr. Soper gives more details of his first contact with yellow fever, which occurred during the period when The Rockefeller Foundation was engaged in the attempt to eradicate the disease from the Americas, in Part VIII, Selection 33. *Ed.*]

Tonight I shall outline for you my ideas of yellow fever in 1920, based on the statements of the most famous North American who has been engaged in yellow fever control, and on personal contact with the Brazilian effort of that time, directed by men trained in the school of Oswaldo Cruz, and contrast these ideas with those we have been forced to adopt up to the present. I shall also present the data responsible for some changes of orientation and shall outline briefly the extent of present control measures and the program for the immediate future.

The clinical and epidemiological pictures of yellow fever accepted by most Brazilian and American workers in 1920 were of the utmost simplicity. In 1920 yellow fever was a disease easily diagnosed on the basis of sudden onset, fever, headache, black vomit and other hemorrhagic manifestations, albuminuria, icterus, and anuria, with death occurring, in fatal cases, generally from the fourth to the seventh day. Mortality ranged from 30 to 70 per cent; foreigners were most susceptible to the disease, and natives of endemic areas were supposed to have the disease in early childhood,

* Excerpts from a translation of a paper read by Dr. Soper before the National Academy of Medicine, Rio de Janeiro, Brazil, November 9, 1933.

The observations on which this report is based were made by the Cooperative Yellow Fever Service maintained by the National Department of Health of Brazil and The Rockefeller Foundation. Dr. Soper was the Representative in South America (Rio de Janeiro Office) of the International Health Division of The Rockefeller Foundation.

This article was first published (*17*) in the *Revista de Hygiene e Saúde Pública* (*Rio de Janeiro*) *8:* 37–61, 73–94, 1934. (About 38 pages of the original text have been omitted, including 21 maps, 6 tables, 1 chart, and 3 figures.)

when yellow fever was thought to be very mild. Epidemiological surveys, based on a study of mortality statistics and conversations with the medical profession and local authorities, were considered sufficient indication of the presence or absence of yellow fever in areas under suspicion. Transmission was thought to occur only through *Aëdes aegypti,* and the control of this mosquito in the large cities of endemic areas to result in the disappearance of yellow fever from such areas through the exhaustion of nonimmunes in the smaller centers of population. Yellow fever was essentially an urban disease and depended for its continuance on a domestic mosquito and a constant supply of nonimmunes.

Today we have proof that yellow fever in endemic areas, among native populations, may be a relatively mild disease in most cases, without the clinical symptoms above enumerated; but, paradoxically, some typical fatal cases do occur even in children born to immune parents in endemic areas. Although the diagnosis of yellow fever in classical cases occurring under epidemic conditions is very easy, experience has repeatedly demonstrated that even fatal attacks of yellow fever occurring under endemic conditions away from the large cities are seldom diagnosed.

Today we know that yellow fever has in the past 20 years been much more widespread than reported outbreaks have indicated, and we recognize the need for a thorough resurvey, with modern methods, of all possibly endemic areas on the American continent, even though such areas have apparently been free of the infection for many years.

[There is a later discussion of rural yellow fever transmitted by *A. aegypti* in Part V, Selection 23. *Ed.*]

Today we know that yellow fever can exist for a number of months, or, possibly, even years, as a rural disease. This rural yellow fever may be associated with *A. aegypti* in some areas, but it has also been observed in two different areas in which aegypti could not be found. The control of *A. aegypti* in the larger centers of population is not sufficient, in Brazil at least, to permit yellow fever to die out within a reasonable length of time, owing to failure of nonimmunes in the surrounding areas.

[In large part the differences between 1920 and 1933 were the result of new information obtained by means of the routine histopathological examination of liver specimens obtained by "viscerotomy" and of the mouse protection test for immunity to yellow fever. These two subjects are discussed in Parts III and IV, respectively. *Ed.*]

Events of the past few years have amply shown that the absence of epidemics and of declared cases of yellow fever from an area does not always indicate the absence of the disease from that area. Protection tests in Brazil indicating the past existence of yellow fever at various places during periods when no history of its existence could be obtained at first suggested

1920	1933
Severe clinical disease considered typical	Severe classical case considered atypical in native population of endemic areas
Absence of reported cases indicated absence of disease	Absence of reported cases not accepted as absence of disease
Yellow fever essentially urban and transmitted only by aegypti	Yellow fever may continue at least for a period of months in rural areas, with transmission by aegypti, or even in the absence of this mosquito
Key-center control believed effective in cleaning surrounding area	Key-center control not effective in Brazil

that epidemics of mild nonfatal yellow fever might occur. However, although it has been shown that yellow fever may carry a very low mortality in the native population of endemic areas, the routine examination of liver tissue indicates that silent endemic foci are not silent because of an absence of fatal infection but because of the failure to recognize them. Studies to date indicate, at least for Brazil, that large series of infections without some fatalities do not occur often. On the other hand, it seems that the virus of yellow fever can be maintained for relatively long periods of time with the occurrence of comparatively few infections.

The methods which have been found most valuable and most practicable for studying the distribution of yellow fever—the mouse protection test applied to samples of blood from selected groups of the population of the areas investigated, and the routine postmortem removal of liver tissue— are both independent of the notification of suspect cases of yellow fever. This is highly important, since declared suspect cases are very rare in true endemic areas not having an influx of nonimmune immigrants. The information secured by each of these methods is complementary to, but basically different from, that secured by the other. The first gives a cumulative picture of past exposure to the virus of yellow fever; the second, a current picture of mortality from yellow fever and an indication of the present distribution of the yellow fever virus.

[See Part V, Selection 19, for a detailed description of the findings in the Vale do Canaan. *Ed.*]

For over three decades it has been known that yellow fever is transmitted by *A. aegypti,* and during this period *antimosquito* measures have universally resulted in the disappearance of yellow fever *from the mortality records* of towns and cities where such measures were applied. An unexpected result of the early campaigns was the spontaneous apparent disappearance of yellow fever from large tributary areas as well as from the centers worked.

The cleaning of Havana resulted in the disappearance of yellow fever from Cuba, and the first campaign in Rio de Janeiro resulted in the disappearance of yellow fever from South Brazil. This phenomenon was observed so constantly that satisfactory explanations were hypothesized, on which a whole generation of epidemiologists planned the final elimination of yellow fever from the world through the application of antiaegypti measures in a relatively few arbitrarily selected key centers of population lying within the known endemic areas. The application of control measures to the key centers of North Brazil, however, did not result in the disappearance of yellow fever from Brazil, and the second campaign in Rio de Janeiro did not result in its disappearance from the states of Rio de Janeiro and Minas Gerais.

Just as the inability of key-center control to eliminate yellow fever from a large endemic area could be demonstrated only through the application and consequent failure of that method, so can the possible importance of rural yellow fever be evaluated only by studies subsequent to the cleaning of all cities and towns. The more intense the antimosquito service in an area, the more significant become the results of epidemiological studies based on protection tests and viscerotomy.

Brazil has recognized yellow fever as a national problem, but in the light of present knowledge of the disease, yellow fever must be recognized as an international problem. Findings of the past few years in Brazil, Colombia, Bolivia, and Africa show that thorough surveys with modern methods of all previously endemic areas are necessary for an adequate understanding of the yellow fever problem. In South America yellow fever may truly be said to be a continental problem in which all countries have a vital interest. Even Uruguay, Argentina, and Chile, where conditions suitable to continued endemicity do not exist, have suffered in the past and Argentina was obliged to organize a defense service in 1932 against the threatened importation from the lowlands of Bolivia. With increased means of rapid transportation in many parts and with an air service now in operation which circles South America in 13 days, yellow fever at any point in South America is of interest to every country on this continent.

The continental program should include

1. Antilarval services in all principal cities and in all ports in tropical America. This measure should prevent the future widespread dissemination of virus and should greatly reduce the possibility of its international spread.

2. Protection test surveys to outline the recent distribution of yellow fever. This will undoubtedly be found much greater than is now believed.

3. Routine collection and examination of liver specimens from rapidly fatal febrile cases from all parts of possibly endemic areas. Smaller towns and rural areas are especially important.

4. Careful study of all places shown to be infected by the examination of liver tissue, with special reference to the possibility of vectors other than *A. aegypti* and of vertebrate hosts other than man.

5. Antilarval services in all towns and villages in and about known infected areas.

I have not attempted to discuss tonight any details of the recent important laboratory work in yellow fever or the possibilities of yellow fever control at some future time through vaccination; nor have I made any attempt to cite by name those responsible for the work herewith reported, which has been possible only through the full cooperation of the laboratory, the control service, the authorities, and many interested friends and colleagues.

It is fitting, however, that special tribute be paid to the memory of Dr. Nelson C. Davis, Director of the Laboratory of the Yellow Fever Service in Baía from its inauguration in 1928 until his death last October 20. Our knowledge of yellow fever has been greatly enriched through his tireless work of the past 5 years, and many of the data presented here tonight represent either his personal contribution or work done under his direction.

These are the notes regarding yellow fever in Brazil which I thought might be interesting to my colleagues who are devoting themselves to other problems of hygiene and medicine, and who cannot, therefore, follow closely the developments in this field. I thank you for your kindness in coming to hear me tonight and I shall always treasure pleasant memories of this occasion. Especially must I thank this learned Academy, which has honored me by permitting the use of its tribune for the presentation of these notes to my Brazilian colleagues and friends.

Selection 5 | Present-Day Methods for the Study and Control of Yellow Fever*

MODIFICATIONS IN AEGYPTI CONTROL

In dealing with urban yellow fever it has long been known that it is not necessary to exterminate the aegypti mosquito but only to reduce its density below the "critical index" for a given place to cause the disease to disappear from that place. The critical point, below which yellow fever may not be expected to continue, is not constant for all places or for all times at the same place but will vary according to many interrelated factors, such as the size of the community, the percentage of the population immune, immigration of nonimmunes, and bombardment by infective cases from without. Experience over many years showed that generally the critical index had been reached when careful house to house inspection revealed aquatic forms of the mosquito on not more than 5 per cent of the premises visited. Experience in many campaigns also showed that whereas it was relatively easy to obtain an aegypti breeding index of 5 per cent or less, the reduction of this index to a figure approaching zero was prohibitive in cost. In the light of this experience campaigns were organized to reduce aegypti breeding to well below 5 per cent, but further reduction was considered impractical. However, about 1928 Dr. D. B. Wilson, working in Parahyba, Brazil, noted that as the aegypti index is reduced through control measures, an analysis of the aquatic forms found shows that there is a critical breeding index below which inspectors on a weekly cycle of visits continue to find each week a few foci of the earlier larval forms of aegypti but practically never encounter the later pupal preadult states. Since the period of development from egg to adult is somewhat greater than 1 week and since adults can only come from pupae, it is clear that the foci found and destroyed each week are not involved in the production of the adults necessary for the reseeding with eggs of the containers which develop

* The studies and observations on which this report is based were made under the auspices of the International Health Division of The Rockefeller Foundation in cooperation with the Government of Brazil. The report covers the work of numerous colleagues on the staff of the International Health Division and the staff of the Cooperative Yellow Fever Service of Brazil. Dr. Soper was the Representative in South America of the International Health Division (Rio de Janeiro office) of The Rockefeller Foundation.

This is an excerpt from pages 666–673 of the published article (27). (See also the excerpts from pp. 661–666 in Part III, Selection 15.) This excerpt is reprinted by permission from the *American Journal of Tropical Medicine 17:* 655–676, 1937. Copyright © 1937, The Williams & Wilkins Company, Baltimore, Maryland.

larvae. Since the aegypti mosquito is a short-lived insect, the continuation of the species throughout a long period of time in a city where no pupal foci are being found must be due, in the absence of a constant importation of eggs or adults from outside the control area, to the failure to discover and destroy certain well-hidden breeding places which continue to produce adults.

This line of reasoning caused Dr. Wilson to introduce the "mother-focus" or "producing-focus" squads. The function of these squads is to supplement the work of the regular inspectors by searching for and elimi-nating the pupal foci too well hidden to be found by these men. Their efforts were at first oriented by the location of such secondary larval foci as were reported by the regular inspectors and by the complaints from householders that mosquitoes were disturbing them. The work of the squads was helpful in cleaning up many aegypti-infested areas, but it was not completely successful, owing to the failure of the regular inspection service to find secondary foci in certain places where pupal foci existed. The tendency of many householders to clean up ahead of the inspector on the day of his visit was undoubtedly an important factor in limiting the usefulness of this service. Complaints of householders proved of little value, since such complaints were generally based on the presence of mosquitoes other than aegypti.

The final reduction of aegypti indices to a figure approaching zero was accomplished only after the introduction of the hand capture of the adult aegypti to orient the work of the "mother focus" squads.

Repeated experience had shown that inspectors' reports, on which the calculation of the aegypti index is based, were often untrustworthy. Some-times this was due to the bad faith of the inspectors, and careful reinspec-tion by special inspectors, and even doctors, was the rule. Although such reinspection generally revealed some missed foci, it was not a proper check on conditions, since it was but a repetition, with the technique of the original inspection, and often missed most of what had been honestly missed by the first inspection. In seeking a method of checking the aegypti index, a page was borrowed from the malariologist's handbook and, in 1930, the capture of adult aegypti in the homes was instituted. Hand cap-ture of adults has proved unexpectedly to be the most sensitive indicator of the presence of and density of aegypti yet found. Having proved its worth in checking the work of the regular inspectors, Dr. E. R. Rickard soon found it to be invaluable in those places where the aegypti index was already low. Through a careful analysis of the distribution of adult aegypti by houses, with special attention to relative density of the two sexes, it has been found possible, in most cases, to localize hidden breeding within a radius of 25 or 30 yards.

The use of the hand capture of aegypti to orient the work of the mother-focus squad was followed by reduction of aegypti breeding to a point previously considered impossible at reasonable expense. Breeding indices in cities and towns throughout Brazil have been brought to less than 0.1 per cent and have remained at this low level during several years. It is no exaggeration to say that in numerous important cities the aegypti mosquito has been exterminated, it being possible to show in many cases in which occasional foci are found that importation from areas not under control has occurred. In many cities previously heavily infested with aegypti the finding of a single focus of breeding of this mosquito is an event of almost as great interest to the control service as the finding of a case of yellow fever would have been in previous times.

The use of hand capture of adults for the localization of breeding is not of great value until the situation is well in hand and the easily found foci have been eliminated; it should really be considered as the secret service section which helps "wipe up" the residual foci not reached by other means.

Experience has shown that once a community has been thoroughly cleaned it can be kept at much less expense than is required to maintain a low index of from 1 to 5 per cent. Furthermore, friction with the public and within the service is greatly reduced, since the work itself is much easier and more satisfying.

Once the aegypti index has been reduced to less than 0.1 per cent for some weeks the cycle of house visits may be increased from 7 to 14, 21, or even 28 days in the larger cities. In the smaller cities services may be, and often are, discontinued for long periods of time without danger. Experience has shown that, where the cleanup of a district has been complete, quarterly visits of the hand capture squads, inspecting every third house, can be relied upon to signalize the reappearance of aegypti before the danger point of production is again reached. On reinspection of towns in which antimosquito measures have been suspended for some time, falsely low breeding indices will often be reported because of the tendency of the people to clean up just in advance of the inspector's visit; but this cleanup does not influence the adult index obtained by the capture squad.

The use of a cycle of inspection greater than 7 days is justified only after the aegypti mosquito has truly been brought almost to extinction; the use of lengthened cycles under other circumstances must lead to disappointing results.

While the exceptional results obtained in aegypti control are attributed by those in the service to the use of hand captures to orient the mother-focus squads, other factors may have been in part responsible. Undoubtedly of great importance has been the practice, introduced in 1931, of routine application of a mixture of diesel and fuel oils to all water containers in which mosquito breeding is observed. The routine oiling has been found to be very efficacious in preventing the "repeating" focus. This measure is a disagreeable one but is particularly good in that it places the responsibility for breeding directly on the person charged with the care of the guilty container; part of its value is thought to be due to the destruction of eggs on the walls of the container, which occurs when the container is thoroughly cleaned, as it must be, before going back into household use.

Routine oiling of foci is a measure of great value at all times in the campaign but should not be used without due warning to the public, except in case of an emergency such as exists when yellow fever is already known to be present in a community. Fish, which were at one time so widely used, have proved to be a very expensive method of permanent control except in cisterns and large surface tanks which cannot be readily sealed but are easily accessible to inspection.

It is to be greatly regretted that the same reduction cannot be made in culex breeding as has been secured in aegypti breeding by the use of mother-focus squads, adult capture squads, and the routine application of oil. A study of the curves of aegypti and culex indices in many cities, based on the percentage of premises where inspectors have found foci, shows clearly that the application of these methods causes a steady decline in the aegypti breeding to a practical zero level not subject to seasonal fluctuation but that the culex breeding continues to fluctuate with the variation in rainfall and temperature. Because of the public clamor against pestiferous mosquitoes, the yellow fever control service is unable to take full advantage of the economies which the practical extinction of aegypti would otherwise make possible.

Selection 6 | The Organization of Permanent
Nationwide Anti-Aëdes Aegypti
Measures in Brazil*

FRED L. SOPER, D. BRUCE WILSON, SERVULO LIMA,
AND WALDEMAR SÁ ANTUNES

HISTORICAL INTRODUCTION

When the medical historian of the future comes to write the chapter on yellow fever, he will be obliged to devote considerable space to the developments of the decade and a half from 1926 to 1940. This short period showed how impossible of fulfillment was the dream of final eradication of yellow fever, but it saw great advances in our understanding of the etiology, epidemiology, and prophylaxis of the disease, including the discovery of animal susceptibility, the rediscovery of the virus origin, the demonstration that mosquitoes other than *Aëdes aegypti* can and do transmit the virus, the development of the protection test for determining immunity, the organization of viscerotomy for the diagnosis of unsuspected fatal cases, the proof that unrecognized yellow fever has been widespread in large silent endemic areas of South America and Africa, the demonstration that the disease exists in many countries of South America as one of jungle animals, independent of the distribution of *A. aegypti* and of man, and finally the modification of the yellow fever virus in such a way as to make mass vaccination practicable. These outstanding developments have tended to overshadow the more prosaic improvements in the organization of measures against the aegypti mosquito in Brazil which have transformed expensive temporary aegypti-reduction campaigns for the eradication of yellow fever into economical permanent services for the species eradication of *A. aegypti* itself from the infested areas.

When the period under consideration began, those active in the study

* This report is based on the work of the Cooperative Yellow Fever Service maintained jointly by the Brazilian Government and the International Health Division of The Rockefeller Foundation for 11 years, 1929–1940. Dr. Soper was the Representative in South America (Rio de Janeiro Office) of the International Health Division of The Rockefeller Foundation; Dr. Wilson was a staff member. Doctors Servulo Lima and Sá Antunes were senior officers in the Cooperative Yellow Fever Service.

This excerpt comprises pages 1–9 of the 137-page book (47) published by The Rockefeller Foundation, New York, 1943. (Figure 1 has been omitted.)

and control of yellow fever anticipated its early disappearance from Northeast Brazil, the only recognized endemic region remaining in the Americas. All other foci of aegypti-transmitted yellow fever had disappeared in the face of antimosquito campaigns organized by The Rockefeller Foundation in collaboration with the national governments concerned. The 1926 outbreak of yellow fever in the Brazilian states of Paraíba, Pernambuco, Baía, and Minas Geraes, which occurred in spite of the antimosquito campaigns carried out in the principal population centers since 1923, was the first clear-cut recognized failure of such campaigns to rid any region of yellow fever (see Fig. 2).

The period under discussion ended in 1940 with the seventh and last of a series of annual shifting epidemics of jungle yellow fever (1934–1940) which swept the forested areas of southern Mato Grosso, Goiás, Minas Geraes, São Paulo, Paraná, Santa Catarina, Rio Grande do Sul, Rio de

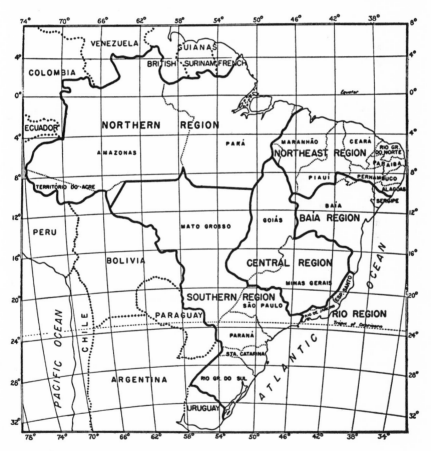

Figure 2. Map of Brazil, showing regional organization of antiaegypti work.

Janeiro, and Espírito Santo, involving also Paraguay and almost certainly part of the Province of Misiones, Argentina. Jungle yellow fever had also been registered, quite independently of this epidemic sweep, in southern Baía, in eastern Minas Geraes, in Maranhão, and at widely scattered points in Amazonas, Pará, and Acre. During this decade and a half aegypti-transmitted yellow fever was reported for all Brazilian states except Rio Grande do Sul, Santa Catarina, and Espírito Santo, but even these states had seen cases on board ships arriving in their principal ports. But several of the observed outbreaks were secondary to jungle yellow fever, and available data indicate that epidemiologists were justified in believing in 1926 that the only area of permanent aegypti-transmitted endemicity lay in Northeast Brazil, between and including the states of Baía and Piauí. There is ample evidence, including the confirmation of several imported cases of jungle yellow fever in the Federal District in 1938, suggesting that the Rio de Janeiro outbreak of 1928–1929 and the subsequent wide distribution of aegypti-transmitted yellow fever in 1928 and 1929 were due probably to an invasion by virus from jungle areas. If this be true, the Rio de Janeiro outbreak of 1928 was but another in the series of transfers of jungle yellow fever virus to towns and cities, followed by aegypti-transmitted outbreaks, which included those of Socorro, Colombia, in 1929; Guasipati, Venezuela, in 1929; Santa Cruz de la Sierra, Bolivia, in 1932; Teófilo Otoni, Minas Geraes, in 1935; Cambará, Paraná, in 1936; Buena Vista, Colombia, in 1937; and Senna Madureira, Acre, in 1942. Today even those who were at first most skeptical of the existence and importance of jungle yellow fever are forced to recognize the permanent threat of invasion from this source hanging over towns and cities which permit high densities of aegypti breeding to persist in these days of rapid transportation linking all parts of the Americas.

In 1931–1932 it was shown that the permanent aegypti-transmitted endemicity of Northeast Brazil was different from that observed elsewhere in the Americas, in that it was based in part on the rural distribution of *A. aegypti*, which was able to maintain yellow fever virus in the rural populations for long periods after the elimination of yellow fever from the larger centers of population. This rural endemicity was responsible for the failure of previous campaigns to eradicate yellow fever from Northeast Brazil, where jungle yellow fever does not occur. Rural endemicity persisted until control measures were applied throughout large rural areas. These measures were crowned with success, and since August 1934 no focus of yellow fever infection has been found in Northeast Brazil. In fact, no aegypti-transmitted yellow fever has been seen in Brazil since 1934, with the exception of a few isolated outbreaks appearing in conjunction with local outbreaks of jungle yellow fever. All such aegypti-transmitted outbreaks have been overcome before secondary foci of aegypti-transmitted yellow fever have developed. The National Yellow Fever Service of Brazil, however, recognizes that all outbreaks of aegypti-transmitted yellow fever are unnecessary and refuses to be satisfied with the past record. In spite of the development of an effective vaccine which is being widely used to protect populations exposed to the jungle infection, a nationwide antiaegypti service is maintained to prevent the transmission of the virus by *A. aegypti.*

The period 1926–1940 showed that temporary key-center antiaegypti campaigns would not eradicate yellow fever from Brazil; but it witnessed the development of methods whereby the domestic vector itself may be eradicated, after which permanent sentinel services can easily prevent reinfestation with this species. Whereas in 1926 antiaegypti measures were being applied in a clumsy, expensive, and comparatively ineffective manner in a few cities of Northeast Brazil at the expense of the International Health Division of The Rockefeller Foundation, the year 1940 saw the return to government control at government expense of a streamlined National Yellow Fever Service operating throughout the entire country, conscious of its direct responsibility for the occurrence of any aegypti-transmitted yellow fever, and *willing to declare its program to be the eradication of A. aegypti from Brazil.*

The eradication of *A. aegypti* from such a large and highly favorable habitat as Brazil is not so utterly impossible as it must appear to those who have combatted this mosquito with methods which failed to wipe out the species in the communities worked. Once eradication has been attained in the large centers of population (Figs. 3 and 4) it soon becomes apparent that ease in keeping these centers free of infestation depends on the absence of the mosquito from the towns, villages, and even rural districts of the tributary regions. Fortunately, the difference in expense between maintaining a safe density of *A. aegypti* in a city and keeping the same city completely free of this species is so great that the cost of clearing contiguous areas of the mosquito to protect a zero index is more than justified over a period of years. Thus any program of species eradication tends to expand automatically to include even the smallest and most distant places, until the entire region is cleared of the species.

It will undoubtedly seem to many that the methods described in the following pages are unnecessarily detailed, that entirely too much record-keeping is involved, and that undue attention is given to checking the work reported. The answer is in the results obtained. Detailed records and maps pay for themselves many times over if they are studied and if they are used to orient an ever-shifting strategy of campaign against the *A. aegypti.* Human nature being what it is, the expenditure of 25 to 30 per cent of the labor budget for checking the work done has proved sound practice in species eradication work.

The methods described must be considered as the accumulated experience of many workers. The Yellow Fever Service operating in Brazil under the auspices of The Rockefeller Foundation since October 1923 was amalgamated with the Yellow Fever Service of the National Department of Health in January 1932, and the consolidated service was able to take advantage of the ideas and methods developed by The Rockefeller Foundation under the influence of Gorgas and by the Brazilians under the influence of Oswaldo Cruz. In addition, the Service has not hesitated to borrow administrative procedure from purely business sources and has had many useful suggestions for modifications from its own subordinate personnel. There are probably few details of the methods described, including the search for hidden producing foci, the routine oiling of foci, and the capture of adult mosquitoes, which have not been used before. The real

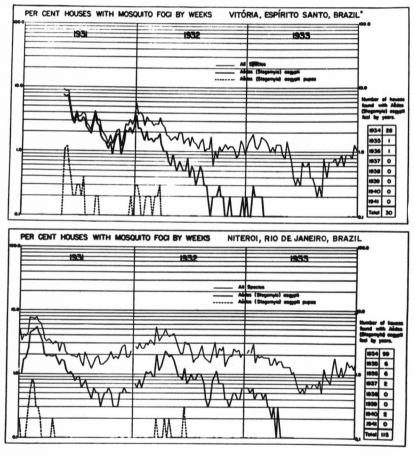

Figure 3. Results of aegypti eradication programs in the cities of Vitória and Niteroi in South Brazil

contribution which has been made has been the application of these methods in such a way as to attain species eradication of *A. aegypti*. Herein lies the greatest achievement of the Cooperative Yellow Fever Service of Brazil.

ANTIAEGYPTI TECHNIQUE

Following the unexpected outbreak of yellow fever in Rio de Janeiro in 1928, the Brazilian Government, realizing that the control of yellow fever is a national rather than a local problem, took steps which resulted in bringing under one administrative head, on January 1, 1932, all responsibility for the investigation and control of this disease throughout the country. These steps were:

1. Assuming early in 1929 partial financial responsibility for the Yellow Fever Service operating since 1923 in North Brazil under the auspices of the International Health Division of The Rockefeller Foundation.

2. Extending on December 1, 1930, the zone of operations of the Cooperative Yellow Fever Service to include all Brazil, except the Federal District.

3. Amalgamating on January 1, 1932, the Yellow Fever Service of the National Department of Health, operating in the Federal District, and the Cooperative Yellow Fever Service.

On May 23, 1932, Federal Decree No. 21434 was issued giving the Yellow Fever Service adequate authority to carry out measures for the prevention of mosquito breeding and to investigate possible yellow fever cases occurring throughout Brazil. No legal provision was made in this decree for

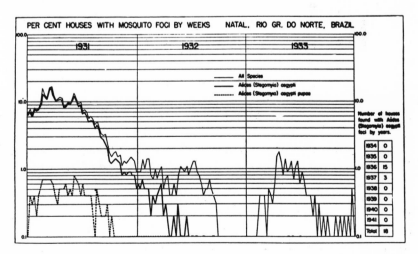

Figure 4. Elimination of aegypti mosquitoes from Natal, in Northeast Brazil.

administrative detail, which was left to be worked out according to local conditions, and subject to such modifications as might become necessary.

While it may be possible to organize small health services on the basis of word of mouth instructions, all details of established techniques must be written down for ready reference if uniform work is to be done on a national scale. The description of the technique of antiaegypti work which follows is an adaptation of corresponding sections of the *Administrative Manual of the Yellow Fever Service of the Ministry of Education and Health of Brazil* as they were at the end of 1939. The Brazilian Yellow Fever Service is not static; modifications of technique are being tested constantly, and those found useful are adopted. And so it is that the Service Manual, in evolution since 1930, continues in a loose-leaf mimeograph form which is easily altered.

In the field of yellow fever control, to an even greater extent than in many other fields of public health administration, the literature on administrative details of the work is inadequate. In the special case of antiaegypti work, all of the few reports available refer to emergency urban campaigns carried out for the purpose of getting rid of yellow fever, rather than to permanent programs for the eradication of the vector.

An essential difference between an emergency campaign and a permanent one is the attitude which must be taken toward cost. At the time of a yellow fever epidemic, or under threat of importation of the infection from nearby epidemic areas, adequate funds are easily obtained to prevent a public calamity, and the health officer is judged not by the amount of money spent but by the immediate results of the campaign. Once the threat of yellow fever passes, however, government authorities and the health officer begin to consider the question of expense, which is indeed heavy in comparison with other important health measures. The director of an emergency campaign must know how, regardless of cost, to reduce the density of *A. aegypti* rapidly to a point where yellow fever transmission becomes impossible, whereas the director of a permanent antiaegypti service must be able to prevent aegypti breeding at such a low cost that the expenditure can be carried by the annual budget. The experience of the Yellow Fever Service in Brazil shows that aegypti breeding cannot be controlled economically by the time-honored methods of simply reducing the intensity of such breeding; only when species eradication, beginning in the larger centers, is carried to the smaller towns, villages, and even rural districts of the surrounding areas, which would otherwise reinfest the larger centers, can *A. aegypti* be controlled at little cost. Fortunately a technique has been developed which makes possible the complete eradication of the aegypti mosquito at a reasonable cost from urban, village, and rural areas.

The Brazilian manual is based on Brazilian conditions, which are sufficiently varied to include most of the problems to be found in other parts of the Americas. No attempt has been made to adapt the techniques described to African and Asiatic conditions, under which certain special problems are encountered.

Theoretically, antiaegypti measures should be easy, since the breeding foci of this mosquito are generally limited to artificial water containers in, and in immediate proximity to, human habitations. In practice, the discovery and elimination of the final traces of aegypti breeding are often difficult, not only because of the instinctive wiles of the aegypti mosquito, but because of the public relations and personnel problems inherent in any attempt to apply routinely even the simplest measures in hundreds of thousands of homes scattered over all Brazil.

The reduction of aegypti breeding to a point where yellow fever disappears from the towns and cities worked is relatively easy, as the dramatic results of early campaigns testify, but the complete eradication of the species in a given place is made difficult by the instinctive ability of the female aegypti to lay her eggs in every hidden inaccessible water container, by the ability of the aegypti egg to withstand desiccation for several months, and by the constant transportation of the species from unworked to worked areas (imagoes by boat and train, and larvae and eggs in portable water containers, such as the universally used clay water jars). However, local species eradication has been accomplished in all the large cities intensively worked in Brazil during the past decade, and wide regions, including several entire states, have been cleared of aegypti.

In using the technique described, it must be borne in mind that the work in any given place should undergo regular evolution and requires different types of organization for its various stages. Many of the methods, such as those of the Vacant House and Roof-Gutter Services, are necessary in the early stages of the campaign while the aegypti density is high but can be discontinued later; others, such as those of the Adult Capture and the Producing Focus Services are of little value as long as considerable aegypti breeding continues to exist but become invaluable during the final cleanup of an area. The most advantageous application of the technique is possible only when a careful current analysis of the progress of the work is used as the basis for timely modifications. The initially large staff required to eradicate the aegypti mosquito from infested areas can be reduced to the relatively small number needed to prevent reinfestation only after careful analysis of the situation. The numerous report forms, maps, and charts of the Service are used not only as a check on the work done, but also as a guide to when and how the program may be modified to meet changing conditions.

The permanent campaign against *A. aegypti* falls naturally into three quite distinct phases:

1. The initial cleanup campaign for the elimination of the easily accessible aegypti foci. This phase is similar in all respects to the early emergency yellow fever campaigns which rid localities of yellow fever but not of the vector species.

2. The discovery and elimination of the final hidden, inaccessible breeding places responsible for maintaining the species in the face of intensive antiaegypti measures.

3. The permanent maintenance of a sentinel service to discover and eliminate any reinfestation which may occur. (Reinfestation in the early months of the sentinel service may be either "internal," due to returning to active use of dry containers with viable eggs, or "external," due to importation of the vectors from infested areas, as already described. Later reinfestations come only from external sources.)

The initial cleanup campaign is always costly, as is the maintenance of the service needed to guarantee the low indexes obtained. The sentinel service to discover early any reinfestation which may occur after zero indexes are secured is inexpensive, and its cost declines progressively as the danger of reinfestation disappears. The interval between adult capture surveys can be increased with safety as the cleaning of contiguous areas proceeds. Only species eradication permits permanent aegypti control at low cost, and no effort should be spared to clear tributary areas as widely as possible.

The stage is set for the second phase of the campaign when well under 5 per cent of the houses inspected are found with aegypti foci and when only secondary, nonproducing foci without pupae are found. But even secondary foci may disappear in well-worked areas before complete eradication occurs. The capture of adults is the most sensitive index of the presence or absence of *A. aegypti* in a neighborhood and is an essential weapon in the final cleanup. Negative reports should not be taken to mean eradication until careful search has been made for adult mosquitoes. Adult aegypti in nature are on the average short lived, and secondary foci or numerous adults in a neighborhood always indicate recent nearby pupal foci.

The final elimination of hidden inaccessible aegypti foci is achieved by

1. Oiling or destruction of all water containers in which mosquito breeding is occurring. (Rapid pouring out or drawing off of water is almost useless; fish are expensive and are used only where no other method of control is possible.)

2. Capturing adult mosquitoes to ascertain persistence of aegypti and to locate hidden pupal-producing foci.

3. Searching out pupal-producing foci in neighborhoods where aegypti mosquitoes persist in the face of routine control measures.

Although Brazil has had since 1932 a rather drastic yellow fever regulation (Decree 21434 of May 23, 1932), its application would be impossible in the absence of the whole-hearted support of the Brazilian public. The Brazilian householder has come to recognize in the Yellow Fever Service employee who enters his home a person who has no political or police objective, does not receive tips, applies the same measures impartially in all the homes under his jurisdiction, and is himself under careful supervision not only by his superiors but also by the householder, through a cumulative record which he leaves in each home, listing the time of each visit and the conditions found.

The local director of the service is always accessible to the public, and mosquito complaints receive prompt attention. The householder, under these circumstances, generally accepts the impositions of the Service and seldom is it necessary to have recourse to legal measures except in those cases where the recommendations of the Service involve the spending of money in structural modifications. The owner is held responsible for any mosquito breeding due to structural defects, the householder for conditions which are independent of the building itself.

As in all administrative work the principal problems of the Yellow Fever Service are those of selection, training, and supervision of personnel. The doctor entering the Service is given an intensive course of training, not only in the field work of the inspector but also in the statistical and accounting sections of the Service. At the end of his period of training the doctor is examined by officers of the Service on his knowledge covering a long list of questions which are given to him when he begins his training.

The inspector is carefully selected: he must be free of physical defects and must present a satisfactory police certificate. He is thoroughly trained and examined before being given independent responsibility. Everything is done to maintain a high esprit de corps. The inspector works in uniform, bears a numbered badge with the federal seal, and is instructed that he is an inspector, a teacher, and a sanitary policeman, but never a "cleanup servant," as was too often the case in previous campaigns. The inspector works with confidence based on detailed written instructions and a full knowledge of the legal basis of the Service he represents; he works with interest because he knows his work will be checked and that he individually will be given credit, or will be blamed, in accordance with the results he achieves.

The Yellow Fever Service operates on the basis of individual responsibility, fixed by written instructions which can be altered only in writing, and checked through detailed reports of work done. Work worth doing is worth recording; records are so planned as to serve the double purpose of facilitating a rapid and easy checking of the work and of giving a picture of the aegypti situation in the areas in which operations are in progress. Records are so dovetailed, one with another and with the respective summaries, that they can be analyzed rapidly by the director. Routine work is reported on printed forms, and in addition doctors, and at times other supervisors, prepare narrative diaries. Full use is made of maps and charts; all houses and even blocks are numbered as an aid to specific fixing of responsibility for work done. Adequate provision is made for checking all field work. It is not enough to outline a given program and assign it to well-trained employees; the director of a service must assume the responsibility for knowing that the work is done. No large administrative service carries on long automatically, and provision has been made in the Yellow Fever Service for the routine collection, summarizing, and presentation of the data needed by the director to follow and check the work accomplished.

The central administrative office of the Yellow Fever Service is in the Federal District, Rio de Janeiro. Regional offices, subordinate to the central office and responsible for the administration of the work in the corresponding regions (see Fig. 2), are maintained in Belém, Pará, for the northern region; in Recife, Pernambuco, for the northeast region; in Salvador, for the Baía region; in Belo Horizonte, for the Minas Geraes region; and in São Paulo for the southern region. Various administrative divisions, styled sectors, divisions, and posts are formed within the region according to the number of doctors available, the presence or absence of *A. aegypti,* and the facility of transportation. Of these divisions, only the sector has a fully equipped statistical and accounting office.

The basic administrative unit is the zone, which consists of a group of city blocks, or a rural area, all the houses of which can be visited by one inspector at regular intervals, following an itinerary defined by the director. The unit next in importance is the district, comprising generally five or six zones so grouped as to permit, during each cycle, a careful checking of all zones by a single district inspector.

The zone inspector's work constitutes the basis of, and is the most important element in, the campaign against the aegypti mosquito. The following section, "Instructions for Inspectors of the Yellow Fever Service," is a translation of a book of instructions prepared for the use of zone and district inspectors in Brazil. It contains a description of the essential points of the duties of the zone inspector and of his supervisor, the district inspector, and the principal regulations covering their work.

Selection 7 | Proposal for the Continental Eradication of *Aëdes aegypti**

It is necessary, however, to point out the advantages of permanent measures against *Aëdes aegypti* everywhere in the Americas, not the programs of Gorgas and Oswaldo Cruz to eliminate yellow fever from selected localities by means of control measures, but the modern antiaegypti measures, of demonstrated effectiveness during the past decade, that are designed to eradicate the species. Although the initial cost will be high, the aegypti-eradication program in the Americas is entirely feasible and eventually will pay large dividends on the capital invested. Inasmuch as species eradication is not easy, requiring adequate legislation and meticulous administration, the eradication of aegypti on a continental scale could be executed more rapidly and more efficiently if there were a general international agreement regarding the campaign. Then there could be simultaneous application of eradication measures under uniform standards, with the training of personnel for the campaign done in countries where eradication has already been achieved.

Our recommendation for the future is merely a repetition, with slight modification, of the recommendations of 1938, in which we said:

"We believe that a reasonable (yellow fever) program for the continent can be based on these three measures: antilarval campaign, viscerotomy, and vaccination.

"(1) The antilarval campaign should be organized on a permanent basis in the principal ports and cities where aegypti is present, especially in those regions suitable for the appearance of jungle yellow fever."

[Paragraphs (2) and (3) omitted; they dealt with viscerotomy and vaccination.]

Today we recommend that the antiaegypti campaign be organized in every place where this mosquito is present in order to eradicate the species from this continent.

There will be those who are opposed to a continental aegypti-eradication campaign, because of its very high cost and the immediately available advantages to be obtained if the same funds were used in other health problems. These critics should review the history of antimosquito measures in

* Translation of an excerpt (pp. 1216–1222) from "Febre Amarela Panamericana, 1938 a 1942," a report by Dr. Soper as an invited guest from The Rockefeller Foundation to the XIth Pan American Sanitary Conference, Rio de Janeiro, Brazil, September 7–18, 1942. The entire report *(43)* was reprinted in Portuguese in the *Boletín de la Oficina Sanitaria Panamericana 21*: 1207–1222, 1942. (Another excerpt from this report, entitled "Complications of Yellow Fever Vaccination," appears in Part VI, Selection 27.)

Brazil, especially here in the beautiful city of Rio de Janeiro. After the victorious campaign of Oswaldo Cruz, 1903–1908, all of south Brazil was practically free of yellow fever for two decades, but eventually the expensive antiaegypti measures were abandoned in favor of health problems that were more urgent. With the reappearance of yellow fever in 1928, Prof. Clementino Fraga had to expend great effort during 15 months to organize a force of 10,000 men to control the disease once again. During 2½ years more than $10,000,000 U.S. were spent, a sum more than sufficient to pay for a program of eradication in the next 10 years in all Brazil, in case it were necessary for such a long period. Brazil will not again tolerate the neglect of antiaegypti measures and will be pleased to participate in the eradication of the species.

Editorial: Continental Eradication
of *Aëdes aegypti**

Although yellow fever was a serious urban and maritime scourge to the
Americas during the eighteenth and nineteenth centuries, the demonstration in 1900 by Reed and his fellow workers that the Finlay theory of transmission by *Aëdes (Stegomyia) aegypti* was correct, together with the
subsequent organization of antimosquito campaigns in Cuba, Panama,
Mexico, Brazil, the United States, and other countries, brought about its
rapid decline. These campaigns resulted practically in the disappearance
of yellow fever, not only from the centers worked, but also from large surrounding regions. The last urban outbreak of yellow fever in the United
States occurred at New Orleans in 1905 and in the Caribbean area in the
early 1920s. So effective was the fight against it that a whole generation of
health workers has grown up in the United States, Mexico, Central America, and the islands of the Caribbean without any experience in yellow
fever.

An entirely unexpected outbreak of urban yellow fever in Rio de
Janeiro in 1928, after a period of 20 years during which the disease had not
been known in the neighborhood of Brazil's beautiful capital, led to an
intensification of research and control measures which have resulted in
demonstrating that yellow fever is fundamentally a jungle disease of
animals, transmitted by forest mosquitoes. This jungle infection is at times
present in parts of Panama and all the South American countries except
Chile and Uruguay. The disease is easily acquired by individuals who work
or travel in the forests, and these in turn are able to infect the *A. aegypti*
mosquito in urban areas, thus initiating the regular epidemic cycle. Since
there are no practical measures for the elimination of jungle infection, this
potential urban threat is permanent and is not limited to cities near the
infected forests, since all cities of the Americas are now within direct striking distance of the disease by means of rapid air travel.

Experience has shown that antiaegypti measures are so costly and so
difficult that they generally are not kept for long at a high level of efficiency
where the threat of yellow fever is not immediate. There are in the Americas today many cities where yellow fever was previously present, in which
A. aegypti is not controlled adequately for the prevention of outbreaks
should the virus of the disease be accidentally imported. The Yellow Fever
Service organized by the Brazilian Government and The Rockefeller
Foundation in Brazil demonstrated that complete eradication of *A. aegypti*

* This article (53) is from the *Boletín de la Oficina Sanitaria Panamericana* 26:
898–899, 1947. Dr. Soper was Director of the Pan American Sanitary Bureau.

is possible. After eradication, aegypti does not reappear when control measures are discontinued unless reintroduction of the species from uncleaned areas occurs. No foci of aegypti infestation now are known in the Brazilian Amazon or in all of South Brazil, and only a comparatively small area of Northeast Brazil is known to be infested. *Aëdes aegypti* was eradicated from Bolivia several years ago, and eradication programs are well advanced in Peru and in British Guiana. The countries which are eradicating aegypti are anxious that neighboring countries should join in the campaign to avoid the danger of future reinfestation. At the XIth Pan American Sanitary Conference, meeting in Rio de Janeiro in September 1942, Bolivia introduced a resolution which was approved by the Conference, reading as follows:

After considering the results obtained in Brazil, Peru and Bolivia in regard to the eradication of *Aëdes aegypti,* the Eleventh Pan American Sanitary Conference resolves to extend its congratulations for this sanitary achievement which is a guarantee against the spread of yellow fever, and at the same time, the Conference requests the Governments of the countries where this vector is found, to organize eradication projects based on the plans adopted in Brazil.

At the meeting of the Directing Council of the Pan American Sanitary Organization in Buenos Aires in September 1947, the following action was taken on the initiative of Brazil:

The Directing Council resolves: (1) to entrust to the Pan American Sanitary Bureau the solution of the continental problem of urban yellow fever, based fundamentally on the eradication of *Aëdes aegypti,* without prejudice to other measures which regional circumstances may indicate, and (2) to develop the program under the auspices of the Pan American Sanitary Bureau, which, in agreement with the interested countries, shall take the necessary measures to solve such problems as may emerge in the campaign against yellow fever, whether they be sanitary, economic or legal.

Argentina, Paraguay, and Uruguay are making funds available for the organization of eradication services in the River Plate Valley in 1948, and it is hoped that Venezuela, Colombia, and Ecuador will join in an effort to eradicate aegypti from the northern part of South America. The Pan American Sanitary Bureau is organizing a special technical staff to coordinate eradication programs in different countries, and it is hoped that all areas in the Americas where aegypti is to be found can be brought into this program in the near future.

In matters concerning national health, the borders of each nation extend as far as the point of origin of all vehicles used for the transportation of persons, animals or things, be it by air, land, or sea. The fight against disease, today more than ever, is truly of international concern and requires the constant vigilance and common efforts of all countries.

Aegypti and Gambiae: Eradication
of African Invaders in the
Americas*

Aëdes aegypti and *Anopheles gambiae* originated in Africa. Each is
adapted to breeding in conditions found universally throughout the
tropics and subtropics; aegypti prefers all kinds of artificial water containers, gambiae, shallow sunlit pools without vegetation. Aegypti arrived
probably with the first European navigators toward the end of the fifteenth
century; gambiae came to north Brazil early in 1930.

How does it happen that I have a reputation of always talking about
aegypti, rather than hookworm disease, yellow fever, malaria, *Haemagogus
spegazzini,* other vectors of jungle yellow fever, *Anopheles gambiae,* typhus,
Pediculus corporis, or some other problem which has occupied my attention in the past?

The answer is to be found, in part, in the very special place that aegypti
has in the history of preventive medicine: (1) aegypti is the first proved vector of a virus disease, (2) aegypti was the first victim of a successful antimosquito campaign for disease prevention, (3) the eradication of aegypti
from several Brazilian cities in 1933 was an important landmark in the
rehabilitation of the eradication concept in the prevention of communicable diseases, (4) the eradication of aegypti led to the eradication of
gambiae, first from Brazil and later from Egypt, and (5) of even greater importance, the evolution of the program for the eradication of aegypti in the
Americas has demonstrated the power of growth and expansion inherent
in eradication projects.

The Pan American Health Organization program for the eradication of
aegypti is the first example of collaboration of all of the nations in a
region in the permanent solution of a common threat.

All of this justifies my harping on the subject of aegypti, but the real
stimulus to garrulity has been the continued failure, since 1947, of the
United States to participate in the program for the eradication of aegypti
in the Western Hemisphere. Fortunately, this stimulus is disappearing—
this talk may well be the prologue to silence on my part, at least on aegypti.

* Dr. Soper was a Special Consultant, Office of International Health, Public
Health Service.

This excerpt is reprinted from the article *(109)* in the *Proceedings* of the 50th
Annual Meeting of the New Jersey Mosquito Extermination Association and the
19th Annual Meeting of the American Mosquito Control Association, Atlantic
City, New Jersey, March 12–15, 1963, pp. 152–160. (About 2 pages of the original
article have been omitted; they dealt with gambiae.)

Returning to Brazil from Toronto (in 1933), I learned, from aegypti incidence charts, that this mosquito was no longer found in a number of Brazilian port cities! Field investigation confirmed the fact that local eradication had indeed occurred.

I would like to tell you the eradication of aegypti came as the result of a carefully conceived and masterfully executed plan of eradication; nothing could be further from the truth.

During the first three decades of antiaegypti campaigns, none had ever attained species eradication. Gorgas, Oswaldo Cruz, and other early workers observed that yellow fever disappeared long before aegypti did; that, as a matter of field experience, a reduction of aegypti house breeding to 5 per cent resulted in the disappearance of yellow fever. Thus, reduction below the 5 per cent threshold of transmission became the limited objective of yellow fever programs. The only serious attempt to eradicate aegypti had occurred in Northeast Brazil in 1928.

Hoping to find a permanent solution to Brazil's baffling yellow fever problem, Dr. M. E. Connor authorized the attempt to eradicate aegypti in the city of Parahyba, then having a population of some 35,000. This prolonged attempt brought the breeding index down to a fraction of 1 per cent but never to zero. Failure to eradicate was attributed to an innate instinct of self-preservation of the aegypti and to the law of diminishing returns, which prevented the suppression of an irreducible minimum of aegypti breeding. This conclusion had not been seriously challanged; the measures which resulted in eradication of aegypti in 1933, in a few Brazilian cities, were those which seemed logical in 1930 in developing an efficient and trustworthy aegypti-control program.

Let us now go backward from 1933 and the observation of aegypti eradication to my first meeting with aegypti, 13 years before; aegypti and I first met up in Recife, Pernambuco, Brazil, in March 1920. The aegypti, larvae and adults, were in the hands of Dr. Servulo Lima, the chief of the Federal Yellow Fever Commission; I was a neophyte on the staff of The Rockefeller Foundation, newly assigned to Northeast Brazil. The offer of Foundation collaboration in the yellow fever program, made at that time, which would have brought Servulo Lima and me together, was rejected, since the aegypti index was low, yellow fever was disappearing, and victory was already apparently in sight. Neither Servulo nor I could imagine then that more than a decade later we would join hands in the creation of a truly national yellow fever service, dedicated to the eradication of aegypti throughout all Brazil.

Although the Foundation participation in yellow fever work in Brazil began 3 years after my meeting with Servulo Lima and with aegypti, I spent the decade, until 1930, in administering hookworm disease programs in Brazil and in Paraguay and in general administration in the Rio de

Janeiro Foundation Office. In the hookworm disease campaigns, I came to know the value of detailed record keeping, the importance of continued visualization of accumulating data, and, above all, the necessity of checking in the field the validity of operational reports.

In 1928, yellow fever suddenly reappeared, one might say out of nowhere, in Brazil's beautiful capital, which had been free of it for 20 years. This invasion came after a 12-month period during which only one case had been diagnosed in the Western Hemisphere!

The next year, 1929, to add insult to injury, cases of yellow fever occurred within 200 meters of the Yellow Fever Office in Recife, Pernambuco! And Recife had been under the protection of the Rockefeller Foundation antiaegypti campaign for more than 5 years! Investigation revealed, of course, that the reported aegypti index of 0.8 per cent was highly fictitious; the first 100 houses inspected by an outside group found an index of 26.0 per cent.

I became personally responsible for the Rockefeller Foundation's yellow fever operations in Brazil in June 1930; I hesitated somewhat before accepting the appointment, since it meant directing a service in which I had had no direct experience.

As a hedge against my ignorance, I spent some 3 months in the field before taking the responsibility for operations. During this period I took maximum advantage of the opportunity to let the inspector (that is, the guarda) at the end of the line, educate me. I did not work with the doctor, or the supervisor, or the chief inspector, but with the man who was carrying out the actual house inspection and who was taking measures against aegypti, when found. I made it a point to start the day's work when the guarda did, to work with him throughout the day, doing everything which he did, including the preparation of the daily work sheet. If the guarda climbed upon a roof to inspect roof gutters, I also climbed the roof. (On more than one occasion, I had difficulty in getting down, not having eyes on my feet to guide them to the top rung of the ladder under the overhanging eave.) My program of education began in Belém at the mouth of the Amazon and continued from city to city along the coast of North Brazil. The climate was hot and humid, and always, the guarda, who had only one day with me, seemed to be overzealous in my education; I had the impression he did twice as many houses in his day with the new chief of the service as he did while working alone. The pace set was such that in less than 3 months, without ever missing a meal and without being ill, I lost 27 pounds of body weight. The loss of body fat was marked not only by the flopping fit of my suit, but also by the looseness of both hat and shoes. I report this not to have you commiserate with me at this late date; I cite it as an important factor in the eradication of aegypti. There were days, while these 27 pounds were melting away, when I was so tired and hot that had I not been under the eye of the guarda, I might well have been tempted to abandon the house visit, hie me to a coffee house or beer joint, and calmly falsify the house-visit record! If this could be my reaction to my self-appointed temporary task, how easily could it be the reaction of the guarda to whom the routine weekly visit, week after week, to the same houses, was merely a means of livelihood.

Gorgas and LePrince are each credited with the dictum that, in order to fight mosquitoes, one must learn to think like the mosquito; this dictum was changed, in the case of aegypti: "If you want to get results in the battle with aegypti, you want to think like the guarda, who is, in the final analysis, the only person attacking aegypti directly."

As my integrity had been guaranteed by the presence of the guarda, so I attempted to evolve means of guaranteeing the integrity, at all times, of the guarda; and of the chief inspector, and of the supervisor, and of the director of the service!

Remembering the fictitious aegypti index of Recife in 1929, and noting that the only concrete object purchased with the funds expended for aegypti work was the breeding index report, I attempted to make this report as trustworthy and as certifiable as the financial report of expenditures in its purchase.

In reorganizing the aegypti service in 1930 and the following years, each city and town worked was mapped; the number and kind of buildings in each block registered; blocks were assembled into zones of approximately the same work load; the blocks were numbered, not only on the map, but the number of the block was painted at each corner of each block, together with an indication of where work began in the block; also indicated was the way the inspector was to work around the block and where the block ended. The inspector was furnished with a map of his zone and with an itinerary by block numbers in the order in which the blocks were to be visited throughout the week. The inspector carried a flag to be conspicuously posted outside the house during his visit; inside the house, generally in the bathroom, was a house-visit register, where he recorded the date and hour of his visit and any significant observations. All this was done to make it easy to follow the inspector's work and to guarantee his integrity!

[Additional details about the development of the methods used for the eradication of *A. aegypti* in Brazil are given in Part VIII, Selection 33, in which Dr. Soper discusses the rehabilitation of the eradication concept. *Ed.*]

The inspector was held responsible for always being on duty unless he had reported off duty—if not found within 10 minutes, a satisfactory explanation had to be forthcoming to avoid the loss of the day's pay. The guarda who failed to die in an explosion in the Nichteroy Arsenal because of absence from duty was discharged on reporting alive for duty the next day. This rigorous regime was softened by a 10 per cent margin in basic wages, plus an opportunity to earn a bonus of up to 25 per cent each month according to the percentage of aegypti breeding missed and found by the supervisors.

The weakness of the aegypti service, even when carefully checked, was that the guarda and supervisors were both using the visual search for aquatic forms of aegypti as a measure of its presence. In 1930 I proposed to check the validity of reported breeding indices, through adult capture squads searching for adult mosquitoes. This proposal was opposed by the service chiefs, one of whom alleged it would cost at least $50 for each aegypti caught in his city. I expressed the hope it would cost $1000 each, since the higher the cost, the cleaner the city; I was hoping for negative evidence.

The adult capture squad proved to be useful for checking indices as planned, and unexpectedly important in pinpointing the presence of hidden breeding on which aegypti depended for its continued existence at low incidence levels. The discovery and elimination of these hidden foci is believed to have been largely responsible for abrogation of the law of diminishing returns and the disappearance of the irreducible minimum in aegypti breeding.

As already stated, aegypti eradication was not planned, but followed careful administrative work plus the independent check on results through adult captures.

In 1930, when the reorganization of the aegypti program began, the Rockefeller Foundation Yellow Fever Service was limited to North Brazil; the states of Espírito Santo, Rio de Janeiro, Minas Gerais, and São Paulo each had its own service; the Federal Department of Health had the responsibility for the Federal Capital, Rio de Janeiro. Following the 1930 Revolution, the Foundation was asked to extend its operation to all Brazil, except the capital city. In 1931, Servulo Lima, the chief of the Yellow Fever Service in Rio de Janeiro, suggested the amalgamation of this service with the larger effort; the union took place January 1932. Servulo and I later collaborated with others in drafting a National Yellow Fever Regulation, which became law on May 23, 1932. The Regulation was most important in the development of an effective National Yellow Fever Service for all Brazil.

Jungle yellow fever, a permanent source of virus for the reinfection of cities with aegypti, was discovered in 1932, the year before aegypti eradication was first observed. In the immediately following years, jungle yellow fever was confirmed for Bolivia, Colombia, Venezuela, and a number of states in South Brazil. Repeated observations were made of the invasion of cities and towns from nearby infested forest areas. It became obvious that the only permanent guarantee to the urban populations of the continent would come through the eradication of aegypti. The first suggestion of eradication in Brazil was accepted as a wild dream of an irresponsible spender. We should remember that the residual insecticides were unknown, that efficient antiaegypti work was based on visiting every house weekly and on eliminating aegypti breeding through destruction, oiling, or fishing of the guilty container. (Emptying proved inadequate; small larvae and viable eggs often remained.)

In spite of all difficulties, aegypti eradication did progress. Fortunately, it was more economical to clear aegypti from the suburbs than it was to maintain permanent aegypti control in the large cities; once the suburbs were clean, it was feasible to clear smaller towns and even rural areas, where infested, rather than to keep limited zones free. With greatly reduced forces in cleared areas, continuous expansion of operations was possible without great increase in staff and budget.

There were many difficulties, some disappointments, and an occasional unexpected reward. One unexpected dividend related to the small town of São Luiz de Quitunde in Alagoas. I first came to São Luiz in 1921, arriving in a dugout canoe, fleeing from a bedbug-infested hotel at the nearby Santo Antonio da Barra.

The hotel at São Luiz proved to be clean, its beans and rice palatable, and I felt the trip well worthwhile. But in answer to my query, "Tem mosquitoes?" came the standard reply, "Não tem, não!" And as I went to my room, I saw, as I knew I would, the rain barrel in the inner patio with hundreds of aegypti wrigglers. (The hotelkeeper was not untruthful, simply immune, following lifelong exposure, to any irritation from the bites of aegypti.)

Seventeen years later, I had a thrill one morning in Rio de Janeiro, a thousand miles away, from reading in the Correio da Manhã, a leading newspaper, a news items from São Luiz de Quitunde announcing that the guarda of the Yellow Fever Service had visited São Luiz and had found it infested with aegypti! This in 1938; in 1921 it would have been news if a guarda had visited any town or village in Alagoas and had not found aegypti! Although I was sorry to learn São Luiz had been reinfested, I was delighted that public education had come to the point of making infestation with aegypti newsworthy!

A real difficulty encountered in promoting the eradication of aegypti in Brazil and in South America was the disrepute into which the concept of eradication had fallen. A big boost in its rehabilitation was the eradication of *Anopheles gambiae* from Brazil in 1939–1940.

During World War II, continued progress in the eradication of aegypti was made in Brazil, and by 1947 Brazil's major preoccupation was with reinfestations of aegypti coming across her borders. Instead of attempting to negotiate with each of her ten neighbors, all infested with aegypti, regarding the prevention of the exportation of aegypti to Brazil, Brazil chose to bring the problem to the attention of the Pan American Sanitary Bureau, of which I had become Director early in 1947. The Directing Council of the Pan American Health Organization approved a resolution calling on all the countries of the Americas to cooperate through the Pan American Sanitary Bureau in the eradication of aegypti.

Work began immediately in Paraguay with the support of Brazil and Argentina, and has been extended as opportunity permitted to other countries. In 1961, progress was such that the Pan American Directing Council called on all countries still infested to eliminate aegypti within 5 years, that is, by 1966.

In 1962 on the mainland of the Americas, aegypti was found only in the United States; in Venezuela, which has a well-advanced eradication program; and in Netherlands Guiana. (The cities of Cúcuta, Colombia, and Georgetown, British Guiana, previously cleared of aegypti, have been reinfested.)

The program that has grown and expanded from observations made during the early weeks of Franklin D. Roosevelt's first administration has merited the following paragraph in John F. Kennedy's Health Program Message to the Congress of the United States of February 7, 1963:

A problem of particular significance in the Western Hemisphere is that of yellow fever. Many countries of the Americas have conducted campaigns to eradicate the mosquito which carries yellow fever, but the problem of reinfestation has become a serious one, particularly in the Caribbean area. We have pledged our participation in a program to eradicate this disease-carrying mosquito from the United States, and the 1964 budget provides funds to initiate such efforts. This will bring this country to conformity with the long established policy of the Pan American Health Organization to eliminate the threat of yellow fever in this hemisphere.

I trust that each of you may live so long as to see similar approaching fruition of your most cherished professional programs.

| The Eradication of *Aëdes aegypti*:
A World Problem*

The concept of eradication is quite modern; it had to await recognition of the specificity of communicable diseases and demonstration of the means of prevention. Local and national eradication of animal diseases began in the last two decades of the nineteenth century and has been popular with veterinarians ever since. International eradication, however, awaited a mechanism for the coordination of national campaigns in regional and global programs.

The concept of eradication as applied to communicable diseases and disease vectors implies permanent nonrecurrence in the absence of all preventive measures. This definition, modified by the phrase "unless reintroduction occurs," applies also to local, state, national, and regional eradication as necessary steps toward world eradication.

Aëdes aegypti is a variable biological group, officially consisting of *A. aegypti,* neotype (Mattingly et al., 1962), *A. aegypti* variety *queenslandensis* (Theobald, 1901), and *A. aegypti* subspecies *formosus* (Walker, 1848).

The neotype and var. *queenslandensis* are closely related to human habitations and are not known to occur as wild free-living forms; the ssp. *formosus* is essentially a wild forest mosquito not associated with human habitations.

Discussion of eradication of *A. aegypti* is necessarily limited to the neotype and var. *queenslandensis.*

Yellow Fever Eradication Fails

In Havana in 1900–1901 the specificity of yellow fever was proved and means of prevention demonstrated; in 1913 the creation of The Rockefeller Foundation provided a mechanism for coordination of national campaigns; in 1915 the Foundation became committed to cooperation with yellow fever countries in its eradication from the earth.

Early yellow fever campaigns led to disappearance of the disease in large endemic centers in a matter of weeks after reduction of aegypti breeding

* Read at the Ninth International Congress for Microbiology, July 24–30, 1966, Moscow, USSR. Dr. Soper was a Special Consultant, Office of International Health, Public Health Service.

This article *(118)* is reprinted with permission from the Proceedings of the Ninth International Congress for Microbiology, Moscow, July 24–30, 1966, *Symposia,* pp. 599–605.

below the threshold required for continued transmission; once these centers were cleared, yellow fever burned itself out and spontaneously disappeared from the towns and villages of tributary zones.

The plan of eradication called for the temporary reduction of *A. aegypti*, the only known vector, in the endemic centers until the disease disappeared forever from man, the only known vertebrate host.

The Foundation effort succeeded in eliminating the last endemic aegypti-yellow fever in the Americas in 1934; but this elimination did not guarantee "permanent non-recurrence in the absence of all preventive measures." Reintroduction could and did occur from previously unrecognized epizootics of jungle yellow fever.

The discovery of yellow fever without *A. aegypti* (1932) and the development of the concept of jungle yellow fever as a disease of forest primates (1935) was followed by observation of the introduction of virus from forest to town with reestablishment of the aegypti–man–aegypti cycle of transmission.

PANAMERICAN *Aëdes aegypti* ERADICATION

The gradually unfolding picture of jungle yellow fever as a widespread and permanent threat to towns and cities forced reconsideration of prevention of urban yellow fever.

Aegypti control, in the pre-DDT period, was very expensive, requiring weekly visits to all houses in the control area. Money and men for control programs were easily had during outbreaks of yellow fever but were often taken away once the immediate threat ended.

The difficulty of keeping up a permanent defense against aegypti-transmitted disease was revealed by the absence of antiaegypti measures in Rio de Janeiro when yellow fever reappeared there in 1928. In Rio, free of yellow fever since 1908, the antiaegypti service had been permitted to deteriorate, and finally was abandoned, early in 1928, when plague, newly arrived in the city, was given first call on available manpower.

Another revelation of inefficiency of long continued aegypti-control programs came the following year in Pernambuco. Investigation there, following the appearance of yellow fever after 5 years of continuous Rockefeller Foundation aegypti control, disclosed actual aegypti-breeding indexes many times higher than those reported. Experience elsewhere has repeatedly confirmed the difficulty of maintaining permanent antiaegypti services and, when maintained, of keeping them efficient.

Beginning in 1930, the attempt was made to so organize the Cooperative Yellow Fever Service in Brazil that its reported aegypti index would be as certifiable as its bank balance; this attempt led in 1933 to the complete disappearance of *A. aegypti* from a number of isolated port cities. This complete local elimination came without any measure not previously used; it came rather from complete coverage, careful supervision, impartial larviciding of all infested containers, and the checking of low-incidence larval indexes by hand capturing of adult mosquitoes.

Eradication was not initially the result of planning for eradication; it occurred unexpectedly, as a reward of excellence of operation.

[A summary of the administrative procedures of the Cooperative Yellow Fever Service, maintained jointly by the Brazilian Government and The Rockefeller Foundation, 1929–1940, was published at the request of Sir Malcolm Watson, a pioneer in antimosquito campaigns. Residual insecticides have simplified the problem, but the essentials remain. See the excerpt in Selection 7. *Ed.*]

Finding *A. aegypti* eradicable did not lead immediately to a drive for countrywide eradication. The first intraservice proposal to eradicate *A. aegypti* in all Brazil was made in 1934; the reaction among experienced yellow fever workers, Brazilians and Americans alike, was one of incredulity, of disbelief in their capacity for such an enormous task.

In spite of this reaction, the Cooperative Yellow Fever Service began to work quietly toward eradication without, however, an official commitment. This was done without increased staff and budget, by first reducing in numbers and then removing all aegypti inspectors from "eradicated" cities and using the manpower thus released to work the suburbs, towns, villages, and even rural areas of the interior.

As the cleared area became greater through peripheral expansion, the threat of reinfestation declined proportionately. Eventually, occasional checking of eradicated areas by mobile units was found adequate to prevent unsuspected runaway reinfestation. Thus eradication proceeded at a regular pace without any great increase in cost and staff.

At the beginning of 1940, the Federal District (Rio de Janeiro, now the State of Guanabara) and six other states were completely free of *A. aegypti;* the eradication effort was nationwide and many cities and towns in other Brazilian states were no longer infested. At this point The Rockefeller Foundation withdrew; the antiaegypti eradication effort was carried forward by the National Yellow Fever Service. This Service became committed officially, in 1942, to the complete eradication of *A. aegypti* from all Brazil.

("Article 10: Incumbent upon the Section of Stegomyia Control shall be: (a) the study and preparation of plans for the control of the stegomyia mosquito (*Aëdes aegypti*) by the field services, looking toward the complete eradication of this species. . . .")

The introduction of DDT in 1947 speeded up the final clearing of the northeastern states, where residual rural infestation existed. By the end of

1949 all known infested areas were free, but another 5 years of detailed searching was needed for elimination of a few residual foci. The Pan American Health Organization (PAHO) certified Brazil free of *A. aegypti* in 1958, a full quarter of a century after the first observation of eradication.

In the meantime, in the 1930s, attempts had been made to get aegypti-eradication programs in Bolivia, Colombia, Cuba, Ecuador, Paraguay, Peru, the United States, and Venezuela. Of these, only that in Bolivia prospered; Bolivia, with but a limited initial infestation of *A. aegypti,* became the first country to report eradication, in 1941.

In 1942 Bolivia proposed, at the XIth Pan American Sanitary Conference, that the American nations eradicate *A. aegypti.* The Conference requested "the governments of the countries where this vector is found to organize eradication projects based on plans adopted in Brazil." Little or nothing was done to comply with this request. Historically, however, the Bolivian initiative is the first indication of the expansive pressure naturally developed by a successful eradication effort.

By 1947 eradication in Brazil had proceeded so far that reinfestation across national boundaries was a serious problem. Brazil followed the 1942 Bolivian precedent and proposed, for its own protection, the continental eradication of *A. aegypti.* The Directing Council of the newly reorganized Pan American Health Organization did not merely request individual nations to act but entrusted "to the Pan American Sanitary Bureau the solution of the continental problem of urban yellow fever, based fundamentally on the eradication of *Aëdes aegypti. . . .*"

The Council went further and resolved that the Pan American Sanitary Bureau, "in agreement with the interested countries, shall take the necessary measures to solve such problems as may emerge . . . whether they be sanitary, economic or legal."

The action of the Council is a landmark in international health; it recognizes the right to protection from reinfection or reinfestation from a neighboring country; it sets a precedent for the nations of a region accepting a joint commitment to specific action of each nation within its own borders; and it firmly fixes the position of the international health organization as the coordinating agency for molding national efforts into regional programs.

The PAHO eradication effort has led to the certification of freedom from *A. aegypti* of the following countries: Argentina, Bolivia, Brazil, British Honduras, Chile, Costa Rica, Ecuador, El Salvador, Guatemala, Honduras, Mexico, Nicaragua, Panama, Paraguay, Peru, Uruguay, and the Canal Zone. Of these, only El Salvador is known to have been grossly reinfested; reinfestation has delayed the certification of British Guiana, Colombia, and Trinidad.

Fortunately, most of South America, the countries of Central America, and Mexico eradicated *A. aegypti* without having to face the problem of resistance to residual insecticides. Resistance has been an important factor in delaying eradication in Venezuela and in several of the West Indies; it has led to the interruption of eradication efforts in several places, including the Dominican Republic, Haiti, and Jamaica. The situation in the Caribbean is admittedly unsatisfactory.

On the other hand, the United States, itself not immediately threatened by jungle yellow fever virus, initiated its eradication effort in 1963, covering the southern states, Puerto Rico, and the Virgin Islands.

The *A. aegypti* situation at the end of 1965 is shown in Map 1; dengue fever appeared in the Caribbean in 1963 and spread in the following years

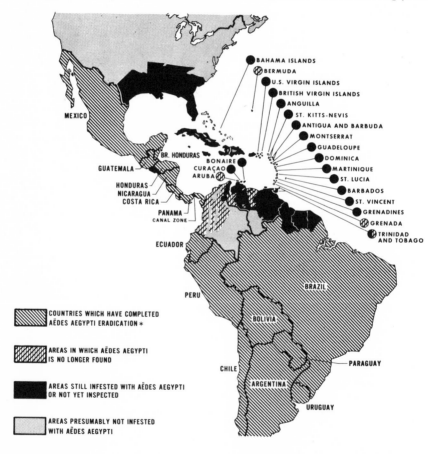

COUNTRIES WHICH HAVE COMPLETED
AËDES AEGYPTI ERADICATION ∗

AREAS IN WHICH AËDES AEGYPTI
IS NO LONGER FOUND

AREAS STILL INFESTED WITH AËDES AEGYPTI
OR NOT YET INSPECTED

AREAS PRESUMABLY NOT INFESTED
WITH AËDES AEGYPTI

∗ ERADICATION CARRIED OUT ACCORDING TO THE STANDARDS ESTABLISHED BY THE PAN AMERICAN HEALTH ORGANIZATION

Map 1. Status of the *Aëdes aegypti* Eradication Campaign, December 1965.

to most of the *A. aegypti*-infested areas, except the southern states of the United States. Map 2 shows the distribution of dengue fever during this period; fortunately, it is not the hemorrhagic dengue of Asia.

Aëdes aegypti: A WORLD PROBLEM

Aëdes aegypti is a world problem as an actual and potential vector of various virus diseases and as a source of reinfestation of "eradicated" areas. All infested nations face one or more phases of this problem.

When America completes eradication, its interest will be in eliminating *A. aegypti* from other regions from which reinfestation may come; as long as Pan American eradication is incomplete, concern must continue over threat of urbanization of jungle yellow fever virus and of importation of hemorrhagic dengue virus from Asia.

Africa has the same reasons as the Americas for eradicating *A. aegypti*. Jungle yellow fever is widespread in Africa; its threat to aegypti-infested cities, towns, and villages is permanent. Increasing urbanization in Africa promises to increase the threat of aegypti-transmitted yellow fever; the extensive yellow fever epidemic in Senegal in 1965 emphasizes the difficulty of permanently preventing yellow fever by long-term vaccination programs.

In Asia, hemorrhagic dengue, as a present danger, has been added to the potential threat of the introduction of yellow fever inherent in the presence of *A. aegypti*. Health officers of the Far East for half a century have voiced the fear that improved communications might bring yellow

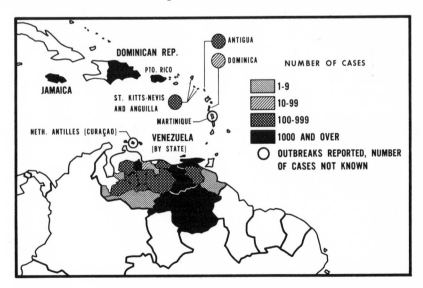

Map 2. Reported cases of dengue in the Caribbean area, 1962–1965.

fever virus to Asia. This fear, voiced by Manson in 1903 because of the building of the Panama Canal, has not waned with the development of rapid air communications. Today Asia has the virus of hemorrhagic dengue to offer Africa and America in exchange for that of yellow fever!

No one can now foresee the extent of the future threat of *A. aegypti* to mankind as a vector of known virus diseases, and none can foretell what other virus diseases may yet afflict the regions where *A. aegypti* is permitted to remain.

RECOMMENDATIONS

1. Recognizing its importance, *A. aegypti* should be studied as a long-term national, regional, and world problem rather than as a temporary local threat to the communities suffering at any given moment from yellow fever, dengue, or other aegypti-borne disease.

2. Adequate laboratory facilities should support field studies to determine:

a. The eradicability of *A. aegypti,* neotype, and var. *queenslandensis* in Africa.

b. The adaptability of *A. aegypti,* ssp. *formosus,* to domestic and urban conditions.

c. The choice of insecticide to be used in different places.

3. Eradicability tests to be significant should be either large or well isolated and have protection against continuing reinfestation; such reinfestation is especially apt to come with the movement of passengers; small boats are particularly dangerous.

4. The world is not ready to undertake the all-out rapid global eradication of *A. aegypti;* on the other hand, it seems futile to attempt permanent local *A. aegypti* control with residual insecticides which may become self-defeating through the development of resistance. Continued effective control of *A. aegypti* requires eradication; local eradication generates expansion at the periphery to prevent reinfestation; such is the life history of eradication in the Americas and such may well be the pattern for Africa and Asia. Each local control effort should be planned as an "island of eradication" in which pressure can be generated for continuing peripheral expansion.

Aëdes aegypti-transmitted yellow fever (referred to herein, for conve-nience, as aegypti yellow fever), long one of the great scourges of the tropical, the subtropical, and even the temperate regions of the Americas, has been brought under complete control in the Western Hemisphere. All yellow fever that was recorded in the years 1900–1931 (Fig. 1) is assumed to be aegypti yellow fever. Only two small and localized outbreaks have oc-curred in the last 28 years, the first at Senna Madureira in the heart of the Amazon Valley in Brazil in 1942, the second in Port of Spain, Trinidad, in 1954. Whether the Americas are to be spared further epidemics of urban yellow fever, sparked from widespread jungle outbreaks of the disease (Fig. 2), depends on the completion of the present well-advanced program for the eradication of *A. aegypti*.

The potential danger is clearly revealed by the 1963–1965 outbreak of dengue in certain Caribbean islands and Venezuela. This outbreak has been dramatically limited to areas still infested with *A. aegypti*. As long as the eradication of *A. aegypti* is incomplete, the continuing threat of rein-festation of areas from which it has been eradicated is very real, as shown by the reinfestations of Colombia, French Guiana, and Guyana [formerly British Guiana]. The most recent break in the advancing eradication pro-gram was the 1965 reinfestation of El Salvador at a time when neighboring countries were not known to be infested. (Initial investigation suggests that this reinfestation came through the importation from the United States of old automobile tires, a favorite breeding place for *A. aegypti* in this mod-ern age.)

The national eradication of *A. aegypti* as a permanent preventative of urban and maritime yellow fever was proposed and unofficially adopted as the objective of Brazil's Yellow Fever Service in 1934. Impossible as this task then appeared, experience was to show that eradication is actually easier than continuing effective *A. aegypti* control. Once a large city is free of *A. aegypti*, it is more economical to clean the suburbs and tributary villages than to maintain permanent control in the city. Continuing pe-ripheral expansion was possible in Brazil with no increase of manpower be-yond that previously used in *A. aegypti* control work in the principal cities.

Aëdes aegypti eradication calls for systematic attack wherever this vector may be found, regardless of the immediacy of disease transmission. This

* Read at the Seminar on the Ecology, Biology, Control and Eradication of *Aëdes aegypti*, Geneva, Switzerland, August 16–20, 1965. Dr. Soper was a Special Consultant, Office of International Health, Public Health Service.

This excerpt is reprinted with permission from the article *(121)* in the *Bulletin of the World Health Organization 36:* 521–527, 1967. (About half of the original text has been omitted.)

policy has been most fruitful in Brazil. Several towns were infected by cases from nearby jungle outbreaks in 1934, 1935, and 1936, but only a single small outbreak has occurred in the last three decades.

The eradication of *A. aegypti* in the Americas is possible because it has

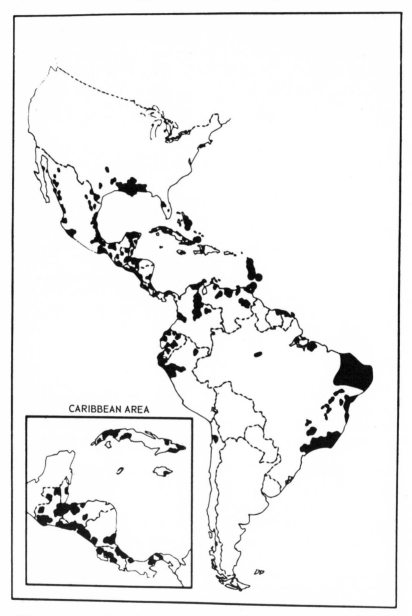

Figure 1. Areas of the Americas in which yellow fever was reported from 1900 to 1931.

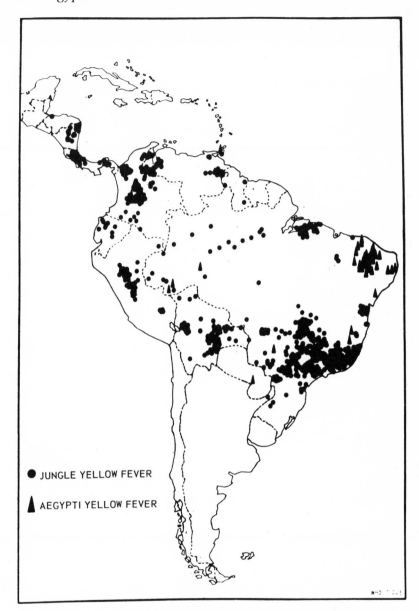

Figure 2. Areas of the Americas in which yellow fever was reported from 1932 to 1955.

never adapted to life in the forest away from human habitation. Apparently this is also true for this vector in other parts of the world away from its original home in Africa, where it still breeds in the forest.

Whether eradication of the domestic *A. aegypti* in Africa would be followed by ready reinfestation with *A. aegypti* from the forest depends on the adaptability of the forest *A. aegypti* to domestic water containers. This has not yet been determined. Until it is, the aegypti yellow fever of Africa can be prevented by measures against *A. aegypti* in the large cities and by vaccination of the population of the interior. Neither method is wholly satisfactory, because neither has a terminal point.

Yellow fever in Africa, previous to the discovery of jungle yellow fever (Fig. 3), was largely limited to West Africa between the Sahara Desert and the Gulf of Guinea, with extension down the coast to the mouth of the Congo River. Since 1932 (Fig. 4) yellow fever has been observed in a projection eastward of the previous range along the coast; this projection has stopped some distance from the coast. Even large outbreaks in the Sudan and Ethiopia lack the characteristics of the aegypti yellow fever of the West African coast and of the Americas.

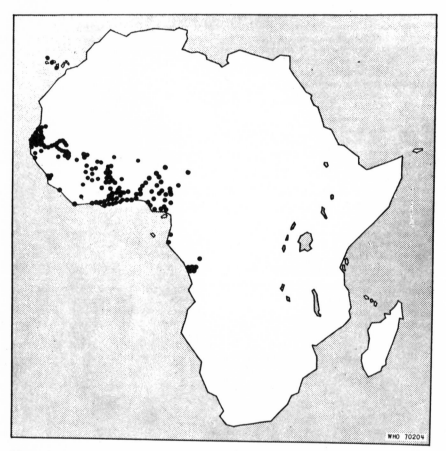

Figure 3. Localities in Africa in which yellow fever was reported from 1900 to 1931.

Yellow fever has never traveled to Asia with man and *A. aegypti* by boat, probably because there has been no epidemic in the port cities of the east coast of Africa. The absence of yellow fever in these cities may not be equally important in preventing the movement of yellow fever by air, however.

Jungle yellow fever in the Americas and in Africa is a permanent source of yellow fever virus, a potential threat to uninfected regions in these days of rapid travel, to all regions infected with *A. aegypti*. Should *A. aegypti* eradication in Asia and the western Pacific be considered because of its transmission of other diseases, freedom from all threat of yellow fever can be cited as an added inducement.

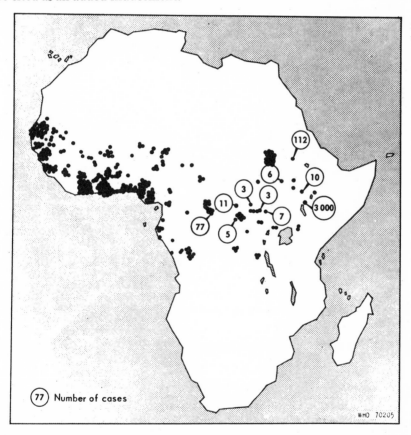

Figure 4. Localities in Africa in which yellow fever was reported from 1932 to 1963.

Selection 12 | Dynamics of *Aëdes aegypti*
Distribution and Density:
Seasonal Fluctuations in the
Americas*

By distribution of *Aëdes aegypti,* one means its geographical range. Density is more difficult to determine; it is inadequately measured by the aegypti index (that is, the percentage of houses with evidence of the breeding of aegypti). Density is affected not only by the number and distribution of infested houses but also by the number and size of available breeding places. Both distribution and density are affected by rainfall and temperature; seasonal fluctuations may be very great.

MECHANISM OF SPREAD OF *Aegypti*

Aëdes aegypti, originally a tree-hole breeder in Africa, owes its worldwide distribution to its adaptation to human habitation, to breeding in artificial water containers, and to traveling with man. Of special importance is the longevity of its eggs.

The sailing ships of the fifteenth to nineteenth centuries, with their open water containers, were extremely favorable for the distribution of *A. aegypti* by sea. It is probable that practically all the seaports of the tropical and temperate zones of the world have been visited repeatedly by *A. aegypti.*

River boats throughout the world are generally favorable to the breeding and transportation of *A. aegypti.* In the tropics and subtropics, the principal river valleys have all been infested, at least up to the first waterfall.

Steam-operated railways have played their part in the distribution of *A. aegypti* away from the seacoasts and river ports. At times, the breeding of *A. aegypti* has been found only in and about the railway stations at interior points.

In its aquatic forms, *A. aegypti* may travel with man in whatever conveyance he may use; it may even travel with him on foot. Religious pilgrims in the semiarid regions of northeast Brazil carry drinking water in small

* Read at the Seminar on the Ecology, Biology, Control and Eradication of *Aëdes aegypti,* Geneva, Switzerland, August 16–20, 1965. Dr. Soper was a Special Consultant, Office of International Health, Public Health Service.

This article (*123*) is reprinted with permission from the *Bulletin of the World Health Organization 36:* 536–538, 1967.

clay pots; these pots have disseminated *A. aegypti* widely through the rural areas of several states of that country.

The adult *A. aegypti* has been observed traveling by passenger automobile in Brazil and has been collected from automobiles crossing the Venezuelan-Colombian border. It travels freely in passenger coaches on trains and was repeatedly found in aircraft arriving in Brazil from Africa in the pre-DDT period.

In summary, *A. aegypti* may travel with man as adult, larva, or egg under almost any conditions. On the other hand, *A. aegypti* is rarely found on the large, modern, ocean-going steamship. Also, there are considerable areas in the interior of South America, suitable for *A. aegypti* breeding, where it has never penetrated. In the Amazon Valley, *A. aegypti* was generally found in the cities and towns below the first waterfall in each tributary, but in many cases it had failed to get around the portage.

In certain instances, local folklore establishes the approximate date of the arrival of *A. aegypti* in important cities in the interior and suggests the mechanism of importation. When yellow fever appeared in Santa Cruz de la Sierra, Bolivia, in 1932, the people declared that *A. aegypti* was a newcomer to their town about 1919. They associated its appearance with the installation of electrical power for the city; they believed the electric lights had attracted this mosquito into the town. In retrospect, it seems probable that the equipment for the power plant became infested with eggs and aquatic forms of *A. aegypti* on its long trip to Santa Cruz through the Amazon Valley.

Similarly, in Bucaramanga, Colombia, the old inhabitants insisted that *A. aegypti* had been unknown in their youth. This mosquito had suddenly appeared, however, about 1908 or 1909, many years before the construction of the railroad, as a new pest in the city. The people, noting a resemblance between this new mosquito and the figure of their archbishop, who visited Bucaramanga about that time, named the mosquito for him. The archbishop had come to dedicate a religious statue recently imported from Italy. Probably this statue offered a suitable breeding place for *A. aegypti* as it was transported up the Magdalena River from Barranquilla.

Aëdes aegypti does not tend to fly for long distances in search of breeding places; expansion of an infested area therefore occurs slowly, except where transportation with man is a factor.

RANGE OF *Aëdes aegypti* IN THE AMERICAS

Early History

The date of arrival of *A. aegypti* in the Western Hemisphere is unknown; it may even have come with Columbus or some of his early followers. That it did arrive fairly early is indicated by records of outbreaks of yellow fever in the sixteenth century.

There was a time when ports along the northern Atlantic seaboard of the United States and even of Canada, suffered summer epidemics of yellow fever. These outbreaks must have depended on spring or early summer importation of *A. aegypti* by boat from the West Indies and later introduction of yellow fever virus. As late as 1878, a widespread epidemic of yellow fever occurred in the Mississippi Valley. For many decades, the traditional home of yellow fever was in the ports of the Caribbean Sea and the Gulf of Mexico, with extension to the Pacific coast of South America.

A great deal is known about the distribution of *A. aegypti* in the yellow fever areas following the demonstration in 1901 that yellow fever can be controlled—can be prevented—by an attack on this mosquito. Following the success of numerous local campaigns, The Rockefeller Foundation undertook the eradication of yellow fever, beginning in 1915. As a result, considerable information on the distribution of *A. aegypti* became available in certain Latin American countries. This information has been greatly extended and completed since 1930, with the attack directed against the *A. aegypti* mosquito itself rather than against yellow fever. Species eradication requires complete survey and coverage of its entire range.

Period Since 1930

In 1930, when the reorganization of the yellow fever operations which led to the program for the eradication of *A. aegypti* began, this mosquito ranged in the Americas from Oklahoma and Tennessee in the United States to Buenos Aires in Argentina and Tocopilla in Chile; it occurred in all countries, territories and islands within this range. Eradication of *A. aegypti* in the Western Hemisphere therefore requires the active participation of all the countries and territories situated there, except Canada and the Falkland Islands.

Within its range, *A. aegypti* was not uniformily distributed, even where temperature and humidity were favorable. Several tributaries to the Amazon were not infested above the first waterfall, and even below this barrier *A. aegypti* was often found only in the larger cities and towns. Isolated homesteads and villages were free of *A. aegypti;* this freedom was apparently due to easy access to river water and lack of need for storage of water for domestic needs.

Throughout its range, *A. aegypti* was generally a domestic mosquito of cities, towns, and villages, but three areas of serious rural infestation were found. These were in the semiarid states of Northeast Brazil, in the delta of the Magdalena River in Colombia, and in the Yucatan Peninsula of Mexico. In these areas, the prolonged dry season leads to extensive storage of domestic water reserves.

Aëdes aegypti breeding was generally limited to human artifacts, but bamboo stems, coconut shells, fallen leaves, and damaged papaya trees proved to be dangerous. Tree holes along city streets and parks were sometimes infested, but tree-hole breeding was never found in the forests away from human habitation. In the Americas, *A. aegypti* does not breed in rain pools on the ground.

There is apparently perfect adaptation of *A. aegypti* to the old automobile tire, whether it is abandoned or is being collected and shipped for recapping, for the making of sandals, or for ships' bumpers.

Present Distribution (1965)

The present known distribution of *A. aegypti* is limited to the northern fringe of South America, to the islands of the West Indies, and to the United States. (Reinfestation in San Salvador, the capital of El Salvador, is reported as of July 1965). The following countries on the mainland of the Americas have been freed of *A. aegypti*: Argentina, Bolivia, Brazil, Chile, Colombia, Costa Rica, Ecuador, Guatemala, Honduras, British Honduras, Guyana, French Guiana, El Salvador, Mexico, Nicaragua, Panama, Paraguay, Peru, and Uruguay. (Guyana and French Guiana have been reinfested since 1963). On the mainland of the Americas, Venezuela, the United States, and the three Guianas are still infested. Cuba, Haiti, Jamaica, Puerto Rico, the Dominican Republic, Trinidad, and the smaller islands of the Caribbean must be cleared before the threat of reinfestation will be over.

SOURCE OF REINFESTATION

Since the eradication effort began in the 1930s, a great deal of work has been done on the epidemiology of *A. aegypti* reinfestation. This has been attributed to direct flight of *A. aegypti* only in closely contiguous areas. Trains, automobiles, and coastal and river boats have been incriminated. The transportation of an infested water container with the effects of a family moving from one place to another has been found guilty. Old tires moved by railroad, truck, and boat have been held responsible.

As far as is known, no country in the Americas has been reinfested from other regions of the world since the eradication effort started.

The only long-distance movement of *A. aegypti* held responsible for a reinfestation has been the apparent movement in old automobile tires from the United States to El Salvador in 1965.

Experience has shown that eradication can be accomplished within a country with a limited staff working progressively from one section to another, using minimal resources to prevent reinfestation of cleared areas.

Seasonal Fluctuations

Seasonal fluctuations of the range of *A. aegypti* do occur at the periphery of its geographical and altitudinal range; exceptionally cold winters may temporarily reduce the infested area to an appreciable degree.

Both the breeding index and the density of *A. aegypti* are affected by temperature and rainfall. In tropical areas, the effect of rainfall alone is quite apparent. In temperate areas, *A. aegypti* may practically disappear during the winter months and slowly increase in density during the spring and early summer. Traditionally, the transmission peak for yellow fever is early autumn.

Drought does not necessarily reduce the range of *A. aegypti* but may reduce its density. The obligatory storage of water during drought periods helps preserve the *A. aegypti* mosquitoes in such areas.

Seasonal fluctuations in *A. aegypti* distribution and density, important as they are to the health officer concerned with epidemic control, lose their importance when the objective is the eradication of *A. aegypti* rather than temporary disease prevention.

Selection 13 | The Routine Postmortem
Removal of Liver Tissue from
Rapidly Fatal Fever Cases
for the Discovery of Silent
Yellow Fever Foci*

FRED L. SOPER, E. R. RICKARD,
AND P. J. CRAWFORD

For more than three decades it has been known that yellow fever is transmitted by *Aëdes aegypti*. During this period antimosquito measures have been applied and have resulted universally in the disappearance of yellow fever from the mortality records of towns and cities in which such action has been taken. An unexpected result of the early campaigns was the spontaneous apparent disappearance of yellow fever from large tributary areas as well as from the centers worked. This phenomenon was observed so constantly that a satisfactory explanation was hypothesized and a whole generation of epidemiologists planned the final elimination of yellow fever from the world through the application of antiaegypti measures in a relatively few, arbitrarily selected, "key centers" of population lying within the known endemic areas. This key-center program did not require detailed studies of the conditions under which yellow fever occurred outside the large cities, since it was assumed that in tributary areas the disease would spontaneously clear up or burn out in a short time in the absence of reinfection from the large cities.

Certain events of the past few years have indicated that the epidemiology of yellow fever is much more complex than it was previously believed to be and have shown the necessity of a thorough study of the conditions under

* The studies and observations on which this paper is based were conducted by the Cooperative Yellow Fever Service maintained by the Brazilian Government and The Rockefeller Foundation, with the active participation of the Bahia Yellow Fever Laboratory of The Rockefeller Foundation. Dr. Soper was the Representative in South America (Rio de Janeiro office) of the International Health Division of The Rockefeller Foundation; Drs. Rickard and Crawford were staff members.

This article (*18*) is reprinted with permission from the *American Journal of Hygiene 19*: 549–566, 1934.

which yellow fever occurs today in the field. Among such events the following may be cited:

1. The failure of yellow fever to disappear from Brazil despite prolonged campaigns of key-center control.

2. The reappearance of yellow fever in Colombia in 1929 without any evidence of reimportation from known infected areas.

3. The demonstration of the occurrence of yellow fever in the absence of *A. aegypti*, first in a rural area of Espírito Santo, Brazil, in March 1932 and later, in May 1933, in the small isolated village of San Ramón, Bolivia.

4. The declaration of a frank epidemic of yellow fever in nonimmune troops from the uplands at Santa Cruz, Bolivia, in March 1932. Santa Cruz, with less than 20,000 population, cannot be considered a key center of population, and, furthermore, lies thousands of miles from any such key center and from any other known focus of yellow fever infection.

5. The confirmation by animal protection tests of acquired immunity to yellow fever in individuals belonging to the younger age groups in areas long believed free of the disease and in districts never known to have been infected.

The difficulties encountered in the study of yellow fever in the native populations of endemic areas cannot be properly appreciated by those whose ideas of the clinical and epidemiological manifestations of the disease have been acquired from the literature of yellow fever, which is largely based either on observations of the disease in groups of newly arrived nonimmunes in the large cities of endemic areas, or on its manifestations in epidemics occurring in nonimmune populations residing outside the truly endemic areas. Classical clinical cases of yellow fever occurring during epidemics among nonimmune troops or immigrants in endemic areas, and in populations living beyond the usual yellow fever zone, are not, generally, difficult to diagnose. The diagnosis of yellow fever, however, becomes rapidly more difficult as the number of classical cases decreases and isolated cases observed in the field in endemic areas can almost never be diagnosed clinically with certainty. Experience in Brazil has shown that the clinical diagnosis of yellow fever is most difficult in those endemic regions where it is most constantly present. As control measures become effective in the larger centers of population, where the movement of nonimmunes is most intense, yellow fever apparently disappears from the surrounding area, but in reality often continues silently in the native population for an indefinite period with but few fatalities, which are readily attributed to malaria, influenza, typhoid fever, and other acute infections.

Various authors have called attention to the occurrence of mild cases in endemic regions and the necessity of recognizing these cases. But the recognition of mild cases in the field is, under present conditions, practically impossible. It is possible, however, to discover some of the occasional fatal cases which do occur, through the examination of liver sections, since characteristic lesions are usually found in this organ. The results of an attempt to discover the active endemic foci of yellow fever in Brazil through the routine examination of liver sections, removed postmortem from febrile cases of less than 10 days' duration, between April 1930 and June 1933, are herewith reported.

HISTORY OF VISCEROTOMY

The possibility of determining, through the examination of autopsy material from a large number of fatal febrile cases, the location of those silent foci of yellow fever responsible for maintaining the endemicity of the disease in North Brazil (that is, the State of Bahia and all states lying north of Bahia) was repeatedly discussed with the public health authorities during 1928 and 1929, but no serious attempt was made at the routine collection of specimens previous to April 1930.

Following the widespread appearance of cases of yellow fever in Brazil in 1928 and 1929, the disease apparently disappeared from all of North Brazil, and no confirmed cases were recorded for this area from July 1929 to March 1930, when an outbreak occurred in Bôm Conselho, Pernambuco, and a suspect case was reported in Belém, Pará. The latter case, although finally declared negative after examination of liver tissue, called attention once more to the possibility of the existence of yellow fever in the Amazon Basin. The city of Belém, at the mouth of the Amazon, as well as the entire Amazon Valley, gives no definite history of yellow fever between 1913 and 1929. In January 1929 several confirmed cases occurred, followed by occasional cases, until July of that year. This outbreak, limited to a total of 12 declared cases, distributed over a period of 7 months and occurring in various parts of the city, was limited to adult foreigners, despite the fact, that, historically, at least, all native-born children under 17 years of age should have been nonimmune and susceptible to the disease. In connection with the suspect case of March 1930, it was noted that there had been a very high mortality reported for malaria during the first trimester of the year and the possibility of a masked outbreak of yellow fever was considered. To help clarify this situation, the state authorities of Pará granted permission on April 9 for the Yellow Fever Service to perform partial autopsies on all fatal febrile cases of less than 10 days' duration. The first partial routine autopsy was secured on April 21, 1930, and the second on May 10. On May 17 one of us (P.J.C.) accidentally learned of the death of a Brazilian child of 4 years of age from a febrile attack of 6 days' duration in Val de Cães, a small town lying 3 miles from Belém. Since this fell within the class of cases upon which routine autopsies were being performed, a liver section was removed, which resulted in a diagnosis of yellow fever. This was the first indication of the persistence of the disease in the neighborhood of Belém in 9 months. Only on June 21 did a single, isolated, clinically recognized case of yellow fever appear in the city.

The routine collection of liver specimens was begun at Natal, Rio Grande do Norte, in cooperation with the Prophylaxia Rural (the Rural Endemic Diseases Service), early in May 1930 and did much to relieve apprehension regarding the possible existence of yellow fever in the city during a sharp and unusual epidemic of malaria, attributed to the recent introduction of *Anopheles gambiae* on the American continent.

It is interesting to note that the routine collection of liver specimens for the discovery of endemic areas of yellow fever was independently organized almost simultaneously in North and South Brazil. In March 1930 the Yellow Fever Service of the State of Rio de Janeiro, alarmed by the appearance of suspicious lay diagnoses in the mortality records of Santo Aleixo, gave instructions for the autopsy of all bodies presented for burial at this point. The result was a positive diagnosis of yellow fever on the first case so autopsied on March 29. Previous to this diagnosis yellow fever had not been known in the State of Rio de Janeiro for about 6 months. The necessity of investigation of other parts of the state was recognized, and in May an organization was developed for securing liver specimens from sections where it was believed the presence of malaria might mask the presence of yellow fever. For this purpose several local civil registrars were brought together, given demonstrations and instructions as to methods of securing liver specimens, and promised a cash payment for each liver specimen forwarded to the Health Department from fatal fever cases of less than 8 days' duration presenting any of the more common symptoms of yellow fever. To make the cooperation of these registrars effective, all cemeteries were prohibited from permitting burial of bodies unaccompanied by death certificates approved by the local registrar. Since the registrar himself had a financial interest in securing the desired specimen, this method was very effective. About 100 specimens were examined in the State of Rio de Janeiro from the time of the organization of this service in May to the end of August 1930, and to it must be credited the first demonstration of the possibility of securing liver specimens from interior points with nonmedical personnel.

During June, attempts were made to organize routine partial autopsy services in North Brazil, in the states of Sergipe, Alagôas, and Pernambuco. The attempt to organize a practical service for the interior of the latter state led one of us (E.R.R.) to attempt the design of an instrument for the removal of liver tissue without autopsy. This instrument, later christened the "viscerotome" by Dr. Mario Bião, reached a practicable stage of development within a few weeks. It is designed to enable the layman to remove

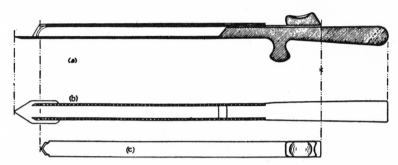

Figure 1. (a) Sectional view of viscerotome with sliding blade in cutting position. (b) Plane view of viscerotome with sliding blade withdrawn. (c) Sliding blade.

sections from cadavers rapidly, without the necessity of handling the body or tissues, and with minimal mutilation of the body.

Description of the Viscerotome

The construction of the viscerotome is shown in Figs. 1, 2, and 3. The instrument consists of but two parts (Fig. 1).

1. A square metal trough having a handle at the proximal end, and one basal and two lateral cutting surfaces at the distal end. The internal surfaces of the sidewalls of the trough have longitudinal grooves with a downward curve just proximal to the lateral cutting surfaces.

2. A sliding blade which operates in the grooves of the trough with a cutting surface at its distal extremity.

When the sliding blade is pushed forward, the curved grooves of the trough cause the distal extremity of the blade to bend downward and come into contact with the floor of the trough (Fig. 2). In this position the viscerotome becomes a four-sided closed punch with three sharp cutting surfaces, which may be forced through the body wall without removing any tissues. Once the point of the instrument has entered the liver, the

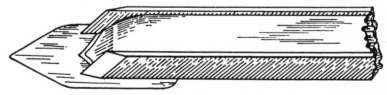

Figure 2. Distal portion of viscerotome showing position of sliding blade during introduction and withdrawal from the body.

sliding blade may be retracted just beyond the curve in the grooves and the instrument thus opened for the reception of liver tissue, with sharp cutting surfaces on the four sides of its lumen (Fig. 3). If the open instrument is forced further into the liver and the sliding blade is again pushed forward the liver section is complete.

The viscerotome has made possible the routine collection of liver specimens by nonmedical personnel, over a wide area, with a minimum of trouble and expense. The removal of sections by the viscerotome does not constitute an autopsy, and is, in fact, hardly more than a simple puncture. The opposition of relatives and friends to autopsy is greatly reduced in the case of viscerotomy, since the operation is very rapid and practically no mutilation occurs. A practiced operator often requires no more than 30 seconds for a viscerotomy. The opening made by the instrument is very small, no skin or muscle is removed, and no sutures are required for closing. The operator need not touch the cadaver with his hands, and the corpse may remain in the coffin almost fully clothed.

In February 1931, viscerotomes were distributed to selected representatives in several towns in the interior of Pernambuco, but, during the following 3 months, the results obtained were negligible. Since the instruments were not placed with the registrars, the viscerotome agents only rarely learned of cases suitable for puncture. Creditable results began to be secured only in June, after the adoption by the State Health Service of a death certificate calling for information regarding the length of final illness and the adoption of regulations prohibiting the burial of any person whose death certificate had not previously been submitted to the viscerotome agent. These were the same measures that had proved effective in the State of Rio de Janeiro in 1930. However, it was discovered that the routine collection of liver specimens, even with the aid of the viscerotome and the control of death certificates and burials, does not carry on automatically, and on June 5 a full-time physician was designated in Pernambuco to direct this service, select representatives, and maintain contact with them, much as a business organization would with its field agents. Once an organization capable of producing satisfactory results had been developed, the program was rapidly extended to other parts of Brazil, and in 1932 to

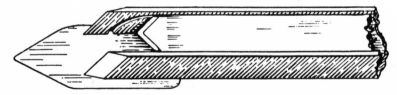

Figure 3. Distal portion of viscerotome showing position of sliding blade during cutting of liver tissue.

Bolivia and Paraguay (Map 1). In June 1933 the Medical Service of the Brazilian Army made the examination of liver specimens in fatal febrile cases of short duration a routine procedure.

The early results of the Viscerotome Service in Brazil were so important that general regulations for this service were included in Presidential Decree No. 21434 of May 23, 1932. A translation of Articles 52, 53, and 57 of this decree follows:

Art. 52. The practice of viscerotomy and routine autopsies is hereby established wherever desired by the (Yellow Fever) Service.

Sec. 1. The (Yellow Fever) Service may delegate authority to local representatives duly instructed in the practice of "viscerotomy," to whom all deaths occurring after less than ten days' illness must be immediately notified.

Sec. 2. In those places where the (Yellow Fever) Service has a representative for the practice of "viscerotomy," permits for burial in cemeteries, chapels, churches, or private burial grounds, may be issued by the civil registrar only on the presentation of death certificates duly visaed by said representative.

Art. 53. Any opposition to the above measures shall be punished by a fine of from 50$000 to 1:000$000 and by the intervention of the police authority

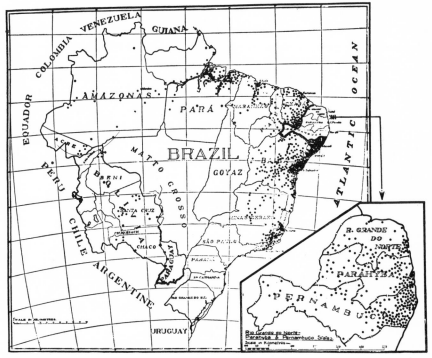

Map 1. Places where viscerotome posts were installed June 30, 1933.

which shall cause the immediate execution of the autopsy or viscerotomy desired.

Art. 57. By "viscerotomy" is understood the puncture of cadavers for the extraction of a section of any organ for diagnostic purposes.

RESULTS OF VISCEROTOMY

Between August 1928, when the Bahia Yellow Fever Laboratory began the examination of tissues from suspect cases of yellow fever, and May 1930, when the first specimen from a routine autopsy arrived, a total of 27 examinations, with 19 positive diagnoses, was made. From May 1930 to June 1933, 28,468 tissues were examined, with 75 positive diagnoses. The growth* and results of the liver collection service are shown in Table 1.

Of the 75 diagnoses of yellow fever made at the Bahia laboratory after the organization of the first routine liver-collection service, only 21 were made on tissues from cases clinically suspected of being yellow fever. The remaining 54 cases came from 43 different places, not known to be infected at the time the pathological diagnoses were made. These were distributed by states, as shown in Map 2.

A scarcely less valuable result of the viscerotome service was the accumulation of thousands of negative specimens from cities and towns engaging in antimosquito campaigns, indicating that the control measures employed were adequate to prevent local outbreaks of the disease.

The tissues received from viscerotome representatives included a small proportion of specimens unsuitable for examination. Since tissues are often secured only at the hour of burial, some show postmortem changes sufficiently advanced to make a diagnosis impossible. Such advanced changes have been found in only 796, or 2.8 per cent, of the total number of specimens received. Occasionally a puncture is unsuccessful and tissue other than liver obtained, and occasionally containers are broken in transit to the laboratory. These two sources of loss accounted for a total of 369 specimens, or 1.3 per cent. Unscrupulous representatives, whose compensation is based on the number of specimens forwarded, have occasionally sent multiple blocks of tissue from the same case under different names, and even blocks of tissue from animal livers. Fortunately, liver specimens usually show individual characteristics, and repeated fraud generally leads to detection in the laboratory. Probable duplication of specimens has been recorded from 36 places involving 118, or 0.4 per cent, of specimens re-

* Previous to March 1933, liver specimens were routinely obtained from cadavers of persons dying of acute illness of not less than 10 days' duration. Cases of death from accident, homicide, sudden death, and puerperal conditions were, naturally, excluded, as were also deaths of infants of less than 1 month of age. From March to June 1933, no punctures were made in infants of less than 6 months of age.

Table 1. Liver Tissues Examined at Bahia Yellow Fever Laboratory August 1928 to June 30, 1933[a]

Source	Before routine collection Aug. 1928–Apr. 1930: 21 months		After routine collection — Total May 1930–June 1933: 38 months		May–Dec. 1930: 8 months		Jan.–Dec. 1931: 12 months		Jan.–June 1932: 6 months		July–Dec. 1932: 6 months		Jan.–June 1933: 6 months	
	Examined	Positive	Examined	Positive	Examined	Positive	Examined	Positive	Examined	Positive	Examined	Positive	Examined	Positive
Brazil														
Amazonas	—	—	568	0	—	—	—	—	16	0	322	0	230	0
Pará	4	3	1,824	2	35	2	300	0	395	0	362	0	732	0
Maranhão	—	—	247	0	2	0	2	0	54	0	63	0	126	0
Piauhy	—	—	175	1	—	—	3	0	16	0	20	0	136	1
Matto Grosso	—	—	7	0	—	—	—	—	—	—	—	—	6	0
Ceará	2	0	7,496	21	—	—	201	5	501	1	3,102	10	3,692	5
R. G. Norte	1	0	2,233	1	19	0	86	0	483	0	609	1	1,036	0
Parahyba	12	10	3,587	6	4	2	63	0	474	1	1,249	3	1,801	0
Pernambuco	1	0	6,363	22	1	0	752	5	1,120	2	2,059	14	2,428	1
Alagôas	2	2	1,624	2	—	—	87	2	346	0	606	0	584	0
Sergipe	5	4	363	1	—	—	1	0	51	0	82	0	229	1
Bahia	—	—	2,501	4	2	0	5	0	127	4	844	0	1,523	0
Minas Geraes	—	—	499	0	—	—	—	—	134	0	166	0	199	0
Esp. Santo	—	—	296	3	—	—	—	—	108	3	110	0	78	0
R. de Janeiro	—	—	504	0	—	—	—	—	105	0	169	0	230	0
Dist. Federal	—	—	2	0	—	—	—	—	—	—	1	0	1	0
Argentina	—	—	9	0	—	—	—	—	—	—	8	0	1	0
Bolivia	—	—	110	12	—	—	—	—	—	—	29	11	81	1
Paraguay	—	—	60	0	—	—	—	—	—	—	1	0	59	0
Total	27	19	28,468	75	63	4	1,500	12	3,930	11	9,803	39	13,172	9

[a]The examination of tissues was carried out by Dr. Nelson C. Davis, Director of the Bahia Yellow Fever Laboratory, except for some months in 1931 when the examination was made by Drs. M. Frobisher, Jr., and H. W. Kumm. Cases reported positive were in most instances submitted by Dr. Amadeu Fialho, of the Pathological Laboratory of the National Department of Health of Brazil, and to Dr. Oskar Klotz, of the Banting Institute, University of Toronto, Canada.

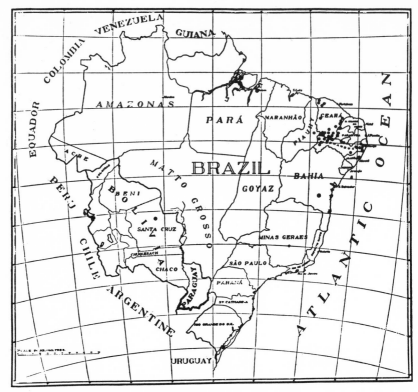

Map 2. Places where yellow fever has been diagnosed through routine examination
of liver tissue, May 1930 to June 1933.

ceived. Dishonest representatives have also collected tissues from nonindicated febrile cases and from cases of more than 10 days' illness. However,
comparative analysis of statistics from different places often reveals the
localities where nonindicated cases are being punctured. On the other

	Places	Cases
Brazil		
Pará	1	1
Piauhy	1	1
Ceará	20	22
Rio Grande do Norte	1	1
Parahyba	2	4
Pernambuco	15	22
Alagôas	1	1
Bahia	1	1
Bolivia	1	1
Total	43	54

hand, the general public sometimes learns that only cases of less than 10 days' illness are being punctured, with the result that more than 10 days' duration is attributed to all fatal illnesses. Here, again, comparative statistics are valuable. In extreme cases, puncture of all cadavers from an area has been temporarily employed to overcome this tendency to falsify the duration of illness.

Discussion

Events of the past few years have clearly shown that the absence of epidemics and of declared cases of yellow fever from an area does not indicate the absence of the disease from that area. Protection tests in Brazil have shown a high percentage of immunity to yellow fever in certain places where no history of the disease is obtainable, and the suggestion has been made that yellow fever may occur in certain epidemics in a mild nonfatal form. Although it has been shown that yellow fever may carry a very low mortality in the native population of endemic areas, the routine examination of liver tissue indicates that silent endemic foci are not silent because of an absence of fatal infections but because of the failure to recognize them. Studies to date indicate, at least for Brazil, that large series of infections without some fatalities do not often occur. On the other hand, it seems that the virus of yellow fever can be maintained for relatively long periods of time with the production of comparatively few fatal infections.

The problem of the distribution of yellow fever may be attacked directly or retrospectively. Retrospective methods of attack include (1) the investigation of mortality statistics and history taking, (2) complement-fixation test, and (3) the mouse protection test. Direct methods of attack include (a) the maintenance of lay investigators in suspect areas, with instructions to investigate all febrile cases, and report daily on temperature, pulse, and albuminuria of cases seen; (b) inoculation into susceptible animals of mosquitoes captured within houses of suspect areas; (c) the exposure of cages of susceptible animals in suspect areas, with autopsy in case of illness and death, or protection test for acquired immunity after a period of exposure; (d) the inoculation into susceptible animals of blood from febrile cases in suspect areas; (e) the autopsy of suspect cases; and (f) the routine partial autopsy or viscerotomy in fatal febrile cases of short duration.*

The methods which have been found most valuable and most practicable on a large scale—the mouse protection test applied to samples of blood from selected groups of the population of the areas investigated, and the routine postmortem removal of liver tissue—are both independent of a notification of suspect cases of yellow fever. This is highly important, since suspect cases

* Viscerotomy is not intended to supplant the complete autopsy recommended for suspect cases which merit the fullest possible investigation.

are very rare in true endemic areas not having an influx of nonimmune immigrants. The information secured by each of these methods is complementary to, but basically different from, that secured by the other. The first gives the cumulative picture of past exposure to the virus of yellow fever; the second, a current picture of mortality from yellow fever and an indication of the present distribution of the yellow fever virus.† The data from the protection test serve to outline the distribution of immunity to yellow fever corresponding to the area of past diffusion of the virus and indicate the area where the organization of the viscerotome service may be most profitable. However, the relationship of past diffusion of the virus to the permanent endemic foci of yellow fever and to the future distribution of the virus is not simple. Numerous articles have been published on the value of the protection test in delimiting endemic areas of yellow fever, and the writers of this article have been among the most enthusiastic in pushing studies on the distribution of immunity to yellow fever, which have resulted in obtaining invaluable information not otherwise available. However, as data on immunity distribution have accumulated, it has become increasingly evident that their application to the problem of yellow fever control is difficult. The distribution of yellow fever in endemic areas is constantly changing, owing in part to changes in living conditions, especially in facilities of transportation, and in part to the building up of a high percentage of immunes in infected places and the gradual growth of new crops of susceptibles in places temporarily free of the disease. No criteria other than the uncertain analysis of the distribution of immunity by age

† A most striking example of the value of combining the results of protection tests and routine liver examinations in field studies is afforded by work done at San Ramón, Bolivia, by Drs. René Valda and Angel Claros under the direction of Dr. A. M. Walcott. Dr. Valda visited San Ramón, an isolated village of 125 people, in September 1932 and was told of suspect cases of yellow fever occurring as early as June of that year. Although canvass of the community failed to reveal larval foci or adults of *Aëdes aegypti,* two of the three blood specimens collected at this time were shown to have protective properties for mice against the virus of yellow fever. In January 1933, reports of further suspect cases were received, and investigation by Dr. Claros in February indicated that two thirds of the population of this small village had, during the previous months, despite the absence of aegypti, suffered from a disease greatly resembling yellow fever. Six of eight blood specimens taken in February proved to possess protective qualities, again indicating the probability of yellow fever in the place. A viscerotome representative was selected in February, but the first case suitable for puncture did not occur until early in May. Examination of this first liver specimen by Dr. Davis resulted in a diagnosis of yellow fever. Confirmation of the continued presence of yellow fever in the absence of aegypti in a small village 11 months after the occurrence of the first suspicious cases is a very important epidemiological finding, made possible only by following up clinical findings and protection test results with routine examination of pathological specimens.

groups exist for the interpretation of immunity statistics in terms of the history of yellow fever in the places studied. Dr. F. F. Russell has stated the difficulty clearly in informing the Yellow Fever Commission that "a recent epidemic in a highly susceptible community, or two or three epidemics at rather long intervals, might give the same percentage of immunes as would be caused if the infection were constantly present in a community large enough to permit the disease to persist continuously." Epidemiologically and for the purposes of control and prevention it is important to know whether localities are in the former or in the latter category.

In this connection it may be noted that epidemics spread by unusual troop movements in 1926, the outbreak of yellow fever in Rio de Janeiro in 1928–1929, and the unusual flux of populations temporarily driven from their homes in Northeast Brazil by the drought of 1931–1932 have all resulted in building up immunity to yellow fever demonstrable by the protection test in areas which may possibly not be of great importance in maintaining permanent endemicity at the present time.

The information secured from the examination of routine postmortem liver tissues, on the other hand, is definite, easily interpreted, and permits investigation of the conditions under which yellow fever occurs in endemic areas. Immediate action can be taken to prevent the further dissemination of the virus from the known infected point. Fatal cases of yellow fever are far more potent arguments for active cooperation of all authorities concerned than are high percentages of positive protection tests. Antimosquito measures have been extended and intensified as a result of diagnoses based on routine liver tissues in silent endemic areas where such control measures could have been justified in no other way. The routine liver collection service has demonstrated that such silent endemic foci are "silent" not because fatal cases of yellow fever do not occur, but because they occur in such small numbers that only pathological diagnoses are convincing.

The negative information accumulated by the liver-collection service is highly important, indicating the probable absence of the virus from large suspect areas apparently differing in no other respect from areas shown to harbor the virus. Negative viscerotome results from all the larger centers of population during the past few years have been particularly comforting to control workers in Brazil.

The organization of the routine liver-collection service is based on the following assumptions:

1. That the existence of yellow fever in a community over a period of months will result in some fatal infections.

2. That the yellow fever liver usually shows characteristic lesions.

3. That fatal yellow fever kills rapidly, its victims rarely surviving more than 10 days.

The advantage of the viscerotome service over other methods for the direct discovery of yellow fever is that it does not depend on the finding of suspect cases or on the ferreting out of febrile illnesses. Illness is easily overlooked, but burial of the dead occurs only after the observance of certain civil and religious formalities which call attention to the fact that a death has occurred. Legal regulations controlling burials bring indicated cases automatically to the notice of the viscerotome representative. Death diagnoses itself, and only a little judicious inquiry is necessary to ascertain if the fatal illness has been of less than 10 days' duration.

The introduction of the viscerotome service is expected to aid greatly in clearing up other public health problems and in accustoming the medical profession and the public to postmortem examinations. The viscerotome service has already resulted in punishing one practising physician for failure to notify a case which he himself believed to be yellow fever. Two interesting cases have occurred in which poisoning and yellow fever were confounded. In the first of these cases the police strongly suspected criminal poisoning, but the laboratory report showed that death had been due to yellow fever. In the second case, in which both yellow fever and criminal poisoning were suspected, the laboratory examination showed that death had not been due to yellow fever. The possibility of mass pathological work on a large scale has been demonstrated and much valuable information regarding the distribution of other diseases producing characteristic liver lesions, such as malaria and schistosomiasis, has been obtained.

Summary and Conclusions

1. The organization of a service for the routine postmortem collection of liver tissue from rapidly fatal febrile cases resulted, between May 1930 and June 1933, in the examination of tissues from over 28,000 livers, and a pathological diagnosis of yellow fever in 54 cases, from 43 places in which yellow fever was not known to be present.

2. A special instrument designed for the rapid removal of liver tissue by laymen without autopsy, to which the name "viscerotome" has been given, is described.

3. The routine liver-collection program has resulted in

a. The demonstration of typical fatal cases of yellow fever in otherwise silent endemic foci.

b. The accumulation of extensive data indicating, as far as negative evidence can indicate, the absence of the yellow fever virus from key centers of population and from hundreds of towns and villages in which antimosquito measures are being applied.

c. The confirmation of yellow fever without *Aëdes aegypti* in a small village 11 months after the occurrence of the first suspect case.

d. The accumulation of valuable data regarding the distribution of diseases other than yellow fever producing characteristic liver lesions.

Recent Extensions of Knowledge
of Yellow Fever*

Lesions of Yellow Fever in the Liver

Before leaving the subject of viscerotomy, attention must be directed to the fact that the diagnosis of yellow fever from the lesions in the liver is not easy, and should preferably be undertaken only by those who have had an opportunity to examine several thousand liver slides, including slides from positive, negative, and doubtful cases. Pathologists with such a background can separate material into three general groups: negative, positive, and doubtful. Under ordinary conditions, not more than one or, at the most, two slides in each thousand may be expected to fall in the doubtful class requiring full investigation for determination of the final diagnosis.

Early workers considered the yellow fever liver as essentially one showing exaggerated fatty degeneration or fatty metamorphosis. To Rocha-Lima must go the credit for calling the attention of modern workers to those characteristics of the yellow fever liver on which a diagnosis may be based. These criteria consist of concomitant lesions of fatty change and necrobiosis. Rocha-Lima believes the fatty changes to be independent of the necrobiosis, since the zones which have the most marked necrobiosis have the least fatty accumulation, and vice versa. Cells with fat tend to have more or less normal staining nuclei and unimpaired vitality. (These are the same cells in which inclusion bodies, not of great importance in the diagnosis of human cases, are to be found when present.) The necrotic cells, on the other hand, are peculiarly granular (Councilman bodies). Rocha-Lima described the division of the lobule into three zones: central, midzonal, and peripheral. The highest concentration of necrotic cells is to be found in the midzone, and the greatest accumulation of fat occurs in the central and peripheral zones. Midzonal necrosis, as such, is not characteristic of yellow fever, but the predominance of necrosis in the midzone is important when the necrosis is of the hyalin type and is scattered irregularly throughout the tissue, necrotic cells, or groups of necrotic cells being surrounded by others not necrotic. Together with the fatty and necrotic changes, there is an absence of extensive hemorrhage and of extensive in-

---

* Report submitted to the Pan-African Health Conference held at Johannesburg, South Africa, November 20–30, 1935. Dr. Soper was the Representative (Rio de Janeiro office) of the International Health Division of The Rockefeller Foundation.

This article was originally published (*23*) in the *Quarterly Bulletin of the Health Organization of the League of Nations 5:* 19–68, 1936. This excerpt is from pages 55–56 of the original article.

flammatory reaction. The trabecular structure remains unaltered, and there is no collapse of the lobule in spite of the extensive necrosis. There is an absence of karyorrhexis and pyknosis.

The lesion on which a diagnosis of yellow fever can be made, then, may be described as a complex one, consisting of a special hyaline type of necrosis scattered throughout the lobule but with its greatest intensity in the intermediary zones of the lobule, occurring in the presence of a marked fatty accumulation in the central and peripheral zones and in the non-necrotic cells among the zones of extensive necrosis and marked by the absence of hemorrhage, inflammatory reaction, and collapse of the lobular structure. The difficulty in applying this syndrome to any given liver increases as the changes become maximal and minimal in extent.

It is believed by pathologists who have made a special study of the subject that the yellow fever lesion, when fully typical, is characteristic and pathognomonic, and the experience of the Viscerotomy Service in general supports this conclusion. However, experience in submitting duplicate slides of suspicious cases to several competent authorities has shown that, while they agree as to the diagnosability of the yellow fever liver, widely divergent opinions may be expressed as to the specificity of the lesion in a given preparation. In such cases it is necessary to make a full investigation in the field and arrive at an "administrative" diagnosis outside the laboratory.

Selection 15 | # Present-Day Methods for the Study and Control of Yellow Fever*

Fatal Yellow Fever Survey

Viscerotomy

Although early investigators had given careful descriptions of the microscopical changes found in the liver in fatal yellow fever, and more recent workers had called attention to the importance of these changes in establishing the diagnosis in fatal *suspect* cases, it was not until 1930 that the routine collection and examination of liver tissue was established for the diagnosis of *unsuspected fatal yellow fever* in an attempt to clear up the enigma of "silent" endemic areas.† It became apparent almost immediately that the silent endemic areas of Brazil are not characterized by the absence of fatal cases. This is true both for areas of aegypti-transmitted yellow fever and for areas of jungle endemicity.

Viscerotomy is a routine measure applied in all cases of death within 10 days or less after onset of final illness except in cases of suspect yellow fever which merit full autopsy. The liver survey for the discovery of unsuspected fatal cases is based on the fact that in yellow fever the liver usually shows characteristic lesions not produced by other acute infectious diseases.

A word of caution must be given regarding the diagnosis of yellow fever from the examination of liver tissue. Unlike the protection test, in which the interpretation depends upon an objective fact—the number of mice which survive the test—the diagnosis of yellow fever from an examination of the liver depends upon a subjective analysis of a complex lesion. For this

---

* Dr. Soper was the Representative in South America (Rio de Janeiro Office) of the International Health Division of The Rockefeller Foundation.

This excerpt is reprinted by permission from the article (27) in the *American Journal of Tropical Medicine 17*: 655–676, 1937. Copyright © 1937, The Williams & Wilkins Company, Baltimore, Maryland. This excerpt is from pages 661–666 of the published article. (See also the excerpt from pp. 666–673 in Part II, Selection 5.)

† The actual collection with the viscerotome of the liver tissue necessary for examination is very simple and rapid, requiring usually only a few seconds or at most a minute or two. After removal the block of tissue is placed in a container with a 10 per cent solution of formalin in normal saline for fixation and is forwarded to the laboratory, where hematoxylin–eosin stained preparations are made for examination.

reason, authorities who agree that the lesion of yellow fever is specific will at times vary in their opinions on a given specimen. Fortunately, it has been possible to determine by other methods the probable validity of most of the positive diagnoses based on liver examination made in South America since viscerotomy was begun. The field investigation of cases has been most valuable in orienting the laboratory on certain cases which were not yellow fever but had very suggestive lesions.

The diagnosis of yellow fever from routine viscerotomy material, which includes much with postmortem degeneration and some that has been poorly fixed, should preferably be undertaken only by those who have had an opportunity to examine several thousand liver tissues, including positive, negative, and doubtful specimens. With such preparation it is believed that false positive diagnoses will be rare. Nevertheless, the reasonable public health official will carry out a complete investigation in the field with all available methods before accepting the statement from the laboratory that yellow fever is present in any part of the district for which he is responsible. •

The most difficult part of viscerotomy is the building up of a field organization with efficient local representatives for the routine collection of liver tissue. The distribution of viscerotomes to doctors throughout areas to be investigated, with the request that specimens from interesting cases be sent into the laboratory, fails utterly to produce results. Good results have been obtained by securing legislation giving control over cemeteries and burials, followed by the appointment of carefully selected representatives, many of whom are laymen, as local viscerotomists. Since the viscerotomist cannot function unless he learns of all deaths in his district soon after they occur, legislation provides that each death certificate must be submitted to him for approval before going to the local registrar who issues the burial permit. Provision is made on the death certificate for a statement of the duration of final illness, which is not, however, binding on the viscerotomist if he has any reason to suspect a fraudulent statement to avoid viscerotomy.

In Brazil several types of viscerotomy organization have been tested, with varying results under different conditions. It has been found advantageous to have full-time viscerotomists in some of the larger cities,* whereas, in others, viscerotomy has been entrusted to the officials responsible for verifying the cause of death. In the smaller communities, and viscerotomy is especially important in small communities, this service is practically always entrusted to a local resident on the basis of a small fee for death certificates forwarded and a correspondingly larger fee for each liver specimen submit-

* Viscerotomy has been suspended in many of the larger cities *where efficient antiaegypti measures are enforced,* after several years of experience had shown that such cities produced no locally infected cases of yellow fever.

ted; a special grand prize is awarded when the first liver with yellow fever lesions is received from each district. Such a system of payment is open to abuse, of course; representatives desiring to increase their income may be expected to puncture bodies other than those of persons dying after 10 days or less of illness and even to submit duplicate and at times quintuplicate specimens from the same liver under different names. At times, liver which is not human in origin has appeared in the laboratory, even liver with nucleated red blood cells! However, such abuses can be discovered, since accumulated experience has shown the approximate percentage of deaths which should occur after short illness in the absence of epidemics, and the microscopical appearance of the individual liver is so characteristic that duplicate specimens from the same liver can usually be recognized as such.

Viscerotomy is limited in its application to fatal cases; but in spite of this and its other defects, it has proved to be the most useful method of locating actual outbreaks of *unsuspected yellow fever*. This statement applies to both the aegypti-transmitted and jungle types of the disease. Even in isolated districts where travel difficulties have prevented the replacement of viscerotomists who have failed during several months to forward specimens, viscerotomy has repeatedly revealed yellow fever. The viscerotomist may be indifferent under normal conditions, but when deaths begin to occur in the neighborhood which may possibly be due to yellow fever, his interest is often stimulated to the point of producing action. In a number of cases the first specimen received from a representative some time after his appointment has resulted in his winning the grand prize offered for the first positive specimen from his district.

Viscerotomy is a valuable sentinel service pointing to spots of active infection where fatal cases are occurring. The consistently negative results in the cities and towns where antiaegypti measures are in force have been important in showing that urban endemicity is not continuing in the face of control measures.

Attention has been called to the differences in age and sex distributions of immunity to yellow fever revealed by the protection test survey in areas of aegypti-transmitted and jungle yellow fever. Equally significant differences are revealed in the age and sex distributions of fatal cases diagnosed by liver examination (Fig. 4). In native populations of rural endemic areas where transmission is by aegypti, fatalities tend to be concentrated in the younger age groups and equally divided between the sexes. In jungle districts, however, fatalities are concentrated in adults, with marked predilection for males. Limited observations on urban yellow fever suggest that fatal cases in the native population of the towns of highly endemic regions will be largely in the youngest age groups, such deaths as do occur in adult life being limited to immigrants from nonendemic regions or from areas of jungle yellow fever where immunity is not acquired early in life.

[Additional information about viscerotomy, and the results obtained with it, may be found in Part V, Selection 23, particularly Table 1, Graph 1, and Map 7.—*Ed.*]

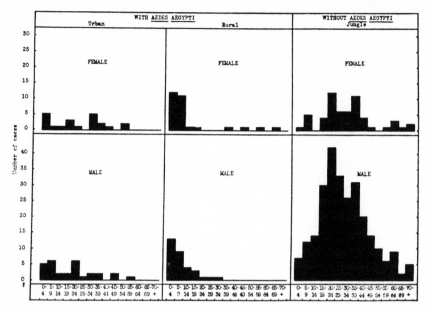

Figure 4. Distribution by age and sex of fatal cases of urban, rural, and jungle yellow fever in Brazil, Colombia, and Bolivia, confirmed by examination of liver tissue between January 1, 1930, and June 30, 1936.

Part IV | Serological Studies of Human Yellow Fever
in South America

Selection *16* | Studies of the Distribution of
Immunity to Yellow Fever in
Brazil

1. Postepidemic Survey of Magé, Rio de Janeiro, by Complement-Fixation and Monkey-Protection Tests*

FRED L. SOPER, M. FROBISHER, JR., J. A. KERR,
AND N. C. DAVIS

Before the successful maintenance of the yellow fever virus in the laboratory and the development of the protection test with *Macacus rhesus* monkeys, which facilitates the postconvalescent diagnosis of yellow fever, individual suspected cases of this disease could be positively diagnosed only after examination of tissues removed at autopsy. Conclusions regarding the distribution of the disease, therefore, depended on knowledge of the case-fatality rate and the factors which might cause such fatality rate to vary. But experience has shown that, in both epidemic and nonepidemic periods, even fatal cases of yellow fever often pass unnoted and that during epidemics deaths due to other causes are frequently attributed to yellow fever.

* The studies and observations herein reported were conducted with the support and under the auspices of the International Health Division of The Rockefeller Foundation. Dr. Soper was the Representative in South America (Rio de Janeiro office) of the International Health Division of The Rockefeller Foundation; Drs. Frobisher, Kerr, and Davis were staff members. The authors are indebted to the directors of the official health services of the states of São Paulo and Rio de Janeiro for cooperation facilitating the studies. For assistance in the collection of specimens they are indebted to Drs. S. Ferreira Pinto, Mario Bião, A. Andrade, Waldemar Rocha, Frederico Motta, Carlos Del Negro, and Domingos Bellizi. They are indebted to Dr. H. Aragão for timely assistance in preparing serum for transport to the laboratory.

This excerpt is reprinted from the article (*13*) in the *Journal of Preventive Medicine 6*: 341–377, 1932. (About 16 pages of the original text have been omitted, including 13 tables and 4 figures.)

The difficulties encountered in the diagnosis of nonfatal cases are such that in the absence of epidemic conditions clinicians are unwilling to declare even moderately severe cases. The apparent case-fatality rate varies, therefore, through errors in the clinical diagnosis of both fatal and nonfatal cases.

Furthermore, although the fatality of yellow fever is known to vary widely, the factors determining such variation have never been demonstrated. Carter cites yellow fever mortality rates ranging from 4 to 25 per cent in extensive outbreaks, and up to 85 and even 98 per cent in certain "closed-group" epidemics. Variations in the virulence or dosage of the yellow fever virus might help to explain variations in the severity of individual cases or differences between one epidemic and another, but they cannot clarify variations in attack rate and severity in different groups living under identical conditions.

Practically all authors are agreed that in outbreaks of yellow fever in endemic areas the highest attack and fatality rates are to be found among foreigners, especially those who have recently arrived. (The term foreigners, as used in this article, refers to individuals born in areas not subject to endemic or repeatedly epidemic yellow fever.) The disease would appear, from the descriptions given, to exemplify, *par excellence,* Cobbett's general statement: "Peoples are more resistant to the attack of the infectious diseases of their own countries and districts than to that of foreign diseases with which neither they nor their ancestors have been accustomed to come in contact."

The relative freedom of natives and long-time residents in endemic areas from the ravages of yellow fever has been generally attributed to a specific immunity acquired through mild attacks in early childhood or to a partial immunity built up from repeated hypothetical subinfective doses of the virus. In regions having a large Negro population native immunity has also been attributed to racial factors. But until recently no method for testing the distribution of immunity was available, and acquired immunity without diagnosed attack could not be distinguished from natural resistance to infection or from absence of exposure.

Although it has long been recognized that recent arrivals from areas in which yellow fever is nonendemic form the group most highly susceptible to the disease, the equally important observation that yellow fever in native populations of endemic areas may be a very elusive disease, even among white adults, has not been sufficiently emphasized. In a place where the disease is permanently endemic it has been almost hopeless to expect diagnosis in natives of the place. The epidemiologist engaged in tracing the distribution of yellow fever has therefore been forced largely to supplement with hypotheses the meager scientific information secured from such fatal cases as were followed by autopsy. How faulty such hypotheses, based for the most part on negative findings, may be in endemic areas with little movement of foreigners, is strikingly revealed by the reappearance of yellow fever in the Department of Santander, Colombia, in 1929 after an apparent absence from the country for 5 years and with no evidence pointing to recent reintroduction of the disease from without. Past experience in Brazil has also repeatedly demonstrated that the absence of declared suspected cases of yellow fever from an area does not necessarily mean that the disease itself is absent. Periods of many months without confirmed cases in all Brazil have frequently occurred, only to be followed by more or less extensive outbreaks in the absence, apparently, of any reintroduction from outside sources.

Announcement of the infection of rhesus monkeys with yellow fever virus (March 1928) and publication of details of the protection test occurred just as authorities in Brazil were beginning to discover isolated cases of yellow fever, which presaged its wide, known distribution in the country in 1928, 1929, 1930, and 1931. From April 1927 to March 1928, no cases of the disease had been confirmed in all Brazil. (Confirmation during this period was possible only by autopsy, as other laboratory methods were not yet available.) Early in March 1928, however, a positive diagnosis was made at autopsy in Estancia, Sergipe (Fig. 1). In April a fatal case occurred at Timbaúba, Pernambuco. And on May 16 an autopsy was performed in Rio de Janeiro on a soldier dead from the disease. No connection was ever established between any two of these three widely separated cases. Further cases are not known to have occurred in either Estancia or Timbaúba during many succeeding weeks of observation when no control measures were being applied. In Rio de Janeiro, epidemiological studies failed to reveal the original case or even the original focus of the disease in Rio de Janeiro. The facts collected demonstrated the existence of at least four distinct foci in Rio de Janeiro in the first half of May (Villa Militar, São Christovão, Saúde, and Catumby), but no relationship was ever established between any two of these foci.

It is impossible to state how long yellow fever had been present in Rio de Janeiro before being diagnosed in May 1928, although a superficial study of general and specific death rates indicates that the disease was probably not an important cause of death in Rio de Janeiro in January, February, and March but may have been so as early as the first week in April. The impossibility of digging out the past ramifications of the disease in Rio was explained on the basis of the supposed occurrence of a large proportion of mild cases at the begining of epidemics. After the recognition of the disease, great anxiety was felt for the safety of the city because of the large nonimmune element in the population, composed of foreigners, Brazilians from nonendemic regions, and natives of the city born since the end of Oswaldo Cruz's memorable campaign in 1908. Later events justified this

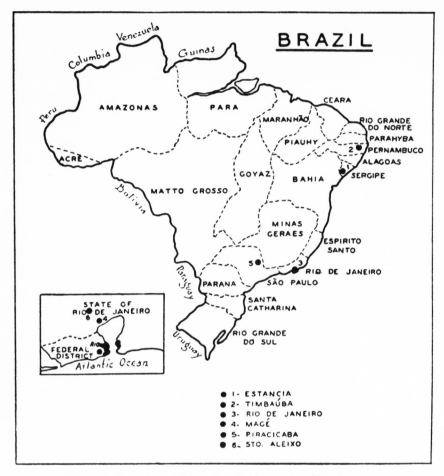

Figure 1. Location of the six localities mentioned in the text.

anxiety regarding foreigners and Brazilians from nonendemic regions, but contrary to expectation, there was not an appreciable number of cases among natives of Rio under 20 years of age. Of 125 officially recognized cases in 1928, 97, or 77.6 per cent, occurred in foreigners, although according to the latest census (1920) only 20.8 per cent of the population are foreigners. Furthermore, 18 of 28 cases (64.3 per cent) occurring in Brazilians were in persons who had resided in Rio de Janeiro less than 5 years. This failure of Rio de Janeiro to produce in two decades a highly susceptible native population was at first attributed to the fact that the disease predominated in sections of the city, Saúde and Catumby, largely filled with foreigners. While it is true that, with the spread of the disease later to other parts of the city, a significant increase was noted in the percentage of cases occurring among Brazilians, foreigners continued to suffer dispro-portionately to their numbers, and some observers suggested that yellow fever may have been more or less constantly present, previous to 1928, in mild or at least undiagnosed form, thus maintaining a high degree of im-munity in the native population. But this hypothesis is not reasonable, because Rio de Janeiro has had a constantly shifting foreign population and has, moreover, long been the Mecca of the Portuguese immigrant; this highly susceptible material would undoubtedly have given rise to explosive outbreaks in the past had the virus been present in sufficient quantity to immunize the local population.

One of us (F.L.S.) observed at close range the Rio de Janeiro yellow fever outbreak of 1928–1929 and early came to the conclusion that information of value might be secured if it were possible to carry out protection tests on a group of native-born residents living in known infected zones of the city. As reasonable certainty existed that yellow fever had not been endemic in Rio de Janeiro on a large scale since 1908, natives less than 20 years of age found to have a specific immunity would most probably have a recently acquired immunity. Plans were made for a series of protection tests, and in January 1929 work was begun with Dr. Hugo Muench in Braz de Pinna, a suburb of Rio de Janeiro. The press of other services, however, made it necessary to discontinue this study. Before the project could be undertaken anew, yellow fever was reported in the nearby town of Magé (Fig. 1) in the State of Rio de Janeiro, where during February, March, and April, a small epidemic of 22 cases with 13 deaths occurred. Magé offered a much more concrete problem than did Braz de Pinna and was chosen as the site of the present study in the belief that the results might be applied with profit to the interpretation of the observed distribution of yellow fever fol-lowing the reintroduction of the virus into Rio de Janeiro, an old endemic center, after an apparent absence of 20 years.

After the work in Magé had been begun (June 1929), the first report of promising results with the complement-fixation test for yellow fever was published. In view of the low cost of this test, it was decided to examine a much larger number of persons in Magé than would have been possible with the more expensive protection test, and provision was made for a series of control tests with sera from a noninfected center. Piracicaba, São Paulo (Fig. 1), lying outside the endemic yellow fever zone, was selected for the collection of sera (1930) for the control series. Later (1931) an oppor-tunity occurred to secure a control series of sera from another known post-epidemic focus of yellow fever at Santo Aleixo, a small town near Magé.

The data secured from these investigations are the basis of the present report, which gives (1) comparative results of complement-fixation tests in Magé and Santo Aleixo, both lying in a previously endemic area and both the seats of recent epidemics, and of similar tests in Piracicaba, São Paulo, believed to have been free of yellow fever for many years; (2) comparative results of complement-fixation tests in Magé, 4, 16 and 22 months after a known epidemic of yellow fever; (3) comparative results of complement-fixation and rhesus protection tests in Magé; (4) an analysis of yellow fever immunity distribution in the population of Magé in 1929, as indicated by complement-fixation and rhesus protection tests.

SOURCE OF MATERIAL

Magé

In June 1929 a house-to-house canvass was made in the central part of Magé, and epidemiological data were collected regarding 1521 people living in 348 houses. During this survey 36 suspected cases of yellow fever were added to the official list of 22. Some of these were relatively mild cases and would not have suggested yellow fever under other circumstances. The distribution of the officially recognized cases and the additional suspected cases is roughly the same. At this same time (June 1929) thick blood smears were taken from 932 residents of the study area to obtain the malaria index, and in July and August 1929, blood samples of 10 to 30 cc for complement-fixation tests were secured from 676 persons, 2 to 81 years of age, living in the area. In July 1930 second blood samples were secured from 88 persons who had furnished samples in 1929; and in January 1931 additional samples were taken from 34 persons who had furnished specimens on one or both of the previous occasions.

Santo Aleixo

In January 1931 blood samples of 10 to 30 cc were secured from 70 persons living in Santo Aleixo and Andorinhas, most of whom were less than 20 years of age (see Fig. 1).

Piracicaba, State of São Paulo

As a control on the results of complement-fixation tests in Magé, 120 blood samples were secured in September 1930 from persons of all ages living in Piracicaba, a busy town of some 25,000 residents in the interior of the State of São Paulo. Piracicaba is situated about 140 miles from Santos at an altitude of more than 500 meters above sea level, and yellow fever is not known to have been present there during the past 35 years (see Fig. 1).

METHODS

All samples for tests were taken in vacuum venules, which are indispensable where many specimens are to be collected in homes and shops. The sera, after separation, were drawn off aseptically, placed in sterile tubes or ampoules, and sent to the laboratory for as early examination as possible.

The complement-fixation test was made, using an antigen prepared from the liver of monkeys infected with yellow fever. The technique of this test has been adequately described elsewhere.

The protection test consisted in injecting 3 or 4 cc of serum intraperitoneally into rhesus monkeys, one serum to each monkey. Within 5 minutes each animal received an infective dose of citrated blood of an animal in the early febrile stage of yellow fever, usually infected with the Asibi strain of virus. A control animal which received no serum was given a similar dose of infective blood at the same time as each group of test animals. Rectal temperatures of all animals were taken twice daily. Autopsies were performed on animals that died, and the gross and microscopic pathological findings were recorded. Interpretation of tests on monkeys surviving febrile attacks was difficult, but after weighing evidence for and against protection, partial protection, and nonspecific reactions, most of these tests could be recorded as positive or negative.

SUMMARY AND CONCLUSIONS

1. Complement-fixation tests on postepidemic blood samples taken from 300 persons in Magé and Santo Aleixo and on 101 samples from Piracicaba, lying outside the yellow fever zone, show a highly significant difference between the percentages of positive reactions in the postepidemic samples and in the samples from the nonendemic area. The conclusion is drawn that the complement-fixation test may be useful in field studies of yellow fever, especially in outlining areas recently epidemic.

2. A small number of comparative results of complement-fixation tests on the same individuals in Magé at intervals of 4, 16, and 22 months after an epidemic of yellow fever indicate that there is a tendency, especially in the first year after infection, for the titer of the complement-fixing bodies in the blood to decrease.

3. Comparative results of complement-fixation and rhesus protection tests with 76 sera indicate that positive complement-fixation tests will generally be confirmed by positive protection tests and that negative protection tests will usually be confirmed by negative complement-fixation tests. However, an appreciable number of sera giving protection showed negative results with the complement-fixation technique. These findings indicate that complement-fixing antibodies demonstrable by present methods are less constantly produced than are protection bodies and are less permanent.

4. The combined results of complement-fixation and protection tests given in this report are interpreted as indicating that, at the time of known outbreaks of yellow fever in Magé and Santo Aleixo, relatively large per-

centages of the local populations were acquiring a specific immunity to the yellow fever virus without apparent attacks of the disease. A statistical analysis of the available data failed to show that such invisible acquisition of active immunity was related in any way to age, sex, or race. No data are presented to indicate what factors are responsible for this ability of the population of these two towns, lying in previously endemic areas, to acquire active immunity with low fatality rates.

5. The possibility of low fatality rates with many unnoted infections in natives of endemic or previously endemic yellow fever areas, without regard to age, sex, or race, must be taken into consideration in any future attempt to study the distribution of the yellow fever virus.

Studies of the Distribution of
Immunity to Yellow Fever in
Brazil.

II. The Disproportion between
Immunity Distribution as
Revealed by Complement-
Fixation and Mouse-Protection
Tests and History of Yellow Fever
Attack at Cambucy, Rio de
Janeiro*

FRED L. SOPER AND ALVARO DE ANDRADE

The postepidemic distribution of immunity to yellow fever in the population of Magé, Rio de Janeiro, as measured by the complement-fixation
and protection tests, indicated that the number of persons acquiring immunity to this disease during an outbreak may greatly exceed the number
of clinical cases observed. Recently, the mouse protection test has largely
supplanted the monkey protection test and has made possible more extensive studies of immunity distribution than were formerly feasible. As a
control for the widespread studies of immunity distribution which are
being undertaken throughout Brazil, and which are based on relatively

* The work on which this report is based was undertaken as a part of a larger
field study of the epidemiology of yellow fever in Brazil being made by the Cooperative Yellow Fever Service maintained by the Brazilian Government and The
Rockefeller Foundaton. The laboratory tests were divided between the New York
and Bahia yellow fever laboratories, both supported by The Rockefeller Foundation. Dr. Soper was the Representative in South America (Rio de Janeiro office)
of the International Health Division of The Rockefeller Foundation; Dr. de Andrade was an official of the Malaria Service of the State of Rio de Janeiro, Brazil.
    This excerpt is from the article *(14)* in the *American Journal of Hygiene 18:*
588–617, 1933. (About 18 pages of the original text have been omitted, including
13 tables and 3 charts.)

small samples from a large number of towns, it was deemed necessary to make an intensive survey of some single community where the history of yellow fever was known. The town of Cambucy, State of Rio de Janeiro, was chosen for this purpose. Fortunately the history of yellow fever in this community is similar to that in Magé, so data for the two towns can be compared. The results of epidemiological and immunity distribution studies in Cambucy, which are reported in the following pages, confirm the observations made at Magé that reintroduction of the yellow fever virus into native populations of previously endemic areas may produce widespread immunity with few typical cases of the disease. But such widespread immunity may be far from uniform in its distribution within even small population groups.

DESCRIPTION OF CAMBUCY

Cambucy, a small town with a population of less than 1000, is situated on the Parahyba River, in the northern part of the State of Rio de Janeiro, about 80 kilometers from Campos, a city of almost 50,000 population, and one of the most important sugar producing centers of Brazil. Cambucy lies outside the heavy sugar producing zone and depends for its existence largely upon the production of coffee in the hilly region north of the Parahyba River. It is only 50 meters above sea level and has a warm, humid climate. The Leopoldina Railway connects Cambucy with both Rio de Janeiro and Nictheroy, which may be reached via Campos in only 11 hours, and via Tres Irmãos and Portella in 13 hours.

The census taken as a part of the present study revealed a population of 823, of which 42, or 5 per cent, were foreign born. Ninety-one persons were born in Brazil of foreign parents, and 44 others reported having one foreign parent. From these figures it appears that the population of the town is about 85 per cent native stock. Despite this fact, however, the racial distribution found was white, 500; black, 135; mulatto, 187; Indian, 1. Females predominated over males in the ratio 110:100.

HISTORY OF YELLOW FEVER IN CAMBUCY

No written record of the occurrence of yellow fever in Cambucy prior to the epidemic here described has been found, but it is believed that the disease must have been present in the town repeatedly during the long period of endemicity in the Federal District and the State of Rio de Janeiro, from 1849 to 1908. How long it may have persisted in this area after the final success of the memorable campaign of Oswaldo Cruz in Rio de Janeiro is unknown, but no autochthonous cases were reported from the entire state during two full decades from 1908 to 1928. The last case of yellow fever reported from Campos during this early endemic period occurred in 1906.

In May 1928 yellow fever was found in the Federal District, and in the following months of 1928 it appeared in the nearby points of Nictheroy and São Gonçalo. During 1929 it was present in the Federal District until July and was reported from many places (including Magé, the scene of the preceding study) in the State of Rio de Janeiro. The entire northern part of the state, in which Campos and Cambucy are situated, failed to report locally infected cases during 1929. From September 1929 until late in March 1930, no cases were reported from the State of Rio de Janeiro, but between the end of March 1930 and July, five towns reported the disease. Four of these, Cantagallo, Itaocára, Portella, and Campos, lie in the northern part of the state and are in relatively close contact with Cambucy. This flareup was followed by months of respite, during which detachments of nonimmune revolutionary troops from Minas Geraes were moved through this region, apparently without becoming infected. During the last week of November, however, a fatal case, confirmed by autopsy, occurred in Cambucy, and a total of 13 clinical cases, with 5 deaths, was registered before the middle of February 1931. Other suspected cases, with at least one death, occurred in the nearby rural districts.

Description of Control Localities

As a control for the results of mouse-protection tests in Cambucy, two towns were selected in which the transmission of yellow fever had never been reported: Friburgo, in the State of Rio de Janeiro, and Guapé, in the State of Minas Geraes.

Friburgo lies about 100 kilometers north of the city of Rio de Janeiro, on the branch line of the Leopoldina Railway, which connects Portella with the federal and state capitals. It is well within the previously endemic area but has apparently always been protected from yellow fever epidemics by its location at 850 meters above sea level. A typical clinical case of yellow fever was observed in Friburgo in 1931, but it did not give rise to any registered locally infected cases, and a mosquito survey at that time failed to reveal the presence of *Aëdes aegypti*.

Guapé is situated in the southern part of Minas Geraes, at an altitude of more than 600 meters above sea level and has no easy contact with known endemic areas. Although occasional epidemics of an undiagnosed fever of short duration have been reported from this town, it is not known to have suffered from yellow fever.

Materials and Methods

Early in February, while yellow fever was still present in Cambucy, a complete census was taken of the population of the community, including, in addition to the usual census data, information as to place of birth and history of recent illness. Blood specimens were secured during February and March from 659 of the 823 persons listed in the census. Unsatisfactory results were obtained in a large proportion of the mouse protection tests made on these specimens, owing to the technical difficulties encountered in the early days of this test. For this reason and because of a desire to measure the rate of loss of complement-fixing bodies, a second collection of blood specimens was made in November and December, in which 598 specimens were obtained.

The first series of blood specimens collected during and immediately after the epidemic was divided. One portion was forwarded to the Yellow Fever Laboratory in New York for the mouse protection test, and the other portion was sent to the Yellow Fever Laboratory in Bahia, Brazil, for the complement-fixation test. The second series of specimens went to the Bahia laboratory, where both mouse protection and complement-fixation tests were performed.

In September 1931, 105 blood specimens were collected in Friburgo from persons between the ages of 2 and 20 years who had resided in the community continually since birth. At the same time, 136 specimens were collected at Guapé, largely from persons of the earlier age groups, although some were obtained from members of the older groups who had never resided outside this area. All sera from Friburgo and Guapé were forwarded to the Bahia Laboratory for the mouse-protection test.

The complement-fixation and mouse-protection tests were carried out by the workers who originally described these tests. The complement-fixation test was performed with antigens prepared from the livers of monkeys infected with yellow fever. No recent modifications have been made in this test. The procedure in the mouse protection test consisted of the intraperitoneal injection of virus fixed for mice and of the serum being tested for protective antibodies, and the intracerebral injection of an inert irritant. Six animals were used for each serum tested, and each run was carefully controlled for virulence of virus used. The few monkey protection tests reported were carried out in accordance with the method previously described.

DISCUSSION

In considering the information on laboratory tests presented above, and their relationship to declared history of recent illness, the intrinsic differences and limitations of complement-fixation and protection tests should be remembered. The complement-fixing antibodies are apparently less constantly produced and are certainly less permanent in character than are the protective antibodies. Complement-fixing antibodies appear more tardily than do protective antibodies and apparently increase over a period of some weeks, only to decline rapidly. This does not mean, however, that all positive complement-fixation tests can be attributed to recent illness, since Frobisher and Davis have shown independently that reexposure to the virus is sufficient to produce an increase in the concentration of complement-fixing antibodies in the blood of monkeys previously immunized, whose complement-fixing titer had fallen very low. The finding of any considerable percentage of positive complement-fixation results in a given population, then, should be interpreted as probably indicating that this community has recently harbored the virus of yellow fever, but does not necessarily imply a recently acquired immunity to the disease in every case. On the other hand, the finding of a high percentage of positive protection tests gives no indication of the time of immunization, except in sera from the younger age groups. Although the protective antibodies are apparently constantly produced and permanent in character, the test for their presence is a biological one, and, as such, subject to occasional variation. The mouse protection test has, then, an important advantage over the monkey protection test in that the result is not based on a single animal but on several. The comparative results of monkey protection and other tests are shown for a small series of persons in Table 14. The monkey protection results are lower than were anticipated on the basis of the other results for the same group. All positive monkey tests were confirmed by mouse tests, but the mouse test disclosed five positives apparently missed by the monkey test.

The percentage of positive complement-fixation results in Cambucy was unexpectedly low in comparison with that in Magé. While this may be due to variation in antigens used, the definite association of complement-fixation results with history of recent illness and the variation shown in the percentage of positives at different periods following suspicious attacks, suggests that the factor of time alone may well account for the difference between the postepidemic results in Magé and in Cambucy. In Magé, specimens for complement-fixation tests were collected 3 and 4 months after the peak of the epidemic, and the percentage of positive

Table 14. Results of Rhesus Monkey Protection Tests Compared with History of Recent Illness and Complement-Fixation and Mouse Protection Tests

Monkey protection test	History of recent illness			Complement-fixation test			Mouse protection test		
	Positive	Negative	Total	Positive	Negative	Total	Positive	Negative	Total
Positive	13	1	14	9	5	14	14	0	14
Negative	11	4	15	6	9	15	5	6	11
Total	24	5	29	15	14	29	19	6	25

results (42.0) was more than twice that (19.9) found in specimens taken during and immediately after the epidemic in Cambucy. That a higher percentage might have been expected some weeks later in Cambucy is indicated by the high percentage (55.6) of positive results in cases with history of attack from 6 to 10 weeks previously.

No significant difference was found between the percentage of immunes observed in Magé with the monkey protection test (55.3) and the percentages found in Cambucy with the monkey protection (48.3) and mouse protection (59.3) tests.

Both Magé and Cambucy failed to show significant differences in the percentage of positive complement-fixation results for the age groups above and below 20 years, but they did show significant differences in the results of protection tests for these groups. Hughes and Sawyer have recently demonstrated that physiological maturation phenomena are not responsible for the increased immunity observed in the older age groups. Hence, if yellow fever was actually absent from Cambucy during two decades previous to the present outbreak, the residual immunity in the older age groups may be roughly calculated from the formula

$$x + r(100 - x) = y,$$

where r is attack rate in group 19 years of age and under and y is the percentage of immunes in group 20 years of age and over:

$$x + 0.515(100 - x) = 65.3.$$

Therefore, it is estimated that approximately 28.5 per cent of the present population over 20 years of age has immunity which was acquired prior to the present outbreak. This compares with 41 per cent calculated for Magé by the same formula, using monkey protection results. If due allowance is made for this preexisting immunity in Cambucy, and their respective immunity rates are applied to the groups above and below 20 years of age, the calculated number of persons recently immunized in the total population of Cambucy is 363. This is an increase of 31 per cent over the number of persons giving history of recent illness (277).

Although Cambucy must surely have been visited repeatedly by yellow fever prior to 1908, only six persons reported having had the disease before the 1930–1931 outbreak. Including the cases in the present outbreak, then, there are but 19 clinically recognized cases in the community on which to base an immunity of approximately 60 per cent in a population of more than 800.

At the beginning of the present study in February 1931, the mild grippe-like epidemic which had been observed by local clinicians since October 1930 could not be definitely identified as yellow fever. In fact, a similar widespread illness noted by local physicians in Magé prior to the discovery of yellow fever in that town in 1929 was not studied because it did not measure up to the criteria on which diagnosis of yellow fever is usually based. (In Magé the illness was thought to be malaria, an opinion later shown to be erroneous. In Cambucy, where malaria is not endemic, the febrile outbreak was believed to be grippe.) Had the results of complement-fixation and monkey protection tests made on sera from Magé not indicated a much higher degree of population immunity than could be expected on the basis of known yellow fever, this outbreak of "grippe without respiratory symptoms" in Cambucy would have received scant attention. Although yellow fever was known to have been present since November, the number of classical cases was so small that it was hard to believe that these were not sporadic cases occurring in a population largely immunized by previous attack.

The high degree of association found between history of recent illness and positive mouse protection and complement-fixation results, and the striking variation of the complement-fixation results at different periods after indicated dates of recent illness, may be interpreted as strong evidence that the widespread immunity observed in Cambucy was for the most part acquired during the 6 month period from October 1930 to March 1931.

The distribution of history of illness by months and blocks shows a remarkable relationship to the distribution of known cases of yellow fever and to the distribution of immunity to yellow fever as shown by the mouse protection test; and one cannot escape the conviction that the Cambucy epidemic of yellow fever of 1930–1931 was composed of several hundred mild infections and less than a score of clinically recognized cases. An attempt to attribute all immunity in the age group below 20 years to the observed epidemic, meets a discrepancy between history of recent illness (28.6 per cent) and results of mouse-protection tests (51.5 per cent). It would seem then that this outbreak of yellow fever in Cambucy either was not the first since 1908, or was characterized by a large number of truly subclinical infections, which either produced no symptoms or symptoms so mild as to be completely overlooked by the families concerned. Considering available information, the latter hypothesis appears more acceptable than the first.

This large percentage of mild subclinical infections is very interesting in the light of the racial distribution of the population of Cambucy. No significant difference was found among the percentages of different racial groups reporting recent illness; neither was there a difference in the percentages of men and women reporting recent illness, although statistics of yellow fever outbreaks generally show appreciably higher numbers of cases among men than among women.

Although the total number of persons in Cambucy shown to be immune to yellow fever greatly exceeded the number giving a history of recent illness, there was found to be a marked correlation between a high percentage of immunes and a high percentage of persons with history of recent illness. For example, two areas, A and B, may be outlined in which the percentage of persons found to be immune to yellow fever by the mouse protection test is very high (90.4) in comparison with the percentage of immune persons outside these areas (47.0). The percentage of persons in these areas giving a history of recent illness (46.7), although much lower than the percentage of immunes, is much higher than the percentage of persons outside the areas with history of recent illness. It should be noted that the distribution of immunity in Cambucy is far from uniform; the percentage of immunes varies greatly in different parts of the town. Caution must be observed in drawing general conclusions regarding the percentage of immunes in a given population from the results of immunity tests on a sample of the population.

SUMMARY AND CONCLUSIONS

An epidemiological survey of yellow fever was made in Cambucy during and after a small epidemic in this previously endemic area, which had been considered free of the disease during two decades. This survey, based on history of illness and complement-fixation and mouse protection tests, if interpreted in the light of past history of yellow fever in the area, indicates that the distribution of immunity in Cambucy bore very little relationship to the recognition of classical cases of the disease, but was highly correlated with the distribution of recent cases of so-called "grippe without respiratory symptoms." This epidemic of grippe was characterized by fever, headache, and body pains, and to a lesser extent by nausea, vomiting, and icterus.

A considerable number of persons, on the other hand, even in the younger age groups, were found to be immune to yellow fever, without history of previous illness, indicating that immunization may often occur without illness sufficiently severe to register in the memory of the individual or his family.

The observation made at Magé and Santo Aleixo that the acquisition of immunity to yellow fever by the native population of a previously endemic region from which the disease has been apparently absent for 20 years may be accompanied by very few classical cases was confirmed in Cambucy.

The results of control mouse protection tests on sera from two non-infectible areas are presented, confirming the freedom of this test from any appreciable percentage of falsely positive results.

This survey has thrown further light on the period at which complement-fixing antibodies are most commonly demonstrable after an attack. A significantly higher percentage of positive results was obtained during the period from 6 to 10 weeks after the attack than either before or after this time. Second complement-fixation tests performed some 8 months after first tests showed great reduction in complement-fixing antibodies, but nevertheless the results of these two tests were highly associated.

Certain evidence is presented suggesting that the mouse protection test may be a more sensitive indicator of immunity to yellow fever than the monkey protection test. Results of mouse protection tests, results of complement-fixation tests, and history of recent illness were found to be closely associated.

The distribution of immunity to yellow fever may be far from uniform even in small communities.

The results of the present study indicate that epidemiological investigations, unsupported by laboratory tests and autopsies, are bound to be falsely comforting in endemic yellow fever areas in which there is little movement of foreigners.

Acknowledgments

The collection of the large number of duplicate specimens at Cambucy was made possible only through the whole-hearted cooperation of Dr. Vicente Dantas and Dr. Ulysses Lannes, who gave freely of their time and influence in aid of the present study.

The authors also acknowledge their indebtedness to the following members of the staff of the Yellow Fever Service: to Dr. D. B. Wilson, Dr. Gastão Cesar, and Dr. Eleyson Cardoso, for collecting specimens in Friburgo, and to Dr. Amaral Machado for collecting specimens in Gaupé. The protection tests in New York were performed by Dr. W. A. Sawyer and Dr. T. P. Hughes and those in Bahia by Dr. Wray Lloyd and Dr. Henrique Penna. All complement-fixation tests were performed by Dr. Martin Frobisher, Jr.

Selection 18 | The Geographical Distribution
of Immunity to Yellow Fever in
Man in South America*

The first attempt to study the distribution of immunity to yellow fever in South America was begun early in 1929 using the monkey protection and complement-fixation tests. The results indicated that even when yellow fever is known to be present in a community, the percentage of the population acquiring measurable immunity to the disease may be much higher than would be expected on the basis of diagnosed cases. The introduction of the mouse protection test afforded the means of confirming these results in 1931, when it was conclusively shown that yellow fever may be, at least among the native population of previously endemic areas, a disease of low mortality, as only a few classical cases occurred during a period of extensive immunization of the general population.

In 1931, during the course of an entomological field trip in the Amazon Valley, R. C. Shannon collected, at the request of Dr. W. A. Sawyer, a small series of sera from children living at various points, including Manáos, Porto Velho, and Iquitos, all previously important centers of yellow fever infection but long considered free of this scourge. Although

* This report gives the results for South America (Brazil, Paraguay, Bolivia, Chile, Peru, Ecuador, Colombia, Venezuela, British Guiana, Dutch Guiana, and French Guiana) of the world survey of yellow fever immunity distribution begun in 1931 by the International Health Division of The Rockefeller Foundation with the cooperation of the governments concerned. Dr. Soper was the Representative in South America (Rio de Janeiro office) of the International Health Division of The Rockefeller Foundation.

The immunity survey of South America has not been the work of an individual or of a small group of individuals but represents the combined efforts of many colleagues who have traveled extensively throughout the continent collecting sera for examination and of the groups of laboratory workers in the New York and Bahia yellow fever laboratories who have been responsible for the testing of these sera. The field collections have been greatly facilitated by the whole-hearted collaboration of national and colonial authorities, public health officials, teachers, and others who have disinterestedly aided in this work. Special mention must be made of the continued support given to these studies by Drs. F. F. Russell and W. A. Sawyer, under whose direction they have been made during the period 1931 to 1936.

This excerpt is reprinted by permission from the article (25) in the *American Journal of Tropical Medicine 17*: 457–511, 1937. Copyright © 1937, The Williams & Wilkins Company, Baltimore, Maryland. (Tables 1 through 29 and Maps 2 through 16 have been omitted from this excerpt.)

the mouse protection test had not yet reached its present high degree of accuracy, the results clearly indicated that some immunization was occurring throughout the valley in the complete absence of observed outbreaks of the disease. However, the percentage of children found with positive protection tests in these cities was small in comparison with that obtained in the study of a known infected center in the same year mentioned above. This low percentage of immunes in the Amazon Valley was very intriguing and could not be explained with the knowledge then available.

Following the discovery in 1932 of yellow fever occurring in a rural area in the absence of *Aëdes aegypti,* a study of the distribution of immunity in this infected area showed that a much lower percentage of the rural population, especially children, had been immunized than was to have been expected on the basis of urban studies, taking into consideration the known duration and extent of the outbreak.

The studies thus begun in Brazil were extended to Bolivia and Paraguay in 1932, when, on the eve of the war for the Chaco, yellow fever unexpectedly appeared at Santa Cruz de la Sierra, Bolivia, in the very heart of the continent. The occurrence of suspect cases in Ecuador and Colombia in 1933 led to similar studies in these countries. In the same year Dr. W. A. Sawyer, who was interested in the completion of a world survey of the present distribution of yellow fever endemicity suggested that the rest of South America be studied. Venezuela, the Guianas, and Peru were accordingly surveyed, and specimens were taken at a couple of points in northern Chile. Only Argentina and Uruguay have been omitted from the present study. Reasonable certainty exists that these countries have not been visited by aegypti-transmitted yellow fever during the present century.

The present investigation, extensive as it is, is only a beginning in the study of the epidemiology of yellow fever in South America. However, enough is already known of the general problem to justify publication of available results without danger of unduly jeopardizing the commercial interests of any nation. These results conclusively show that the problem of yellow fever control is one involving the interests of the entire continent.

Collecting and Testing of Material

The collections of blood specimens for the present survey were made in most cases by members of the staff of the International Health Division of The Rockefeller Foundation or by medical officers attached to the cooperative services maintained by The Rockefeller Foundation and the various interested governments. Special mention must be given to the work of Dr. A. M. Walcott, who made the collections in Chile, Peru, the Amazonian portion of Ecuador, and the Guianas, in addition to part of the collections in Venezuela and Bolivia. Especially difficult trips for the collection of specimens were made also by Drs. Gastão Cezar, Jr., J. Paternoster, Mario Alcantara, and A. W. Burke in Brazil; by Drs. L. Patiño Camargo, Arthur Vergara-Uribe, Jorge Boshell, and Alfredo Correa-Henao in Colombia; by Drs. J. E. Elmendorf and Antonio Anzola-Carillo in Venezuela, and by Drs. Angel Claros and R. Valda in Bolivia. In addition, collections were made by Drs. E. R. Rickard, F. A. Machado, P. J. Crawford, Eleyson Cardoso, Alvaro de Andrade, Oswaldo Novis, N. Tavares, J. Serafim, Jr., Jose F. Pinheiro, H. W. Kumm, Milton Pessoa de Mello, D. Silva-Lima, Virgilio Oliveira, C. S. Manso, S. Faro, and E. P. Salgado, in Brazil; by Drs. Mario Bião, and Jose Ynsfrán in Paraguay; by Drs. J. Illingsworth I., E. Sayago S., Eleutherio Constante-Freire, and F. L. Soper in Ecuador; by Drs. R. I. Chacon and Briceño Rossi in Venezuela; and by Drs. E. R. Rickard, George Bevier, and I. Moreno-Perez in Colombia.

Collections of specimens from the frontier regions of the Uapés and Japurá rivers were possible only through the invaluable collaboration of the high officials, both Brazilian and Colombian, who formed the special commission for permanent demarcation of the international boundary.

Special mention must be made of the collaboration of Drs. D. B. Wilson, Servulo Lima, Waldemar Sá Antunes, and a host of other colleagues in the Yellow River Service who, while not directly responsible for the collection of specimens, have handled the many administrative details necessary in connection with such collection.

Space does not permit of more than a general note of appreciation to the innumerable officials, health officers, physicians, school teachers, and others whose aid has been indispensable in collecting the material for the present immunity survey.

Actual collections in the field have generally been made in 30-cc venules. In the beginning the sera were separated and pipetted off and placed in ampoules for shipment to the laboratory. During the latter stages of the study the separation of serum was made directly from the original venule to a smaller one and the latter was then sent to the laboratory. The latter method actually reduces costs when collections are being made at long distances from the laboratory and also lessens breakage and chance contamination.

When the present survey was begun, nothing was known of the existence of jungle yellow fever. The collection of blood specimens for the survey was therefore limited to the towns and cities of the areas studied. In each community studied, specimens were obtained, whenever possible, from 100 persons born and continuously resident in the place, one half of these persons being less than 10 years of age. The plan of collection was that not more than two persons from any family were to be bled, and when two were bled from the same family one was to be less than 10 years of age and the other over 10 years of age. In practice, these suggestions, simple as they are, were difficult to follow. Collections were often made in schools, and full information regarding the past of the individuals was not obtainable. In some cases, especially among the Indian tribes investigated, only an approximate age could be entered. In certain districts population movement has been so great, because of seasonal work, seasonal floods, and occasional droughts, that very few families have been found who have been constantly resident in one place over a period of years. In spite of these difficulties, however, it is believed that the data herewith presented give a good general idea of conditions throughout the area studied.

The mouse protection tests on which this report is based were performed in the yellow fever laboratories in the International Health Division of The Rockefeller Foundation in New York and Bahia.* Among those who have carried the burden of this work, special mention is due Drs. W. A. Sawyer, Wray Lloyd, J. A. Kerr, Henrique Penna, Loring Whitman, S. F. Kitchen, Mr. Harry Burruss, and Senhor Antonio Sotero Cabral. Although the earlier results, obtained at a time when difficulties were still being encountered because of resistant strains of mice, weak virus preparations, and epidemics of various kinds among the experimental animals, are not so clear cut as those obtained during later years, no reason was found for modifying any of the essentials of the technique of the mouse protection test during the course of the present studies.

Discussion of Results

The results of the protection test survey of South America have been tabulated by states and countries, and corresponding maps have been prepared. Map 1 is a general map of South America showing the relationship to each other of the areas covered by Maps 2 to 16.

The classification of the population groups studied as urban or rural is somewhat arbitrary and not entirely satisfactory. The urban group includes many living in small villages and settlements as well as those in organized towns and cities. The rural group includes those living in both heavily and scantily populated agricultural districts, as well as those from jungle areas.

* The Yellow Fever Laboratory at Bahia, installed in 1928 in a building lent for the purpose by the Government of the State of Bahia, was maintained by the International Health Division until the end of 1934, at which time it became an integral part of the Yellow Fever Service of the National Department of Health of Brazil, supported by the Government of Brazil and The Rockefeller Foundation.

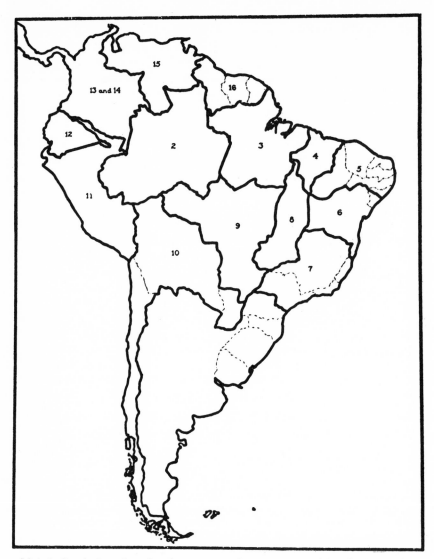

Map 1. South America, showing states and sectors covered by the immunity
survey, with area numbers.

Brazil

State of Amazonas (Area 2)

The results obtained in the State of Amazonas were entirely unexpected
and are not in keeping with the known history of yellow fever previous to
the beginning of this study. Historically, Manáos, the capital of the state

and its most important center of navigation, was first infected with yellow fever in 1856 and remained an important focus of infection until about 1912, when the disease disappeared from the city and apparently from the entire Amazon Valley as the result of antimosquito campaigns organized in the three endemic centers, Belém, Manáos, and Iquitos. During the past 20 years only one case of yellow fever, imported from Pará in 1929, has been diagnosed in Manáos, and no outbreaks had been reported elsewhere in the state previous to the present study. In spite of this absence of visible yellow fever during such a long period of time, the results of the protection test indicate that the disease had maintained its endemicity throughout most of the state. Notable exceptions to this endemicity, however, are the two most important cities in the state, Manáos and Itacoatiára. *The low percentages of immunes found in these cities indicate conclusively that they have not served during recent years as important distributing centers of infection.* Of special interest are the relatively high percentages of immunes recorded for the Indian population of the Uapés region where the *Aëdes aegypti* mosquito is not found.

That the endemicity of the Amazon region does not depend on a mild harmless strain of virus is indicated by the discovery, through viscerotomy, of fatal cases during the period covered by the present study of yellow fever at three widely separated points in the state: Lauro Sodré, 1933; Fonte Bôa, 1934; and Lábrea, 1936.

Territory of Acre (Area 2)

The positive protection test results recorded for Acre in the complete absence of large cities in the region and with no recorded outbreaks during many years might cause doubt of the validity of the protection test were it not for the confirmation through viscerotomy of active fatal infection in the region, namely, at Rio Branco in 1933, at Cobija, Bolivia, just across the frontier from Brasiléia, in 1936 and at Xapury in 1937.

State of Pará (Area 3)

The city of Belém (Pará), the gateway to the Amazon, was first reported to have yellow fever in 1850 and continued to have known outbreaks of the disease until 1912, when the city was cleaned through antimosquito measures. No cases were then reported from the entire state until 1929, when the city of Belém was apparently infected through maritime contact with infected capitals further south. At the beginning of 1930 there was no reason for thinking that the infection still persisted in the state. In May of that year, however, viscerotomy revealed that it was still present in the neighborhood of Belém, and a few scattered cases occurring in the presence of aegypti were identified, the last of which, seen in August 1931, had apparently been infected in Bragança.

In spite of this scanty history during two decades, the immunity survey shows that the infection has been widespread during the past 15 years. Especially noteworthy is the fact that much lower percentages of immunes were recorded for Belém, the only large city and principal port, than for a number of other towns. The highest percentages of immunes were recorded for Bragança, where no recent history of infection was obtained except for the single case already mentioned.

That the yellow fever endemicity of this region does not depend on key-center distribution of the virus, as suggested by the history of the disease in Belém and the low percentages of immunes found, is confirmed by the discovery through viscerotomy of fatal cases of jungle yellow fever close to Curralinho in 1934 and 1935, at Oriximiná in 1935, and at Santa Izabel between Belém and Bragança in 1937. That urban cases have not been recorded may well be due to the organization of antiaegypti measures in all the principal towns of the state.

The negative results from Rio Curipí and Clevelandia are interesting, since this is one of the few primitive areas investigated failing to show immunes. The failure to find aegypti in São João do Araguaya and Conceição Araguaya suggests that the few instances of immunity found among adults are due to infection away from these towns, either in the jungle or in towns where aegypti do occur.

State of Maranhão (Area 4)

During more than two decades no cases of yellow fever were known to have occurred in Maranhão. Only after the organization of viscerotomy was a positive case found at Picos in 1935. Investigation failed to determine whether this case was urban or jungle in origin, but an extensive outbreak of jungle yellow fever was uncovered in the region of São João de Patos during 1936. The failure to find aegypti at Carolina is associated with very low percentages of immunes, as was noted for the nearby towns of São João Araguaya and Conceição Araguaya, Pará.

Northeast Brazil (States of Piauhy, Ceará, Rio Grande do Norte, Parahyba, Pernambuco, and Alagôas) (Area 5)

Except for an interval of about 2 years (1921–1923), more effort has been devoted to the study and control of yellow fever since 1919 in the six states here grouped in the region Northeast Brazil than in any similar region during the same period.

In the Amazon region the immunity survey led the way in calling attention to regional endemicity, but in Northeast Brazil viscerotomy was responsible for showing that yellow fever continued widespread throughout the interior of this part of the country in spite of the antiaegypti measures applied in what were thought to be the key centers for the maintenance and distribution of the infection. Fatal cases were found in each of the six states during the 5-year period 1930–1934.

Investigation showed that a large part of the interior of Northeast Brazil had a widespread distribution of the urban vector of yellow fever, aegypti, throughout rural districts. No evidence of jungle yellow fever was found in this region, and since the introduction of antiaegypti measures in infected rural districts viscerotomy has failed to reveal positive cases in such districts. Viscerotomy disclosed interior foci of infection until August 1934, but for almost 3 years now it has not unearthed a single positive case in Northeast Brazil.

The protection test results from Northeast Brazil are especially interesting, since they show how thoroughly native populations of endemic areas where aegypti is the vector may be subject to immunizing yellow fever infections early in life without the occurrence of severe epidemic outbreaks. Viscerotomy has likewise shown that the majority of fatal infections occur under such circumstances in the younger age groups.

States of Bahia and Sergipe (Area 6)

Bahia has long been considered the southern limit of yellow fever endemicity in Brazil, although the local authorities have often attributed the reappearance of the disease in Salvador, the capital, to reinfection from the north, especially from Sergipe. Many interior towns along the railways and along the São Francisco River are known to have suffered from outbreaks of yellow fever in 1926, but during the past decade, in spite of repeated investigations and the organization of viscerotomy, no cases have been diagnosed outside the narrow coastal plain of Sergipe and the corresponding region of Bahia as far south as Ilhéos. *In contrast with Northeast Brazil, no evidence of rural endemicity due to aegypti has been found in either Sergipe or Bahia, but the existence of jungle yellow fever has been demonstrated in Bahia in the heavily forested region about Ilhéos.*

State of Minas Geraes (Area 7)

During the course of the present study most surprising facts have been uncovered regarding yellow fever in Minas Geraes. During the period previous to 1908 when yellow fever was known to be endemic in the city of Rio de Janeiro, occasional summer outbreaks of the disease were recorded in nearby cities of Minas Geraes. Not until 1926 were cases again recorded in the state, and then the infection came up the São Francisco River as far as Pirapora but is not known to have extended above this point. During the Rio de Janeiro epidemic of 1928–1929 a number of imported cases were diagnosed at various points in the state, but only at Corintho did a local outbreak occur (1929). This was followed by a self-limited outbreak recorded at nearby São Hypolito 6 months later.

[*Corrigendum:* In early 1931 yellow fever was found at various points in the eastern portion of the state along the railroad line from Recreo to Manhuaçú. This was a direct extension of the urban epidemics which occurred late in 1930 and early in 1931 along the railroad line between Campos, Rio de Janeiro State, and Recreo. These outbreaks responded to antiaegypti measures, the last case occurring in May 1931. The clearing of this railroad line is considered as the terminal point of the aegypti-transmitted yellow fever in South Brazil seeded from the Rio outbreak of 1928–1929, the official onset of which was in May 1928.]

During a period of 5 years no outbreaks of yellow fever are known to have occurred in the state, but in 1935, 1936, and 1937 viscerotomy has revealed the presence of infection in the western, southern, and extreme eastern parts of the state. In the west many counties lying between the Rio Grande and the Rio Parnahyba and others contiguous with the boundary between the State of Minas Geraes and the states of São Paulo and Goyaz have had serious outbreaks of jungle yellow fever. No cases in this area have been attributed to urban aegypti transmission and no indication of the presence of the disease in the region was given by the protection tests on blood specimens collected in Uberlandia and Araguary early in 1935, although these towns are in the heart of the infected district. In the east aegypti-transmitted urban yellow fever appeared in Theofilo Ottoni in 1935 after protection test surveys of this community made in 1931 and early in 1935 had shown very low percentages of immunes among children, although the aegypti density was high. Retesting of 33 children previously negative showed that 20 of them had acquired demonstrable immunity during the outbreak of 1935. The town of Figueira had a series of aegypti-transmitted cases in 1936. The conclusion based on epidemiological considerations that these outbreaks were probably due to invasion of the towns by jungle virus from nearby districts is supported by the finding of 12 immunes among 20 cebus monkeys captured near Figueira and by the diagnosis through viscerotomy in 1937 of a case of jungle yellow fever contracted about 20 kilometers from Theofilo Ottoni. (Theofilo Ottoni was the object of special observation following reports in 1931 of suspect cases. No evidence of the disease was found until after the second survey in 1935, when a sharp outbreak occurred. The 1936 results are from post-epidemic studies on children previously shown to be nonimmune.)

State of Espirito Santo (Area 7)

Yellow fever apparently disappeared from the State of Espirito Santo following the sanitation of Rio de Janeiro, which was completed in 1908. In 1917 an outbreak was recorded in Victoria, the capital city, but no further incidence of aegypti-transmitted fever has been observed up to the present time, not even during the Rio de Janeiro epidemic of 1928–1929. In 1932 the first outbreak of rural yellow fever without aegypti to be described occurred in the Valle do Chanaan. This outbreak was apparently self-limited, and viscerotomy has failed to reveal fatal cases in the state during the past 4 years.

State of Rio de Janeiro and the Federal District (Area 7)

The State of Rio de Janeiro is not known to have harbored the virus of yellow fever during the 20 years previous to 1928. Cases were diagnosed, however, almost immediately following the discovery of the disease in the neighboring City of Rio de Janeiro in May 1928, and during the succeeding 3 years yellow fever was found at more than 40 points in this small state. The survey data presented really represent special study information, since any general survey could only confirm the previously recognized general distribution of the virus in the state.

The negative results from Novo Friburgo confirm the contention that under the conditions obtaining in this state, altitudes of from 2500 to 3000 feet are free of yellow fever. The results from Cambucy, which represent almost the entire population of the town, have been discussed elsewhere. The results in the Federal District and in the nearby suburban parts of the State of Rio—Nictheroy, Nilopolis, Novo Iguassú, São João de Merity, and Caxias—are based on the examination of material collected from carefully selected children who had been under 5 years of age at the end of the outbreak in 1929 and who were still living, when tested, in the house of their birth. These results clearly indicate that although but few infections were diagnosed in children under 5 years of age during the last epidemic, the disease did not fail to attack this age group.

State of São Paulo (Area 7)

The port of Santos was previously a notorious center of yellow fever infection, and occasional outbreaks of the disease were observed in the interior. Following the antimosquito campaigns of the first decade of this century, however, no locally infected cases were recorded within the state until 1935, when viscerotomy revealed the presence of jungle yellow fever in several counties. During 1936 and 1937 yellow fever was an important problem throughout almost the entire state and was even found in these years in the State of Paraná, which is just south of São Paulo and was not included in the present survey because it was thought to be outside the yellow fever zone. Most of the cases recorded have been rural infections occurring in the absence of aegypti, although certain towns in both São Paulo and Paraná have had suspicious outbreaks probably due to aegypti transmission. The protection tests made at four points in the interior in 1935 failed to give any indication of the presence of the infection in the surrounding rural areas. The only immune recorded for the city of Santos proved on further investigation to have been born in Northeast Brazil and probably came to Santos already immune.

State of Goyaz (Area 8)

There is no history of the occurrence of yellow fever in Goyaz previous to 1935. The collection of blood specimens was made to complete the immunity survey and to obtain data bearing on the problem of jungle yellow fever in Matto Grosso. Specimens from several communities in southern Goyaz were collected during the latter weeks of 1934 and the early weeks of 1935. Among more than 500 children less than 15 years of age only six immunes were found, and the youngest of these was 9 years old! Routine collections from southern Goyaz had been already completed, without any information regarding the disease having been obtained, when a chance conversation occurring between the colleague making the collection and an old classmate then practicing in this region led to the investigation of a rural outbreak of fevers occurring some distance from the nearest town. A positive autopsy resulted in the rapid extension of viscerotomy throughout the region, with the discovery of jungle yellow fever over an enormous area comprising the southern one third of the state, contiguous areas in Minas Geraes to the east and to the south, with extension even into São Paulo and later (1936) into Paraná. As far as is known no urban infections occurred, although some of the towns are infested with aegypti. During 1936 and the first 6 months of 1937 viscerotomy failed to reveal fatal cases of yellow fever in Goyaz.

It is interesting to compare the results of the immunity survey in Goyaz, where aegypti-transmitted yellow fever has not been observed but where jungle yellow fever has been widespread, with those of the survey in Northeast Brazil, where transmission is apparently entirely due to aegypti.

State of Matto Grosso (Area 9)

In 1933 three children in Corumbá, Matto Grosso, were found to be immune to yellow fever. Although investigation indicated that two of them must have acquired their immunity within the state, the disease is not definitely known to have existed in Matto Grosso during the present century previous to 1934, when the jungle infection was shown to be present on the planalto east of Cuyabá. This outbreak in the area about Coronel Ponce, Ponte Alta, and Uzina Rio da Casca has been the subject of special studies. During 1936 and the early months of 1937 jungle yellow fever was found to be present in a number of localities of southern Matto Grosso lying roughly between the São Paulo border, the Paraguay River, and the Paraguayan frontier.

The results of the immunity survey of Matto Grosso fail to indicate that there have been any important outbreaks of aegypti-transmitted yellow fever in the recent past, but they do suggest that the jungle endemicity is widespread.

Bolivia (Area 10)

Although there was published in Bolivia in 1887 a description of an epidemic believed by the authors to be yellow fever, this report was never fully accepted and is not known to have made its way into the general literature of yellow fever until after the dramatic appearance of this disease among the troops in Santa Cruz de la Sierra in 1932, just a few months previous to the opening of the War for the Chaco. When the investigation of the Santa Cruz outbreak began it was already known that yellow fever could exist in the absence of aegypti. However, the density of aegypti was high in Santa Cruz and in a number of nearby towns where cases had occurred, and there seemed to be no reason to attribute the infection to other than urban origin, although the source of infection seemed mysterious because of the isolation of this district and the complete absence of nearby cities large enough to be considered permanent endemic foci of aegypti-transmitted yellow fever. In May 1933 yellow fever without aegypti proved to have been present in San Ramón, a small Indian village even more isolated in the lowlands of Bolivia than is Santa Cruz. In 1935, after a period of more than 2 years during which antiaegypti measures were applied in the principal towns of the Bolivian lowlands, yellow fever reappeared in the war zone south of Santa Cruz *as a jungle infection*. A much more serious and widespread distribution of jungle yellow fever was recorded during 1936. During the first 5 months of 1937 a single case of jungle yellow fever was revealed in Bolivia by viscerotomy. The available evidence suggests that yellow fever endemicity in the lowlands of Bolivia is basically jungle endemicity.

Paraguay (Area 10)

Paraguay is known to have had outbreaks of yellow fever during the last century, but infection was always attributed to river transportation from the south. The immunity survey failed to indicate any recent incidence of the disease in the country, although one 19-year-old immune was found. However, early in 1937 the existence of jungle yellow fever was proved in northern Paraguay. Further studies are needed to clarify the yellow fever situation in Paraguay.

Chile

Yellow fever is reported to have been present in Chile, at Tocopilla, in 1912. The results of protection tests at Tocopilla and Arica indicate that these cities at least have not been the scene of undiagnosed outbreaks of the disease during recent years.

Peru (Area 11)

From the standpoint of yellow fever endemicity, Peru is divided by the Andes mountains into two distinct regions, eastern or Amazonian Peru and the Pacific Coast. The history of yellow fever in the Amazon region is similar to that of the State of Amazonas, Brazil. Iquitos and Yurimaguas and other ports on the rivers were known to have yellow fever at times until after the antimosquito campaign which was responsible for the cleaning of Iquitos in 1913. Following this date, although suspicious cases have been recorded in the region, no clearly confirmed case has come under observation.

The history of yellow fever on the Pacific Coast of Peru indicates that infection in this region was due to movement of the virus up and down the coast rather than over the mountains. The last known outbreak occurred in 1921 shortly after the cleaning of Guayaquil, which was apparently the only important endemic focus in the Pacific coast of South America.

The immunity survey results show that in Amazonian Peru, as in other parts of the Amazon Valley, there is a surprisingly high percentage of immunes, even in those towns where aegypti are not found, but that there is an almost complete absence of immunes among children tested on the Pacific Coast. Considering the high aegypti indices of this region, it seems improbable that the 3 immune children found among some 750 tested could have acquired their immunity in the Pacific Coast towns without the occurrence of outbreaks which would have resulted in high percentages of immunity in the children of these towns. The actual existence of yellow fever in Amazonian Peru has been proved by the observation of clinical cases and by autopsy in the Chanchomayo Valley in 1937. (Unpublished observations: Dr. Henry Hanson, Dr. Richard P. Strong.)

Ecuador (Area 12)

Ecuador, like Peru, is divided by the Andes into two distinct regions. Yellow fever is reported to have been present in Guayaquil, the principal port of Ecuador, from its first introduction in 1750 until 1920, since which date no fully confirmed cases are known to have occurred. The immunity survey results herewith reported for the Pacific Coast are based on special studies made to ascertain whether suspicious cases occurring in Guayaquil and certain nearby towns of the coastal plain could be yellow fever. The protection test results fail entirely to substantiate the thesis that yellow fever has been present during recent years in the towns of the Pacific Coast of Ecuador, where the density of aegypti is generally high. The positive results from Amazonian Ecuador are in keeping with results from other parts of the Amazon Valley in Brazil, Bolivia, Peru, and Colombia. They are especially interesting in view of the fact that no aegypti were observed at any point where specimens were collected. This mosquito has apparently not penetrated beyond the head of launch navigation on the Napo River.

Colombia (Areas 13 and 14)

The story of yellow fever in Colombia forms one of the most interesting chapters in the history of the disease, and recent epidemiological findings would be well-nigh incredible were it not for the fact that these findings confirmed by clinical observation, autopsy, immunity tests, and isolation of the virus, afford a reasonable explanation for much that is not otherwise subject to explanation. Colombia is divided by high mountain ranges and plateaus into a number of rather distinct regions, communication between which has been until quite recently difficult and slow. Yellow fever endemicity in the Pacific Coast ports and in the narrow Pacific slope has apparently depended in the past on repeated maritime infection. No cases have been registered in this region since the city of Guayaquil, long considered the most important focus of infection on the Pacific Coast, was sanitated in 1920. Endemicity in the important Caribbean ports and in the river ports of the Magdalena River, the disease having been recorded as far up as Honda, has apparently depended largely in the past on maritime endemicity in the Caribbean region. Since the disappearance of yellow fever in Havana, Panama, and other important ports of the Caribbean, the disease has not been common in the Caribbean and Magdalena River ports of Colombia, the last confirmed outbreak in a port occurring in Cartagena in 1919. However, after a period of 4 years, during which the disease had not been observed in Colombia, urban yellow fever appeared unexpectedly in Bucaramanga, an isolated city in the Magdalena Valley. The source of this infection remained a mystery. After a further period of 6 years, during which yellow fever was apparently absent from Colombia, another urban outbreak occurred in 1929 in the town of Socorro, Santander, a point in the mountains even more isolated from possible known sources of the infection than was Bucaramanga. These two outbreaks are the only ones recorded since 1919 in which transmission of yellow fever has occurred in the presence of aegypti. Early studies of immunity distribution in Colombia led to the conclusion that yellow fever had not been present during recent years in Santa Marta and the river ports, although a few scattered immunes were found among young children along the river. These studies failed to show that the region of Cúcuta in the Catatumbo Valley, previously subject to infection secondary to that in Maracaibo, Venezuela, had been recently infected. The finding of high percentages of immunes in certain rural districts, especially Muzo, of the Magdalena Valley, caused the conclusion to be drawn that there probably existed a rural type of endemicity not dependent on aegypti, similar to the then recently described situation in the Valle do Chanaan in Brazil. The llanos, or tropical savannahs, of Amazonian Colombia which lie in the valleys of both the Orinoco and Amazon rivers, take no part in the previous history of yellow fever except for a suspect outbreak along the Meta River in 1886.

Although no cases of yellow fever have been confirmed for the lower llanos, the results of the immunity survey of the Uapés and Caquetá river points, when considered together with results from the contiguous areas of the State of Amazonas, Brazil, indicate that the disease is endemic in this region, as in many parts of the Amazon Valley. Yellow fever was first confirmed by autopsy for the upper llanos at Restrepo, near Villavicencio, in 1934. The disease continued under observation during 1935, 1936, and 1937 entirely as a jungle infection, no aegypti having been found in the towns and cities of the region. In the Magdalena Valley, investigation has proved the existence of a large endemic area of jungle yellow fever lying east of the river and north of Honda. Cases confirmed by autopsy or viscerotomy were found in 1933, 1934, 1935, 1936, and 1937. The identity of the disease in the Magdalena Valley and in the llanos has been amply established by clinical observation, autopsy, immunity tests, and isolation of the virus. The finding of one young immune in Quibdó suggests that the Pacific Coast of Colombia may not be entirely free of the yellow fever virus.

Venezuela (Area 15)

The principal Caribbean ports of Venezuela together with Ciudad Bolívar, the chief port of the Orinoco River, apparently formed part of the Caribbean maritime endemic region and have not had important outbreaks of yellow fever since the disease began to disappear from this region.

Yellow fever was last recognized in Venezuelan ports in 1914, when Puerto Cabello, La Guayra, and Ciudad Bolívar were infected. Maracaibo last reported the disease in 1911. Venezuela had long been considered free of yellow fever infection when, in 1929, a series of suspect cases were reported from the isolated towns about Guasipati and Tumeremo, well south of the Orinoco River, in the valley of the Cuyuni River. Autopsies were performed and positive diagnoses obtained from pathologists, but the epidemiology was not clear and the cases were always considered doubtful by the authorities. During the collection of specimens for the present study, it was learned that a few cases had been observed in the region of Carapito the diagnosis of which was not perfectly established. The examination of autopsy material collected a full 12 months previously at Quiriquire (1933) resulted in a confirmation of the diagnosis of yellow fever.

The protection test results for Venezuela are surprisingly negative in comparison with those from several other regions of South America with equally scant history of recent infection. These results do, however, permit the conclusion that the outbreak in the Cuyuni Valley was really yellow fever and that the source of infection could not have been the principal ports of the Orinoco River, as was at first suggested. The low percentage of positives found in the younger age groups in La Guayra, Caicara, Quiriquire, and San Fernando suggest that the virus of yellow fever in Venezuela is not limited to the Cuyuni Valley but, together with other negative results, must be accepted as strong evidence that outside of the Cuyuni Valley there have been no recent important outbreaks of *urban* yellow fever in Venezuela.

British Guiana, Dutch Guiana, and French Guiana (Area 16)

The principal ports of the Guianas apparently long formed part of the Caribbean region of yellow fever endemicity. The last report of recognized cases in Paramaribo and Cayenne was made in 1909, and suspect cases occurred in the same year in Georgetown. That this may not have been the last appearance of the infection however is indicated by the finding in 1934 of one immune of 15 years of age in Dutch Guiana, one of 21 years of age in British Guiana, and one of 24 years of age in French Guiana. This conclusion is borne out by the results of an independent immunity survey of Dutch Guiana by Kotter, who reports immunity in three immigrants who had been in the country only since 1912, 1913, and 1920 (!), respectively. However, the large number of negative results obtained by Kotter and in the present study indicate that there have been no important urban outbreaks of the disease in recent years. Further studies are indicated to determine the presence or absence of jungle yellow fever infection in the Guianas.

CONCLUSION

The immunity survey of South America shows that yellow fever continues endemic in vast areas of Brazil, Bolivia, Peru, Ecuador, Colombia, Paraguay, and Venezuela long considered free of the disease. Much of this endemicity depends upon the persistence of the disease in sparsely populated jungle districts where *Aëdes aegypti* does not exist. That the immunity found is not due to infection with mild attenuated strains of the virus is amply proved by the fatal cases confirmed by liver examination in all but a few of the Brazilian states, in Bolivia, in Paraguay, in Peru, in Venezuela, and in the Magdalena and Orinoco valleys of Colombia during the course of this survey. Concurrent studies have more than confirmed the results of the immunity survey and have revealed in a number of places jungle infection the existence of which was not suspected from the results of the immunity survey of the towns. The negative results for the Guianas should not be interpreted to mean that the virus of yellow fever is entirely absent from these colonies but only that the disease has not invaded the cities in recent years.

SUMMARY

1. The reported incidence of yellow fever is no safe index of its occurrence in endemic zones.

2. Although visible urban and maritime outbreaks may decline and even cease entirely for a time, there is a vast, previously silent reservoir of infection in the interior of South America.

3. Yellow fever infection due to *Aëdes aegypti* has been much more widespread in the interior of Northeast Brazil than was believed, even though this area had long been under special observation. Aegypti-transmitted fever in this area did not spontaneously disappear following the organization of anti-aegypti campaigns in the principal centers of population.

4. Yellow fever endemicity, instead of being limited to the coast of northeast Brazil as was believed, extends to all of Brazil except a few of the southern states, to Bolivia, Paraguay, Peru, Ecuador, Colombia, and Venezuela, involving many districts in which *A. aegypti* does not exist.

5. Widely varying percentages of immunes have been found in proved endemic regions, depending upon whether transmission is due to *A. aegypti* or occurs in the absence of this mosquito.

6. There is no evidence of recent yellow fever outbreaks in any of the important Pacific or Caribbean ports of South America.

Part V | The Discovery of Jungle Yellow Fever and
Studies of Its Epidemiology

Selection 19 | Yellow Fever Without *Aëdes aegypti*. Study of a Rural Epidemic in the Valle do Chanaan, Espirito Santo, Brazil, 1932*

F. L. SOPER, H. PENNA, E. CARDOSO,
J. SERAFIM, JR., M. FROBISHER, JR.,
AND J. PINHEIRO

Following the demonstration by the American Army Commission of the transmission of yellow fever by *Aëdes aegypti*, these investigators and other workers carried out a limited number of experiments in which other species of mosquitoes were tested as possible vectors of the disease. These experiments gave uniformly negative results. The necessity of using human volunteers in this early work prevented a thorough canvass of the field, and it was not until more than a quarter of a century later that successful inoculation of animals with yellow fever virus led to the testing of a number of different mosquitoes. Bauer and Philip in Africa and Davis and Shannon in South America have shown that several species of mosquitoes may transmit the virus from animal to animal in the laboratory and that other species not yet shown to transmit the virus may harbor it in a living state for a period equal to the usual incubation period in *A. aegypti*. Wide variations in facility and regularity of transmission have been reported for the different species studied.

Among epidemiologists and students of yellow fever the disease has long

* The studies and observations on which this paper is based were conducted by the Cooperative Yellow Fever Service maintained by the Brazilian Government and The Rockefeller Foundation, with the active participation of the Health Department of the State of Espírito Santo, Brazil, and the Yellow Fever Laboratory of The Rockefeller Foundation at Bahia, Brazil. Dr. Soper was the Representative in South America (Rio de Janeiro Office) of the International Health Division of The Rockefeller Foundation; Drs. Penna, Cardoso, Serafim, and Pinheiro were officials of the Cooperative Yellow Fever Service; and Dr. Frobisher was a staff member of the Foundation.

This excerpt is from the article *(15)* in the *American Journal of Hygiene 18:* 555–587, 1933. (Five tables and two maps have been omitted, but the original text is complete.)

been considered essentially an urban one, with aegypti necessary for its transmission in nature. The dramatic disappearance of yellow fever from all the notorious centers of distribution on the American continent, following the application of measures directed against the reproduction of aegypti, seemed to confirm the belief that this species was the only one of importance in the production of natural infection. Yellow fever has never failed to disappear from the morbidity and mortality records of cities and towns shortly after the reduction of aegypti breeding, and the absence of this species from a locality was often accepted as sufficient evidence that yellow fever did not exist there.

Beginning in April 1930, an attempt was made to determine the distribution of yellow fever in Brazil, through the routine histological examination of liver specimens from persons who had had fatal febrile infections of less than 10 days' duration. This attempt resulted in the diagnosis of yellow fever in certain isolated cases in rural areas where subsequent field investigations failed to reveal other cases of the disease, and suggested that aegypti probably could not have been responsible for transmission.

This report is devoted to a strictly rural epidemic of yellow fever, occurring in the Valle do Chanaan, Espírito Santo, Brazil, from January to April 1932, in which aegypti can be definitely ruled out as the vector. The results of epidemiological and entomological surveys of the Valle do Chanaan are herewith presented.

THE INFECTED AREA

The Valle do Chanaan (spelled Vale do Canaan in later papers) is a delightful and picturesque valley or group of valleys lying between the town of Santa Thereza and the Rio Doce, in the central part of the State of Espírito Santo. This state, one of the smallest in Brazil, has an area of about 45,000 square kilometers and an estimated population of only ½ million. It lies almost entirely between the eighteenth and twenty-first degrees of south latitude, on the Atlantic coast. Its location with regard to Rio de Janeiro and Salvador, State of Bahia, both of which were formerly important distributing points for yellow fever, is shown on Map 1. The bulk of the population is concentrated in the southern half of the state. The capital and principal seaport, Victoria, has a population of 40,000, and is a port of call for foreign ships from many nations engaged in the coffee trade, as well as for the vessels of several national lines engaged in coastwise freight and passenger service. The Leopoldina Railway links Victoria with Rio de Janeiro, which may be reached in 20 hours (Map 1). A second railway line, the Victoria and Minas Geraes, runs north and northwest from Victoria, striking the Rio Doce at Collatina and following the river for some distance into the State of Minas Geraes. The surface of the State of

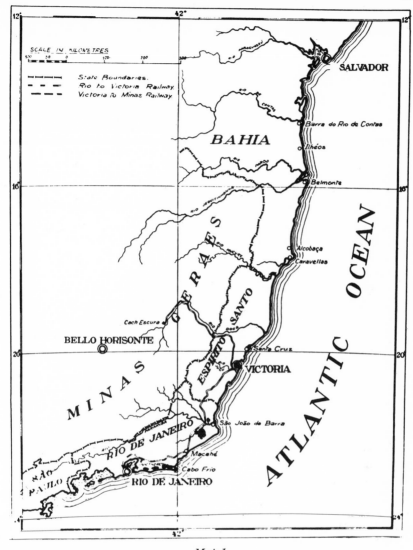

Map 1

Espírito Santo is very irregular, and some sections are mountainous, although no really high altitudes occur within the state.

The Valle do Chanaan (Map 3) is formed by the Rio Santa Maria do Rio
Doce and its tributaries, where a mountain range falls away from Santa
Thereza toward the Rio Doce. The most striking characteristics of this
area, immortalized for future generations of Brazilians by Graça Aranha in
the romance *Chanaan,* are the narrowness of its valleys and the steepness
of its slopes. The automobile highway connecting Victoria and Collatina

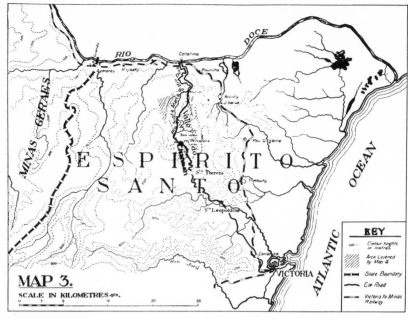

Map 3

climbs through Santa Thereza to strike the head of the valley at an altitude of over 700 meters. From this vantage point, the Valle do Chanaan is indeed striking, presenting a fairyland picture of steep green hillsides, and narrow well-watered valleys with homes scattered at short distances along the streams. The highway descends rapidly into the valley and traverses it at an average altitude of less than 200 meters above sea level. The numerous streams of the valley, although they usually descend over rocky beds, are occasionally flanked by small swamps of the type so often found in mountainous districts.

The official census of 1920 showed a population of 18,298 in the Municipo of Santa Thereza, which has a total area of approximately 793 square kilometers. A consideration of the resultant coefficient of 23 inhabitants per square kilometer does not convey an adequate idea of the density and distribution of the population in the Valle do Chanaan. This valley is a heavily populated rural area having no villages or towns of importance. The land is divided into relatively small holdings; and since practically all homes are built along the streams, the distance from any house to its nearest neighbor is seldom more than a few hundred meters. The area was colonized during the latter decades of the past century by Italian and German immigrants, and these stocks still predominate. The principal export crop of the region is coffee, in the care and gathering of which all members of the family generally participate. The only points of concentration of population in the valley are São João de Petropolis and Patrimonio de Santo Antonio, with about 50 houses each. The absence of towns has given rise to a system of names for different parts of the valley, which is very difficult for the newcomer and apparently somewhat uncertain for the native. A few places are referred to by the name of the patron saint of the local church, but the great majority take the name of nearby streams. At times a rather vague distinction is made between the mouth of the stream, the stream itself, and its headwaters. Considering the mountainous character of the country, this system often results in places hours apart by horseback travel being referred to by the same name. Off the main highway, travel is slow and difficult and is properly indulged in only on foot or on horseback.

HISTORY OF YELLOW FEVER IN ESPÍRITO SANTO

Considering its strategic position between Rio de Janeiro and Bahia, Espírito Santo could not but have a long and funereal yellow fever history during the period from 1849 to 1908, when the disease was endemic both to the north and to the south. With the development of European colonization, Victoria became notorious as a yellow fever center, and at least one foreign government took measures during the last decade of the nineteenth century to prevent emigration of its nationals to Espírito Santo. With the disappearance of yellow fever from southern Brazil following the early antimosquito campaigns, Victoria reported no cases of the disease for several years, but finally it suffered from a sharp outbreak during 1917 and 1918. Two suspected cases occurred in Santa Leopoldina in 1925, but these were not confirmed by the official investigation; and no yellow fever was reported for the entire state during 13 years (1919–1931). With the reappearance of yellow fever in 1928 in Rio de Janeiro, only 20 hours from Victoria either by boat or by rail, the State Health Department of Espírito Santo organized control measures and maintained them until April 1931, when the administration of the antimosquito service passed to the Cooperative Yellow Fever Service maintained by the National Department of Health and The Rockefeller Foundation. In December 1930, in preliminary discussions with one of us (F.L.S.) of the possible continued endemicity of yellow fever in Espírito Santo as an explanation of the failure of this state to produce visible autochthonous cases of the disease during the years 1928, 1929, 1930, and 1931, when it is known to have been present in the neighboring state of Rio de Janeiro, Dr. Alvaro Mello, Director of the State Health Service, mentioned the Municipio of Santa Thereza, of which the Valle do Chanaan is a part, as a suspected area. As a result of this discussion the attention of the Yellow Fever Service in Victoria was called to this county, but many months passed during which no suspicious cases were recorded. In January 1932, Dr. A. M. Walcott visited the State of Espírito Santo to organize the service for the routine collection of liver specimens from patients with fatal fever cases of short duration. In discussing the distribution of this special service, the object of which is the discovery of otherwise unknown foci of yellow fever, Dr. Mello again mentioned Santa Thereza as an area requiring investigation. Dr. Walcott visited the town of Santa Thereza, lying more than 600 meters above sea level, found no aegypti, and decided against installing a liver-collection service. Driving to the top of the pass beyond Santa Thereza he looked down upon the beauties of the Valle do Chanaan, hundreds of meters below, but, like Moses of old, who gazed upon but did not enter the Land of Canaan, Walcott turned back. Santa Thereza and the Valle do Chanaan were logically struck from the list of places needing further investigation. Subsequent events were to prove that yellow fever had been present in the Valle do Chanaan when this decision was made.

YELLOW FEVER IN THE VALLE DO CHANAAN

On March 3, 1932, Dr. Arnaldo de Andrade, representative of the State Health Service for Santa Thereza, reported a suspected case of yellow fever. This case proved fatal and an autopsy was performed by Dr. Andrade and Dr. Americo Oliveira. Examination of liver tissues by Drs. Amadeu Fialho and N. C. Davis resulted in a confirmation of the clinical diagnosis.

Field investigations, which were begun immediately, resulted in a second positive autopsy a few days after the first and in a third positive autopsy on March 26. The presence of yellow fever in the Valle do Chanaan was further demonstrated by the fact that Dr. Davis was able to establish the virus in *Macacus rhesus* at the Bahia Yellow Fever Laboratory, by the injection of serum from a patient in this area from whom a blood specimen was taken on April 3. The places where yellow fever was shown, by autopsy and by animal inoculation, to exist are widely separated. Actually, because of the difficulties of travel, these infected points are much more isolated than they would appear to be on a map.

Dr. Alvaro Mello, Director of the Health Department, installed hospital facilities in São João de Petropolis. Here Dr. Arnaldo de Andrade attempted to concentrate for study all acute febrile cases occurring in the valley. The authors are deeply indebted to these colleagues for their wholehearted cooperation, without which this study would have been most difficult. It soon became apparent that cases of typhoid and malaria were occurring in the region, as well as cases of yellow fever, which were few in number and widely scattered. Finally, on April 21, the São João Hospital was turned over to the Yellow Fever Service as a laboratory for carrying out transmission experiments.

Our earliest definite clue to the presence of yellow fever in the Valle do Chanaan was the report of three cases, one fatal, which had occurred in the 13 de Agosto Valley, with onset on January 19, 1932. The description of these cases given by the attending physician and by the surviving patients agrees with the classical picture of yellow fever. However, they could scarcely have been the original cases, since all the patients fell ill on the same day. Further evidence that these were not the first cases in the area is furnished by the second known fatal case, which occurred on February 1 in the 15 de Agosto Valley, at some distance from the first fatal case and without any apparent contact with this focus. A less convincing case of 8 days' duration in an employee 22 years of age, who had had no medical attention, was reported by a family in the 5 de Novembro Valley as dating back to the beginning of the summer, in November 1931. In the same month this family lost a 2-year-old child, but they were unable to supply satisfactory details of its illness.

Information was collected regarding a total of 83 suspected cases with 9 fatalities which occurred between January 15 and April 15, and which were scattered over an area of some 50 square kilometers. The epidemic was apparently on the decline when it was discovered, and only 21 cases, with 3 deaths, were observed after the appearance of the first suspected case. This apparent low mortality of yellow fever in a population predominantly white and largely composed of European stocks recently established in this area emphasizes the fact that other factors than race are important in determining susceptibility to yellow fever. It is believed that the number of deaths reported is close to the number actually caused by yellow fever, but it is hard to estimate the number of infections, since difficult travel conditions made repeated visits to suspected cases impossible. The time of onset of cases, by weeks, is shown in Table 2. In considering this information, it must be remembered that conclusions regarding happenings previous to the first week in March are based largely on information furnished by unskilled observers. With cases of typhoid and malaria both appearing in the infected area, it is probable that there are several errors in the data presented.

During the field investigation, various persons stated that this was not the first time that "black typhus" had been present in the Valle do Chanaan but that it appeared at intervals of several years, killing a few persons in the valley and then disappearing. The only definite reference to the previous existence of yellow fever in this region was made by a widow who said that her husband had died of the disease in 1911. One of her two children, who was reported to have had the disease at the same time, was found by the protection test to be immune to yellow fever.

Beginning May 1, 15 days after the appearance of the last observed case of suspected yellow fever, and continuing through the month of June, a

Table 2. Date of Onset of Suspected and Confirmed Cases of Yellow Fever
in the Valle do Chanaan, 1932[a]

	Date	Estimated week of epidemic	Known distribution	
			Cases	Deaths
Jan.	18–24	1	3	1
	25–31	2	0	0
Feb.	1– 7	3	3	1
	8–14	4	5	2
	15–21	5	5	0
	22–28	6	12	1
	29–Mar. 6	7	18	2
Mar.	7–13	8	5	0
	14–20	9	1	0
	21–27	10	4	1
	28–Apr. 3	11	4	0
Apr.	4–10	12	4	0
	11–17	13	2	0
	18–24	14	0	0
	Subtotal	—	66	8
Undated cases previous to				
	March 6	—	17	1
	Total	—	83	9

[a]The data in this table are a summary of those in Table 1, which has been omitted.
Ed.

house-to-house census was carried out, in various parts of the Valle do
Chanaan. During this census, 582 blood specimens were secured from
among 3262 persons residing in 496 houses situated in what may be termed
the suspected area. These specimens were distributed as follows:

1. Four hundred and twelve routine specimens from among 618 persons
living in the first 87 houses visited in the rural areas north and east of São
João de Petropolis, listed under "Routine bleeding" in Table 3.

2. One hundred and sixty-eight specimens from São João de Petropolis,
Patrimonio de Santo Antonio, Pé da Serra, and an area lying south and
east of Dona Marta, and including sections of 15 de Agosto, 13 de Agosto,
and 25 de Julho, listed under "Selective bleeding" in Table 4. The samples
in this group were limited to not more than two from any family, and were
from persons native to the Valle do Chanaan.

As a control on specimens collected from the suspected area, 68 samples,
representing 41 families, were secured from persons born in the zone called
São Jacyntho, lying just outside the known infected zone and close to Mutum, the nearest known source of *A. aegypti*. The results of tests on these
specimens are not significantly different from those in the known infected
area, 13 de Agosto, 15 de Agosto, and 25 de Julho, and they are included

Table 3. Result of Mouse-Protection Test by Age of Donor of Serum and Place of Residence in Valle do Chanaan

Routine Bleeding

Age group (years)	Pagani		P. Pretti and Sta. Maria		S. Bôa Vista, São Bento, São Roque		Dona Marta		Total		
	No. of sera tested	No. of sera protecting	No. of sera tested	No. of sera protecting	No. of sera tested	No. of sera protecting	No. of sera tested	No. of sera protecting	No. of sera tested	No. of sera protecting	Percentage of sera protecting
0– 9	17	1	13	0	28	1	4	0	62	2	3.2 ± 1.5
10–19	16	1	43	0	45	9	17	0	121	10	8.3 ± 1.7
20–29	19	1	32	4	49	10	15	2	115	17	14.8 ± 2.2
30–39	12	4	16	3	32	10	9	0	69	17	24.6 ± 3.5
40 and over	10	3	16	7	9	1	10	5	45	16	35.6 ± 4.8
Total	74	10	120	14	163	31	55	7	412	62	15.0 ± 1.2
Percentage of sera protecting	13.5 ± 2.7		11.7 ± 2.0		19.0 ± 2.1		12.7 ± 3.0		15.0 ± 1.2		

Table 4. Results of Mouse-Protection Test by Age of Donor of Serum and Place of Residence in Valle do Chanaan

Selective Bleeding (see text)

Age group (years)	Pé da Serra		Patrimonio de Santo Antonio		São João de Petropolis		São Jacyntho		13 de Agosto, 14 de Agosto, 25 de Julho		Total		
	No. of sera tested	No. of sera pro-tecting	No. of sera tested	No. of sera pro-tecting	No. of sera tested	No. of sera pro-tecting	No. of sera tested	No. of sera pro-tecting	No. of sera tested	No. of sera pro-tecting	No. of sera tested	No. of sera pro-tecting	Percentage of sera protecting
0– 9	9	0	15	0	13	0	23	3	15	0	75	3	4.0 ± 1.5
10–19	6	0	14	0	12	0	21	0	21	1	74	1	1.4 ± 0.9
20–29	7	0	9	0	7	0	15	1	8	1	46	2	4.3 ± 2.0
30–39	4	0	6	1	5	1	7	0	7	1	29	3	10.3 ± 3.8
40 and over	1	0	2	0	3	3	2	1	4	1	12	5	14.2 ± 6.8
Total	27	0	46	1	40	4	68	5	55	4	236	14	5.9 ± 1.0
Percentage of sera protecting	0		2.2 ± 1.5		10.0 ± 3.2		7.4 ± 2.1		7.3 ± 2.4		5.9 ± 1.0		

in Table 4 under "Selective bleeding," together with results for specimens selected in the same manner in the infected area.

The occurrence of a fatal autopsied case in a man 72 years of age, a resident in the Valle do Chanaan for 45 years, suggested that this area was not highly immunized. The results of mouse protection tests in the valley showed a surprisingly low percentage of immune persons, considering the wide geographical distribution of immunity and the fact that the disease apparently disappeared spontaneously. (All protection tests reported in the present study were made by Dr. Henrique Penna at the Yellow Fever Laboratory of The Rockefeller Foundation, in Bahia.) This situation might well have been due to transmission by some insect vector showing high efficiency in the laboratory but low efficiency in nature because of non-domestic habits, and consequently less contact with the human host than *A. aegypti* has. The very small percentage of immune persons found in the age group 10 years and under and the absence of cases in the small hamlets of São João de Petropolis and Patrimonio de Santo Antonio are both possible of explanation on the basis of field transmission. On the other hand, the age distribution of positives might be interpreted as a result of repeated visits of the disease with a small number of cases during each invasion. Such repeated invasions with few cases would, in the course of time, build up higher percentages of immunity in the older age groups. This fact seems to be confirmed by the study by age groups of the history of suspected illness among positives who probably acquired their immunity in the Valle do Chanaan. This study shows a much higher percentage of young than of old positives, among those having a history of recent attack.

ENTOMOLOGICAL INVESTIGATIONS

Inspectors sent to the area immediately upon the report that yellow fever existed there failed to find *Aëdes aegypti* breeding in the Valle do Chanaan or in the town of Santa Thereza. (Among the first foci collected in São João de Petropolis, one contained larvae classified as *A. aegypti* by Dr. A. Lutz. Most careful search failed to reveal other foci of the same mosquito. It is not known whether this focus represented an accidental one brought in from nearby points where *A. aegypti* is common or was really from some other place and forwarded in a mislabeled container.) Detailed studies carried out during many weeks by highly trained workers failed to reveal larvae or adults of this mosquito. Nearby towns showed high indices of aegypti breeding but no recognized cases of yellow fever. The comparative findings regarding the prevalence of aegypti on first inspection, for different points in the Valle do Chanaan and for nearby apparently uninfected towns, are given in Table 6 [omitted]. This table, in the absence of positive autopsies and transfer of virus to rhesus monkeys must have resulted in the denial of the existence of yellow fever in the Valle do Chanaan.

The absence of aegypti from the Valle do Chanaan probably depends on several factors, among which may be mentioned (1) the small number of water containers inside the houses, as a result of the location of practically all homes on the banks of small mountain streams or rivers, which obviates entirely the necessity of storing water for domestic purposes; (2) the almost complete absence of artificial water containers outside the homes; and (3) the relatively brusque changes in meteorological conditions, probably the result not so much of the altitude of the valley as of its formation and its relationship to the surrounding mountains. Unfortunately, adequate meteorological data are not available. The limited observations made during the present study at São João de Petropolis were begun only after the epidemic was over. That weather conditions can change rapidly here is well shown by the data for June 4: temperature, maximum 40°C, minimum 15°C; relative humidity, maximum 94 per cent, minimum 42 per cent. That the area is not suitable for aegypti breeding is emphasized by the low percentage of houses (3.2) with larvae of this species in Mutum, the nearest point where larvae were found.

Early attempts to determine the common mosquitoes of this area by the capture of adults inside the houses at various hours of the day and night were almost fruitless. Occasionally one to four mosquitoes might be found in a house, but at no time during the present studies were appreciable numbers of any species of mosquito captured inside houses. The first reaction to this failure to find mosquitoes in the houses was to hypothesize transmission by some blood-sucking parasite other than the mosquito. Search of houses for such insects, however, failed to produce suggestive results, except that the possibility of the implication of *Phlebotomus* spp. was presented. Triatoma, bedbugs, fleas, and ticks were not commonly found during the months of this study.* Accidental transmission through parasites of domestic animals seems impossible, since the number of such animals is small.

Only when adult mosquito captures were undertaken with animal bait outside of, but close to, houses, did the wealth of mosquito life become apparent. The number of mosquitoes of different species found outside the houses proved to be in marked contrast to the scarcity of mosquito life in the houses. During March, April, and May extensive adult captures at all hours of the day and night, supplemented by the collection of larvae and the identification of foci, were made at 11 points where local transmis-

---

* N. C. Davis has recently reported extensive transmission experiments with *Argas persicus* (Oken) , *Amblyomma cajennense* (Fabricius) , *Rhipicephalus sanguineus* (Latreille) , and *Boophilus mircoplus* (Canestrini) with negative results by bite and by injection of eggs of infected females. The virus was shown to survive for periods of 6 to 28 days in individuals of the various species studied. H. Aragão subsequently reported transmission with *Amblyomma cajennense* (Fabricius) by bite and (personal communication) by emulsion of eggs from infected females.

sion of yellow fever had almost certainly occurred. As a control on this work, less exhaustive investigations were made at 21 other houses, most of which had produced suspected cases of yellow fever. These investigations failed to produce any adults or larvae of aegypti. The following species of mosquitoes and *Phlebotomus* spp.* were captured or identified from larvae secured in the Valle do Chanaan:

Aëdes scapularis, fluviatilis, serratus, terrens, fulvus, jacobinae, leucoce-laenus, rhyacophilus, sp. n. to be described by Dr. A. da Costa Lima
Mansonia titillans, juxtamansonia, chrysonotum, albicosta, fasciolata, indubitans
Microculex imitator, pleuristriatus, and unidentified species
Culex corniger, nigripalpus, conservator, surinamensis, coronator (Moch-lostyrax) various species, *(Melanoconion)* various species, and other unidentified species
Anopheles tarsimaculatus, argyritarsis, albitarsis, bachmanni, darlingi, brasiliensis, fluminensis, intermedius, maculipes, minor, (Kertezia) cruzii, (Chagasia) fajardoi
Psorophora cingulata, ciliata, cilipes, ferox, lutzii
Wyeomyia oblita, bromeliarum, tripartita, pallidoventer, unidentified species
Dendromyia personata, melanoides, mystes, unidentified species
Megarhinus violaceus, fluminensis
Uranotenia geometrica, lowii, pulcherrima
Joblotia digitata
Haemagogus equinus
Limatus durhami
Isostomyia, unidentified species
Miamyia, unidentified species
Sabethoides, unidentified species
Phlebotomus intermedius, fischerii, migonei

Although the insect fauna collected was extensive, additional species should be encountered in surveys conducted earlier in the summer, when the temperature is higher and the rainfall heavier.

In view of the work that had already been done on transmission with various species of mosquitoes in the laboratory, the following species were chosen from among those captured, for further consideration as possible vectors in the 1932 outbreak in the Valle do Chanaan: *Aëdes fluviatilis, A. scapularis, A. serratus, A. terrens, Mansonia* (all species), *Psorophora* (all species), and *Phlebotomus* (all species). *Phlebotomus* was included in the

* The authors are indebted to Drs. A. Lutz, A. da Costa Lima, and N. C. Davis for valuable assistance in identifying insects from the Valle do Chanaan.

list because no work had been reported on this insect. The comparative incidence of adults and of larvae of the above-mentioned species, found at 11 points where there is reasonable certainty that local transmission of yellow fever occurred, suggests that *A. scapularis* may well have been the vector during the outbreak studied. *A. scapularis* was found at all 11 places, *A. fluviatilis* at 5, *A. serratus* and *A. terrens* at 1 place each, *Mansonia* (all species) at 8 places, *Phlebotomus* (all species) at 6 places, and *Psorophora* (all species) at 3 places. Adult captures with animal bait at these eleven points included 224 *A. scapularis,* 12 *A. fluviatilis,* 652 *Mansonia* spp., 1486 *Phlebotomus* spp., and 12 *Psorophora* spp. However, uncommonly swampy conditions existed at one place of capture (No. 11), and repeated catches were made here to secure *Phlebotomus* spp. for transmission experiments. Leaving out the figures for No. 11, the totals for adult captures become *A. scapularis* 208, *Mansonia* 176, and *Phlebotomus* spp. 210. *A. scapularis* proved to be a ready and vicious biter, especially so from 5:00 to 10:00 P.M. and 4:00 to 7:00 A.M.

In many families reporting suspected cases of yellow fever during the present epidemic, apparently only one, or, at most, two individuals had attacks. The one outstanding exception to this general rule was the Vago family, living on the Serra da Bôa Vista, which reported 7 cases with 3 deaths during January and February. Special studies made about this home to determine, if possible, wherein its mosquito fauna might differ from that of other parts of the infected area, were rewarded by the discovery of millions of larvae and pupae of *A. scapularis* in a nearby swampy depression. (Eight hundred larvae and pupae of *A. scapularis* were counted in 100 cc of water dipped from this swamp.) No other focus of similar extent and productivity was found in the entire region during the present study.

Transmission experiments were attempted by Dr. Martin Frobisher, Jr., with *Phlebotomus* spp. that had been captured both inside and outside the houses, but great difficulty was encountered in maintaining these insects alive in the laboratory and in inducing them to feed a second time. A few unsuccessful attempts were made to infect monkeys directly with mosquitoes of various species captured at points where cases of yellow fever had recently occurred.

DISCUSSION

The events leading to the discovery of yellow fever in the Municipio of Santa Thereza in 1932 are almost dramatic in their sequence: the suggestion of the Health Director for the State, in 1930, that this municipio be investigated for the presence of the disease, although he was unable to adduce any concrete basis for such suggestion; the reiteration of this suggestion a year later, when the liver-collection service was being organized; the visit of an experienced field investigator to this municipio and his decision to exclude it from the liver-collection program as "unlikely yellow fever territory"; the declaration of suspected cases; the confirmation of these cases by autopsy and infection of rhesus monkeys.

The discovery of yellow fever in the Valle do Chanaan was to a large extent fortuitous. The local health officer had seen yellow fever during the Rio de Janeiro epidemic of 1928–1929 and was familiar with the typical mild cases as well as with the classical picture presented by medical textbooks. Fortunately, he did not know that *Aëdes aegypti* was not prevalent in the Valle do Chanaan. Had the confirmation by autopsy been limited to a single case, certain doubts must have remained in the minds of most students of the disease; but three clinically typical cases at widely separated points, all positive by microscopical examination, can leave no reasonable doubt of the diagnosis of yellow fever. Moreover, additional confirmation exists in the reproduction of the disease, with typical lesions of yellow fever, in rhesus monkeys, with blood drawn from a patient with a suspected case on the second day of illness.

Had a report of yellow fever, even though supported by pathological diagnosis based on microscopical examination of tissues, been made under similar conditions, previous to the laboratory studies consequent to the establishing of the virus of yellow fever in laboratory animals, it would have been indeed difficult to find any yellow fever epidemiologist willing to accept the possibility of an outbreak of yellow fever in the Valle do Chanaan. Yellow fever was believed to be an urban disease which was transmitted by aegypti and was expected to obey the epidemiological rules based on this belief. Even with the mental preparation for rural yellow fever provided by the knowledge that nondomestic species of mosquitoes had proved to be efficient vectors of the virus in the laboratory, the writers found difficulty at first in accepting the diagnosis of yellow fever in the Valle do Chanaan. The failure to find aegypti in the zone producing suspected cases; the wide scattering of relatively few cases over a large rural area; the absence of suspected cases from the small hamlets in the Valle do Chanaan; the failure to find cases in towns in the surrounding area with high indices of aegypti breeding, even after the alarm had been given; and the concurrent appearance of cases of both malaria and typhoid in the Valle do Chanaan were all factors which made the epidemiological diagnosis of yellow fever difficult. Although typical clinical cases of yellow fever were observed, any epidemiological investigation unsupported by laboratory methods must have failed to convince investigators that yellow fever was present in the infected area.

There are various indications, including the definite report of a death from this disease, that yellow fever had visited the Valle do Chanaan previously, although absolute proof is, of course, lacking. The age distribution of immunity, as shown by the protection test, tends to confirm this belief, although it might be argued that those of the older age groups had naturally, in the past, had more opportunity for casual infection outside this area. In any case, the percentage of immune persons found was surprisingly low, considering the distribution of the epidemic and the length of time it was known to have lasted.

It is frankly admitted that the vector or vectors of yellow fever in the Valle do Chanaan have not been established. The epidemiological findings suggest that the guilty vector or vectors are not house-limited mosquitoes. The evidence points rather to infections occurring in the field, and to the possible transfer of infection from one house to another by the vector, as well as by the human host. The presence of *Phlebotomus* spp. inside the houses as well as outside is significant in the absence of other insects, and studies of the possible role of these insects as vectors are needed. The low percentage of immune persons disclosed by mouse-protection tests indicates, we believe, that yellow fever disappears through failure of the insect host rather than through failure of the human host. This failure of the insect host was probably due to changes in meteorological conditions affecting either its breeding, its flight range and activity, or the length of time necessary for the development of infectivity.

The most logical explanation which can now be given of the epidemiology of yellow fever in the Valle do Chanaan is that the virus of yellow fever is from time to time introduced from nearby silent endemic areas where aegypti is present. Once introduced, the disease is transmitted by some relatively inefficient but widespread vector.

Another possible hypothesis, which must be considered in the future, is that there may be some long-lived, relatively inefficient vector, possibly seasonal in its activity, capable of transmitting yellow fever. The existence of such a vector would give a satisfactory explanation for continued suspicion of this area and would also account for the appearance of apparently isolated cases in other areas, not satisfactorily explained on the hypothesis of mosquito transmission. It should be remembered that the State Health Department had vague suspicions regarding yellow fever in this area more than a year before the appearance of the first case now definitely considered to have been yellow fever. The intervening winter temperatures of the Valle do Chanaan are believed to be sufficiently low to have prevented the persistence of the virus in this area on the basis of mosquito transmission.

In considering the role of the insect vector in the epidemiology of yellow fever, it must be remembered that in the laboratory wide variations have been found in the ability of different species to transmit the disease. Certain species, the outstanding example of which is aegypti, seem to show a high percentage of exposed mosquitoes infective after an incubation period of 10 to 12 days at ordinary tropical temperatures. Apparently, some species are less efficient as vectors, only a small percentage of the mosquitoes effecting transmission. Other species apparently require a longer period of incubation before becoming infective, and still others have not been tested because of their refusal to take repeated feedings in the laboratory. In considering any insect as a possible vector of yellow fever, thought must be given to its breeding and feeding habits as well as to its actual ability to transmit the disease in the laboratory. From a consideration of published laboratory experiments on the ability of various species of mosquitoes to transmit yellow fever, and of the results of adult captures and larval collections at many points in the Valle do Chanaan, it is believed that *A. scapularis* was the most probable vector among the various mosquitoes captured and studied. This mosquito was widespread and proved to be a vicious biter. However, the possibility that *A. fluviatilis* may have been in part responsible, cannot be entirely discounted, since it is apparently a more efficient vector in the laboratory than is *A. scapularis.* Many parts of the Valle do Chanaan possess suitable natural breeding places for *A. fluviatilis,* although but few adults were captured with animal bait. The finding of this species in ant rings indicates that it may be a facultative artificial deposit breeder.

Various species of *Anopheles* and *Culex* were found in abundance in the Valle do Chanaan, but they were not given serious consideration as possible vectors, since all previously published reports indicated that species of these genera had not been incriminated. Kerr has recently shown that *Culex thalassius* may become infective after an incubation period of more than double the usual period required by *Aëdes aegypti.** However, any factor which prolongs the period of incubation in the insect host, will, of necessity, greatly reduce the efficiency of that host as a vector, since the mortality of mosquitoes in nature is known to be very high.

In considering the possibility of intermediate vectors, other than mosquitoes, only *Phlebotomus* spp. were found in sufficient numbers and so distributed as to be open to suspicion. Further laboratory tests are needed to determine the relationship of this insect to yellow fever transmission.

As a result of the observations in the Valle do Chanaan, certain conceptions of the epidemiology of yellow fever will have to be revised. Natural infections are not always acquired by the bite of an infected aegypti, and it has been shown that a local epidemic of several months' duration may be

---

* N. C. Davis has recently succeeded in transmitting yellow fever by the bite of *Culex (Culex) quinquefasciatus* (Say) and *Psorophora (Janthinosoma) ferox* (Humboldt). (Unpublished communication.) [The disappearance of yellow fever from urban communities that were freed of *A. aegypti,* while *C. quinquefasciatus* remained in undiminished numbers, indicates strongly—even if it does not prove— that *C. quinquefasciatus* is not able to maintain yellow fever virus in man in the absence of *A. aegypti. Ed.*]

maintained without the intervention of this species. Yellow fever is not necessarily an urban disease. Villages whose populations are largely non-immune may have no outbreaks of the disease, although situated in infected rural areas. Yellow fever is not necessarily a house disease, nor is it necessarily transmitted by house mosquitoes. It may persist in a rural community for months and disappear spontaneously, through some failure of the intermediate host, leaving a large percentage of the local population nonimmune. Although spontaneous disappearance apparently occurred in the Valle do Chanaan, it has been shown that an entirely rural epidemic, not transmitted by aegypti, did maintain itself for at least 3 months; therefore the possibility of regional rural endemicity must be considered. It must also be emphasized that this slowly burning rural epidemic disappeared spontaneously through no failure of the human host. How long an epidemic of this type may maintain itself under more favorable meteorological conditions cannot be stated. The possibility of a long-continued rural regional endemicity, more or less independent of movement of population, must not be overlooked in the future. One of the most surprising findings of the present study is the low percentage of positive protection tests in combination with the widespread dissemination of the disease. May it not be possible that a slowly burning epidemic of this type is more serious from the standpoint of final elimination of yellow fever from an area than is the rapidly explosive type, which burns itself out quickly and disappears from failure of the human host?

The finding of yellow fever without aegypti comes as a distinct disappointment to those workers who, in the face of repeated laboratory demonstrations of the infectibility of other species, took consolation in the words of Carter. After admitting the possibility of other vectors being found for yellow fever, Carter stated: "Owing to the invariable disappearance of yellow fever when this species (*Aëdes aegypti*)—and this species alone—is sufficiently controlled, it seems quite certain that in the Americas no other mosquito associated closely with man is a vector."

But, in the case of a widespread rural epidemic in which the transmitting agent is not a house mosquito breeding in artificial containers, the accepted methods of yellow fever prophylaxis, so universally and so dramatically successful for three decades, are not applicable. Possibly other methods, similar to those already used in combating malaria, may be adapted to the control of the rural vectors of yellow fever, once these have been identified and their habits studied. Should further investigation reveal large rural endemic areas, little hope is entertained for the development of economically feasible prophylactic methods.

From the point of view of the general problem of yellow fever control, it is impossible to estimate the importance of the present findings. Generalizations must be very guarded, because the conditions in the Valle do

Chanaan are believed to be exceptional, at least, for the yellow fever zone in Brazil. This epidemic was apparently self-limited, and it is possible that there are no rural regions in America which are truly endemic for yellow fever. Future studies of the distribution of yellow fever should include entomological surveys and protection tests with the sera of persons born and residing constantly in rural areas, as well as routine examination of liver tissue from all persons dying in suspected areas after a fever of short duration.

Summary and Conclusions

Yellow fever was discovered in the Valle do Chanaan, Municipio of Santa Thereza, Espírito Santo, Brazil, early in March 1932. This finding was confirmed by examination of tissues from three persons dying of the disease, and by infection of a rhesus monkey (*Macaca mulata*) with blood from an early case. Field studies indicated that

1. Yellow fever was, during at least 3 months, widespread in a strictly rural district in which *Aëdes aegypti* was not found, even after a thorough and prolonged search begun 6 weeks before the apparently spontaneous disappearance of the disease from this district.

2. Of the species of mosquito incriminated by laboratory experiments as potential vectors of the yellow fever virus, only *Aëdes (Ochlerotatus) scapularis,* Rondani, and *Aëdes (Taeniorhynchus) fluviatilis,* Lutz, exist throughout the infected area in sufficient numbers to merit consideration as being possibly responsible for the epidemic. Of these, *A. scapularis* was found much more frequently, both as larva and as adult, and is believed to be the more dangerous species.

3. Despite this epidemic and despite rumors of previous invasions of yellow fever in the Valle do Chanaan, immunity to the disease, as indicated by the mouse-protection test on sera from several hundred residents, widely disseminated geographically, was limited to a surprisingly low percentage of those tested. On the basis of this low percentage of immune persons, the spontaneous disappearance of yellow fever in this area is attributed to inefficiency of the insect vector rather than to failure of the human host.

| Report on the Problem of Yellow
Fever in South America*

In 1930 it was already known that several mosquitoes other than *Aëdes aegypti* could transmit the virus of yellow fever from animal to animal in the laboratory. However, it was not until March 1932 that yellow fever was proved to exist under such conditions that *Aëdes aegypti* could be eliminated from consideration as the vector. The first recorded outbreak of yellow fever without aegypti occurred in the Valle de Canaan, Espírito Santo, Brazil, and was apparently limited during a period of 4 or 5 months to the strictly rural parts of this beautiful, productive, and densely populated valley. No evidence of cases occurring in the villages of this valley was obtained. The identity of the disease was established by clinical observation, by autopsy, by the protection test, and by the reproduction of the disease in Indian monkeys inoculated with the blood of an early case.

That the Amazon Valley might not be so innocent of yellow fever as its record of the past 20 years had led the whole world to believe was first suggested by the absence of reported cases in the native population of Pará in 1929, at which time cases were occurring among residents of foreign birth. Positive protection test results on children living at widely separated points in the Amazon Valley in Brazil and Peru gave additional weight to this suggestion in 1931. Rude confirmation came in March 1932 with the entirely unforeseen outbreak of the disease in Santa Cruz de la Sierra, Bolivia, a town of some 20,000 inhabitants, lying well toward the periphery of the Amazon Valley. Had further proof been required of the fallacy of the key-center theory of the maintenance of yellow fever endemicity in South America, the evidence given by the outbreak in Santa Cruz, hundreds of leagues from all known recent foci of the disease, would have been conclusive.

Studies in Bolivia have resulted in the proof of the previous existence of the disease at other towns in Bolivia where its presence had not been observed clinically, and have given added weight to the suggestion that the Santa Cruz outbreak was the result of Amazon Valley endemicity. These studies also resulted in the second observation, confirmed by clinical histories, by protection test, and by histological examination of liver tissue,

* Dr. Soper presented this report to the IXth Pan American Sanitary Conference, Buenos Aires, Argentina, November 14, 1934, at a time when "jungle yellow fever" had not yet been named. He attended the Conference as a specially invited Representative of The Rockefeller Foundation.

The text herewith is a translation of pages 99–105 of the *Actas* of the Conference (published only in Spanish) by the Pan American Sanitary Bureau (*19*).

of yellow fever existing in the absence of aegypti. The small village of San Ramón, with a population of only 125 persons, presenting conditions quite different from those in the Valle de Canaan, apparently maintained the virus of yellow fever over a period of many months in the complete absence of aegypti. The San Ramón outbreak of yellow fever was quite important in suggesting that Amazon Valley endemicity may be independent of and much more extensive than the distribution of aegypti.

Further surveys for determining the distribution of immunity to yellow fever through the protection test in the Amazon regions of Brazil, Peru, and Colombia, during 1932, 1933, and 1934, have given further confirmation of the existence of acquired immunity to yellow fever among children at practically all points investigated. The Viscerotomy Service has during the last year furnished livers, on which positive diagnoses of yellow fever have been made by competent pathologists, from Rio Branco, Acre; from Lauro Sodré, close to Leticia; from Fonte Bôa, between Leticia and Manáos; and from São Sebastião, on the Ilha Marajó, Pará. These cases have been uncovered in the complete absence of declared suspect cases of yellow fever. Apparently, we are just beginning to uncover the story of yellow fever in the Amazon Valley. Careful investigation has shown that the cases found at Lauro Sodré and São Sebastião occurred among families scattered along the river bank at some distance from any town or village and in complete absence of aegypti.

Strange and unforeseen as were some of the facts regarding yellow fever in the Amazon Valley, noted above, the climax of the unexpected in the epidemiology of this disease was reached in April of this year when an unusual, rapidly fatal disease attacking by preference adult field laborers in a very sparsely populated rural district at Coronel Ponce, 180 kilometers from Cuyabá, the capital of Matto Grosso State, Brazil, was shown by autopsy and protection test to be yellow fever. The known infected area lies just on the divide between the Amazon Valley and the River Plate Valley, and is quite free of aegypti. That the virus was probably not introduced into this rural area from silent foci of the disease in the three nearest towns of any size is indicated by the absence of positive protection tests on children in Cuyabá, Poxoréu, and Lageado.

The rural population is so small in number and so widely scattered that it is difficult for those who have visited the area to believe that some vertebrate host other than man is not involved. Coronel Ponce is so isolated from other known foci of yellow fever that no reasonable explanation of the source of the infection has yet been found by the investigations now in progress in Matto Grosso.

The behavior of yellow fever in Colombia during the past few years has been no less interesting and intriguing than in Brazil and Bolivia. The 1929 outbreak in Socorro, which followed a period of 6 years during which no cases of yellow fever were known to have occurred in the country, called attention to the probable persistence of the virus in Colombia. Although the Socorro outbreak occurred in the presence of abundant aegypti, protection test studies failed to indicate that the infection of Socorro had come from other urban centers in the Magdalena Valley, where this mosquito abounds, nor was any evidence found that yellow fever had been present in recent years in the river ports.

Protection test studies in 1931 and 1932 did, however, confirm the rumor, often started by the laity and as often denied by the yellow fever experts sent to investigate, of the existence of yellow fever in the region of the famous emerald mines at Muzo, Colombia. As far as can be ascertained, aegypti do not exist in this region at the present time, but clinical cases of yellow fever have been reported at short intervals over a period of many years. Protection tests revealed immunity in convalescent cases and later in a high percentage of routine blood samples on children living in the rural areas of Muzo. Positive autopsies were secured in 1934, but the mode of transmission and the apparently perennial source of the virus have not been discovered. Considering the sparseness of population and the comparative isolation of this region, it seems impossible that such a short-lived vector as the mosquito should be capable of maintaining the infection year after year. During 1933 an outbreak of yellow fever was confirmed by autopsy in the County of Caparrapí, not far from Muzo. This outbreak was strangely similar to that in Matto Grosso, Brazil, in that reported cases occurred only in rural field laborers and in the absence of aegypti. As in Matto Grosso, the people themselves were convinced that the disease was contracted in the fields.

In September 1934, just 2 months ago, a rural epidemic, clinically resembling yellow fever and with a high mortality, was reported from Restrepo, close to Villavicencio, Colombia. Field investigation has resulted in the full confirmation of the diagnosis of yellow fever by repeated autopsies and by positive protection tests. This outbreak is important since it is rural in character, has attacked mostly field workers in an area where aegypti do not exist, and is topographically very isolated from all other known foci of the disease. Restrepo lies on the eastern slope of the Andes, in the valley of the Meta River, a tributary of the Orinoco River, and is separated from Muzo and the Magdalena Valley by the high Andes.

The health authorities of American ports were alarmed by the report of suspect cases at Santa Marta, Colombia, in 1930, and at Guayaquil, Ecuador, in December 1932 and April 1933. Careful investigation of the Santa Marta situation failed to convince the investigators that they were dealing with yellow fever, and protection tests on children showed that the disease had not been widespread in this area in recent years. The situation in Ecuador is still under investigation but final negative conclusions are anticipated. Although both of the initial suspect cases were autopsied, conclusions could not be drawn, since various competent pathologists, to whom the tissues were submitted, failed to agree on a diagnosis. Studies in Ecuador during the past 15 months have resulted in the collection of further tissues on which pathological agreement cannot be obtained. Protection tests, however, on a large number of children from various points have been uniformly negative, and no explosions of the disease are known to have occurred in towns from which suspect livers have been received, although these towns have high aegypti indices and a nonimmune child population. Clinical histories have not been conclusive but have brought out the interesting fact that all but one of the various suspect cases reported had been given anthelmintic treatment shortly before death. Studies are being continued on the Pacific Coast which may well result in the conclusion that this area is probably free of yellow fever at the present time.

During the 5-year period under discussion, the presence of yellow fever in epidemic form has not been confirmed for any important port on the American continent, nor has any evidence of international exchange of yellow fever virus been found.

Urban yellow fever transmitted by aegypti has apparently declined rapidly and no outbreaks in towns of over 3000 population have been recorded during the past 2 years on the American continent.

On the other hand, we are forced to admit that in spite of the enormous amount of work which has been done in yellow fever control in the past the disease still exists, as detailed above, in the rural areas of Northeast Brazil, in various widely separated points in the Amazon Valley, in the Magdalena Valley, and in the Orinoco Valley in Colombia. Furthermore, we must admit that the factors responsible for persistent endemicity of rural and sparsely populated areas are unknown. Likewise, methods of control applicable to areas where aegypti is not the responsible vector have not been devised.

Today all responsible health authorities on the American continent in the areas possibly exposed to yellow fever infection should be familiar with the following facts:

1. Antimosquito measures directed principally against the aquatic forms of *Aëdes aegypti* are effective in the elimination of and prevention of urban outbreaks of yellow fever.

2. Although urban yellow fever does not long continue in the face of effective antilarval measures, the cleaning of urban centers does not necessarily result in the disappearance of the disease from tributary areas.

3. Yellow fever may persist for relatively long periods of time in areas distant from any large centers of population which might serve as constant sources of the virus.

4. Yellow fever may occur in nature in rural areas either associated with *A. aegypti* or in the absence of this mosquito.

5. Rural areas may be infected with yellow fever without any evidence

of the disease having originated in or passed through nearby towns and cities, even though such towns and cities have a high aegypti index and a large nonimmune population.

6. Yellow fever may occur in very sparsely inhabited regions where aegypti are not found and where the number of people is so small as to emphasize the need of a full investigation of the possibility of vertebrate hosts other than man. Cases have been observed under conditions suggesting that they might be accidental occasional cases occurring in the course of an epizootic somewhat as human cases of plague occur accidentally in the course of epizootics of this disease.

7. Yellow fever may recur at irregular intervals over a period of years in a relatively sparsely populated area under conditions suggesting the existence of long-lived vectors other than mosquitoes.

8. The absence of reported clinical cases in either towns or rural areas, even though the reporting be honestly done, does not necessarily indicate the absence of yellow fever nor even the absence of fatal cases of yellow fever.

9. Although the percentage of severe and fatal cases in the native population of endemic areas may be small, observation indicates that the existence of yellow fever in a community over a period of months will generally result in some fatal infections, which can be revealed by the routine examination of liver tissue from all rapidly fatal febrile cases.

10. The presence or absence of yellow fever in suspect areas can best be studied by the mouse protection test and the routine examination of histological preparations of liver tissue from the bodies of all persons dying within 10 days of onset of any febrile illness.

Selection 21 | Rural and Jungle Yellow Fever: A New Public Health Problem in Colombia*

In announcing the subject of today's discourse, I did not intend to give the impression that the problem is new or that it is limited to Colombia. It is only the recognition of the problem which is new and Colombia is only one of several South American countries where it is known to exist. Future investigation may be expected almost certainly to reveal similar problems in various parts of Africa and possibly in Central America and Mexico.

First recognized and described on the American continent almost 300 years ago, yellow fever has continued to be the most dreaded scourge of the American tropics and subtropics until the present day. International quarantines have been common and commerce has suffered much more from yellow fever than from any other disease of equal importance as a cause of death.

Following the demonstration in 1900 that the virus of yellow fever could be transmitted by *Aëdes aegypti,* it was assumed, on the basis of negative experiments with other species of mosquitoes, only a few of which were made because of the dangerous nature of human experimentation, that this mosquito was the only vector of the disease. Campaigns for the control of this mosquito organized thereafter in the large endemic centers such as Havana, Panama, and Rio de Janeiro, gave such striking results in the reduction of urban and maritime yellow fever, a reduction in no wise limited to, but extending far beyond, the endemic centers worked, that no doubt remained but that *Aëdes aegypti* was the only vector of importance, and about 1915 plans were made for the elimination of yellow fever from the American continent, and possibly from the world, through the organization of antimosquito campaigns in the few known remaining endemic centers. During the next 10 or 15 years these campaigns were so successful that yellow fever ceased to be a major preoccupation among health officers

* Translation of a lecture *(21)* by Dr. Soper given before the Faculty of Medicine of Bogotá, Colombia, April 5, 1935, and originally published in the *Revista de Higiene (Bogota) 4:* 47–84, 1935.

The observations on which this paper is based were made under the auspices of the International Health Division of The Rockefeller Foundation and of the Departamento Nacional de Higiene of Colombia. Dr. Soper was the Representative in South America (Rio de Janeiro Office) of the International Health Division of The Rockefeller Foundation.

throughout the Americas. That the threat of yellow fever continued to exist however, so that antimosquito measures might not be relaxed with safety in previously endemic areas even after the apparent absence of the disease for many years, was shown by the unexpected outbreak in Rio de Janeiro in 1928 and even more unexpected outbreak in Socorro, Colombia, in 1929. That the international dread of yellow fever also persisted was amply proved by the costly quarantine restrictions placed by other countries on vessels touching at Brazilian ports in 1928 and 1929. Although the source of the virus producing the Rio de Janeiro outbreak was never traced, it was assumed to have been the interior of north Brazil, where yellow fever was known to persist.

The isolation, however, in both time and space, of the Socorro outbreak from other known outbreaks of the disease, prevented the formulation of any satisfactory hypothesis as to its origin, on the basis of the then accepted epidemiology of yellow fever. Let me remind you that the epidemiology of yellow fever was, during many years and until quite recently, one of the best examples of a closed argument in all medicine. It is true that doubts continued to be expressed as to the cause of yellow fever, but the epidemiology of the disease was so delightfully simple and so marvelously supported by the results of control measures that none could doubt. Doubts first began when the string of victories registered during a quarter of a century in Havana, Panama, Rio de Janeiro, Iquitos, Manáos, Pará, and Guayaquil, among which are some of the most glorious won by man in combat with any disease, was interrupted by the failure of yellow fever to obey the accepted epidemiological rules written down by man for its behavior. Yellow fever refused to disappear from Brazil in spite of conscientious antimosquito measures over several years in all the important key centers; yellow fever reappeared in Colombia at Socorro after an apparent absence from the land during 6 years with no evidence of reimportation and with no known source of virus!

RECENT LABORATORY PROGRESS

However, just as the simple problem yellow fever used to be was becoming the complex one it is today, a great advance was made when in 1927 the virus of yellow fever was brought from the field to the laboratory. The virus was first established in rhesus monkeys and later, as a neurotropic strain, in mice.

It was now no longer necessary to employ dangerous human experimentation in the laboratory study of yellow fever and a period of great activity followed in which important advances were made in laboratories located in Africa, Brazil, the United States, England, Holland, and France. It is true that previous to the development of the serum and virus method of vaccination in 1931, the laboratory manipulation of the virus was not without its dangers and a number of laboratory infections occurred, resulting in the loss of valuable lives. The serum-virus vaccination method is based on the results of early protection tests in monkeys in which it was observed that animals inoculated simultaneously with virus and known immune serum did not develop yellow fever either at the time nor later when inoculated with virus alone. The possibility of using this method with humans was considered for several years but was not carried out until the neurotropic strain, still dangerous as a possible cause of encephalitis, but incapable of producing viscerotropic yellow fever, was available. Although this method of vaccination is still too cumbersome for application in the field on a large scale, its introduction has been followed by the complete disappearance of laboratory and field infections among those studying yellow fever.

The combination of field and laboratory studies in recent years has opened up new horizons in yellow fever and the worker in this field is no longer forced to rely entirely on his own judgment but is able to check field investigations against laboratory results, and, I might add, laboratory results against field investigations.

A number of animals in the laboratory have been proved susceptible to yellow fever and others susceptible to infection with the virus of yellow fever followed by the development of antibodies even though no symptoms have been observed. Epidemiological observations in the field seem to indicate the possibility of animal hosts other than man in nature, and extensive studies are now being undertaken to clear up this point.

A large number of mosquitoes other than *A. aegypti* have been shown in the laboratory to be capable of harboring the yellow fever virus over a period of time, and a small number have proved to be efficient vectors of the disease from animal to animal in the laboratory. At the same time, field investigation has amply demonstrated the existence of yellow fever without aegypti and studies are being made to determine what mosquitoes or other blood-sucking forms may be the responsible vectors.

Recent Epidemiological Progress

The development of a highly specific protection test first using monkeys, later mice, for determining whether a person whose blood is being tested has previously been infected with yellow fever or not has been followed by a widespread reconnaissance of the distribution of immunity to yellow fever throughout the world, and many surprising situations unknown to clinicians and public health administrators are being disclosed.

Likewise, methods have been devised for the routine collection and examination of liver tissue from rapidly fatal febrile cases for the detection of silent endemic foci, which have resulted in the discovery of dozens of unknown foci of yellow fever, the collection of valuable information regarding the incidence and distribution of other diseases such as malaria and schistosomiasis, and has revealed the presence of kala azar on the American continent.

Such progress has been made in the study of yellow fever both in the laboratory and in the field that today we recognize that field studies must depend on the laboratory and that the laboratory must depend on the field for material on which to work and for the final explanation of laboratory results.

After checking all methods of investigation against each other, today we possess overwhelming proof based on isolation of the virus, on thousands of protection tests, and on numerous autopsies that in addition to the urban yellow fever of history, of simple epidemiology and easy control, there exists, widely disseminated throughout South America, a rural and jungle yellow fever which occurs quite away from urban centers and in the complete absence of the famous "yellow fever" mosquito, *A. aegypti*.

I limit this statement regarding nonurban yellow fever to South America, although it is reasonable to believe that similar conditions may hold for other parts of the Americas. Direct observations of this nonurban yellow fever have been made only in South America, but recent publications on the distribution of immunity to yellow fever in Africa suggest, to one whose knowledge of that continent is limited very largely to the somewhat lurid tales of adventure read in childhood, that the immunity reported from certain regions in the interior of that continent may well be due to jungle yellow fever.

While there is no reason for believing that this nonurban non-aegypti-transmitted yellow fever represents a recent adaptation of the yellow fever virus to new conditions, its recognition is so recent that the *Early History of Yellow Fever* by Carter, the closest student of yellow fever and yellow fever history in recent times, published posthumously in 1931, contains the following statements: "It is a disease of collections of men, civic rather than rural . . . Yellow fever is essentially a disease of towns and cities; malaria is essentially rural, or at most suburban."

The first proved occurrence of rural yellow fever in the absence of *A. aegypti* was only 3 years ago, in March 1932. Events have moved so rapidly in the meantime, however, that rural and jungle yellow fever occurring in the absence of any known nearby urban outbreaks which could have served as immediately preceding sources of the virus has been proved by autopsy in such widely distributed political units as Bolivia, the Brazilian states of Bahia, Espírito Santo, Goyaz, Matto Grosso, Pará, and Amazonas, and, to come closer home, the Municipios of Caparrapí, Muzo, and Restrepo. I realize that the terms I have used—rural yellow fever, jungle yellow fever, and nonurban yellow fever—are not satisfactory without further explanation but have been unable to devise more satisfactory terms.

Epidemiological Classification of Yellow Fever

Yellow fever as it has been observed in South America in recent years may be epidemiologically classed as follows:

A. Yellow fever with *A. aegypti*
1. Urban yellow fever of the classical type, occurring in cities, towns, and villages in the presence of *A. aegypti* and disappearing when the incidence of this vector is reduced.
2. Rural yellow fever, occurring in strictly rural areas having a high *A. aegypti* index and disappearing when this index is lowered. This type of yellow fever has not been observed in Colombia and has been found only in a section of Northeast Brazil, where climatic conditions, including occasional severe droughts necessitating the storage and transport of water by travelers, have greatly facilitated the spread of aegypti in rural areas.
B. Yellow fever without *A. aegypti*
1. Rural yellow fever, occurring in strictly rural areas in the absence of *A. aegypti* but in the presence of a sufficient density of human population to suggest that the cycle of infection may be a simple one: man to vector to man.
2. Jungle yellow fever, occurring in the absence of *A. aegypti* in rural and jungle areas and at isolated points along certain river banks where the density and the movement of the human population are so low that the suggestion cannot be avoided that human cases found are, to a certain extent, accidents in an epizootic rather than part of an epidemic limited to humans.

It is possible that the epidemiology of rural yellow fever without aegypti and that of jungle yellow fever will be shown after further study to be the same. In any case these differ from the urban and rural yellow fever occurring with aegypti in that cases tend to occur in field workers and that house, or family, epidemics, although they may occur, are rare. It is interesting to record that *all observations so far made of yellow fever without A. aegypti have been in places where clearing of the land of forest and jungle has not been complete.*

All the yellow fever seen in Colombia in the past 5 years has occurred in the absence of *A. aegypti*.

Rural and Jungle Yellow Fever

It is not the purpose of this talk tonight to trace the development of the newer epidemiology of yellow fever farther than is necessary for the understanding of the situation in Colombia. I shall limit my discussion to Muzo and Caparrapí, in the Magdalena Valley, and Restrepo in the Orinoco Valley, although, in passing, I can say that we have evidence of yellow fever in the recent past in Amazonian Colombia, and that, in spite of the negative results of protection tests on children in the city of Santa Marta, the surrounding rural area merits further investigations.

Following the cleaning of Havana and Panama a great decrease was noted in the incidence of yellow fever in Colombia as well as in other countries bordering on the Caribbean. This decreased incidence was noted not only in the Caribbean ports but also in the Magdalena Valley in direct contact with them. In the last 25 years urban yellow fever has been reported only in the following cities and in the years mentioned:

Buenaventura	1915–1920
Bucaramanga	1910–1923
Cartagena	1919
Barranquilla	1912
Socorro	1929

It will be noted that all these outbreaks occurred in maritime ports and hence were attributable to importation of the virus, except those of Bucaramanga in 1910 and 1923 and that of Socorro in 1929. These unexplainable outbreaks in Bucaramanga and Socorro, however, were urban outbreaks occurring in the presence of aegypti and disappeared when anti-larval measures were undertaken. They do not form part of the subject under discussion tonight except in sofar as they may be accepted as secondary to rural or jungle yellow fever and therefore indicative of the constant threat of urban outbreaks as long as high aegypti indices are permitted to exist in the towns and ports of Colombia.

Muzo

The history of yellow fever in Muzo is one of the most interesting in all yellow fever epidemiology and is indeed unique in certain aspects. I know of no other small isolated community which has so continuously, over a quarter of a century, been the scene of repeated suspicious outbreaks. No other community of equal size has been the scene of so much investigation by eminent authorities as has Muzo, but in spite of the uniformly negative opinions expressed during many years, the local authorities have continued to declare suspect cases.

Muzo is a small town of some 350 inhabitants lying in the county of the same name, about 150 kilometers to the north of Bogota. The Municipio of Muzo is reported to have a population of some 4,000 inhabitants, only a small percentage of whom live and work at the Muzo emerald mines, famous as the source, during several centuries, of the world's best emeralds. The activity at the mines varies greatly from time to time, and the number of employees ranges from none at all, during periods of abandonment, to 300 or more miners at the height of activities. When I visited the mines in April 1934 with Drs. Patiño and Bevier it was stated that the total population on the reservation was about 170 people, including in addition to the miners a small administrative staff maintained by the government, and a rather heavy police guard to prevent invasion of the emerald-producing district by outsiders and to prevent the theft of emeralds by employees. Labor for the mines is purposely recruited from rather distant regions to reduce the possibility of theft of emeralds. A large percentage of the laborers come from the region of Ubaté, which is well above the zone in which yellow fever can occur endemically and are, of course, nonimmunes on arrival. There is no fixed term of service, but laborers generally remain for several months at a time. During the period of service the miners are required to live at the quarters provided for them at the mines and only under orders of the Administrator may they live in the the few outlying houses which are on the closely supervised portion of the reservation. The total reservation belonging to the government consists of some 3600 hectares, of which only about 800 hectares are kept under close observation, no one being permitted to enter or leave without a special pass. In general the employees at the mines are not permitted to bring families to the reservation. Once each week, on Saturday evening, they are permitted a few hours away from the reservation. Most of the men spend this time in the town of Muzo. The town of Muzo itself has never been reported to harbor the *A. aegypti* mosquito, the principal urban vector of this disease and, as far as the speaker has been able to ascertain, outbreaks of yellow fever have never occurred there.

I have gone into these details regarding the population at the mines because they are the factors which are believed to be responsible for the repeated reports of suspicious outbreaks. It is probable that conditions in the Muzo area outside the mines are not greatly different from those in many other parts of the same region. It is likewise almost certain that the relatively small number of nonimmune laborers brought in to work the mines has not been sufficient to explain the continued endemicity of yellow fever in Muzo. The number has been sufficiently large, however, to give occasional outbreaks which have been called to the attention of the health authorities largely because of the government's interest in the mines. In other words, it is possible that yellow fever has not been more common in Muzo than elsewhere in the region but that Muzo itself is only a visible example of what may be happening invisibly in many other places in Colombia.

At frequent intervals since 1885 when the first reported outbreak of yellow fever occurred in Muzo, epidemics of a severe type have occurred which have given this place a bad reputation.

It is interesting to review rapidly the reported outbreaks of yellow fever which have occurred in Muzo since the first outbreak of 1885. This outbreak was attributed to infection brought by troops from Honda, where yellow fever then existed. The history of the Muzo outbreaks furnishes a striking example of the great difficulty experienced in making epidemiological investigations before the introduction of modern methods of diagnosis. In 1906–1907 an important outbreak of a suspicious disease occurred in Muzo and was investigated by Drs. Roberto Franco, Gabriel Toro-Villa, and Jorge Martínez-Santamaría, who performed autopsies, made blood examinations, and collected mosquitoes. These authors observed cases of both yellow fever and relapsing fever, but reported an almost complete absence of malaria, and made the only recorded observation of *A. aegypti* in this region.

Thanks to the kindness of Dr. Franco, I have been able to consult his original report and wish to recommend it to all who are interested in field investigation in epidemiology as a very careful piece of work, combining careful clinical records, laboratory investigations and epidemiological observations of the utmost value, at a time when such a combination was rare indeed. From the careful presentation of individual case histories, there can be no doubt that yellow fever was present in Muzo in 1907. The modern tendency of most modern scientific journals to refuse the publication of detailed reports is to be deplored, since recorded observations have a permanent value whereas conclusions based on such observations may need alteration in the light of later observations.

Whereas the careful observations made and recorded by Dr. Franco and his colleagues convince me that yellow fever was present, they also suggest to me that there may have been a mistake in the identification of *A. aegypti*, which at that time was known as *Stegomyia calopus*. The point is of sufficient interest, since the recorded observation of *A. aegypti* in 1907 at Muzo has become widespread in the literature, and since the original of Dr. Franco's report is available to only a few readers, to justify the presentation of the original statement here [p. 189 in translation]:

In an effort to see whether the ideas which we had formed regarding the nature of these fevers would conform or not to the concepts generally accepted at the present time in regard to yellow fever, which concepts we have just summarized, we suggested that collections of mosquitoes be made in the vicinity of the workers quarters and also close to the places where they work. Near the buildings of the mine (sleeping quarters and administrative offices) mosquitoes were very rare, only a few specimens being found with considerable difficulty, while in the forest and undergrowth they were found in abundance. Less than 5 per cent of these specimens were anophelines; the great majority were "culicidios" and many of these belonged to the genus *Culex*. *Stegomyia calopus* (=*A. aegypti*) is present, but we cannot consider it to be the most common mosquito. There also exists in abundance a culex which is brilliantly adorned with bands of silvery and golden scales on the thoracic region and with brilliant patches of similar scales on the head and abdomen. This mosquito is so elegant and so beautiful that only the best jewelers of most refined and artistic tastes could imagine anything equal to it. It seems similar to the species described in Japan as *Culex aureo estriatus*.

These mosquitoes bite during the daytime, and although dawn and twilight may be the preferred hours of feeding, inoculation may take place at any time during the day. This is demonstrated by *the predominance of cases among those laborers engaged in the cutting and clearing of forest for the opening of roads and for the conduction of water to the saw mill, etc.*

It is interesting to quote here also from the conclusions of this report [p. 195 in translation]:

1. The epidemic which we studied at the Muzo mines in 1907 consisted of yellow fever and an associated fever of spirochetal origin. These two entities exist endemically in this region, which is subject to epidemics which are produced and maintained by the frequent arrival of susceptible individuals from the cold uplands.

2. The yellow fever (observed here) has certain peculiarities from an etiological point of view:

    a. It is contracted in the forest and not in the neighborhood of the houses.

    b. It is transmitted by *Stegomyia calopus* (= *A. aegypti*) and probably also by other culicines.

    c. Inoculation takes place during the daylight hours, which are spent by the workers in places where the transmitting mosquitoes predominate.

It is indeed remarkable that these conclusions are in entire accord with our own based on a much fuller knowledge of yellow fever than was available at that time, with the single exception of the presence of *A. aegypt*. From the internal evidence of Dr. Franco's report, even without taking into consideration all later failures to find aegypti at Muzo, we are, I believe, justified in concluding that aegypti was probably not present at Muzo in 1907, since the description of the distribution and activities of the mosquitoes found does not correspond to that of those universally observed for aegypti. Dr. Franco has really given us, a quarter of a century ago, an excellent description of jungle yellow fever, acquired in the forest and believed by him to have been transmitted by a nondomestic mosquito whose habits are described. In the face of this description later students are to be criticized more severely for accepting the classification of this mosquito made in 1907, when the finer points of entomological classification were known to but few, than is the author for having made it.

In 1916 suspect cases were again recorded from Muzo and the region was investigated by no less an authority on yellow fever than General Gorgas. The visit of the Gorgas Commission coincided with a complete dearth of cases but on the basis of a few clinical histories taken and from the fact that a most careful search failed to reveal *A. aegypti* mosquitoes, the conclusion was drawn that yellow fever had not been present but that the cases reported had probably been of malaria.

In 1923 attention was again drawn to Muzo and a careful entomological search made by Hanson and Dunn for *A. aegypti* but without result. In 1924 suspect cases were again recorded, but I have been unable to find any report on investigations at that time.

In 1927 still another outbreak occurred which was investigated by Drs. César Uribe-Piedrahita and George Bevier. These investigators failed to find *A. aegypti* and concluded that the outcry had been caused by cases of malaria.

Epidemics of Yellow Fever, 1930–1934

Toward the end of 1930 another violent epidemic in the Muzo area began which continued for some months and was investigated in 1931 by Dr. Ignacio Moreno-Pérez and other colleagues. Many cases of malaria were observed, confirmed by blood smears, which yielded readily to quinine.

Dr. Moreno-Pérez failed to find any cases suggestive of yellow fever. The following abstract from his report is of interest [p. 329 in translation]:

> It still remains to be explained why a quarter of a century ago, when Dr. Franco's Commission was there, malaria was so rare among the employees and the workmen of the mines, who were, for the most part, recently arrived from the cold highlands, and why today such a high incidence of malaria is observed both in the inhabitants of the village and of the surrounding rural territory and among those who live at the mines. The same holds true for persons who have lived a long time in the region, as well as those recently arrived. On the other hand, recurrent fever (i.e., tick-borne relapsing fever), in spite of the abundance of its transmitting agents, has become very rare, judging by a goodly number of blood examinations during a period of several months. *The same may be said of yellow fever, which apparently has not presented itself in epidemic form,* perhaps due to lack of sufficient immigration. To investigate the endemicity of this disease, blood specimens were taken from 80 persons varying in age from 1 to 80 years; these have been sent to the [Rockefeller Foundation Laboratory in the] Rockefeller Institute for examination by the protection test.
>
> 1. It may be affirmed that in the last 15 years the epidemics which at irregular intervals have appeared in the region of Muzo have not been yellow fever but pernicious malaria.

It should be noted that Dr. Moreno-Pérez states that the epidemics in Muzo in recent years have not been yellow fever but, on the other hand, does not deny the possibility of yellow fever endemicity. The bloods collected by Dr. Moreno-Pérez in 1931 were tested for immune bodies indicative of previous attacks of yellow fever with the result that yellow fever was shown to have been present in Muzo much later than the last reported outbreak diagnosed by Dr. Franco, since several individuals born long after the 1907 outbreak were found to be immune. In addition, it was found at this time that a certain number of children living in the rural areas were immune. These tests were performed, however, in the early days of the mouse-protection test before the method had been used on a sufficiently high number of sera to prove its specificity. Consequently it was decided that as many of the positives as possible should be repeated the following year. Drs. J. A. Kerr and Luis Patiño-Camargo visited Muzo in 1932 and secured second specimens from some of the positive cases and a small number of other individuals. It is interesting to note that although these authors at the time of their visit to Muzo and afterward scouted the possibility of yellow fever in Muzo, since no *A. aegypti* nor suspicious cases could be found, the results of the protection tests in 1932 confirmed the work done in 1931. All of you are probably familiar with the report by Drs. Kerr and Patiño. I wish to quote from this report [p. 13 in translation]:

The fact that the greater part of the persons shown to be immune to yellow fever are inhabitants of the rural region, and the absence of *Aëdes aegypti* in the village of Muzo and in the mines, every time that this mosquito has been sought, with the only exception of the findings of Dr. Franco, are good proof in support of the belief that yellow fever has been endemic among the rural population of the county of Muzo. Moreover, it may be supposed that the epidemic among the workers of the mines in 1907 was probably only an incident in the endemicity of the region. It does not seem very probable that the county of Muzo with its population of only 3000 to 4000 persons takes in all the endemic region. This county is only one of various contiguous counties which have similar climates, topography, and population, and which together probably form the endemic region.

[and p. 21 in translation]:

Considering the epidemiology of yellow fever in the region of Santander, the results of our studies in Muzo are of great interest due to the similarity between the rural parts of this county and those of the region of Santander. We believe that the finding in Muzo that a great portion of the rural population is immune, in proportion to the increase in age of the persons examined, is good proof that yellow fever has been endemic in this rural region.

Among the conclusions of these authors (1933) are the following [p. 23 in translation]:

Yellow fever has been endemic during many years in the rural part of the county of Muzo, cases of this illness having presented themselves as recently as in the year 1921.

It would be wise to consider the region of Santander as a dangerous focus of yellow fever from which the disease might be spread to the highly infectible low-lands of the country.

It may be of interest to note that I had an opportunity in May 1933 to look over the English manuscript of the report of Drs. Kerr and Patiño and took a decided stand against these conclusions, although they were based in part on the, at that time, recent report on the first observed rural epidemic of yellow fever occurring in the absence of *A. aegypti,* of which I was one of the coauthors.

I wrote a lengthy letter to Dr. Kerr pointing out what I felt to be the weak points in the argument in favor of rural endemicity in this part of Colombia and was able to convince him that the report should not be published with such dangerous conclusions. The proposed publication in English was canceled but fortunately my objections arrived too late to prevent the publication here in Spanish. A few months later I had the opportunity of visiting Colombia for the first time, found conditions to be quite different from what I had always imagined, and readily admitted that I had probably been wrong in opposing these conclusions. Recent happenings have proved that I was wrong and that yellow fever continues endemic in the rural regions of Muzo up to the present time.

During 1932 and 1933 no highly significant outbreaks requiring extensive investigation were reported from Muzo. However, in January 1934, a series of cases, seven of which were rapidly fatal, occurred among about 100 workers at the mines. Vague reports were heard of other cases in the surrounding country. As so often happens, most of the workmen fled and the cases ceased, only to reappear again in March, when a number of workmen were back on the job. Drs. Patiño and Bevier and myself visited the mines in April 1934, and learned that the beginning of active operations had been accompanied by a few suspect cases in June 1933 but that nothing further had occurred until January, at which time the deaths mentioned had occurred. Then, in March, four more deaths were known to have occurred, two at the mines, one in Muzo and one in Coper, the two latter occurring in workmen who were fleeing from the disease. We were able to secure blood for a protection test from the only known survivor of this epidemic and a liver specimen from one of the fatal cases. The laboratory gave positive reports on both specimens. At the time of our visit in April no domestic mosquitoes were found and no suspect cases of illness could be learned of in the entire region. In June, however, almost 2 months after our visit came a third series of suspect cases during the year. Dr. José Jesús Castillo has described the circumstances of this outbreak as follows [in translation]:

In the month of May of the current year (1934), landslides caused by the heavy rains blocked the main ditch bringing water to the hydroelectric plant. This ditch comes down from the nearby mountains following a course cut in stone for some 13 kilometers. Fifteen workmen, recently arrived from the cold highlands, were sent to clear the ditch. They slept at a camp called "Guamito," which consisted of nothing more than a wattle house located 6 kilometers from the buildings of the mines and situated at an elevation of 200 meters more than that of these buildings.

After remaining at the camp for 15 days, the workers returned to the mines, five of them very severely ill, especially the more youthful ones who were working for the first time in the region.

Of these five cases, all of which presented typical clinical symptoms of yellow fever, two were fatal and were both confirmed by liver examination. Two others were confirmed by protection test results. The house in which these men slept was located in a small clearing with four other houses located in a wild and almost uninhabited region.

No other cases were observed at this time among workmen at the mines nor among another group of 15 men working on the same ditch much lower down, who slept at the police station at the back entrance to the reservation.

Following this series of five cases, nothing suspicious was observed during 4 months. In October, however, Dr. Aquiles González observed a rapidly fatal case of only 3 days' duration in a workman who had been for some time engaged clearing away the forest at a point some 3 kilometers from the mine. This man was known to have had previous attacks of malaria and his final illness was so diagnosed. However, a liver specimen removed after death was found to contain the typical lesions of yellow fever. No other cases were observed at the time among the men at the mines nor among the three people living in the same house with this case. This isolated case could never have been diagnosed yellow fever without the aid of the laboratory. Since October no suspicious cases have been reported.

When the final proof by autopsy of the existence and continued endemicity of yellow fever in Muzo in 1934, during which year four apparently isolated series of cases occurred in January, March, June, and October, is added to the proofs and reports of other years, little room is left for doubt as to the permanent endemicity of this region. Muzo itself may not be more important than other counties. Most likely it is part of a much larger area forming an endemic focus in which the same constant history of suspect outbreaks is not obtained because the same importation of fairly large groups of workmen from the uplands at frequent intervals does not occur. In no other place has the same continuity of suspect cases been observed, and Muzo requires a full and complete field study, with adequate collaboration from the laboratory.

All investigations made in Muzo beginning with that of Dr. Franco in 1907 indicate that yellow fever is not transmitted there by domestic mosquitoes. The evidence points rather to field infections and to the possibility of vertebrate hosts other than man existing in the forests. It is interesting to note that monkeys are quite common* in the Muzo area and have been found to be common in all regions so far investigated on this point where jungle yellow fever has appeared.

Yellow Fever at Caparrapí

Although much more recent and not so widely publicized, the recent suspect outbreaks at Caparrapí are almost as interesting as the ones at Muzo in that they may more truly reflect what is probably occurring over a wide area than do the series of cases occurring under the special conditions which exist in Muzo. Also, because of its greater proximity to the towns on the Magdalena River, the Caparrapí endemic presents a more immediate threat to the commerce of the country.

The region lying between Muzo and Puerto Liévano is very hilly, with steep mountain slopes and changes in altitude of from 200 to 1500 meters within very short distances. Strange to say, practically all the towns of this region are situated on the tops of the ridges, so that a study of reported altitudes and of such meteorological data as may be available from the towns is of little or no value in giving an idea of conditions in the surrounding veredas.

The municipality of Caparrapí is a very extensive one with some 13,000 inhabitants. The town of Caparrapí, with a population of about 1800 and at an altitude of 1270 meters, is located only about 20 kilometers from El Dindal, one of the stations on the railroad between Utica and Puerto Liévano. An investigation of suspect cases of yellow fever in the municipality of Caparrapí was made by Dr. Augusto Gast in March 1933. At this time Dr. Gast did not see any cases but investigated an epidemic which had occurred in December 1932 and January and February 1933 at Azauncha, some 35 kilometers north of Caparrapí. Thirty-seven cases with 12 deaths were uncovered. This epidemic had been diagnosed as pernicious malaria, although local conditions were not highly favorable to anopheline production. No definite decision was made at the time regarding the character of this outbreak.

In June of the same year another investigation was made because of suspicious cases occurring on the hacienda Tatí among men working in the Pitás Valley, somewhat closer to Caparrapí and much nearer the railroad than is Azauncha. To quote from Dr. Gast's report [in translation]:

The Pitás Valley is known as a dangerous region because people who stay there invariably become sick. For this reason all houses so far constructed in this valley

* *Editorial Note:* Information obtained in later years revealed that monkeys were not common in the humid tropical forests of the Muzo area, in spite of their prevalence in such forests in other parts of the Magdalena Valley and elsewhere in Colombia.

have been abandoned. Recently some workmen have been cultivating the land along Pitás Creek for the purpose of sowing corn. These workers come down to their fields on Monday and on Saturday return to their houses, which are situated on high land. They carry down their food and take shelter in the abandoned houses. All the persons attacked by the recent epidemic were laborers who had been working along the banks of the Pitas, with the exception of one man who had not left Buenavista but who lived in company with another man who had acquired the disease in Pitás. Another interesting detail is that not one woman nor child has suffered from the disease.

The epidemic occurred in the rural regions to the southwest and to the west of the village and distant by one day's travel from Caparrapí.

The region is formed by a series of three ranges running from north to south and at an approximate altitude of 1200 meters. The ranges are separated by deep and narrow valleys. The higher regions consist of coffee plantations and are well populated. The valleys are used for the cultivation of corn and sugar cane and are traditionally considered unhealthy. Only when agricultural necessity requires it are these valleys temporarily inhabited.

A total of 11 deaths in the month of June were attributed to this fever. An examination of blood smears from 36 persons showed 10 carriers of *Plasmodium vivax* and 2 of *P. falciparum*. At the time the investigation was completed the diagnosis was still in doubt, and this outbreak was proved to be yellow fever only by autopsy and protection test results. Of nine sera from suspect cases in the June epidemic, eight were frankly positive and the other probably positive. A liver tissue obtained from the partial autopsy in June was examined by Dr. Oskar Klotz, who stated: "The liver lesion is not that of malaria. The lesions in this case are very interesting and remind us of the Santa Marta cases of a few years ago. Whatever the diagnosis of this case from Caparrapí, the same can be given for the Santa Marta cases. Hence I have ventured the diagnosis 'possibly yellow fever' as I do not know what else I may call it. If the Santa Marta cases were not yellow fever then this also it not yellow fever, and its classification is yet undetermined."

In the face of these results, and another autopsy reported below, there can be no doubt that the Caparrapí epidemic of June 1933 was yellow fever and we have ample reason for believing that the previous epidemic in January and February was of the same nature. I would like to call your attention once more to the difficulty which is constantly encountered in differentiating between jungle yellow fever and malaria. This difficulty, I believe, in great part explains the fact that jungle yellow fever passed for so many years without being described.

I do not wish to go into the discussion here tonight of the Santa Marta cases of 1930–1931 further than to say that in spite of the full and careful investigations which were made in the town of Santa Marta and the results of which have been published, with the conclusion that the cases reported were not yellow fever, I consider the possibility of endemic yellow fever in the Santa Marta area an open one. At the time the Santa Marta investigation was made, nothing had been published regarding the possibility of rural and jungle yellow fever and hence the investigation of Santa Marta was carefully limited to the town itself, where sufficient *A. aegypti* were found to justify the assumption that widespread transmission must have occurred had cases come into Santa Marta in the infective stage of the disease. Likewise, I do not wish to enter into a discussion of the value of the examination of the liver in the diagnosis of yellow fever, except to state that it is most useful, when due weight is given to the clinical history and field investigation, in differentiating yellow fever from other rapidly fatal febrile conditions. The statement of Dr. Klotz, regarding the Caparrapí liver, was made in ignorance of the results of protection tests on cases from the same epidemic. In the light of these results, the remarks of Dr. Klotz are highly important, not only from the standpoint of Caparrapí, but also with reference to the Santa Marta region.

After the results of these first laboratory examinations were known further studies were undertaken in the municipality of Caparrapí.

Dr. Horacio Gómez collected 59 bloods, 15, or 25 per cent, of which proved to be positive by the mouse protection test. An analysis of the distribution of these positives by age groups is very important, not only from the standpoint of local epidemiology, but also as an indication of the need for great care in the use of the age distribution of immunity in a community as an indication of the date of the last appearance of the disease therein.

Among 46 bloods taken from children living in Caparrapí and in the veredas, 20 of which were from children living in houses in which cases were known to have occurred, only 4 positives were found, all in the latter group. One of these was a boy of 15 years, who later stated that he had the disease in the first suspect outbreak at Azauncha, in January 1933. This result tends to confirm the conclusion that this first epidemic was really yellow fever. The other 3 positives, found under 20 years of age, were all children in the same family, whose father had died during the 1933 epidemic. In contrast with these results, however, are the negative results with the sera of two children who had lived through the same epidemic in a house where 3 fatal cases occurred. It would seem, then, that although a series of cases may occur occasionally in the same house, suggesting house infection, rural and jungle yellow fever is not essentially a house disease such as the urban type tends to become.

In comparison with 4 positives in 46 tests, or only 9 per cent positives, in the age group below 20 years, 9 positives, or 70 per cent, were reported in 13 tests on sera from the age group above 20 years. The only two women in this group were negative. These results, together with the 8 positives in 9 tests reported earlier, considered together with the positive diagnosis by liver examination, justifies the conclusion that yellow fever has existed for some time in the Caparrapí district as an endemic disease, largely transmitted in the field or jungle and limited almost entirely to field laborers.

On the other hand, had these sera come to the laboratory unaccompanied by a history of recent events, the only reasonable interpretation which could have been given to these results would have been one we know to be false—that a widespread epidemic of yellow fever had passed through Caparrapí more than 20 years ago, immunizing a large percentage of the population, even in the younger age groups, and had then disappeared, not returning in the interval. This is another striking demonstration of the need of close collaboration between laboratory workers and field investigators in the study of yellow fever.

Although no important series of cases has been observed since June 1933 up to the present time, Dr. Horacio Gómez autopsied an isolated suspicious case, which became sick while working in a place called Hoya Palacio and died in the town of Caparrapí itself in February 1934. Dr. Klotz made a clear-cut positive diagnosis on the tissues from this case. This result is added proof that the disease being studied is yellow fever and that yellow fever can continue for months and possibly years in isolated communities. More than a year has passed now since this last confirmation, but it will be no surprise to learn that the virus still continues in this region.

Jungle Yellow Fever in the Orinoco Valley

The experience in both Muzo and Caparrapí demonstrates the futility of temporary and rapid field investigations unsupported by laboratory tests. Although such investigations of so-called outbreaks of "fiebre perniciosa" may result in proving the existence of malaria, relapsing fever, or typhoid fever, autopsies and protection tests should always be made to determine whether yellow fever may not also be present and be responsible for part of the heavy mortality. The present epidemic in the country about Restrepo might easily have been overlooked, since numerous cases of both malaria and relapsing fever have been observed concomitantly with the outbreak of yellow fever. This outbreak is less important than those of Muzo and Caparrapí as a threat to commerce because of its isolated position on the eastern slope of the Andes at the edge of the llanos, but epidemiologically is fully as interesting. There have been no reports of yellow fever elsewhere in the entire Orinoco Valley for many years. The only reference I have found regarding yellow fever in this region refers by a strange coincidence to exactly the same area which now occupies our attention. The reference is as follows: "In 1886 the communities along the Meta River were decimated by epidemics of some disease which spread up the Orinoco River and its branches as far as Cumaral (about 40 kilometers from Villavicencio). However, the clinical records are so meager that there is doubt as to the diagnosis. It is possible that a type of pernicious malaria may have become epidemic as occasionally happens in those vast and unhealthy regions, or that relapsing fever was mistaken for yellow fever." The site of the village of Cumaral is reported to have been moved at that time in an attempt to move away from the disease.

Since July of last year (1934) suspicious cases of pernicious fever which did not conform to his requirements for a diagnosis of either malaria or relapsing fever were noted by Dr. Jorge Boshell, who was representing the National Department of Health in Villavicencio, on the other side of the river from Restrepo. These cases were first observed in the veredas Caibe, Sardinata, and Caney, not far from Cumaral and Restrepo. Cases were largely limited to field workers from the mountains, who were working in the rice harvest. The definite diagnosis of yellow fever was somewhat delayed since no *A. aegypti* could be found and Dr. Boshell was not yet familiar with the fact that yellow fever could occur without this mosquito. The inhabitants of the region insisted that they did not know a mosquito conforming to the description of the aegypti, and were not bitten by mosquitoes in their homes but were attacked by a vicious-biting, "blue" mosquito in the fields. Likewise in the towns of Restrepo, Cumaral, Villavicencio, and Medina no aegypti have been found. The definite diagnosis was finally established through the autopsy in September of three fatal cases and the demonstration of protective antibodies in the blood of 20 of 28 suspects and contacts bled. In November, the disease had spread to, and seemed limited largely to, the houses along the Guacavía River. Along this river, at this time, yellow fever seemed to be a house disease and cases were observed to occur among several members of the same family, women and children being affected as well as the men who worked in the fields. In December 1934 and January, February, and March of this year, cases have been observed in other veredas lying much closer to Restrepo and in the vereda Retiro, which lies roughly between Restrepo and Villavicencio. No cases have, however, been reported from the right bank of the Guatiquía River. Likewise, cases have again been observed in the veredas first known to be infected. These cases of the past few months have been mostly in men, who were working in the fields in the clearing of the forest in preparation for this year's crops. Certain clearings have given repeated cases and those who have worked in the area feel that, with the exception of the cases along the Guacavía River in November, most infections have been acquired in the field. A rather complete study of the blood-sucking fauna of the region is being carried out by Dr. Paulo Antunes of the Instituto de Higiene of São Paulo. Dr. Antunes has found, just as the people told Dr. Boshell in the beginning, that the most common mosquito in the region is the "blue" mosquito, *Haemagogus equinus,* which is found to be a vicious biter in the field, even when the men are actively at work, attacking by preference around the feet and ankles.

It may be of significance that the earliest cases known in the region occurred in the most recently settled section where the people are living most closely in contact with the rain forest. Here, as in certain other places in South America where studies are going forward, it would appear that, quite contrary to the observations for urban yellow fever, the greatest danger of jungle yellow fever is where the human population is least but is in most intimate contact with jungle life. At least 4 species of monkeys, known locally as Socay, Tití, Maicero, and Araguato, are common in the forests about Restrepo, and one cannot avoid the thought that possibly one or all of these species, as well as possibly other vertebrates of the forest, may serve as animal hosts of the virus.

In this connection I might mention again that the region about the Muzo mines abounds in all forms of wild life and that monkeys are very common there. It has proved very difficult in Restrepo as elsewhere to capture wild monkeys for the purpose of getting blood for protection tests. However, protection tests have been attempted on six specimens from this region of which four have been positive, one was inconclusive, and the other proved to have been contaminated in collection. These results are very suggestive but, of course, need numerous controls from the same and other regions before they can be definitely interpreted.

Epidemiologically the Restrepo outbreak of jungle yellow fever is very important, since it is occurring in the entire absence of *A. aegypti,* this mosquito not being found even in the larger towns of the area. It would be hard to find a more isolated point in which to demonstrate that jungle yellow fever persists in and of itself and is not secondary at present to endemic urban centers of this disease.

Discussion

I have referred in my title to rural and jungle yellow fever as a problem, and I wish to emphasize that it is a very complex problem with many unknown factors. The extent of infected regions of Colombia is unknown. The different species of mosquitoes which may be involved in transmission in Colombia and their relative importance have not been determined nor is it clear whether other blood-sucking forms than mosquitoes are involved in its transmission. The existence of long-lived vectors would help explain the continuance of the infection from one outbreak to another but are not necessary if natural infections occur in other vertebrate hosts in the jungle. Although there is some evidence suggesting the existence of animal reservoirs an immense amount of work remains to be done before their existence

LIBRARY
HOLY CROSS JUNIOR COLLEGE
NOTRE DAME, INDIANA

can be considered proved, and even though evidence should be accumulated indicating that monkeys do take part in the epidemiological picture, other vertebrates must, likewise, be studied and proved, or eliminated from consideration, one by one.

Many Factors Still Unknown

It is clear that as long as the above factors are unknown, it will be difficult to plan control services directed against jungle yellow fever. Unfortunately the serum-virus vaccination using the neurotropic strain of virus which has proved so efficacious in protecting individuals is still considered unsafe for use without the administration of large amounts of immune serum. The development of a modified virus which can be safely used without serum is an urgent necessity. In the meantime, we are forced to admit that control measures applicable to jungle yellow fever are as yet unknown. Although the presence of yellow fever in Muzo was proved a year ago, nothing has been done there to prevent the further spread of the disease except disinsectization of the sleeping quarters of the men. In Caparrapí, where the existence of yellow fever has been known for the past 18 months, no measures of prevention have been taken and none have been recommended. Likewise in Restrepo, observers have been in the field since last October but have done nothing toward the prevention of the disease. These observers have watched the disease spread from one section to another, studying the cases clinically, performing numerous autopsies, collecting insects, and taking bloods for protection tests, but have been unable to advise the inhabitants and authorities of the region as to how the disease can be avoided.

I have attempted to present briefly the problem of rural and jungle yellow fever in Colombia as we understand it today without going into details of other equally interesting situations elsewhere on the continent. Before stating briefly plans for future studies and recommendations for prevention it is only fair that I should point out the possibility, probably a remote one, that the virus of jungle yellow fever may have been so modified by continuous passage through vectors other than *A. aegypti* that it is no longer easily transmitted by this most common urban vector. The fact that very few visible outbreaks of urban yellow fever have occurred in the past 20 years in the entire Amazon Valley, in spite of the fact that both protection tests and autopsies have proved that the disease has continued widespread in this area, might be adduced as an argument in favor of such an alteration of the virus. On the other hand, the number of cases occurring in an outbreak of jungle yellow fever at any one time is always small in comparison with the numbers observed in active urban epidemics. The dissemination of urban yellow fever from one small town to another, except when there is some large distributing center with many cases, furnishing many sources of infection is disappointingly slow and irregular, in spite of the fact that the infection is acquired and redistributed in houses and hotels and that every nonimmune traveler or visitor is a potential distributor of the infection. On the other hand, travelers and visitors do not go to the fields and jungle, where as you have seen, observations indicate that jungle yellow fever is acquired. Furthermore, the sick person, who remains in bed with jungle yellow fever, is generally of no importance in the production of secondary cases, since house vectors are not believed to be common and the sick man does not return to the field during the period of infectability. These observations not only help to explain the rarity of urban outbreaks secondary to rural outbreaks, but also argue most strongly in favor of the existence of vertebrate hosts in nature other than man.

Urban and Jungle Viruses Identical

There are, however, further facts arguing for the identity of the virus of urban and jungle yellow fever and against the hypothesis that the virus of jungle yellow fever is not readily transmitted by *A. aegypti,* including the following:

1. In the laboratory, the yellow fever virus adapted to *A. aegypti* is readily transmitted by several other mosquitos.

2. Epidemics with and without *A. aegypti* have been observed in Bolivia apparently as part of the same outbreak.

3. The most reasonable explanation of the Bucaramanga and Socorro epidemics is that the source of virus was in nearby areas of jungle endemicity.

4. Cross protection tests of known immune sera and with the viruses from urban and jungle yellow fever are positive.

5. The clinical course of urban and jungle yellow fever is the same.

6. The pathological picture in the human produced by urban and jungle yellow fever is essentially the same. (Dr. Klotz was quoted above as classifying the first Caparrapí and the Santa Marta livers together as possibly somewhat different from others. However, his diagnosis on the second Caparrapí liver was a straight "positive yellow fever.")

Although a recent attempt to establish the virus of Restrepo in the laboratory failed, there are already four strains of yellow fever isolated in nature in the absence of aegypti in Brazil, available for studies now being undertaken to determine whether jungle yellow fever is always readily transmitted under favorable urban conditions. An answer to this question will be available in the very near future.

RESPONSIBILITIES AND RECOMMENDATIONS

Even though it should be proved that modifications have occurred in the virus making it less suitable for urban life, the evidence of Bucaramanga and Socorro would suggest that reverse modifications would also be possible. From the point of view of the health officer, then, the question is purely academic, since the threat is present in either case.

Yellow fever was one of the subjects given special consideration at the IXth Pan American Sanitary Conference in Buenos Aires in November of last year. Dr. Jorge Bejarano, the Colombian delegate to this conference, sat on the committee responsible for drawing up the final recommendations in regard to the study and control of yellow fever made by this conference to the governments of the 21 American republics represented, all of which have suffered in the past from epidemics of yellow fever. These recommendations read as follows [in translation]:

Recommendations of the IXth Pan American Sanitary Conference regarding yellow fever:

The IXth Pan American Sanitary Conference, after considering recent work on yellow fever, recommends to the countries of the continent the following program of studies and prophylaxis:

1. Systematic investigation of the distribution of immunity to yellow fever among the inhabitants of all tropical countries and regions of the continent to establish the geographical distribution of the disease in recent years.

2. Systematic histopathological investigations (collection by viscerotomy and examination of specimens of liver from persons dying of febrile disease of less than 10 days of evolution) in all regions previously considered endemic, and in those in which the investigation of the protective power of the blood indicates the presence of or recent existence of the disease.

3. Organization of permanent antilarval services which will guarantee a minimal or zero aegypti index in all cities of the continent.

4. Establishment of similar services in all infected localities and in the nearby regions.

5. Adoption of regulations which facilitate and guarantee the efficiency of antilarval and viscerotome services. Regulations similar to those adopted by Brazil, Bolivia, and Paraguay are recommended.

6. Trimestral reports to the Pan American Sanitary Bureau concerning the organization of antilarval campaigns and respective aegypti indices.

7. Determination of supplementary methods for the campaign in rural regions in which antilarval methods may be ineffective or impractical.

8. Preventive yellow fever vaccination in susceptible persons traveling through or into endemic regions, and of rural populations in such regions where yellow fever is known to exist and the campaign against the transmitter is difficult or impossible.

9. Founding of special laboratories for the study of yellow fever. Those countries which do not have specialized laboratories or institutes should make agreements with neighboring countries or with private institutions of international nature for carrying out the necessary investigations.

The responsibility of the public health agencies of those countries where jungle yellow fever exists is twofold: first, urban populations must be protected from yellow fever transmitted by *A. aegypti*; and second, some means must be devised for the protection of rural populations and those who go into the jungle to develop the rich economic possibilities of the sparsely inhabited regions. I make no mention of the responsibility of a country to avoid the dissemination of the yellow fever virus to other countries, since the protection of urban populations, especially those of maritime, fluvial, and air ports, is undoubtedly at the same time the greatest single measure for reducing the possibilities of international spread of yellow fever through shipping and air traffic.

The protection of urban populations against yellow fever is today a problem of administration only. The technique is known and the results are sure. Experience has repeatedly shown in Colombia, as elsewhere, that, although ample funds for control can be secured from the national treasury in the presence of an urban outbreak of yellow fever (especially if this outbreak occurs in an important port), as soon as the immediate danger disappears and the outcry ceases, funds are curtailed and antimosquito activities reduced or abandoned. The finer points of modern technique in urban yellow fever services are all devoted to the cheapening of antimosquito measures to the point where they may be maintained on a permanent basis at a reasonable cost. Such great progress has been made in reducing the cost of antilarval work in recent years that urban yellow fever can no longer be considered a public health problem but rather an administrative crime. In regard to the development of control measures for jungle yellow fever it must be admitted that until much more is known regarding the distribution of this disease and the factors responsible for such distribution, intelligent plans cannot be made for its control through the control of either vectors or vertebrate hosts. Basic studies necessarily preliminary to such work are just in the initial stage in various parts of South America. I am happy to report that in accord with the traditional policy of collaboration of the government of Colombia and The Rockefeller Foundation in problems relating to yellow fever, first established by those most eminent hygienists, Drs. Pablo García-Medina and W. C. Gorgas, a special Yellow Fever Study Service has been organized in the Sección de Saneamiento Rural of the National Department of Health.

The program of this study service includes

1. The determination of the distribution of yellow fever in the recent past in urban, rural, and jungle areas through the protection test on random blood samples from children in different parts of the country.

2. The discovery of active but silent foci of yellow fever, urban or rural, through the routine collection of liver tissue by viscerotomy on all fatal

febrile cases of less than 10 days' duration throughout possibly endemic areas.

3. The investigation of suspect outbreaks when such outbreaks become known.

4. The organization of special intensive field study units equipped with laboratory facilities at such points as may seem to be of greatest interest, to determine what biological factors are responsible for jungle endemicity.

The success of this service depends upon close and intimate collaboration with adequately equipped laboratories. At present this study service is being served by the Yellow Fever Laboratory of the Rockefeller Foundation in New York and by the Laboratory of the Brazilian Yellow Fever Service in Rio de Janeiro. I am happy to report that the Honorable Minister of Agriculture, whom we thank for his presence here today, is considering with Dr. Arturo Robledo, the Director of the National Department of Health, and with Dr. Bernardo Samper, Director of the National Laboratory of Hygiene, plans for organization of a Yellow Fever Section at the Laboratory. Such a section should not only be invaluable in the study of yellow fever, but should eventually result in the development of important studies in other virus diseases and in medical entomology.

Much work is being carried out in the yellow fever laboratories of America and Europe on the problem of a safe and simple method of efficient vaccination. Attempts are being made to avoid present dangers and difficulties either through the production of an attenuated, yet still active virus, or through the production of sera with antibodies in such high concentration that only minimal doses need be applied. It is not too much to expect important advances in the near future. This field of vaccine and serum production is surely a legitimate field of activity for the National Laboratory of Hygiene.

Selection 22 | Jungle Yellow Fever—A New Epidemiological Entity in South America*

DISCUSSION

As stated in the beginning, the epidemiological picture of jungle yellow fever is quite different from that of the classical yellow fever transmitted by *Aëdes aegypti.* Jungle yellow fever attacks by preference persons who, for one reason or another, come into contact with the jungle, whereas infection in the case of yellow fever transmitted by the domestic vector *A. aegypti* generally takes place within the house. These statements are supported by the data presented in Tables 1 and 2 [omitted], which show that the cases of jungle yellow fever in the Valle do Chanaan occurred almost exclusively in male adults and that in the same valley the existing immunity is likewise almost entirely limited to the same population group, whereas immunity to yellow fever in a group of Brazilian towns where transmission occurs through *A. aegypti* is much more frequent and more uniformly distributed throughout all age groups of both sexes.

An analysis of the age and sex distributions of the fatal cases diagnosed by liver examination occurring in Brazil, Colombia, and Bolivia from 1930 to September 1935 (Table 6) confirms the differences in incidence of yellow fever transmitted by aegypti and of that met in the absence of this mosquito.

It is noted that the fatal cases of rural yellow fever with aegypti were limited largely to children, involving both sexes equally, whereas jungle yellow fever eliminated by preference male adults at those ages when a man's capacity for field work is at its best. Among females also the fatalities from this form occurred mostly in adults, just at the period of greatest

* This paper is based on studies and observations made under the auspices of The Rockefeller Foundation and the governments of Brazil, Bolivia, Colombia, and Venezuela. It is a summary of investigations in which local authorities, epidemiologists, and laboratory workers have collaborated. Unfortunately, it is not possible within the limits of this paper to make special mention of all those participating in these investigations. Dr. Soper was the Representative in South America (Rio de Janeiro Office) of the International Health Division of The Rockefeller Foundation.

Excerpts (pp. 125–141) from a translation of a paper (22) read before the National Academy of Medicine, Rio de Janeiro. Brazil, October 17, 1935, and published in English in the *Revista de Hygiene e Saúde Pública (Rio de Janeiro)* *10:* 107–144, 1936.

Table 6. Urban, Rural, and Jungle Yellow Fever[a]

Age group (years)	With *Aëdes aegypti*						Total with *A. aegypti*	Without *A. aegypti*		Total without *A. aegypti*
	Urban			Rural				Jungle		
	Males	Fe-males	Total	Males	Fe-males	Total		Males	Fe-males	
0– 4	5	4	9	13	12	25	34	2	1	3
5– 9	4	1	5	9	11	20	25	4	1	5
10–14	1	—	1	4	1	5	6	5	—	5
15–19	2	3	5	3	1	4	9	6	1	7
20–24	5	1	6	1	—	1	7	15	7	22
25–29	1	—	1	1	—	1	2	11	3	14
30–34	2	5	7	1	—	1	8	8	4	12
35–39	2	2	4	—	1	1	5	6	3	9
40–44	—	1	1	—	—	—	1	7	3	10
45–49	1	—	1	—	1	1	2	2	—	2
50–54	—	2	2	—	—	—	2	1	—	1
55–59	1	—	1	—	1	1	2	1	—	1
60–64	—	—	—	—	—	—	—	3	1	4
65–69	—	—	—	—	1	1	1	—	—	—
70 and over	—	—	—	—	—	—	—	1	1	2
Total	24	19	43	32	29	61	104	72	25	97

[a]Distribution by age and sex of cases occurring from 1930 to September 1935 in Brazil, Colombia, and Bolivia confirmed by examination of liver tissues.

productivity. From an economic point of view, then, this jungle yellow fever deserves the closest attention of the authorities.

Table 6 also shows that the fatal cases of urban yellow fever, fortunately relatively few in number, do not seem at first glance to have any characteristic distribution. But it will be noticed that the distribution in the age groups from 1 to 14 years is similar to that of rural yellow fever with aegypti for the same age groups, and that in the age groups above 15 years the distribution is similar to that for jungle yellow fever. The secondary grouping of cases in urban areas between 15 and 40 years of age is attributed to the fact that this is the period during which individuals, both foreigners and nationals, who have not been immunized in childhood, begin to travel and to flock to the towns where infection can occur. The incidence of urban yellow fever in endemic areas then would appear to be composed of two distinct elements, the incidence among children born in the area decreasing from year to year as immunity is acquired and the incidence among adults who come into contact with the virus through moving into infected areas. This yellow fever of young adult life in the cities gives many classical cases and *comprises the group of cases upon which, before the advent of viscerotomy and the mouse-protection test, almost all statements of incidence and epidemiology were based.*

The distribution by age and sex of fatal cases of rural yellow fever with aegypti and of jungle yellow fever is given in Table 6. It is apparent that there are not great differences in the age and sex distribution when the disease is transmitted by aegypti, but that in the case of jungle yellow fever, although the age distribution in the two sexes is similar, the number of cases among females is much smaller than that among males.

Although the first observation of yellow fever without aegypti under conditions permitting a definite diagnosis, did not occur until 1932, there are two descriptions of yellow fever from former times to be mentioned which, in the light of present knowledge, undoubtedly refer to yellow fever without aegypti.

The first description of this kind which has come to my notice is the report by Camó and Ortiz of an investigation made in 1887 among the Catholic missions along the foothills of the Andes south of Santa Cruz de la Sierra, Bolivia.

A description is given of cases observed at Abapó, El Espiño, Muchirí, and Masavi, in exactly the same region in which yellow fever without aegypti was encountered in 1935, which, considering the fact that the senior author was familiar with this infection as it occurred in Cuba, is convincing evidence that the disease seen by them was yellow fever. Yellow fever had never previously been reported for this entire region and was not to be again diagnosed here until 1935, although, as mentioned previously, cases had occurred in 1932 in Santa Cruz de la Sierra.

Quite naturally these early authors do not report on the presence or absence of aegypti in this region, since it was only some 13 years later that the transmission of yellow fever by this mosquito was first demonstrated. They realized that their diagnosis would be criticized and probably not accepted, as indeed it was not, since no reference to this report apparently reached the international literature until after the finding of yellow fever in Santa Cruz in 1932. To quote [in translation]: "Without doubt many authorities will be unwilling to admit the presence of yellow fever isolated in the heart of Bolivia far from the places in which yellow fever generally exists and without known routes of penetration from without." These words describe fittingly the difficulties of accepting the same diagnosis in this same area 45 years later. That this last outbreak should not have been entirely unexpected however is suggested by the fact that the 1887 epidemic was apparently not the first. To quote again [in translation]:

The older inhabitants state that Abapó was stricken some 20 years ago by a disease which presented these same symptoms and which Dr. José Lorenzo Sanchez, who was then in charge of the local parish, called yellow fever. Likewise this year it was a priest who announced the true name of this disease. The virtuous Señor Sarrazona, the priest of Abapó, who was to be one of the first to pay tribute to the scourge, styled it, as a good Spaniard would, Vómito Negro.

The second description is that by Franco, Martinez-Santamaria, and Toro-Villa of a mixed outbreak of relapsing fever and yellow fever at the emerald mines at Muzo, Colombia, in 1907.

The careful clinical observations then recorded do not permit any doubt that yellow fever was present and these authors left epidemiological notes which point conclusively to jungle yellow fever and which read as follows [in translation]:

a. It is contracted in the forest and not in the neighborhood of the houses.

b. It is transmitted by *Stegomyia calopus* and probably also by other culicines.

c. Inoculation takes place during the daylight hours, which are spent by the workers in places where the transmitting mosquitoes predominate.

Except for the statement that *"Stegomyia calopus"* (=*Aëdes aegypti*) was present, the description of yellow fever as given for Muzo in 1907 can stand as a true description of the jungle yellow fever observed in Muzo in 1934. That the classification of mosquitoes found at Muzo as *S. calopus* was a mistake is clearly indicated by the description of the habits of the mosquitoes encountered in 1907 and by the failure of numerous investigations there between 1916 and 1935 to reveal this mosquito.

In addition to these descriptions, there is the reference by Dr. Adolpho Lutz (1930) to two outbreaks many years before in São Paulo reputed to have occurred in the absence of aegypti.

The brief references of Lutz are very interesting since they describe so closely the conditions under which jungle yellow fever has been recently found and justify their quotation here [in translation]:

The first of these outbreaks, of which I know only from the reports of others, occurred in an Indian village on the Rio Verde. In the other case which I investigated personally, yellow fever was found in some huts built in the midst of the forest and inhabited by laborers. These men were clearing the forest in preparation for the construction of a railroad which was to join Funil to Campinas. I examined several huts from which had come cases of yellow fever, without finding any trace of the larvae or adults of *Stegomyia* (=*Aëdes aegypti*), although forest mosquitoes were present. This observation is especially interesting since it has lately been shown in Africa that transmission may occur through other mosquitoes than the domesticated stegomyia. This latter will always be among us the most important vector, and *the transmission by other species should be rare and exceptional,* but the determination of other species which may transmit the virus is nevertheless an interesting problem.

Unfortunately as shown by the observations presented here "the transmission by other species" is not as "rare and exceptional" as Dr. Lutz and all of us believed until recently.

The discussion of jungle yellow fever this evening has so far been limited to defining jungle yellow fever and describing actual outbreaks which have been observed in the past 3½ years—outbreaks all of which have been confirmed by examination of liver tissue removed at autopsy or by viscerotomy. This limitation, or rather this emphasis on the results of the examination of liver tissue, has been made because most authorities are as yet more ready to accept the evidence of such examinations than the evidence of immunity tests and isolation of the virus, rather than because these latter methods are any less reliable than is the examination of pathological material. However, there is already available a wealth of information from protection test surveys which not only confirms the data presented here tonight, but also greatly extends the limits of the known endemic region. The data presented here should, then, be considered not as a representation of what has happened during the period under consideration, but merely as what has been uncovered by comparatively inefficient methods of investigation, ably seconded in many cases by local officials and by chance.

Two years ago your attention was called to the possibility of the existence and transmission of yellow fever under natural conditions without *A. aegypti*; tonight data have been presented indicating the existence of a widespread jungle endemicity of yellow fever in the absence of this mosquito.

It is realized full well that the data so far available regarding jungle yellow fever raise more questions than they settle. It must be admitted that an enormous amount of work remains to be done before complete and satisfactory answers can be given to the following questions:

1. What are the component factors in the cycle or cycles which enable jungle yellow fever to continue in the absence of *A. aegypti* and a dense human population, both previously considered essential to yellow fever endemicity?

The answer to this first question can be reached only after much hard work has been done at many points and covering a wide variety of possible vertebrate hosts and invertebrate vectors. The possibilities of the existence of animal reservoirs of virus as distinguished from animal hosts subject to natural infection with the early development of specific immunity, and of long-lived invertebrate vectors with possible passage of virus from generation to generation, in contrast to such relatively short-lived temporary vectors as mosquitoes, must be considered.

Some of the accumulated evidence suggests that jungle yellow fever usually occurs in man as an accidental infection, secondary to an epizootic or enzootic in the lower animals, very much as human bubonic plague occurs secondary to plague in rats and other animals. Other data, such as that from Muzo, suggest a highly localized endemicity continuing over many years and the possibility of conservation of the virus in invertebrates similar to that demonstrated for Rocky Mountain spotted fever. If only a partial answer to the question stated above were required, very suggestive evidence might be presented for jungle yellow fever in man as secondary to yellow fever in monkeys with transmission by mosquitoes, especially *Aëdes scapularis, Haemagogus* spp., and various other jungle species of mosquitoes.

The arguments in favor of such an assumption are as follows: Jungle yellow fever has so far been observed only in districts where incomplete clearing of the jungle has occurred and where monkeys are present. A large number of the species of South American monkeys have been tested and practically all have been found susceptible to infection, with the development of demonstrable protective antibodies in the blood.

Although Dr. Davis found positive protection tests in a few monkeys bought in Bahia on ships coming from North Brazil, the results of tests made in 1935 on the sera of 15 monkeys of various species from the Museu Goeldi in Belém, and of about 50 monkeys also of various species bought in North Brazil, were all negative.

Similar tests, however, made on animals captured in zones admittedly infected with jungle yellow fever, produced very different results.

Monkeys, either shot or captured for the purpose of determining naturally acquired immunity, in Colombia, in Matto Grosso, and in Minas Geraes, have given some positive protection test results along with some to be expected negatives as shown in Table 8.

It is interesting to note that in Colombia and in Matto Grosso, where the few animals tested were obtained by colleagues of the Service themselves at places known to be infected, the monkeys were nearly all immune. The animals from Minas Geraes, which, on the contrary, were captured on a larger scale by persons residing in the infected area, indicate that an irregular distribution of immunity, similar to that found in man, may be expected among monkeys.

But this demonstration that some monkeys are naturally infected in the jungle does not necessarily prove that they are any more important than is man himself in the epidemiology of jungle yellow fever nor does it preclude the possibility of other and possibly more important animal hosts. Likewise, a high density of certain species of mosquitoes, even though proved capable of transmitting the virus, does not necessarily indicate that these mosquitoes have any part in maintaining permanent endemicity, but only suggests that they may be a factor in the temporary visible phase of yellow fever activity.

It should be recalled that the proof in 1900 of the transmission of yellow

Table 8. Results of Mouse Protection Tests with Sera from
Monkeys Captured in Colombia, Matto Grosso, and Minas Geraes

Captured in	Species	No. exam.	No. pos.
Restrepo, Intendencia de	*Callicebus ornatus*[a]	4	3
Meta, Colombia	*Saimiri sciureus*[a]	1	1
Planalto region of Matto Grosso, Brazil			
Ponte Alta	*Pseudocebus apella* (L.)[b]	1	1
Deputado	*Pseudocebus apella* (L.)[b]	1	1
Furriel	*Pseudocebus apella* (L.)[b]	3	3
Minas Geraes, Brazil			
Mun. Araguary (Vendinha)	*Hapale penicillata* (Goeffr.)[b]	2	0
Mun. Araguary, Faz. Patrona	*Pseudocebus apella* (L.)[b]	1	1
Mun. Campina Verde Faz. Rio Verde	*Pseudocebus apella* (L.)[b]	1	0
Mun. Patos (Capellinha de Chumbo)	*Pseudocebus apella* (L.)[b]	1	0
Mun. Patos, Faz. Alberto	*Pseudocebus apella* (L.)[b]	1	0
Mun. Patos, Faz. Bananal	*Pseudocebus apella* (L.)[b]	57	8
Mun. Patos. Faz. Pantano	*Pseudocebus apella* (L.)[b]	20	0
Total		93	18

[a]Identified in October 1935 by G. H. H. Tate, Assistant Curator of South American Mammals of the Department of Mammalogy of the American Museum of Natural History, New York.

[b]Identified by Prof. Alipio de Miranda Ribeiro, Chefe da Secção de Zoologia, Museu Nacional, Rio de Janeiro, Brazil.

fever from man to man by *A. aegypti* was regarded as a complete answer to the problem of yellow fever endemicity and was accepted as such for more than a quarter of a century; today we know that the answer was only a partial one and we should therefore not deceive ourselves by again being satisfied with an explanation which covers only a part of the problem which now faces us.

Existing conditions necessitate broad plans for studies which may lead to the complete solution to the problem. This solution cannot be obtained in the laboratory alone, by studies of the susceptibility of various animals to the yellow fever virus and of the transmitting capacity of certain hematophages; it will require also studies *in loco,* under natural conditions, at different places over long periods of time. Even then results, when positive, must not be accepted as eliminating other complementary possibilities.

2. Why does the widespread dissemination of jungle yellow fever not result in more frequent visible outbreaks and in the development of a high percentage of immunes in towns and cities with *A. aegypti* throughout the area of jungle endemicity?

Before the existence of jungle yellow fever was recognized, it was difficult to accept at their full value the positive results of protection tests from different parts of South America and Africa indicating that yellow fever had recently existed in certain districts in which it had either never been recognized or had not been recognized during the lifetime of some of those whose protection tests were positive.

The argument most frequently advanced against the possibility of permanent yellow fever endemicity in the Amazon Valley, before the conditions here related had been observed, was that if it had continued to exist in the region it would surely have appeared at least among foreigners coming into the valley and would have been recognized by clinicians familiar with the disease from the days of its endemicity. A similar argument has been advanced for Colombia, where it seemed impossible that yellow fever could have persisted in the valley of the Magdalena River, without making its appearance from time to time at some of the river ports where aegypti are abundant.

These apparently valid arguments, however, do not correspond to actual observations. In addition to the facts presented tonight, there are already available the results of a study of the distribution of immunity to yellow fever in the Amazon Valley which limited time does not permit me to place before you. These results prove clearly that the native population, far from the cities and the more civilized regions, is more exposed to yellow fever infection than are inhabitants of the large cities themselves. It can no longer be denied that yellow fever has been widespread for many years in many rural, fluvial, and jungle regions in South America, without the production of frequent urban outbreaks of the disease, although, as previously stated, the identity of jungle and urban yellow fever has been amply proved by clinical observation, by pathological and immunological evidence, and by a comparison of the behavior of jungle and urban strains of virus in laboratory animals.

Many experiments have been reported showing that a number of non-urban mosquitoes can transmit the urban virus, and more recent work has shown that aegypti can transmit the freshly isolated jungle virus. In addition, there are epidemiological observations strongly suggesting that certain outbreaks of urban yellow fever have been due to the introduction of virus from nearby jungle areas. The 1929 outbreak in Socorro, Colombia, an isolated town in the interior far from the coast and of difficult access from the exterior, is the only aegypti-transmitted outbreak of the disease observed in that country in 12 years. Jungle yellow fever has recently been shown to be endemic, however, in various parts of Colombia and even in the Magdalena Valley. It is difficult to avoid concluding that the Socorro outbreak had its origin in jungle yellow fever.

In the same year a suspect outbreak occurred at Guasipati and El Callao in the valley of the Cuyuni River in Venezuela. At the time, the health authorities were not convinced of the specific nature of this outbreak because of the isolation of these towns from all contact with suspect yellow fever areas, and the entire absence of suggestive cases in any of the towns on the Orinoco River, particularly Ciudad Bolívar, from which the region might most logically have been infected. Studies of immunity distribution by the protection test have confirmed the existence of yellow fever in Guasipati and El Callao during the past decade and the absence of the disease during recent years in Ciudad Bolívar and other Orinoco river towns. The infection of these isolated points, then, is logically attributed to the jungle.

Both jungle and urban yellow fever were observed in Bolivia in 1932–1933 and jungle yellow fever again in 1935, under conditions suggesting that the virus is interchangeable. Within the past few months, a most suggestive situation has developed in Theophilo Ottoni in the State of Minas Geraes. Theophilo Ottoni is a town of 8000 inhabitants lying in a rather heavily populated district of Minas which is somewhat isolated from contact with other sections of the state. In this connection it is interesting to note that the most usual practice in traveling from Bello Horizonte, the capital of Minas Geraes, to Theophilo Ottoni is to go along the seacoast via Rio de Janeiro and Caravellas and then inland. At the request of the State of Minas health authorities, the Yellow Fever Service investigated certain suspect cases in Theophilo Ottoni in 1931 but failed to find any reason for accepting the diagnosis of yellow fever. Protection tests done with sera collected in 1931, and again in March 1935, likewise failed to indicate that yellow fever had been of any great importance in the city in recent years: and viscerotomy during 1932, 1933, and 1934 gave no indication of yellow fever either in the city in question or in the area. In the meantime, effective anti-aegypti services had been organized in Caravellas and the other port towns which might have been considered as possible sources of urban virus for the infection of Theophilo Ottoni. In spite of these precautions, and in the absence of other observed outbreaks in the region, viscerotomy resulted in a positive diagnosis of yellow fever in Theophilo Ottoni in a case dying in May 1935, and investigation revealed an active aegypti-transmitted outbreak of recent development which was later confirmed clinically, by autopsy, by protection tests, and by animal inoculation. The evidence is very suggestive that this outbreak, the first in some 3 years in all Brazil, in which representatives of the Yellow Fever Service have had an opportunity to study a series of cases of urban aegypti-transmitted yellow fever had its origin in a jungle virus brought to town.

Admitting, then, that jungle yellow fever forms a constant threat to areas where the aegypti density is high, the culmination of this threat in frank urban outbreaks must depend on the operation of the usual laws of mathematical probabilities on the factors which permit of the urbanization of the jungle virus. In this connection it must be noted that even urban yellow fever, in which high concentrations of virus are built up in infected houses, so long as the supply of nonimmunes is adequate, through the fact that the sick generally spend the period of infectivity in direct contact with the transmitting agent, *A. aegypti,* a house mosquito, is often not highly explosive. Those who have come in contact with yellow fever only in the course of active epidemics in large centers of population with a high density of aegypti and a large percentage of nonimmunes, epidemics which have taken weeks or months to build themselves up to peak activity, often fail to realize that yellow fever can be a very slow moving and irregularly distributed disease, even when conditions appear to favor its spread. An active focus may be observed in a small town when careful investigation in nearby towns, with high aegypti indices, and intimate connection with the infected town, reveal no other centers of infection. A small section of a large city even may have an active focus and no cases be found in other parts of the same city. Yellow fever, then, is a disease which, except under ideal epidemic conditions, may be expected to spread very slowly.

As a jungle disease yellow fever attacks especially field workers and those coming in direct contact with the jungle. It would appear from observations in the field that there are no important domestic vectors in the jungle area and that the human case spending the infective stage of the disease in the house does not build up a concentration of virus in the house, nor, being out of contact with the jungle during this period, does he act as a source of virus for future human infections. It is believed that one of the most important factors in preventing the transfer of jungle yellow fever to the towns is the actual mechanical physical separation of jungle virus from the aegypti mosquito in the towns.

Although the yellow fever patient is often very sick from the onset, his first symptoms, really alarming symptoms required to spur the jungle or rural resident, accustomed more often than not to frequent malarial attacks, to seek medical attention in town, seldom occur earlier than the third day, which is generally considered the last day of infectivity for mosquitoes. Thus, by the time a case of jungle yellow fever is brought in for treatment, the danger of infecting aegypti in the town is generally past. It would appear that the occasional town resident traveling through infected jungle areas may be a greater potential danger for the infection of towns and cities than is the resident of such areas himself. This danger has been minimal in the past because until recently very few adults living in exposed towns were nonimmunes. With the freedom of the cities from yellow fever, however, this danger undoubtedly grows greater as the number of susceptible adults in urban districts increases.

The history of urban yellow fever in the past indicates that it has been by preference, except in a few of its largest centers of distribution, epidemic rather than endemic in character. The disease has shown a tendency to burn itself out in a town or even in a group of towns and not return until chance again brought the virus to the town after the development of a new group of nonimmunes. That many urban communities need constant and rather heavy bombardment with infective cases for the maintenance of endemicity is indicated by the disappearance of yellow fever from most of the towns and cities of the Caribbean region following the elimination of the disease in two endemic centers, Havana and Panama, a disappearance confirmed by results of protection tests in the younger generation.

Enough is not yet known regarding jungle yellow fever to permit drawing a final conclusion, but there is a suggestion that jungle yellow fever may be the more natural form of yellow fever endemicity and that urban aegypti-transmitted yellow fever has always been an exotic form maintained with more difficulty than is the jungle type.

3. What control methods can be used to best advantage in the prevention of jungle yellow fever: those directed to the reduction of vertebrate hosts, to the elimination of invertebrate vectors, or to the artificial immunization of the rural and jungle populations of endemic regions?

It is clear that the application of control methods to reduce the density of vertebrate hosts and invertebrate vectors cannot be considered until much more work has been done to determine the respective hosts and vectors of importance in the districts to be worked. If monkeys should prove to be the only vertebrate hosts of importance, biological studies may lead to some satisfactory method for their destruction in certain limited areas, their destruction throughout the endemic region being impossible so long as large areas of jungle remain. The cost of methods of control of invertebrate vectors, mosquitoes and others, will undoubtedly be prohibitive in most jungle areas. The most hopeful method of control would seem to be by individual vaccination. In 1931 it was shown that humans could be safely immunized by applying to them the technique of the protection test as developed in 1928, using, however, a neurotropic virus and known immune serum of a high titer. Extensive studies have been carried out since, and it is a pleasure to state that some of the major difficulties of mass vaccination against yellow fever have recently been overcome. A tissue culture virus has been developed with greatly decreased viscerotropic properties and with no increase in neurotropism. At the same time heterologous immune sera have been obtained of such high titers that only small amounts by volume need be used, thus facilitating application on a large scale. Field studies of vaccination with tissue culture virus and these sera are to be made, beginning in the immediate future. It is a pleasure to me to know that these first mass demonstrations with tissue culture virus can be made in Brazil.

When I had the honor two years ago of discussing the subject of yellow fever before this illustrious Academy, I stated it as my belief that the program of control and studies then under way "would lead either to the eradication of yellow fever from the country, or to a knowledge of the factors which render such elimination impracticable."

In the face of facts presented here tonight, I believe the most optimistic among us must agree that the idea of eliminating yellow fever from Brazil has no chance of immediate fulfillment. With the acceptance of this fact, we in no wise depreciate the work that has been done in the glorious campaigns of the past but rather again emphasize the necessity for the organization on a permanent basis of anti-aegypti services in all cities and towns of endemic areas to avoid the necessity for repetitions of such campaigns. There is no question of the necessity for maintaining antimosquito services for the protection of cities, and the time has come when the occurrence of cases of yellow fever due to transmission by *A. aegypti* should be considered as a public health crime reflecting on the competence of health authorities. If efficient control measures against aegypti are maintained in threatened areas, we may look forward to the complete disappearance of aegypti-transmitted yellow fever, which was, incidentally, the only type of the disease known when the program for its elimination was first evolved, and the development of a program of specific individual immunization may be expected to reduce the lamentable mortality due to jungle yellow fever, formerly attributed to malaria and unspecified malignant fevers.

Selection 23 | Yellow Fever: The Present
Situation (October 1938) with
Special Reference to South
America*

The *Annual Report of The Rockefeller Foundation for 1915* contained (pp. 68–72) the following paragraphs:

Prior to the work of Reed and the Army Commission in Havana, yellow fever was regarded as one of the great plagues. For more than 200 years the tropical and subtropical regions of America had been subject to devastating epidemics of the infection, while serious outbreaks had occurred as far north as Philadelphia and Boston and as far away from the endemic centres as Spain, France, England, and Italy.

Sanitarians hold that the endemic foci are the seed-beds of infection, and that if these seed-beds be destroyed the disease will disappear from all other points. Fortunately, these seed-beds are few in number. There are probably not more than five or six endemic foci all told, so that the problem of eradicating yellow fever reduces itself to the problem of stamping it out at these five or six points. The work done by General Gorgas at Havana and Panama, and by Oswaldo Cruz at Rio de Janeiro, has demonstrated that the disease can be exterminated in such endemic centres and has given grounds for the belief that its complete eradication is a feasible undertaking.

Such is the simple declaration of faith which was, for many years, to determine the program of The Rockefeller Foundation in collaborating with the nations of America in combating yellow fever. It was based on the belief that the virus of yellow fever was to be found only in man and in the *Aëdes aegypti* mosquito, neither of which could maintain the virus over long periods of time without the other. Epidemiologically the cycle of infection, *man–aegypti–man,* depends upon the aegypti mosquito feeding on a case of yellow fever during the first few days of illness, surviving 10

* The observations on which this report is based have been made by a large number of colleagues over a period of many years during which the International Health Division has collaborated with the health authorities of the South American countries concerned in the study and control of yellow fever. The observations in Brazil which form the bulk of this report have been made by the Serviço de Febre Amarella maintained jointly by the Ministry of Education and Health and The Rockefeller Foundation. Dr. Soper was the Representative in South America (Rio de Janeiro Office) of the International Health Division of The Rockefeller Foundation.

This article was originally published (*32*) in the *Transactions of the Royal Society of Tropical Medicine and Hygiene 32*: 297–332, 1938.

or 12 days, and then feeding on a nonimmune person. Since there are no human "carriers" of the virus and the aegypti mosquito is incapable of passing the virus through the egg from one generation to the next, the disease could be maintained only by an unbroken chain of human cases for which a considerable supply of nonimmunes was required. The number of nonimmunes needed to maintain the infection was to be found only in the large cities and in such smaller places as had a constant supply of travelers from nonendemic regions. The sanitation of Havana and Panama had resulted in the disappearance of the disease, not only from these two cities, but also from many other cities of the Gulf of Mexico and the Caribbean Sea; the cleaning of Santos, Rio de Janeiro, and Nichteroy had been followed by apparent freedom from yellow fever in all of South Brazil, and antimosquito campaigns in a few of the principal ports of the Amazon Valley had been sufficient to eliminate yellow fever from the statistics of this vast region.

And so it was that The Rockefeller Foundation became actively interested in the yellow fever problem and embarked on what was to have been a program of "complete eradication" of the disease. General Gorgas accepted the direction of the Yellow Fever Commission of the Foundation and personally conducted a reconnaissance of South America in 1916. This reconnaissance indicated that Guayaquil, on the Pacific coast, was the clearest example of an endemic seedbed still remaining on the continent and that there was no evidence of the existence of other endemic foci with the possible exceptions on the Atlantic coast of Salvador, Baía, and Recife, Pernambuco, Brazil.

The active participation of the Foundation in anti-yellow fever measures dates from late 1918, when work was begun in Guayaquil, Ecuador. The campaign in Guayaquil was followed by one in northern Peru in 1920 with the happy result that no cases of yellow fever have been recorded for the Pacific Coast of South America since 1921. (This record held until 1951 when an outbreak of jungle yellow fever occurred at Santo Domingo de los Colorados, Ecuador.) Apparently similar results were later obtained in Colombia, Mexico, and Central America and the *Annual Report of The Rockefeller Foundation for 1925* carried the following statement:

"During 1925 only three cases of yellow fever were reported from all the Americas. These occurred in North Brazil. It is not quite certain that all three were authentic. To one who knows something of the history of yellow fever, this record is striking."

However, in 1926, the movement of nonimmune troops through the interior of Northeast Brazil resulted in a flareup of the disease in several states. This outbreak was brought under control and the last half of the year 1927 was free of known cases. But the optimism of late 1927 and early 1928 was shattered by the discovery of cases in March and April in the states

of Sergipe and Pernambuco. In May came the entirely unexpected declaration of cases in the capital city of Rio de Janeiro, where the disease
had not been seen during 2 decades following the memorable campaign of
Oswaldo Cruz. Rio lies almost 1000 miles from the nearest point at which
cases had been observed during the previous 12 months and no satisfactory
explanation could be made at the time as to how the virus might have
reached the capital city without some trace of its passage having been observed.

The importance of large centers of population as sources of virus for the
infection of towns and ports is strikingly demonstrated by the events of
1929, when during the peak of the Rio outbreak, yellow fever was diagnosed on shipboard at various points along the coast from Buenos Aires to
Belém, Pará, and even up the Amazon River to Manáos, over a total distance of some 4000 miles. The disease was recorded from 42 places in the
State of Rio de Janeiro alone; and even in the state capitals in North
Brazil, where control measures were in operation, and where, for a considerable period of time, no cases had been observed, a few locally acquired
infections were seen. The density of aegypti in these northern capitals was
apparently sufficiently low to prevent the occasional infective case which
arrived from the surrounding endemic regions from giving rise to visible
outbreaks of yellow fever, but was not low enough to withstand the bombardment of virus from maritime contact with an infected coastline fed
by the Rio epidemic.

With the reorganization and intensification of antimosquito measures,
the Rio de Janeiro outbreak terminated in July 1929 and the last secondary
extensions of the disease attributed to it were brought under control in
May 1931. This date may well be taken as marking the end of the influence
of the large key-center seedbed of infection in maintaining and distributing the virus of yellow fever in the Americas up to the present time. Unfortunately there are still a number of cities in the Americas with such high
densities of aegypti breeding that the fortuitous introduction of the virus
of yellow fever might well lead to outbreaks, disastrous not only to these
cities themselves but to many others as well.

The events of 1928 and 1929 forced yellow fever workers to realize that,
although the sanitation of all the larger cities and ports of Brazil—which
might conceivably function as endemic seedbeds of infection—gave a striking reduction in the observed incidence of the disease, complete disappearance from tributary areas did not occur as it apparently had done in
other parts of the Americas where similar measures had been undertaken.
That this failure to disappear completely was not a characteristic of yellow
fever limited to Brazil was suggested by the occurrence in 1929 of two
widely separated outbreaks at isolated points in Colombia and Venezuela
having no possible connection with each other or with the Brazilian out-

breaks of the same year. Studies since 1930 have shown that there were two unknown epidemiological factors which doomed to failure the attempt to rid the continent of yellow fever by sanitation of the endemic seedbeds of infection:

1. Rural yellow fever transmitted by *Aëdes aegypti.*
2. Jungle yellow fever occurring in the absence of *Aëdes aegypti.*

Epidemiologically these two types of yellow fever are quite distinct and up to the present time have not been observed in the same geographical regions.

RURAL YELLOW FEVER TRANSMITTED BY *Aëdes aegypti*

The inconsiderate failure of yellow fever to disappear from Brazil in accord with the rules laid down by epidemiologists for its behavior led, in 1930, to a radical change in the plan of campaign. Since the elimination of yellow fever from the large endemic centers had not resulted in a spontaneous cleaning of the tributary areas, the campaign against the vector, *A. aegypti,* was to be extended to the smaller cities and towns of such tributary areas, working smaller and smaller towns and villages until the disease disappeared. The first extension of the program called for working all towns of 2000 population and over in those districts of Northeast Brazil, lying between the São Francisco and Parnahyba rivers, which had a definite history of previous outbreaks of yellow fever. It was felt that the cleaning of this region, long considered to be the last stronghold of endemicity on the American continent, was an essential preliminary step to more detailed studies of the Amazon region to the north and of South Brazil and Baía.

The introduction of viscerotomy and the routine microscopical examination of liver sections from persons dying after less than 10 days' illness soon showed that a considerable number of fatal cases were regularly occurring in the so-called "silent" endemic area of Northeast Brazil in the complete absence of "visible" outbreaks; and that this "silent" endemic area was much more extensive than had been indicated by the occurrence of previously reported outbreaks. At the same time viscerotomy dispelled, once and for all time, the myth that yellow fever is a mild disease in the children of endemic regions. Viscerotomy by its very nature is limited to the diagnosis of fatal infections; in Northeast Brazil viscerotomy revealed more cases in children under 5 years of age than among persons of any other age group.

It soon became apparent that the working of towns of 2000 population would not result in the elimination of yellow fever from Northeast Brazil, and smaller and smaller towns were worked with satisfactory results as far as the towns themselves were concerned. Viscerotomy, however, still continued to reveal fatal cases occurring in the rural regions where field investigation uncovered a most surprising and unusual distribution of *A. aegypti* in the rural homes, a type of distribution not yet found in any other part of South America. This rural distribution is attributable to the fact that the rainfall in the interior of Northeast Brazil is, in normal years, sharply limited to a few months and during periodic droughts entirely absent. Every family stores as much rainwater as possible to carry over the periods of shortage and thus aegypti everywhere finds suitable breeding conditions when fortuitously distributed by travelers and religious pilgrims who carry its eggs and larvae with them in their waterjars. It is improbable that such a rural distribution of aegypti would be capable of maintaining yellow fever endemicity were it not for the nomadic habits of the people, who move freely from place to place in times of drought and who make religious pilgrimages requiring weeks of travel on foot.

Only after it was apparent that measures limited to cities, towns and villages would not result, within a reasonable period, in the eradication of yellow fever from the interior of Northeast Brazil, was the antiaegypti service extended to the houses of a large rural area, including especially parts of Pernambuco and Ceará States. The results of antiaegypti measures in the rural areas were similar to those obtained in cities and towns and yellow fever rapidly disappeared from the regions worked. Since August 1934, during a period of 4 years, viscerotomy has failed to reveal the existence of yellow fever in Northeast Brazil. [This record still holds in 1969. *Ed.*] Apparently yellow fever in this region, comprising six states with a population of several million people, is entirely dependent on the association of man and the *A. aegypti* mosquito. [Part II of this book is devoted entirely to *Aëdes aegypti* and its role in the epidemiology of yellow fever *Ed.*]

Jungle Yellow Fever Occurring in the Absence of *Aëdes aegypti*

While the work in Northeast Brazil was suggesting that the complete eradication of yellow fever from South America could be accomplished by an extension of antiaegypti measures to small towns and to rural areas, discoveries elsewhere were proving the contrary.

The introduction of the mouse protection test for determining immunity was followed by field surveys which showed that yellow fever continued in the Upper Amazon reaches of Peru and Brazil and the region about Muzo in Colombia long after it had apparently disappeared. The observation in 1932 in the Vale do Canaan (written Valle do Chanaan in earlier papers), Espírito Santo, Brazil, quite outside the known endemic region, of a rural outbreak of yellow fever occurring in the complete absence of *A. aegypti* had led to the gradual unfolding of an unsuspected

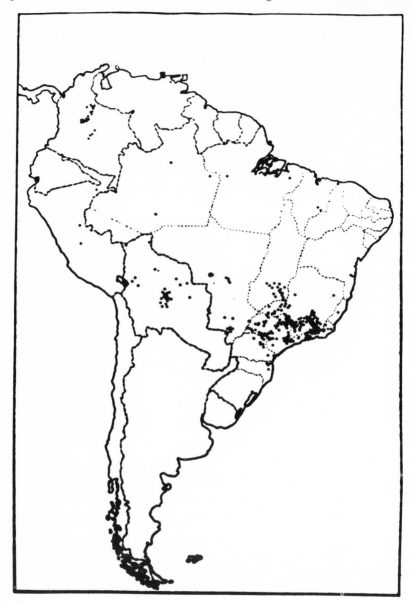

Map 1. South American localities where cases of jungle yellow fever have been diagnosed, 1932–1938.

phase of the epidemiology of yellow fever, a phase entirely out of keeping with all previously held beliefs. Today yellow fever is, in South America, primarily a jungle infection of which *A. aegypti* is not the vector and for the maintenance of which man is generally not an important source of

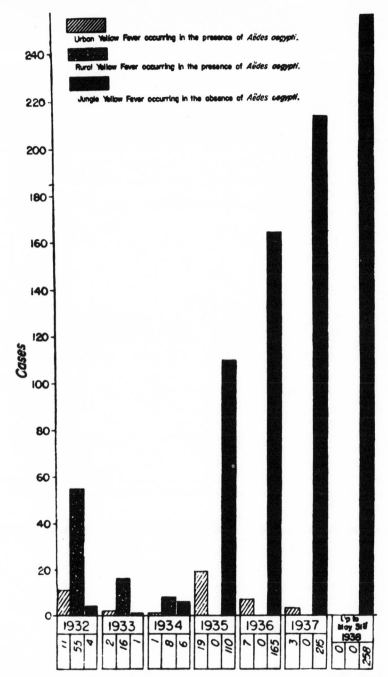

Graph 1. Confirmed cases of yellow fever in Brazil from January 1932 to May 1938.

virus. This jungle disease involves vast areas of the continent where yellow fever was previously never recognized as well as regions apparently free of yellow fever for many years (Map 1). Jungle yellow fever has been shown by viscerotomy to have occurred during the past 6 years in the Brazilian states of Amazonas, Pará, Maranhão, Baía, Espírito Santo, Minas Gerais, São Paulo, Rio de Janeiro, Paraná, Santa Catharina, Goiáz, and Mato Grosso; in Paraguay; in the departments of Santa Cruz, Cochabamba, Beni, and La Paz, Bolivia; in the departments of Junin and Loreto in Peru; and in the departments of Cundinamarca, Boyacá, Caldas, Antioquia, Santander, and the Intendencia de Meta in Colombia. The results of immunity surveys in Venezuela, Ecuador, British Guiana, Dutch Guiana, and Panama leave no doubt that these countries are also involved in the problem of jungle yellow fever.

In any discussion of jungle yellow fever, emphasis must be given to the fact that this term is one of epidemiological significance only. Clinically, pathologically, and immunologically, it has so far been impossible to differentiate jungle yellow fever from the classical aegypti-transmitted variety. Strains of virus isolated from jungle cases differ no more from strains isolated from urban cases than do these latter from each other. Jungle strains can be transmitted in the laboratory by *A. aegypti* just as the urban strains can be transmitted by various species of jungle mosquitoes found in Africa and others found in South America.

The way in which the jungle infection has come to dominate the epidemiological picture in Brazil is illustrated by Table 1 and Graph 1. (In considering the data it should be stated that in general, since 1932, only cases which have been definitely confirmed by viscerotomy, isolation of virus, or the repeated protection test are reported. The data of the table give no measure of the total mortality of yellow fever in the various years but only indicate how much fatal yellow fever came within the scope of activities of the Yellow Fever Service at a given time. Thus the figures for 1936 include, from the State of São Paulo, only 91 cases for which positive liver sections were received, although the state authorities have published reports indicating that about 1000 cases occurred with approxi-

Table 1. Urban, Rural, and Jungle Yellow Fever in Brazil from 1932 to May 1938[a]

Type of yellow fever	1932	1933	1934	1935	1936	1937	1938
Aegypti-transmitted							
Urban	11	2	1	19	7	3	0
Rural	55	16	8	0	0	0	0
Non-aegypti-transmitted							
Jungle	4	1	6	110	165	215	258
Total	70	19	15	129	172	218	258

[a]Since 1937 a single small urban aegypti-transmitted yellow fever outbreak has occurred in Brazil, at Sena Madureira. This was secondary to jungle yellow fever deep in the Amazon Valley.

mately 50 per cent mortality. Yellow fever statistics from regions covered by viscer-otomy should not be compared with those from regions where only the more serious outbreaks are recognized and reported.)

Field observations have, during the past 4 years, failed to indicate that any of the minor aegypti-transmitted outbreaks observed during this period had been due to a previous aegypti-transmitted outbreak, but have suggested in each instance that the town had been invaded by a virus from nearby jungle districts.

Were it not for the existence of the jungle infection yellow fever might have disappeared permanently from the Americas in 1934!

Although the clinical picture of yellow fever is the same whether the infection is acquired in the town or in the jungle, the epidemiology of the two types of yellow fever is quite different. Aegypti-transmitted yellow fever is generally acquired indoors, tends to involve all nonimmunes of all ages living in infected houses, and spreads from place to place along the routes of human travel. The disease is practically limited to man and is easily controlled by reduction of the density of the vector.

Jungle yellow fever, on the other hand, is usually acquired in or at the edge of the forest during working hours by those whose occupation takes them to the woods, and does not tend, in the absence of aegypti, to involve other members of the household living under the same roof with infective cases. Exceptions to this rule generally indicate that the other members of the household also visit the jungle or even that the house itself is in very intimate contact with the forest. The infection of man is apparently an accident occurring in the course of some cycle or cycles of infection in the jungle of which man is not an essential part. The infection apparently spreads throughout jungle areas without relation to routes of human travel. The only reasonable hope of prevention of human cases of jungle yellow fever is based on individual immunization of exposed populations, which has recently become possible on a large scale at a reasonable cost.

(The term "jungle" is not applied to yellow fever in the same sense that the term "selvatic" has recently been applied by some workers to plague. While it is theoretically possible that non-aegypti-transmitted yellow fever may occur quite away from the tropical and subtropical forest, or may be able, under special conditions, to maintain itself with man the only vertebrate host, such cases have not yet come under observation. The term "jungle yellow fever" is used to designate the non-aegypti-transmitted yellow fever occurring always in conjunction with uncleared land as observed in South America since 1932.)

A great deal of work remains to be done before the factors responsible for maintaining the jungle infection can be definitely known. Recent work has resulted in the capture of three species of mosquitoes, *Aëdes leuco-celaenus, Haemagogus capricorni,* and one of the sabethines naturally infected in the woods; and there is a great deal of accumulated evidence, both scientific and hearsay, indicating that monkeys are infected in the jungle and that certain species, notably the howlers (*Alouatta* spp.), die in large numbers at the time human infections are occurring in the forest. It is difficult, however, to fit all observed facts into any simple *mosquito-*

monkey–mosquito cycle of infection and the search is continuing for other factors. Jungle yellow fever occurs under such a wide variety of natural conditions that it seems unreasonable to anticipate finding a single set of factors operative throughout.

Although observations indicate that jungle yellow fever may be permanently endemic in a region such as the Muzo district in the Magdalena Valley of Colombia, where it has been frequently reported during the past 30 years, it has appeared during the past 5 years in South Brazil as a surprisingly severe epidemic wave, spreading apparently from infected regions to noninfected contiguous districts, in a series of annual spurts corresponding roughly to the summer seasons, apparently disappearing during 5 or 6 months of the cool, dry season, only to reappear in nearby areas the next hot season. Such epidemic waves, involving some of the richest and most heavily populated districts of Brazil, emphasize the fact that jungle yellow fever is important, not only as a source of virus for the infection of cities and towns infested with aegypti, but also as a serious public health problem in its own right.

Throughout the epidemic year, July 1, 1933, to June 30, 1934, yellow fever was recognized (Map 2) at only two points reasonably accessible to

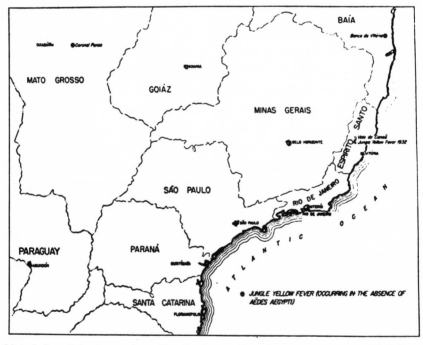

Map 2. Localities in southern Brazil where yellow fever cases were notified from July 1, 1933, to June 30, 1934.

South Brazil: Banco da Victoria, Baía, and Coronel Ponce, Mato Grosso. In both instances the infection was found in the jungle more than 2 years after the last recognized outbreak of yellow fever in South Brazil—that occurring in the Vale do Canaan, Espírito Santo, in 1932. Coronel Ponce is a very isolated point and the discovery of yellow fever there came at a time when the Yellow Fever Service was devoting most of its energies to other parts of the country. Viscerotomy had not yet been organized in Mato Grosso, Goiáz, São Paulo, or the western part of Minas Gerais, and in the light of later events it seems probable that the 1934 outbreak must have been much more extensive than was ever known. A child in a mission school close to Cuiabá, Mato Grosso, received a letter from his mother in Rio Verde in southwestern Goiáz in 1934, telling of a strange disease with symptoms similar to those of yellow fever which had appeared in that district. An investigation of Goiáz begun in December 1934 resulted in finding yellow fever at Itaberaí (Map 3) in January 1935, and a hurriedly organized viscerotomy service revealed the presence of the disease throughout southeastern Goiáz, western Minas Gerais, and even within the borders of the State of São Paulo. It is interesting to note that southwestern Goiáz and the section of Mato Grosso lying directly west of it were not found to be infected in 1935 or in succeeding years. It may well be that the epidemic

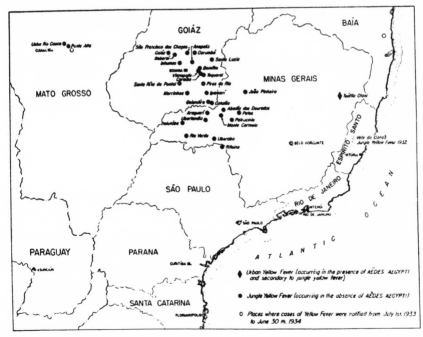

Map 3. Localities in southern Brazil where yellow fever cases were notified from July 1, 1934 to June 30, 1935.

wave had passed through parts of this region in 1934, as suggested by the letter from Rio Verde mentioned above. The year 1935 was also marked by an urban aegypti-transmitted outbreak of yellow fever at Teófilo Otoni for which the source of infection was not found.

In 1936 (Map 4) jungle yellow fever was widespread throughout much of São Paulo State and contiguous areas of the states of Minas Gerais and Paraná. The disease was also shown to be present in southern Mato Grosso and to continue near the points found infected in 1934: Coronel Ponce, Mato Grosso, and Banco de Victoria, Baía. Urban cases occurring in the presence of aegypti were found at Campo Grande, Mato Grosso; at Cambará, Paraná; and at Figueira, Minas Gerais. The outbreak at Cambará was clearly traced to the introduction of the virus by a case infected in the jungle. The origin of the virus for the production of the single case found at Campo Grande and of the outbreak at Figueira could not be traced, although the possibility of Teófilo Otoni having infected Figueira could be pretty definitely excluded.

In 1937 (Map 5) jungle yellow fever failed to reappear at most of the points in São Paulo visited in 1936 but did invade untouched regions, including some of the most heavily populated rural districts, and came very close to the city of São Paulo, with a population of 1,000,000.

Outside the State of São Paulo, which had dominated the picture in 1936, 3 important and threatening extensions of jungle yellow fever occurred in 1937, one toward the south in Mato Grosso, involving northern Paraguay, a second also to the south, along the coastal area of Paraná and Santa Catharina, and a third eastward through southern Minas Gerais. In passing, it should be noted that the infection continued in the region of Coronel Ponce and that jungle yellow fever was found for the first time at Teófilo Otoni. The latter finding is interpreted as giving a reasonable basis for believing that the previous outbreaks in both Teófilo Otoni and Figueira were probably due to introductions of jungle virus, although it must be admitted that logically the reverse interpretation is possible.

During the 1938 epidemic season (July 1, 1937, to June 30, 1938) yellow fever has followed up each of the three threats of the previous season (Map 6). The southern coastal area of Brazil was not so fortunate and serious outbreaks occurred among the German colonists of this region with numerous fatal cases. But even this region was fortunate in comparison with those portions of Minas Gerais and Rio de Janeiro which were involved in the eastward sweep of the disease this year, lying roughly between the cities of Rio de Janeiro and Bello Horizonte.

It is a matter of great satisfaction to those responsible for the organization of antiaegypti measures in Brazil that no cases of aegypti-transmitted yellow fever were encountered during the 1938 Minas Gerais–Rio de Janeiro outbreak. Four cases, 3 of which were fatal, are known to have

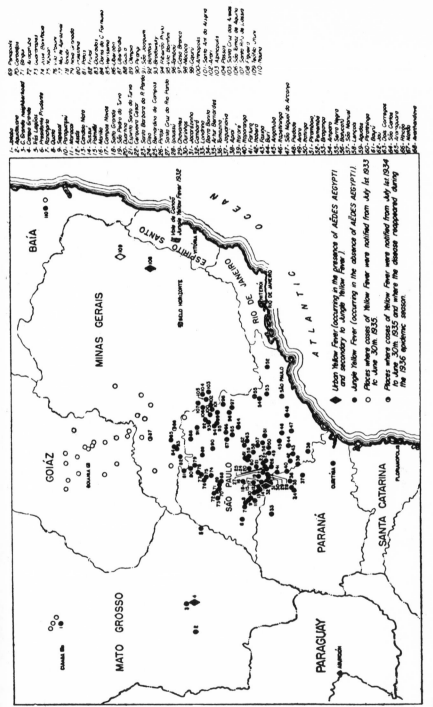

Map 4. Localities in southern Brazil where yellow fever cases were notified from July 1, 1935, to June 30, 1936.

203

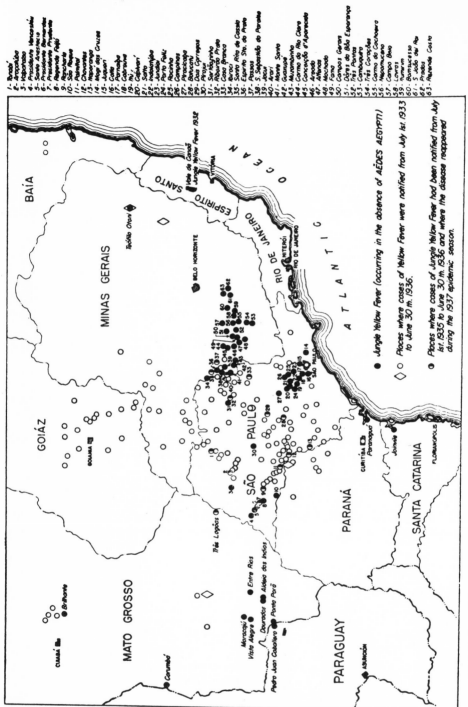

1.- Turabá
2.- Arapoabá
3.- Itapororoca
4.- Presidente Venceslau
5.- Santo Anastacio
6.- Presidente Bernardes
7.- Presidente Prudente
8.- Regente Feijó
9.- Pirapó
10.- São Paulo
11.- Piratininga
12.- Chavantes
13.- Piraçununga
14.- Rios das Cruzes
15.- Avaré
16.- Gália
17.- Piratuba
18.- Cabreúva
19.- Iri
20.- Cabreúva
21.- Sarto
22.- Indaiatuba
23.- Jundiai
24.- Porto Feliz
25.- Rocinha
26.- Campinas
27.- Piraçununga
28.- Boituva
29.- Dois Córregos
30.- Pirajú
31.- Serrinho
32.- Ribeirão Preto
33.- Casa Branca
34.- Buricá
35.- Santa Rita do Passo
36.- Espirito Sto. do Pinto
37.- Pirassununga
38.- S. Sebastião do Paraíso
39.- Jacui
40.- Arari
41.- Monte Santo
42.- Guaçuí
43.- Guaxupé
44.- Muzambinho
45.- Carmo do Rio Claro
46.- Conceição d'Aparecida
47.- Arpoá
48.- Aliança
49.- Machado
50.- Poços de Caldas
51.- Campos Gerais
52.- Três Pontas
53.- Obras de Bôa Esperança
54.- Três Corações
55.- Carmo do Cachoeiro
56.- Cambuquira
57.- Mecanucano
58.- Campo Belo
59.- Lavras
60.- Nunnim
61.- Bomsucesso
62.- S. João del Rei
63.- Prados
64.- Piranha Casta

Map 5. Localities in southern Brazil and Paraguay where yellow fever cases were notified from July 1, 1936, to June 30, 1937.

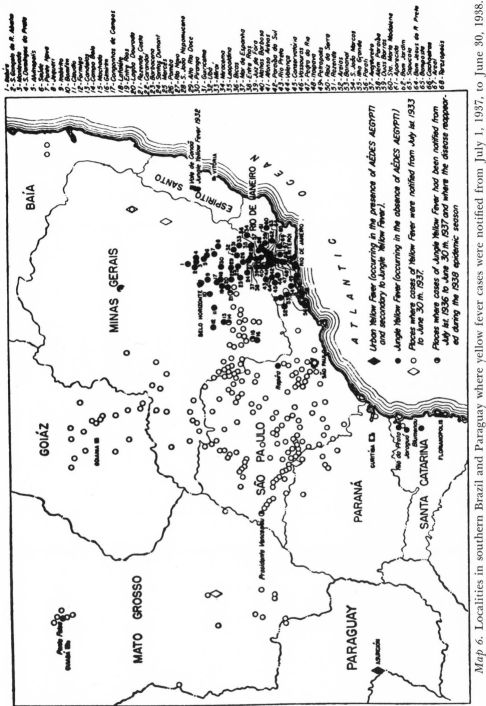

1 - Matão
2 - S. Simpão de R. Aberto
3 - Monlevade
4 - Conselheiro da Preto
5 - Alvinopolis
6 - Salde
7 - Ponte Nova
8 - Aveporé
9 - Indiúma
10 - Guarini
11 - Canela
12 - Gorunga
13 - Campo Belo
14 - Campo Belo
15 - Machado
16 - Guarini
17 - Conquistas de Campos
18 - Lindéira
19 - Entre Rios
20 - Lago Dourada
21 - Rezende Costa
22 - Carandaí
23 - Barbacena
24 - Santos Dumont
25 - Matosinhos
26 - Mercês
27 - Rio Novo
28 - S. João Nepomuceno
29 - Alto Rio Doce
30 - Piranga
31 - Guaricema
32 - Ubá
33 - Mira
34 - Maracena
35 - Leopoldina
36 - Bicas
37 - Mar de Espanha
38 - Entre Rios
39 - São Luiz Borba
40 - Mira Barbosa
41 - Afonso Arinos
42 - Paraiba do Sul
43 - Rio Preto
44 - Valença
45 - Conservatória
46 - Vassouras
47 - Pedro do Rio
48 - Itaipava
49 - Petropolis
50 - Reu do Serra
51 - Rezende
52 - Areias
53 - S. Marcos
54 - S. José dos Marcos
55 - Parati
56 - Bragantina
57 - Além Paraiba
58 - Duas Barras
59 - Sto. Maria Madalena
60 - Aparecido
61 - Bom Jardim
62 - Espacial
63 - Bom Jesus do R. Preto
64 - Bom Jesus do R Preto
65 - Casmbuco
66 - Carangola
67 - Araji
68 - Teresopolis

Map 6. Localities in southern Brazil and Paraguay where yellow fever cases were notified from July 1, 1937, to June 30, 1938.

205

come to the capital city either before onset or during the period of infectivity without giving rise to secondary cases. The observation of these cases suggests that the previously unexplained invasion of Rio de Janeiro which resulted in the 1928–1929 epidemic may well have been due to the introduction of the yellow fever virus by cases infected in nearby jungle areas.

And so we come to the 1939 yellow fever season with the double threat of a continued extension to the south along the coast in Santa Catharina and possibly Rio Grande do Sul and of further extensions in Rio de Janeiro, Espírito Santo, and eastern Minas Gerais.

Yellow Fever Campaign in Brazil

In Brazil, which is somewhat larger in land area than the continental United States, there is a wide variety of conditions influencing the epidemiology of yellow fever, including
1. Cities in the tropics suited to permanent endemicity.
2. Cities in the temperate zone suited to summer epidemics.
3. Rural regions suited to aegypti-transmitted endemicity.
4. Rural and jungle regions in both the tropics and the temperate zone suited to epidemics of jungle yellow fever as well as permanent endemicity.

In spite of this diversity of conditions, the yellow fever campaign in Brazil is based primarily on three factors: viscerotomy, antiaegypti measures, and vaccination. During the past 8 years no provision has been made for (1) quarantine, (2) medical surveillance, (3) fumigation, or (4) isolation of cases. No evidence has been found that any of these traditional methods would have prevented the occurrence of any observed outbreaks.

Viscerotomy

Some will immediately question the inclusion of viscerotomy as a control measure but, since it is essential to know when and where yellow fever is occurring in order to combat it successfully, viscerotomy must be considered a basic part of yellow fever control. Much valuable information regarding the past distribution of yellow fever can be secured from properly interpreted immunity surveys, but positive findings of such surveys are limited to surviving or *nonfatal cases,* which are not highly useful in convincing responsible authorities to spend the funds required for the organization of antiaegypti services and for the manufacture and mass application of vaccine in endemic regions. Viscerotomy, as the term is used by the Yellow Fever Service in Brazil, means much more than the etymology of the word indicates. Viscerotomy refers to the routine postmortem removal of liver tissue for microscopical examination from the bodies of all persons dying less than 11 days after onset of any febrile illness, irrespective of the clinical diagnosis. Most viscerotomists in Brazil are part-time local representatives, generally not doctors, who are paid according to the number of specimens collected. The Viscerotomy Service in Brazil has collected material from more than 140,000 bodies since 1930. The distribution of representatives authorized to collect material during the first quarter of 1938 is shown in Map 7. It is fully recognized that viscerotomy in many rural areas is very deficient and that many fatal cases of yellow fever escape detection each year. Even so, viscerotomy has been the most important factor in the recognition of yellow fever in South America in recent years. [Part III of this book is devoted entirely to the subject of viscerotomy. *Ed.*]

Antiaegypti Measures

Emphasis should be given to the fact that the region of South Brazil which has been discussed was supposedly free of yellow fever from 1908 to 1928 except for an outbreak in Victoria, Espírito Santo, in 1917, and that

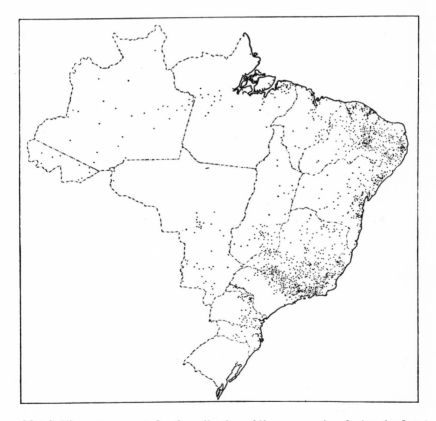

Map 7. Viscerotomy posts for the collection of livers operating during the first quarter of 1938 in Brazil.

the urban yellow fever outbreaks of 1928 to 1931 completely disappeared in the face of antiaegypti campaigns. The necessity of organizing antiaegypti and viscerotomy services in South Brazil threw a great additional burden on the budget of the Brazilian Yellow Fever Service which could be carried only because of improvement and simplification of the antiaegypti work. In 1933, it was observed that the aegypti mosquito had practically disappeared from many of the cities of North Brazil where for years it had been impossible to reduce the house-breeding index of this mosquito below 1 to 2 per cent. The zero indices obtained are attributed to a combination of factors, including the routine application of fuel oil to all larval foci and the use of special squads to search out and destroy the difficult residual breeding foci missed by the regular inspectors week after week. The search for the adult aegypti mosquito has proved to be the most sensitive indicator of the existence and location of residual foci. Once the aegypti index has been brought to zero, it has been found possible to lengthen the cycle of house inspections from 1 week to 2, 3, or 4 weeks, and in many places discontinue routine larval inspections completely. Experience has shown that a quarterly visit of adult capture squads is sufficient to indicate when and where services which have been discontinued should be renewed. The distribution of cities, towns, and villages in which the aegypti mosquito was under control during the first quarter of 1938 is shown in Map 8.

Vaccination

Field vaccination for the control of jungle yellow fever was carried out early in 1936 with a cultured virus and hyperimmune animal serum, but was eventually abandoned because of a number of unpleasant results, including a considerable number of cases of delayed hepatitis of the type first observed and described by Findlay and MacCallum. During the epidemic season of 1937, field vaccination was not attempted but was begun at the end of the season in June, after careful observations on a series of persons vaccinated in the New York and Rio de Janeiro laboratories had indicated that a strain of virus developed in the laboratory of the International Health Division of The Rockefeller Foundation in New York could safely be used without an accompanying injection of immune serum. This strain of virus, known as 17D, has lost much of both its viscerotropic and neurotropic properties, apparently as the result of growth during many passages on chick embryo tissue, from which both brain and spinal cord have been removed. The field work with virus 17D (Map 9) began with a single unit in a region where cases had been occurring a few weeks previously. After some 3000 persons had been inoculated, additional units were placed in the field and the mass vaccination of rural populations in threatened areas undertaken. With the onset of the active yellow fever season in 1938, units were

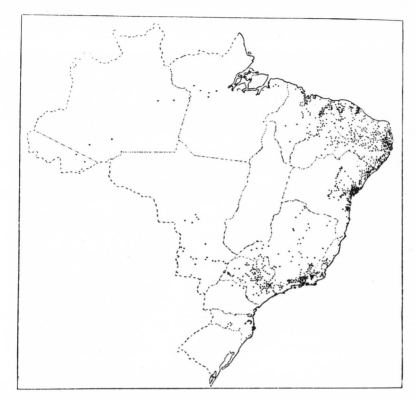

Map 8. Places in which antilarval and adult mosquito capture services were in operation during the first quarter of 1938 in Brazil.

shifted to known infected districts in São Paulo, Minas Gerais, Rio de Janeiro, and Santa Catharina (Map 10). The demand for vaccine exceeded all expectations and a special budget of 2000 contos (over $100,000 U.S.) was granted by the Brazilian Government for a program calling for the vaccination of 1,000,000 persons during 1938.

Both epidemiologically and from the standpoint of laboratory tests for immunity, vaccination has been highly satisfactory. Where vaccination has been carried out in the presence of active outbreaks of the disease, cases have been observed with onset up to 4 or 5 days after vaccination, but by the end of 1 week no further cases appear, although demonstrable antibodies are generally not to be found in the blood of vaccinated persons at this time. Laboratory tests 3 to 4 weeks after vaccination indicate that over 90 per cent of persons receiving living virus have developed demonstrable antibodies. The average duration of postvaccination immunity remains to be determined before any definite program of vaccination and revaccina-

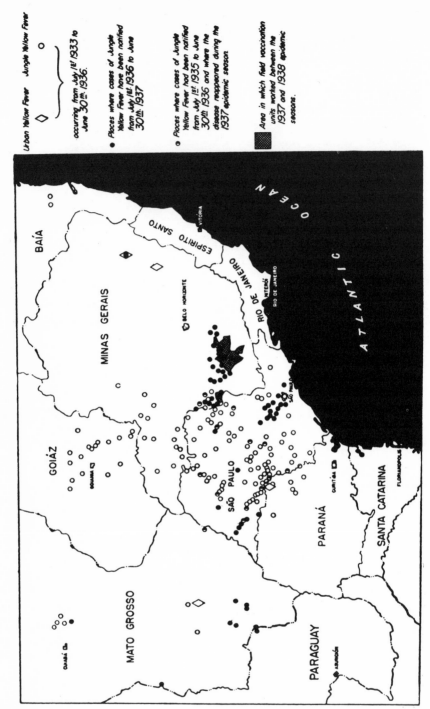

Map 9. Distribution of field vaccination in Brazil in relation to known occurrence of yellow fever (between 1937 and 1938 epidemic seasons).

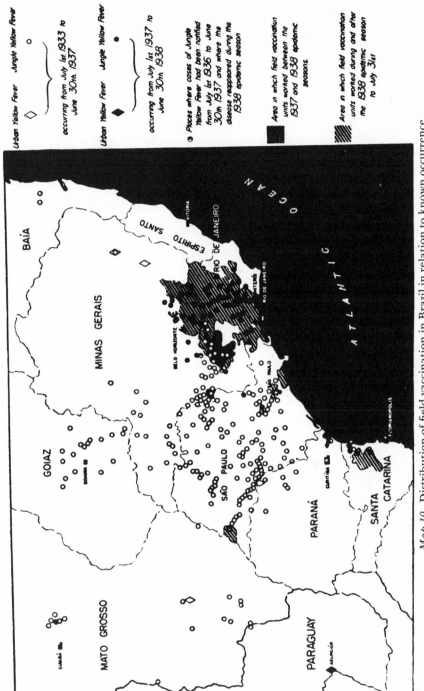

Map 10. Distribution of field vaccination in Brazil in relation to known occurrence of yellow fever (during and after 1938 epidemic season to July 31).

211

tion can be drawn up. In Brazil, field vaccination has largely been used in rural districts to protect against imminent danger and the problem of revaccination has not arisen. Fortunately reactions to the vaccine virus are so mild as to cause no serious difficulty in its acceptance by the people. Extremely gratifying has been the complete absence of postvaccination hepatitis since the introduction of virus 17D in February 1937. [See Selection 27 in Part VI regarding the subsequent occurrence of postvaccination hepatitis in Brazil. *Ed.*] No contraindications to the use of virus 17D have been found and early restrictions have been removed, even very young infants and women in all stages of pregnancy now being routinely vaccinated. Fears have been expressed that virus 17D might regain its virulence by repeated mosquito passage through nonimmunes of virus picked up from vaccinated persons. These fears have been shown to be ungrounded.

An airmail letter just received from Dr. D. B. Wilson, Rio de Janeiro, states that the number of vaccinations in 1938 had passed the 800,000 mark on October 1. The million mark will easily be reached well before the end of the year at a per capita cost of probably between 8 and 9 cents U.S.

Brazil has led the way in accepting yellow fever as a permanent national problem and today possesses a far-flung viscerotomy service to indicate where the disease exists at all times, a widespread antiaegypti service covering all the more important cities, towns, and villages throughout endemic regions, a laboratory capable of producing well over 1 million doses of vaccine yearly and field vaccination units to apply this vaccine where most needed. Colombia, a somewhat smaller country, is proportionally not far behind Brazil, and great interest is being shown in the permanent control of yellow fever in Venezuela, Peru, Bolivia, Ecuador, and Paraguay.

In closing, may I quote once more from the *Annual Report of The Rockefeller Foundation for 1915?*

Great anxiety is felt throughout the Far East on account of the possibility of the introduction of yellow fever into that region as a result of the opening of the Panama Canal. The canal has wrought radical changes in trade relations. Countries and ports between which there had been little or no exchange have been brought into close relation. Pest holes of infection that have been relatively harmless because of their isolation are now on or near the world's highway of commerce and travel. As early as 1903, Manson called attention to the grave risk of conveying infection to the Far East as a result of the opening of the Canal. Dr. S. P. James, of the Indian Medical Service, who was employed by his Government to make a thorough investigation of the subject, reports that the menace is sufficiently great to call for a permanent quarantine force to be maintained in Panama, Hongkong or Singapore, at the expense of the English colonies in the East, and recommends to the Indian Government a systematic attack on the *Stegomyia* mosquito. It is recognized by sanitarians that if the infection should once be introduced into the Orient, with its dense population of non-immunes, the ill resulting from it would be incalculable.

The threat of the Panama Canal to the Pacific and to the Orient has not materialized, probably because the Canal Zone and the adjacent cities have been kept free of the disease. The development of air traffic, however, has conjured up another and possibly more serious threat to India and the Orient from another direction, the endemic regions of Africa, which have been shown to be much more extensive than was previously known. The immediate threat to the Orient can now be handled by vaccination of all crews and passengers of airplanes some days before leaving endemic regions. The more difficult problem to solve is the prevention of an extension of yellow fever from Central Africa to the ports of East Africa from which ports the virus might readily be carried by ships to the Orient.

A consideration of this problem may well lead to a program similar to that of Brazil:

1. Viscerotomy to disclose the actual distribution of yellow fever and to give a measure of its importance as a cause of death among the natives.

2. Antiaegypti measures:

a. In the principal cities of endemic regions, not only for the protection of the local population, but also to prevent the building up of large reserves of virus in the human population, since such reserves are highly explosive epidemiologically.

b. In the principal cities and ports of threatened regions.

3. Vaccination of

a. Travelers.

b. Populations exposed to jungle yellow fever.

c. Populations of towns where for one reason or another antiaegypti measures cannot be carried out.

SUMMARY

The Rockefeller Foundation embarked, in 1915, on a program of eradicating yellow fever from the Americas, by collaborating in the organization of anti-*Aëdes aegypti* measures in the few remaining seedbeds of infection. This program apparently gave expected results for many years in various countries but failed to eradicate yellow fever from Brazil, where two previously unrecognized epidemiological types, rural yellow fever transmitted by *A. aegypti* and jungle yellow fever occurring in the absence of this mosquito, were found to be responsible for maintaining nonurban endemicity. The problem of rural aegypti-transmitted yellow fever has been solved by extension of antiaegypti measures to the rural areas of Northeast Brazil, the only region in South America where this type has been found.

Jungle yellow fever is not limited to Brazil, but also occurs in Paraguay, Bolivia, Peru, and Colombia and almost surely in Ecuador, Venezuela, Panama, British Guiana, and Dutch Guiana.

Jungle yellow fever has been observed in South Brazil as a wavelike phenomenon involving many of Brazil's richest districts in the years 1934 to 1938.

The control of yellow fever in Brazil is based on viscerotomy, antiaegypti measures, and vaccination.

As a result of viscerotomy over 140,000 liver tissues have been examined for lesions of yellow fever since 1930. Costs of antiaegypti measures have been greatly reduced in recent years. Over 800,000 persons have been vaccinated during the first 9 months of 1938 with satisfactory results and without serious complications of any kind.

The threat of extension of yellow fever from present endemic regions of Africa to the ports of East Africa and to the Orient is sufficiently important to call for a consideration of viscerotomy, antiaegypti measures, and vaccination to meet it.

[See Part VIII, Selection 31, for a brief account of the major outbreaks of jungle yellow fever in the Americas from 1939 to 1951. *Ed.*]

The 1964 Status of *Aëdes aegypti*
Eradication and Yellow Fever in
the Americas*

During the first 9 months of 1964 the total of but 84 cases of yellow fever has been reported from the Western Hemisphere. These come from the following countries: Bolivia, 13; Brazil, 6; Colombia, 9; Peru, 54; and Venezuela, 2.

This small number of cases reported from five countries, each of which probably harbors the yellow fever virus continuously, has little relationship to the actual occurrence of yellow fever. While jungle yellow fever may occur in relatively heavily populated and accessible areas, its permanent haunts tend to be isolated and relatively inaccessible. Medical care is often completely lacking and persons sick enough to seek a doctor are too sick to be moved. Yellow fever is generally reported only by microscopic examination of liver tissue removed by viscerotomy after death. Thus, for various reasons, what is reported of yellow fever is but a fraction of the reality.

To evaluate present findings, one should look at yellow fever over the past 30 years. Although there are points such as Ilheós in Brazil, and Muzo and San Vicente de Chucurí in Colombia, where yellow fever virus seems to maintain itself indefinitely, in general yellow fever occurs as an acute self-limited infection of vertebrates moving in smaller or greater cycles of wave-like infection in susceptible populations.

Geographically, we can think roughly of great pools of virus moving rather freely from place to place in the Orinoco, Magdalena, and Amazon Valleys of Venezuela, Colombia, Ecuador, Brazil, Bolivia, and Peru. From these pools we see, from time to time, pseudopodic extensions of virus infiltrating both to the south and to the northwest. The southern epizootic extension may involve the southern part of Mato Grosso, Goias, Minas Gerais, São Paulo, Paraná, Santa Catarina, Rio Grande do Sul, Rio de Janeiro, and Espírito Santo in Brazil; eastern Paraguay; and the Province of Misiones in Argentina. The northwestern extension involves Panama,

---

* Read by J. Austin Kerr at the Symposium on the Eradication of *Aëdes aegypti* in the United States at the Annual Meeting of the American Society of Tropical Medicine and Hygiene, New York, November 5, 1964. Dr. Soper was a Special Consultant, Office of International Health, Public Health Service.

This article was originally published *(113)* in the *American Journal of Tropical Medicine and Hygiene 14:* 887–891, 1965. This short excerpt summarizes the known extent of jungle yellow fever in South and Central America in the 1960s, three decades after it was first recognized there.

Costa Rica, Nicaragua, Honduras, Guatemala, British Honduras, and Mexico.

Historically, yellow fever is known to have been in Central America and Mexico in the period 1918–1924; there is, however, no convincing evidence of it here between that period and 1948. Between 1948 and 1958, yellow fever moved from east of the Panama Canal to all these countries except El Salvador. (In 1956, yellow fever moved up to the Canal Zone but failed to penetrate western Panama, Central America, and Mexico.)

Direct extension of yellow fever to the south from the Amazon Valley to the valleys of the Paraguay and Paraná rivers was first observed during the period 1934–1940. Further invasions of varying extent, never so widespread as the first, have occurred beginning in 1944, 1951, and 1956.

Even with the small number of cases recorded this year, we know that yellow fever virus is present on both sides of the river in the Magdalena Valley and on the eastern slope of the Andes in Colombia, in the lower Orinoco Valley not far from its mouth in Venezuela, and on the eastern slopes of the Andes mountains in Peru and Bolivia, with extension out on the lowlands to the area about Santa Cruz in Bolivia.

In Brazil, with its vast infectable and known infected areas, only six cases have been diagnosed in 1964. These six cases, by their strategic location, show that yellow fever virus is on the march once more from the southern reaches of the Amazon Valley down into the Paraguay and Paraná valleys of southern Brazil in the states of Mato Grosso and Goias. Yellow fever virus is again following the traditional route of invasion followed repeatedly since the early 1930s. The health officers of southern Brazil, Paraguay, and Argentina should be on the alert and should get their exposed populations vaccinated immediately. Fortunately, this entire region of the South American continent is free of *Aëdes aegypti*; hence no risk of urban outbreaks exists.

[As predicted, yellow fever did invade the states of Paraná and Rio Grande do Sul, and the provinces of Misiones and Corrientes, Argentina, in 1965 and 1966. In spite of advance warning, vaccination was intensified only after fatal yellow fever was diagnosed in the area. *Ed.*]

Part VI | Yellow Fever Vaccines and Field Studies
of Vaccination

| Vaccination Against Yellow Fever
in Brazil, 1930–1937*

Two years ago when I presented to this learned Academy the results of
the observations regarding jungle yellow fever, I referred to the possibility
of preventing the disease by means of vaccination. I said at that time that a
modified form of the virus, obtained by means of tissue culture, exhibited
greatly reduced viscerotropism without any increased neurotropism. I
stated also that heterologous immune sera had been obtained with such
high titers of antibody that it was possible to use them in very small quantities, thus facilitating vaccination with serum plus virus on a scale that
previously was not possible. I went on to say that the investigations regarding the feasibility of an intensive vaccination program with the tissue
culture virus referred to above, plus the sera just mentioned, would be
undertaken in Brazil within a few weeks.

At this time I am greatly pleased to be given the honor to present once
more to this illustrious Academy the conclusions drawn from these observations, as well as the preliminary results obtained with another strain of
virus which has been modified in tissue culture to the point at which its
neurotropic and viscerotropic qualities are so greatly attenuated that it can
be used as a vaccine without the concomitant administration of immune
serum.

Before going on I must emphasize that this lecture, as were the two
previous ones I had the honor of making in this hall, is based on the work
of many dedicated colleagues, who are doing their utmost to solve the
problems of yellow fever, a disease of such great importance to mankind.

Having discussed in my two previous communications to this Academy
the studies carried out by the Yellow Fever Service on vaccination against
the disease, I shall attempt to summarize those efforts in Brazil, beginning
with the year 1928. I shall not discuss any of the procedures used in other
countries, nor will I go into the details of all the methods used here, since
these are already available in scientific publications. My communication
today is primarily an attempt to present the practical results that have been
obtained to date.

An effective method of vaccination against yellow fever has been sought

* Translation of a lecture given in Portuguese at the National Academy of
Medicine, Rio de Janeiro, Brazil, November 4, 1937. The original text (*28*) was
published in the *Arquivos de Higiene* (*Rio de Janeiro*) 7: 379–390, 1937.

Dr. Soper was the Representative of the International Health Division of The
Rockefeller Foundation in South America (Rio de Janeiro Office) ; he was also the
Inspector-General of the Yellow Fever Service of Brazil.

by many research workers ever since 1927, when, in West Africa, the Yellow Fever Commission of The Rockefeller Foundation succeeded in bringing the virus into the laboratory and in developing procedures that made it possible to study the disease as an experimental infection. Immediately after the publication of the results obtained in West Africa, Hindle, in England, and Aragão, in Brazil, prepared vaccines from tissues from infected monkeys that contained the virus of yellow fever, using chemical methods for the attenuation of the virulence of the virus in the same manner that had been used for many years with other vaccines. Aragão reported that in 1929 about 25,000 persons were vaccinated in Brazil, but the results were not all that had been desired. Among the vaccinated persons, some 25 cases of yellow fever were observed with some fatalities, which occurred between 5 days and 2 months after the vaccination. One case, that of Dr. Paul Lewis, who was infected in the Bahia Laboratory, occurred 6 months later.

Theiler and Sellards were the first to demonstrate that the combined injection into monkeys of serum and virus produced an active immunity and suggested the possibility of vaccination against the disease by this procedure. The finding was confirmed shortly afterward by various authors. However, the later studies with serum and virus gave irregular results, because methods were not then available for titrating the virus and the antibody content of the serum.

A striking example of irregular results obtained was reported by our esteemed colleague, the late Nelson C. Davis, who tested his own serum in a monkey protection test. Davis acquired a laboratory infection in April 1929, which was proved to be yellow fever by the infection of a rhesus monkey, and thereafter he never reacted clinically during several years when he allowed cages full of infected mosquitoes to obtain their blood meals on him. In the months immediately following that infection, his serum gave the results described below, when inoculated together with Asibi virus into rhesus monkeys in the amount of 0.5 cc of serum per kilogram of body weight of the animal being used:

  May and July—prevented the death of the monkey but not fever
  September—did not prevent the death of the monkey from yellow fever
  October—prevented any signs of infection
  November—permitted a marked febrile reaction but prevented death
  December—prevented the appearance of any signs of infection

These disconcerting results, which were due to the lack of satisfactory techniques for the titration of the virus and of the serum antibodies, indicated that vaccination with fully potent virus and immune serum without any titration could not be used without serious danger; laboratory workers continued to be protected with human immune serum, even though among

them cases of yellow fever occurred within 2 weeks after receiving supposedly effective doses of such sera.

In November 1930 Davis made his first trial of human vaccination with
virus and serum. The test was done on Raymond C. Shannon, entomologist
of the Yellow Fever Laboratory at Bahia. On November 14, 21, and 27
Shannon was given 50 to 60 cc of immune serum, and on those same days
was exposed to the bites of infected mosquitoes.

On November 14, 3 mosquitoes fed on him that had previously received
virus that had been passed 20 times by intracerebral inoculation in mice;
on November 21, 10 mosquitoes fed, 3 of which were carriers of highly
virulent virus and 7 of which had been exposed for a long time to a temperature of 36°C in an effort to attenuate the virus which they were carrying;
and on November 27, 10 mosquitoes infected with fully potent virus fed.
Control animals, fed upon by mosquitoes of the same lots, reacted as follows: on November 14, one nonfatal attack; on November 21, one fatal
and one nonfatal; and on November 27, one fatal attack.

Shannon suffered no noteworthy reaction as a result of these inoculations. The monkey protection test on his serum drawn 2 months later was
negative; but the mouse protection test, more sensitive than the monkey
test done in 1936, revealed complete protection. Shannon left the laboratory immediately after the vaccination and did not have any contact with
the virus from 1930 to 1936, making it probable that the first attempt at
vaccination with serum and virus had been successful.

No further attempts were made to obtain immunization with highly
virulent virus and large doses of immune serum because Theiler had demonstrated the possibility of modifying yellow fever virus by changing the
manner in which it was cultivated. This suggested the possibility of vaccination with virus modified by tissue culture under special conditions.
Theiler demonstrated that yellow fever virus is not only viscerotropic but
also neurotropic, and that the white mouse, which under usual conditions
is not susceptible to infection, is highly susceptible to intracerebral inoculation. He demonstrated that the mice thus inoculated died of an encephalitis without any other lesions, indicating that no organ had been attacked
other than the central nervous system. After many serial intracerebral
passages in mice, the virus lost its capacity to produce visceral lesions in
rhesus monkeys but acquired increased affinity for the central nervous system. Such virus will be referred to as "neurotropic" virus or "virus fixed for
mouse brain." Lloyd, Theiler, and Ricci succeeded later, after prolonged
culture of the pantropic virus in mouse embryo tissues, in producing a
strain which had lost almost entirely its viscerotropism and which did not
reveal any increase in neurotropism. That strain of virus is referred to as
17E. Somewhat later, Theiler and Smith observed that the strain of virus

cultivated by Lloyd in 1934 in tissue culture containing chick embryo tissue from which the brain and spinal cord had been removed had lost a large part of its viscerotropic and neurotropic properties without having undergone any appreciable loss in its antigenic properties. That attenuated virus, known as the 17D strain, is being used at the present time for human vaccination in Brazil to the exclusion of all other types.

This is not to imply that human vaccination had not been done prior to the development of this improved strain of virus. Sawyer, Lloyd, and Kitchen, in May 1931, after appropriate tests in monkeys, began to use fixed neurotropic mouse brain virus together with immune human serum for the protection of laboratory personnel and other small groups of people highly exposed to the infection. Among these was a staff member of The Rockefeller Foundation, one of those assigned to work in Brazil, Dr. D. B. Wilson, who served as guinea pig for the first test on man.

The use of this method was gradually increased, and in the years 1931–1935, 50 persons were vaccinated by that method in South America in spite of the difficulties in obtaining the large quantities of human immune serum required to administer from 0.3 to 0.6 cc of such serum per kilogram of body weight of the person to be vaccinated. Of these individuals, 34 were vaccinated in Brazil at Rio de Janeiro, Bahia, and Recife, 11 in Colombia, and 5 in Argentina. The prevaccination protection tests of 38 of these people showed that they were not immune prior to vaccination, and similar tests after vaccination on all 50 people indicated that 48 had acquired immunity and only 2 had remained negative. The dried virus used in these 2 persons may have been inactivated during the month since the ampoules had left the Bahia Laboratory.

The introduction of this method of vaccination led to the disappearance of the laboratory infections which had been a serious hazard, but it did not make possible the large-scale vaccination of the rural population against jungle yellow fever. Neurotropic virus fixed for mouse brain was never used in Brazil without immune serum, because studies made in the New York Laboratory indicated that it could not safely be used in that manner in rhesus monkeys. Although there seemed to be very little or no possibility of producing typical yellow fever with this neurotropic virus, experience in human vaccination and the studies on rhesus monkeys made it necessary to consider the possibility of encephalitis. To prevent this possibility the amount of immune serum per kilogram of body weight was increased from the original 0.3 to 0.6 cc while this technique was used. The amount of immune serum used was that which would prevent the demonstrable circulation of virus when tested by the intracerebral inoculation into mice of blood serum from the vaccinated persons.

During the period in which these attempts were being made to attenuate the virus in various culture media, other studies were directed toward the production of hyperimmune sera with antibody content so high that a very small dose would be sufficient to protect each vaccinated person. The production of those sera represented considerable progress, but its importance was recently eclipsed by the availability of the attenuated 17D virus, which is being used without any serum.

In the New York Laboratory, Hughes obtained a serum with the concentration of antibodies 15 times greater than the standard human immune serum by injecting goats weekly for several months, by the intravenous route, with large doses of virulent virus from infected rhesus monkeys. Then by concentrating the total globulins and the pseudoglobulins, it was possible to obtain antibody titers 31 to 60 times greater than that of the standard immune serum.

A more effective method for obtaining hyperimmune serum was the result of the observation in 1935 by Whitman that a second dose of virus given to the animals some weeks after their original immunization produced a rapid but temporary increase in circulating antibodies. The hyperimmunization of monkeys was then obtained by the inoculation of large doses of virus 6 to 8 weeks after the immunizing infection. From the blood collected 9 days after the inoculation of the hyper-immunizing dose of virus, sera were obtained with antibody titers 20 to 60 times higher than that of the standard human immune sera.

In October 1935, Dr. Wray Lloyd arrived in Brazil to begin an intensive study of vaccination using 17E virus and heterologous immune serum instead of human serum. As mentioned above, the viscerotropism of this virus had been greatly reduced without increasing its neurotropism. It had been concluded, however, that the attenuation of viscerotropism was not sufficient to justify using the virus without immune serum.

Between October 1935 and April 1936, 44 persons were vaccinated in Brazil with 17E virus cultivated in tissue culture and human immune serum; protection tests of 37 of these persons, done 1 month after vaccination, showed that 35 of them were immune.

The major difficulty in the use of hyperimmune animal serum lay in the accurate determination of the amount of antibody required. The ideal antibody dose to be inoculated is that which prevents the circulation of the virus in the blood without preventing a sufficient multiplication of the virus to produce immunity. Even if information regarding the amount of standard human serum necessary to produce this result were available, the data would not be directly applicable to goat and monkey sera. It must also be kept in mind that heterologous sera are eliminated more rapidly than are homologous sera. In practice, twice as much antibody was administered when animal sera were used as when human sera were given. The results of studies in Brazil indicate that this dose is insufficient with goat serum and excessive with rhesus monkey serum.

Experimental vaccinations were made on 16 persons with hyperimmune goat serum and 17E virus cultivated in mouse embryo tissue culture. All of these were immunized when tested by the mouse protection test, but they all experienced serum reactions ranging from local to general urticaria. In five of these persons there was evidence of the presence of virus in the circulating blood, on the seventh day in one and from day 11 to day 13 in the others. This exceptionally late appearance of circulating virus is believed to be due to the elimination of the antibodies in the heterologous serum before the production of immunity.

In spite of these results, and in the face of a serious situation in Londrina, Paraná, 215 persons were vaccinated there with goat serum and 17E virus between February 25 and March 2, 1936. The postvaccination follow-up of 207 of these persons revealed that 176 of them had suffered serum sickness of various degrees and that 44 had suffered reactions attributable to the virus that was used. Of these latter patients, 13 were sick enough to have to stay in bed one or more days, and there were three cases that were very suggestive of mild yellow fever—but it may be remembered that jungle yellow fever was present in the area at the time. Of 184 persons examined 1 month after vaccination, 24, or 13 per cent, showed no evidence of immunity.

The preliminary studies of the use of hyperimmune monkey serum and 17E virus gave better results than those obtained with goat serum. The serum reactions were limited to slight local urticaria, which was observed in half of the 18 persons vaccinated. Circulating virus was not found in the tests done daily during a period of 2 weeks, and all 18 became immune, as shown by the results of mouse protection tests done 30 days after vaccination.

In view of these favorable results, large quantities of hyperimmune monkey serum were produced and used in additional field studies. From January 1936 to June 1937, 795 persons were vaccinated in Brazil with hyperimmune monkey serum and 17E virus. Of these, 576 were vaccinated in three places in which special studies were done: Anápolis, Goias, 122; Campo Grande, Mato Grosso, 231; and the State of Paraná, 223. The studies at Campo Grande enjoyed the full cooperation of the health service of the Brazilian Army, thanks to the gracious cooperation of General Alvaro Tourinho. During the same period, 219 persons were vaccinated in the Rio de Janeiro Laboratory and in a number of localities in Maranhão, São Paulo, and Paraná.

There was no significant reaction to the serum used, nor to the virus, following the injection of the hyperimmune monkey serum. However, the postvaccination protection tests gave a larger proportion of negative results than had been obtained when human or goat serum had been used, and the antibody titers of the persons vaccinated with monkey serum were lower than those obtained with human serum.

It is probable that both of these results were due to the use of excessive amounts of antibody. The rhesus monkey serum appears to be eliminated much more slowly than the goat serum, and the double dose of antibody administered was perhaps capable of preventing the immunizing effect of the virus in many cases. The importance of this factor is brought out by the fact that 70, or 36 per cent, of 192 nonimmune persons vaccinated with monkey serum at Campo Grande proved to be nonimmune 30 days after vaccination.

A comparison of the results obtained in Brazil with tissue culture virus and various types of immune serum showed that

1. Human serum, although giving the best results, is not practical because of the difficulty in obtaining the large quantities needed.

2. Goat hyperimmune serum gives a high percentage of serum reactions and does not prevent the delayed circulation of virus in the peripheral blood nor the appearance of symptoms of a virus infection; in compensation, a high percentage (84 per cent) of nonimmune persons become immune.

3. Hyperimmune monkey serum in the doses used produces only mild serum reactions and prevents the circulation of virus, but only 65 per cent of the persons vaccinated were immunized.

While the hyperimmune monkey serum did not give all the results desired, its use was discontinued only when 17D virus became available and could be administered without serum. It is very probable that if it became necessary to return to the method of vaccination with serum and virus, further studies regarding the dosage of antibody would make it possible to improve very greatly the results obtained with monkey serum.

Although no significant reaction either to the serum or to the virus was observed during the month after vaccination in the persons vaccinated with monkey hyperimmune serum, it was eventually found that among these persons unexplained attacks of jaundice occurred 2 to 8 months after vaccination.

These attacks, which occurred most frequently 3 to 4 months after vaccination, could be attributed to it only by the fact that they were unduly frequent in some groups of the vaccinated persons. The symptoms usually observed were those of a benign "catarrhal jaundice" and were in no way suggestive of yellow fever. These attacks of jaundice occurred not only in persons whose protection tests revealed immunity prior to vaccination, but also in persons immunized by the vaccine used, and in persons not immunized by the inoculations supposedly linked with the jaundice. Findlay, in London, observed an unusual number of cases of jaundice in persons vaccinated against yellow fever prior to July 1936. The cases occurring in Brazil came to the attention of the Yellow Fever Service only in November 1936. They were limited to vaccinated persons who received two of the six pools of hyperimmune monkey serum. No case of jaundice has been recorded to date in the individuals inoculated with human serum or goat serum or with the other four pools of monkey serum. In Rio de Janeiro, of 81 persons inoculated with serum of the incriminated pools, 8 cases of jaundice occurred. The occurrence of these cases led to an inquiry of the postvaccination history—done in June 1937—of the soldiers vaccinated at Campo Grande in October 1936 with serum of the two suspect pools of serum. This investigation revealed that jaundice had occurred in 61, or 32 per cent, of 191 vaccinated persons at a time during which there was no unusual occurrence of jaundice among the soldiers in the same barracks or in the civilian population of Campo Grande. Accepting the possibility that the vaccination with serum and virus had some etiological connection with these delayed attacks of jaundice, the distribution of the cases seems to indicate that the jaundice must be attributed to the immune monkey serum and not to the virus. In this regard it is interesting to note in a report from South Africa that horses vaccinated with combined serum and virus against African horse sickness exhibited postvaccination icterus and that the phenomenon was no longer observed when the serum was omitted and only the virus was used.

In 1934, Lloyd, who had succeeded in cultivating pantropic yellow fever virus *in vitro,* using mouse embryo tissues, transferred the 17E strain to cultures of chick embryo tissues from which the central nervous system had been removed, attempting in this manner to decrease the neurotropism of the strain. The substitution of chick embryo tissue for mouse embryo tissue also avoids the possibility, in the course of continuous passages through mice, of an accidental contamination of the yellow fever virus by some other virus pathogenic for man. Theiler and Smith continued the studies of Lloyd and observed, in 1936, that after prolonged culture in chick embryo tissues not only the viscerotropism but also the neurotropism of the strain was greatly reduced. This 17D virus, after a total of 114 subcultures, became attenuated and produced extremely mild reactions when inoculated subcutaneously into rhesus monkeys and acted as an efficient immunizing agent against subsequent inoculations of highly virulent virus. Furthermore, this virus had lost its capacity to produce a fatal encephalitis when injected by the cerebral route into monkeys, even though it was still capable of producing encephalitis in white mice.

The preliminary studies of the use of this 17D virus in human vaccination were done, as usual, on staff members of The Rockefeller Foundation in New York, after which Dr. Hugh H. Smith, in January of the current year, brought it to Brazil for further studies. In the beginning only small groups of people were vaccinated, and these were carefully studied for the presence of virus in the circulating blood and for symptoms of infection. From the fourth to the tenth day after vaccination, the presence of small amounts of circulating virus during one or more days was demonstrated in 12 of the 29 persons observed during 14 days. Among the first 200 persons vaccinated in Rio de Janeiro, only 20 per cent complained of symptoms which could be attributed to the virus. In general, the symptoms were slight headache and backache which occurred 6 or 7 days after the vaccination, accompanied in some cases by a slight febrile reaction. Nobody had to interrupt his normal activities because of these reactions. In Rio de Janeiro, after the inoculation of the 17D virus, postvaccination protection tests were done on 45 persons who were nonimmune at the time of vaccination. Of these, 42, or 93 per cent, showed complete protection, 1 showed partial protection, and 2 no protection. One of these failures occurred in an individual who, after previous vaccination with another strain of virus, failed to produce antibodies; the other person had received only 0.001 cc of the rehydrated virus preparation in a test to determine the amount of virus that would be needed in the routine immunizations.

In June of the current year, large-scale vaccination was begun in Varginha, in southern Minas Gerais, and the measure is being extended to Lavras, Três Corações, and Três Pontas, neighboring counties to Varginha, all situated in the State of Minas Gerais and known to have been infected this year with jungle yellow fever. This vaccination has been largely limited to the rural populations of the coffee plantations. Up to the present time more than 18,000 persons have been vaccinated in southern Minas Gerais. Only in a very small percentage have any symptoms been noted that could have been caused by the virus, and there are no reports of any serious reactions. Protection tests done on 344 persons of this group showed that only 5 continued to be nonimmune after vaccination.

Even though the preparation and the storage of 17D virus presents some difficulties, these are of such minor importance compared with those of the other procedures that in the course of a few months it was possible to vaccinate in Brazil a number of people 20 times greater than had been vaccinated in the 6 previous years. The virus which has been used in this intensive vaccination is the yellow fever virus that has been cultivated since 1934 in chick embryo tissues from which the central nervous system had previously been removed. The vaccine virus is obtained by the inoculation, after rehydration, of the desiccated stock virus into chick embryos inside their shells. The incubation of the embryos thus inoculated results in a concentration of virus much higher than that obtained by tissue culture methods.

After a few days of incubation, the inoculated chick embryos are ground up in 10 per cent normal human serum. The resulting material of high titer is dried in vacuum and sealed in ampoules and then rehydrated immediately before inoculation. It is essential for immunization that the virus be alive when it is inoculated. Experience has shown that the dried virus can be preserved for a long time at low temperatures, and for this reason material is shipped to the field on ice in Thermos jugs. In spite of these precautions, the viability test—done by inoculating into mice a remaining portion of each lot of vaccine immediately after its use—indicated that the material used at one of the plantations was inactive. Protection tests done subsequently on 20 persons vaccinated at that plantation revealed that no immunization had been produced there. As long as the viability of the virus cannot be absolutely guaranteed, the viability test has to be continued.

During the 8 months of use of 17D in Brazil, no case of delayed jaundice has been observed (such as those that had occurred with the vaccinations done with virus and serum), but a somewhat longer period of observation will be necessary before it will be possible to completely eliminate this possibility.

Some may criticize the use of a virus which circulates, as has been proved, although in small amounts, in the blood of some of the persons vaccinated. This possibility was the cause for the delay in vaccinating airline flight personnel in Miami and Brownsville in the United States until the winter of the current year. Laboratory workers, familiar with the difficulties of the transmission of normal yellow fever virus by *Aëdes aegypti* when there are only small quantities of circulating virus, do not consider this to be important. This problem is not limited to the use of virus without serum but may occur with any method of vaccination using live virus. I have already had occasion to mention that even when serum and virus were used in combination, virus was found circulating in the blood of a certain percentage of vaccinated persons, and it is to be expected that this would continue to happen as long as the present difficulties in the titration of the antibodies and the virus continue. Furthermore, it is doubtful that the transmission of 17D virus by the mosquito would be followed by an immediate recovery of its original viscerotropic properties and consequently the possibility of producing cases of classical yellow fever. It would seem to be more likely that, at least during several passages, the virus would maintain its characteristics of a vaccine, behaving like 17D virus that had been inoculated into man directly from tissue culture. In any case, studies have been started here in the Rio de Janeiro Laboratory to determine whether the *A. aegypti* mosquito can be infected when it bites vaccinated persons and, if this does occur, what would happen during serial transmission in rhesus monkeys.

The most carefully controlled studies with this new virus have been carried out in Brazil, but its use is not limited to this country. The Pan

American Sanitary Bureau has taken measures to prevent the international dissemination of yellow fever by airline flight personnel who travel to infected zones. Part of this personnel was vaccinated in Brazil and part in Panama and Peru. Many vaccinations have been done during the last few months in active foci of infection in Colombia. It is probable that about 2000 persons have now been vaccinated in South America outside of Brazil without the occurrence of any untoward incidents.

Additional research may possibly result in the development of one or more strains of virus more satisfactory than 17D for vaccination; however, it appears that 17D strain will make it possible to immunize the rural populations of the infected regions for which no other method of protection is available.

In closing, I must not fail to emphasize that the present method of vaccination must be considered as still under trial and experimentation, and that therefore its use cannot, at present, be generalized without the precautions which are being used. It seemed to me, however, that a method which we felt justified in using for the vaccination in a short time of more than 20,000 persons was worth bringing to the attention of this learned Academy.

To the National Academy of Medicine my sincere thanks for the gracious manner in which once again it has given me the signal honor of bringing to the medical profession news of what has been done in the country, thanks to the cooperation of the Brazilian Government, to solve the problems involved in yellow fever.

SUMMARY

The attempts which have been made over the past 10 years to find a satisfactory method of vaccinating against yellow fever are described. One case is mentioned which was successfully vaccinated by means of the bites of infected mosquitoes after the person had been inoculated with human immune blood serum. The results of the vaccination done in Brazil by the Cooperative Yellow Fever Service are given in detail, including results with the following types of vaccine:

1. 1931–1935: 50 persons vaccinated with human immune serum and virus modified by serial passage in mouse brain.

2. 1935–1936: 44 persons inoculated with human immune serum and tissue culture virus.

3. 1935–1936: 231 persons inoculated with small amounts of hyperimmune goat serum and tissue culture virus.

4. 1936–1937: 795 persons vaccinated with hyperimmune monkey serum and virus attenuated by prolonged passage in tissue culture.

5. 1937: About 18,000 persons in Brazil and 2000 in other countries vaccinated by inoculation of tissue culture virus without immune serum.

The human serum gave good results but could be used only on a small scale. For better results with animal sera, additional research would be necessary. Vaccination without serum, with virus attenuated by prolonged passage in cultures of chick embryo tissues, have proved to be the most practical. The new vaccine, which is still considered to be under study, cannot, for the present, be made available for general use.

| Vaccination with Virus 17D in
the Control of Jungle Yellow
Fever in Brazil*

FRED L. SOPER AND H. H. SMITH

The first attempt to protect an exposed population against jungle yellow fever by vaccination was made in Paraná, Brazil, early in 1936, using hyperimmune goat and monkey sera and a virus modified by culture in mouse embryo tissue (17E). The difficulties encountered were such as to cause the discontinuation of this method in the field, and during the yellow fever season (January–May) of 1937, no attempt was made to protect exposed populations.

Work with another modified virus (17D) developed in the laboratories of the International Health Division of The Rockefeller Foundation in New York, began in Brazil in February 1937. By June, these studies had progressed far enough to justify field vaccination, and the county of Varginha, Minas Geraes, in a region where jungle yellow fever had been found a few weeks previously, was chosen for the first field application of the new vaccine virus. During the next three months, 2746 persons were vaccinated in the field, with satisfactory results, and, in September, routine field vaccination began, which increased the total field vaccinations for the year 1937 to 36,104.

The 1938 yellow fever season in South Brazil began early in January, with an outbreak of jungle yellow fever at Presidente Wenceslau, São Paulo, and shortly thereafter the disease was found at Mathias Barboza, Minas Geraes. Vaccination units were moved into both these districts, and an attempt was made throughout the following months to vaccinate threatened populations wherever yellow fever was found. The 1938 yellow fever

---

* This report is based on work of many colleagues of the Cooperative Yellow Fever Service, jointly maintained by the Ministry of Education and Health of Brazil and the International Health Division of The Rockefeller Foundation. Special credit for the rapid expansion of vaccination in 1938 must go to the Brazilian Government, which furnished the necessary additional funds. Dr. Soper was the Representative in South America (Rio de Janeiro Office) of the International Health Division of The Rockefeller Foundation; Dr. Smith was a staff member.

This article was originally published (*33*) in the *Transactions* of the Third International Congresses of Tropical Medicine and Malaria (Amsterdam), Sept. 24–Oct. 1, 1938, Vol. 1, pp. 295–313, 1938. (Four tables and 1 chart have been omitted, but the text is complete.)

season was an active one, with outbreaks in some of the richest and most heavily populated agricultural districts of Brazil, in the states of Minas Geraes, Rio de Janeiro, São Paulo, and Santa Catharina. The need for vaccine greatly exceeded the initial production capacity of the laboratory and the ability of the field service to apply it. The Brazilian Government opened a special credit of 2000 contos (approximately $100,000 U.S.) to cover the cost of a program for the vaccination of at least 1 million persons during 1938.

From January 2 to July 31, a total of 557,861 persons were vaccinated, and the final figures for the year will almost certainly exceed the preliminary estimate of 1 million. Table 2 gives the distribution of persons vaccinated per month in Brazil, from September 1937 to July 1938, by population groups.

Origin of Vaccine Virus 17D

In December 1933, Lloyd transferred the Asibi strain to tissue culture containing mouse embryo tissue and monkey serum; after 18 subcultures, a second transfer was made to a medium containing whole chick embryo tissue, from which, after 56 passages, it was transplanted to tissue culture containing chick embryo, from which the central nervous system had been removed. After 39 passages in this medium, without central nervous system tissue, this strain of virus, now known as 17D, was tested and found to have lost much of its viscerotropism and neurotropism, while still retaining the property of stimulating the production of antibodies. Virus 17D was first used for human inoculation on November 30, 1936, in New York, with material transferred 227 times in tissue culture since its last previous passage in an animal host. Subcultures used as source of vaccine in Brazil have ranged from the 205th to the 317th.

Table 2. Distribution by Population Groups of Persons Vaccinated in Brazil, September 1937 to July 31, 1938

Population group	Sept.–Dec. 1937	Jan.–July 1938	Total
Farms and hamlets	16,530	397,809	414,339
Military units	1,105	23,730	24,835
Schools	994	34,348	35,342
Labor gangs	368	39,183	39,551
Cities and towns	14,361	53,337	67,698
Miscellaneous	—	9,454	9,454
Total	33,358	557,861	591,219

Results Obtained with Virus 17D

The points on which a method of vaccination for general use as a public health measure should be judged, may be grouped under the following headings:

1. Ease of manufacture of standard product.
2. Ease of application under field conditions.
3. Safety and comfort of persons vaccinated.
4. Safety of persons not vaccinated.
5. Antibody production.

Ease of Manufacture of the Standard Product

The titer of virus in tissue culture material is much below that obtained by growth in the developing chick embryo. The vaccine virus is maintained in tissue culture free of central nervous system tissues, to avoid any possible reversion to type, but for the preparation of vaccine, tissue culture is inoculated in the allantoic sac of the 6-day old chick embryo. After further incubation for 4 days, at a temperature of 37°C, the embryo is removed, triturated, and suspended (10 per cent) in inactivated human serum diluted with equal amounts of distilled water. The filtrate of this suspension, which is the vaccine material, is distributed in ampoules, frozen, dried in vacuum, sealed, and stored at about 2°C. In addition to the usual bacteriological controls for sterility, each lot of vaccine is titrated for virus content by intracerebral inoculation in serial dilutions in white mice, and is inoculated intracerebrally into a rhesus monkey, to test for possible increase in either viscerotropism or neurotropism.

Although laboratory studies indicate that a much smaller dose may be sufficient, between 350 and 800 MLD for mice are now being allowed for each person vaccinated in Brazil. On this basis the Rio de Janeiro Laboratory is producing some 120,000 doses of vaccine per month, at a total cost, including overhead, excepting rent, of less than $3000 U.S., or 2.5 cents U.S., per dose.

Ease of Application under Field Conditions

Virus 17D, even when dried and sealed, is susceptible to ordinary temperatures and to direct sunlight; the vaccine leaves the Rio laboratory, packed with ice and salt, in wide-mouthed Thermos flasks and is thus kept chilled until the moment of rehydration. Even after rehydration with distilled water the ampoule is kept on ice, and the vaccine is finally diluted in physiological saline solution in the syringe itself immediately preceding inoculation. To determine the viability of the virus used, mice are inoculated intracerebrally with the remaining vaccine after the last person has been inoculated.

Experience shows that a vaccination unit, consisting of three persons— a doctor, a technical assistant, and a secretary-chauffeur—can, under optimum conditions, register and inoculate from 1000 to 2000 persons a day. (The use of three "Forsbeck" needle racks by each unit is advisable, to avoid unnecessary delays in waiting for needles to cool after boiling. It is believed that certain irregular results of postvaccination protection tests are due to failure to cool needles after boiling, with consequent inactivation of the vaccine virus.) The actual cost of applying vaccine in Brazil in 1938 has not exceeded, including initial cost of automobiles and equipment, 7 cents U.S. per capita. The actual field operating expense has dropped from 5.5 cents U.S., per capita, in January, to 3 cents U.S. in June. However, the per capita cost of application must increase rapidly in sparsely populated regions and in areas where transportation is difficult.

Safety and Comfort of Persons Vaccinated

Since the beginning of work with virus 17D in February 1937, a conscientious search has been made among vaccinated groups for evidence of

1. Severe reaction at site of inoculation.
2. Sensitization to foreign protein.
3. Serum sickness.
4. Virus reaction, visceral and neural.
5. Delayed jaundice.
6. Infection with other viruses.

Special attention should be called to the distribution of vaccinated persons by population groups (Table 2). Employees of the Yellow Fever Service, of the airlines, the population of large coffee fazendas, inmates of schools, laborers and highway construction gangs, and members of military units, all form very useful groups for observation. Even where it has not been possible for physicians of the Yellow Fever Service to make personal observation, fazenda owners, military medical officers, school directors, and other responsible persons have given information as to the severity of postvaccination reactions.

The sum total of observations on vaccinated groups may be stated briefly as follows: For the 18-month period, during which almost 600,000 persons were vaccinated, there is no evidence of severe reaction at the site of inoculation, of sensitization to foreign protein, of serum sickness, of delayed jaundice, or of infection with other viruses. [However, see Selection 27 regarding the subsequent occurrence of postvaccination hepatitis and encephalitis in Brazil. *Ed.*] A number of cases have received second and third inoculations of 17D without any evidence of sensitization to chick embryo protein.

The type of relatively mild reaction which is observed seems to be a general, not neural, reaction to the virus itself, after an incubation period of generally from 5 to 8 days.*

The symptoms most frequently noted are headache, backache, body pains, weakness, and malaise, lasting from a few hours to a couple of days. The reaction to virus 17D is not severe enough to have any influence against its general acceptance by the people. Fazenda owners, and others responsible for large groups, generally report from 5 to 8 per cent reactions, with not more than 1 to 2 per cent of the reactions severe enough to cause loss of time from work. A person-to-person canvas, however, will result in 20, 40, or even 50 per cent of individuals questioned reporting at least a slight headache, but the number of severe reactions does not increase correspondingly. The most severe reactions reported are those related to each other by members of the foreign colony in the capital city of Rio de Janeiro!

Considering the number vaccinated, it seems truly remarkable that many more conditions occurring after vaccination have not been credited to the inoculation. Experience has failed to reveal any contraindications to the use of virus 17D, early restrictions have been entirely removed, and children of all ages and women in all stages of pregnancy are routinely inoculated.

Safety of Persons Not Vaccinated

In using a living virus for vaccination, the possibility of such living virus being picked up from the bloodstream by some insect vector, and sooner or later reverting to its original virulence, must be considered. Such return to virulence of a yellow fever vaccine would have to depend upon the following factors:

1. Circulation of virus in the bloodstream in quantities sufficient to infect the insect vector.

2. Ability of the infected vector to transmit the vaccine virus.

3. Ability of the vaccine virus to revert to a virulent state.

Experimental work indicates that sufficient virus does not circulate to infect the traditional vector, *Aëdes aegypti*, and that even when this mosquito has been infected by special methods it does not readily transmit the

---

* So far, only one case has been reported, in which symptoms of involvement of the central nervous system were attributed by the attending physicians to inoculation with virus 17D. Case E.R.C., observed by Drs. Raul Azevedo and Deolindo Couto, Rio de Janeiro, to whom we owe thanks for details of this case, developed signs of meningeal involvement 1 month after vaccination with Lot 136 of virus 17D, the estimated virus used being 220 MLD for mice. Complete recovery occurred, and studies are now in progress to determine, if possible, the nature of the infection.

17D virus, even after prolonged incubation. Attempts to infect aegypti by postvaccination feeding on humans and on rhesus monkeys, which have been shown to circulate more virus than do humans, were failures, no virus being demonstrated in the mosquito by either feeding on monkeys or inoculation into mice. The immersion of aegypti larvae in high concentration of virus did result in the production of infected adult mosquitoes, as demonstrated by mouse inoculation; such infected aegypti failed completely to transmit virus to susceptible animals, even after prolonged incubation periods.

The difficulty of getting virus 17D to circulate in appreciable quantities with regularity, has, so far, prevented conclusive experiments with the jungle vectors of yellow fever, only a few of which have very recently been definitely incriminated. The same difficulty has prevented the carrying out of a large series of animal passages, to determine the ability of virus 17D to revert to its original type; the relative stability of the virus in tissue culture, embryo passage, and in mouse brain passage, suggests that such reversion to virulence, if it did occur at all, would be slow in appearing. This opinion is strengthened by the results of other workers, who have not been able to transmit a tissue culture virus with aegypti or to reconvert it to virulence by direct liver-to-liver passage.

Antibody Production

The rhesus monkey, which is more highly susceptible to yellow fever than is man, becomes fully resistant to virulent strains, such as Asibi, following inoculation with virus 17D. Similar tests on humans have not been made, but the wide use of virus 17D this year, among exposed populations, during active outbreaks of jungle yellow fever has resulted in a mass of field observation almost as conclusive as laboratory experiments. Local physicians and other observers report a sudden reduction in observed cases in infected districts shortly after mass vaccination, and cite instances in which individuals who failed to be inoculated later contracted the disease in infected forests, while vaccinated members of the same labor gangs escaped. Field experience suggests that the protective effect of vaccination begins not later than 1 week after inoculation, although laboratory tests fail to show demonstrable antibodies at this time. While it is probable that a much larger number of cases of yellow fever must have occurred among persons infected before vaccination, only eight of these have been reported: four in Minas Geraes, three in Santa Catharina, and one in São Paulo. Onset in two was on the same day as vaccination, in the other four, between the first and fourth days following. Two of the three fatal cases in this group were confirmed by viscerotomy, and a virus, quite different from the vaccine virus, was isolated from one of the nonfatal cases.

Two additional cases of postvaccination yellow fever have been found; one mild case with onset 30 days, and one fatal case with onset 6 weeks after vaccination. These cases had received virus from lots 95 and 117, both of which gave irregular results, as measured by the protection test. It is possible that neither received active virus.

The mouse-protection test has been used since 1931 for determining the presence of yellow fever antibodies in the blood serum of persons and animals. It is customary to inoculate six mice with highly neurotropic virus and with the serum to be tested. Results are read as a fraction showing the proportion of mice living on the fourth day (denominator), which survive to the tenth day (numerator) after inoculation.

Seven readings are possible, of which only two, 6/6 and 5/6, are, in analyzing critical immunity surveys, considered definite evidence of previous infection with yellow fever; 4/6 and 3/6 results are considered inconclusive; and 2/6, 1/6, and 0/6 as negatives. It has been noted in immunity surveys that bloods from regions where yellow fever has never been present give remarkable clear-cut negative readings, whereas bloods from endemic regions give an appreciable number of inconclusives, as well as positives and negatives. The majority of these inconclusives are probably from individuals who have at some time been exposed to yellow fever infection, and are, almost certainly, not apt to ever again develop clinical yellow fever. It seems reasonable at the present time to read mouse-protection test results as indicating full protection, partial protection, and no protection, without attempting to interpret too rigidly these readings in terms of reaction to yellow fever infection, further than to assume that those showing full protection are, at the moment tested, adequately protected against fully virulent virus. Postvaccination results, when compared with prevaccination results (Fig. 1), suggest that virus 17D does produce some measurable antibody formation in almost 100 per cent of persons receiving 50 MLD or more of living virus. It has been noted that in many postvaccination protection tests, in which the final reading is: 2/6, 1/6, or even 0/6, the average length of survival of inoculated animals is from 1 to 2 days longer than for similar negative tests in unvaccinated groups. This suggests that sufficient antibody is present to definitely delay the action of virus inoculated in animals.

Figure 1 gives the results of pre- and postvaccination tests on the same individuals, including both laboratory and field groups, during the preliminary phase of observation, before routine field vaccination began. (Vaccination of these groups was carried out under the direct supervision of Dr. H. H. Smith, who, with Drs. Henrique Penna and Adhemar Paoliello, has published a report covering observations on the first 60,000 vaccinations in Brazil.) Attention must be called to the fact that on one occasion, the virus was apparently inactive before inoculation began, since all of

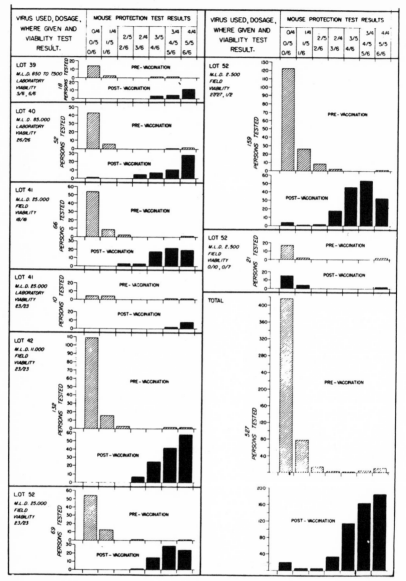

Figure 1. Immunity to yellow fever before and after vaccination with 17D virus.

the persons tested failed to give evidence of antibody development, and the inoculation of the remaining vaccine into mice failed to cause any deaths.

Table 4 [omitted] covers a special investigation to determine the results obtained with different dosages of virus and to evaluate the viability test as an indication of efficiency of the preceding vaccination. The groups bled for this special study were selected as probably representative of the poorest work of the season and included groups receiving the lowest doses of virus used during the height of the yellow fever outbreak, working with newly trained personnel, far from headquarters. The results indicate that doses as low as 50, 85, and 100 MLD per person are adequate to give satisfactory results. They also indicate that the viability test, in and of itself, is not a safe indication of the efficiency of the vaccination. For example, lot 117 of virus 17D was used and tested in five groups, of which only one gave satisfactory results, the viability tests for which, 0/5, 1/5, and 1/4, were poor. Postvaccination mouse-protection tests on a number of persons from vaccinated groups are proving a better method of checking the work of field units than is the test for viability of the remaining vaccine.

Figure 2 gives a general summary of all postvaccination protection test results for work with virus 17D in Brazil. The results show that with standardized methods of vaccine production and with adequate supervision of the administration of virus in the field, highly satisfactory results can be obtained.

Anticipated Results of Vaccination

Admitting that the individual can be protected by vaccination, the epidemiological results of vaccination must vary with the conditions under which infection occurs. Where man is an essential element in the cycle of infection, responsible for maintaining the virus, as in urban aegypti-transmitted yellow fever, artificial immunization of the bulk of the population should effectively protect the remaining nonimmunes. It is probable that occasional mass vaccination will be found more economical and practicable in certain regions, for breaking the cycle of infection, man–aegypti–man, than is the traditional maintenance of antimosquito services for the prevention of aegypti breeding.

In considering jungle yellow fever, however, in which man is, apparently, not an important factor in maintaining the virus, vaccination should alter the epidemiological picture, mostly by preventing the infection of vaccinated persons, and, only in a very minor degree, by reduction of the source of virus for forest vectors.

Vaccination promises to be a great aid in preventing the transfer of yellow fever infection from one place to another by the human host; the long-distance transfer of virus, by modern methods of rapid transportation, can be prevented by vaccination, as can also the introduction of virus from jungle to urban areas. Since the jungle infection, apparently, exists independent of the human population, and spreads from place to place by other than human carriers, vaccination cannot be expected to completely eradicate yellow fever.

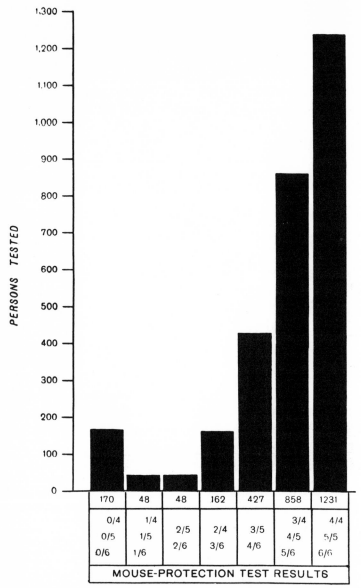

Figure 2. Postvaccination mouse protection test results on 2944 persons
inoculated with 17D virus.

SUMMARY

During the period September 1937 to July 1938, over ½ million persons
were inoculated with the modified yellow fever virus 17D. Vaccination with
this virus was widely used throughout the 1938 epidemic of jungle yellow

fever in South Brazil. Field observations indicate that vaccination becomes effective within a week after inoculation. Reaction to vaccination is relatively mild, and no contraindications have been found. The results of approximately 3000 mouse-protection tests are presented, showing that a high percentage of persons vaccinated develop demonstrable antibodies. [See Part V, Selection 23, Maps 9 and 10, and the accompanying discussion of the progress of the vaccination program in Brazil in 1938. *Ed.*]

| Complications of Yellow Fever
Vaccination*

The number of vaccinations against yellow fever done in the Americas up to the time of the previous Conference (1938) reached a total of 10,000 in Colombia and 60,000 in Brazil, with the number in Brazil reaching 1,000,000 before the end of 1938. At the previous Conference it was stated that tests had shown that 85 to 90 per cent of the persons vaccinated had acquired demonstrable immunity, and that the majority of vaccinated persons suffered no reaction attributable to the vaccine.

Unexpected complications occurred during the large-scale vaccination with attenuated 17D virus in Brazil in 1939, 1940, and 1941. The extensive vaccination done late in 1938 and early in 1939 in the State of Espírito Santo, ahead of the epidemic wave that was advancing, failed to protect some of the persons vaccinated against an attack of yellow fever, and some fatalities were observed in this group of people. Later studies revealed that even though the viability tests indicated that the vaccine had contained living virus, only about 20 per cent of some groups of people had been immunized. Apparently the 17D virus in the higher passages used for the preparation of the vaccine had undergone further changes. A return was made to lower passages, and the subsequent lots of vaccine gave satisfactory immunization. But late in 1939 and in 1940, again in the State of Espírito Santo, the vaccination program encountered difficulties when postvaccination icterus caused 22 deaths in 1000 cases studied. In spite of the fact that there was an irregular distribution of the cases of icterus by geographic areas, by vaccine lot, and even by the same lots of vaccine, field studies revealed no constant factor, except the vaccine itself, that could be held responsible for this irregularity. In view of the reports in the literature of similar outbreaks of icterus following the use of measles immune serum, and in view of the fact that the postvaccination icterus was observed in some persons who were shown to be immune to yellow fever before vaccination, and in others who continued to be nonimmune after vaccination, it appears logical to conclude that the vaccine virus was not responsible for the icterus but that this probably was associated with the (human blood) serum used in the preparation of the vaccine.

* Translation of an excerpt (pp. 1214–1216) from "Febre Amarela Panamericana, 1938 a 1942," a report by Dr. Soper as an invited guest from The Rockefeller Foundation to the XIth Pan American Sanitary Conference, Rio de Janeiro, Brazil, September 7–18, 1942. The entire report (*43*) has been reprinted in Portuguese in the *Boletin de la Oficina Sanitaria Panamericana 21*: 1207–1222, 1942. (Another excerpt from this report, entitled "Proposal for the Continental Eradication of *Aëdes aegypti*," appears in Part II, Selection 6.)

The method of preparing the vaccine was changed during the second half of 1940, omitting the use of serum, and no undue occurrence of icterus has been observed among 347,000 persons vaccinated with vaccine prepared in the Rio de Janeiro Laboratory during the last 2 years. However, this proves nothing, because after the first observation of postvaccination icterus in Brazil in 1936–1937, 1,677,332 persons were vaccinated prior to the occurrence of the cases registered in 1939–1940. While the etiologic agent appears to be a virus with a long incubation period, no virus has been isolated nor has it been possible to produce the disease experimentally in animals. The vaccine from the Bogotá Laboratory was widely used in Colombia and Peru without any incident; however, more than 28,000 cases of postvaccination icterus, with 62 deaths, occurred during the present year in the Armed Forces of the United States following the use of the vaccine from the New York Laboratory.

In 1941, using a highly antigenic vaccine that was prepared without any human serum and which was not producing any jaundice, the vaccination program was proceeding calmly when some cases of encephalitis occurred after vaccination in certain groups of vaccinated persons. These cases were very few in number, compared to the number of individuals vaccinated, and could have escaped observation in a large-scale vaccination program. Of the 55,000 persons vaccinated in the area where the most extensive studies were made, only 273, or 0.5 per cent, had reactions classified as exceptionally severe; 199 of these persons presented symptoms indicating that their central nervous systems had been affected. Fortunately, there was knowledge of only one fatal case. Later studies in the field and laboratory seem to indicate that this encephalitis was not caused by a concurrent epidemic or by a contamination of the vaccine but by a slight modification in the vaccine virus itself. After changing to another substrain of 17D virus for the production of the vaccine, no further cases of encephalitis were observed.

After these three years of difficulties in Brazil—1939 with vaccine of low antigenicity, 1940 with postvaccination icterus, and 1941 with postvaccination encephalitis—we hope that the principal difficulties of the 17D yellow fever vaccine have been overcome. Let us not forget, however, that large-scale vaccination has become possible primarily because of the variation with attenuation of the virus of yellow fever that has occurred. Continuous vigilance must be maintained to prevent any variations which would impair the production of a high degree of immunity without danger.

Based on past experience, we see no reason to abandon the program of mass immunization of all the population exposed to jungle yellow fever and of all those who need to travel in areas in which there is a risk of yellow fever. However, the use of vaccine in the control of yellow fever should occupy more or less the same place that typhoid vaccine has in the control of typhoid fever. No sanitary authority would desire to substitute typhoid vaccination for the supply of pure water and food, so we must not accept the yellow fever vaccine as a substitue for the eradication of *Aëdes aegypti*. The vaccine provides individual protection for the person who cannot be protected by more general measures.

The duration of immunity after vaccination seems to be long-lasting; studies made on sera collected in 1941 from persons vaccinated in 1937 have revealed no appreciable decrease in antibody titers.

Part VII | The Eradication of *Anopheles gambiae* from Brazil and Egypt

Selection 28 | *Anopheles gambiae* in Brazil, 1930 to 1940*

FRED L. SOPER AND D. BRUCE WILSON

ACKNOWLEDGMENTS

A special note of recognition is due to those persons who were responsible for approving the program and budgets of the Malaria Service of the Northeast for the years 1939 and 1940, at a time when there was very little concrete evidence of the possibility of species eradication. It is a pleasure to place at the head of the list the names of Dr. Getulio Vargas, the President of Brazil, and of Dr. Gustavo Capanema, the Minister of Education and Health, both of whom took a personal interest in the Malaria Service of the Northeast and never failed to meet its demands, which must at times have seemed excessive.

To Raymond B. Fosdick, President of The Rockefeller Foundation, to Dr. W. A. Sawyer, Director of the International Health Division, as well as to the individual members of the Board of Scientific Directors of the International Health Division,† sitting in New York, special credit must be given for their willingness to assume the responsibility for granting large sums of money to what at times, and from a distance, must have seemed an impossible project.

Mention has already been made of the action of Dr. Barros Barreto who, as Director of the National Department of Health, was responsible for recommending to his government the organization of a cooperative project under the auspices of the International Health Division. Special mention must be made of the kindly dignified interest and collaboration of Dr. Samuel Libanio who, during the most critical stages of the campaign

* Dr. Soper was the Representative for South America (Rio de Janeiro Office) of the International Health Division of The Rockefeller Foundation; Dr. Wilson was a staff member of The Rockefeller Foundation and Director of the Malaria Service of the Northeast.

This excerpt comprises only about 100 pages of the 262-page book (*45*) published by The Rockefeller Foundation, New York, 1943.

Additional detailed data regarding the eradication of gambiae from Brazil are contained in the publication "Campanha contra o '*Anopheles gambiae*' no Brasil, 1939–1942," published by the Brazilian Government (*46* in the Bibliography).

† The Board of Scientific Directors which approved the budget for 1940 consisted of the following members: Wilbur A. Sawyer, M.D.; Ernest W. Goodpasture, M.D.; Stanhope Bayne-Jones, M.D.; Harry S. Mustard, M.D.; Thomas Parran, M.D.; Lowell J. Reed; Felix J. Underwood, M.D.

against the *Anopheles gambiae* mosquito, from June 1939 to April 1941, occupied the directorship of the National Department of Health.

Brief reference has been made during the present report to the work of Dr. Evandro Chagas and the group of colleagues working under his direction. In the untimely death of Dr. Chagas, in November 1940, Brazilian epidemiologists lost a leader and we of the Malaria Service of the Northeast, a valued friend and collaborator.

It is a pleasure to record the collaboration of the Oswaldo Cruz Institute of Rio de Janeiro and of the Institute of Hygiene of São Paulo, both of which graciously loaned staff members for the work of the Malaria Service. During several months of 1939, Drs. Oliveira Castro and Gilberto Freitas of the Oswaldo Cruz Institute were members of the laboratory, and Dr. Paulo Antunes, of the Institute of Hygiene, took an active and important part in the administration of the field work from April 1939 to July 1941.

An entirely individual and personal expression of gratitude is due Dr. M. A. Barber, who in the course of an extended trip through Latin America in 1939, was pressed into service as a volunteer worker, without salary, during the months of May, June, and July. Dr. Barber made valuable contributions to the success of the Service through the demonstration of the simpler methods of Paris green application and of many refinements of laboratory techniques for the study of both mosquitoes and parasites. Dr. Barber's field work, under a tropical sun, in investigating the relationship of gambiae to malaria in the frontier zones, put to shame the physical resistance of much younger men. To Dr. Barber the Malaria Service of the Northeast owes the coinage of the most poignant criticism of its early months—that it was not getting the desired results because, as a "shade-loving service," it failed to contact the "sun-loving larvae" of gambiae.

R. C. Shannon, who made the original observation of gambiae on the American continent in 1930 and surveyed Northeast Brazil for extensions of its range at the end of the dry season in the same year and with Gastão Cesar de Andrade made the 1938 dry season survey, returned to the infested area in August 1939 and once more gave the Malaria Service his valuable collaboration. His knowledge of gambiae's dry season biology was based on prolonged, careful observations in the field projected against his unexcelled background of observation of the biology of other anopheles in various parts of the world.

The authors take great pleasure in putting on record the names of the colleagues who took part in the work of the Malaria Service of the Northeast and only regret that it is not possible to put on record the individual efforts of thousands of others who risked malaria infection and who worked under very difficult conditions to carry out the measures on which the success of the campaign against gambiae depended. Among these thousands, as among the doctors of the Service, were many who had proved their dependability by long years of loyal work in the Yellow Fever Service campaign against *Aëdes aegypti*.

Of the names which are listed below, it is impossible to pass over without particular mention those of Drs. Mario Franca and Oswaldo Silva, who as assistants shouldered extraheavy responsibilities.

A special place must be given to the name of Dr. Manoel Ferreira, the Director of the Antimalaria Service, who recommended that it be discontinued to make way for the Malaria Service of the Northeast. Dr. Ferreira continued as assistant in the new Service for the first 15 months of its existence and only after organizing the Central Laboratory and seeing the Service well on its way to success did he abandon it in favor of urgent personal interests.

The two nonmedical assistants, Snrs. Juarez Corrêa Lemos and Deusdedite Campos Alves, merit special mention; without them the task of the medical staff would have been a great deal more arduous.

Medical Staff of the Malaria Service of the Northeast

Name	Period of Service	
Assistant Directors		
Manoel José Ferreira, M.D.	January 1, 1939	April 5, 1940
Mario Franca, M.D.	January 14, 1939	June 30, 1942
Paulo Cesar de Azevedo Antunes, M.D.	April 23, 1939	August 27, 1941
Oswaldo José da Silva, M.D.	January 27, 1939	June 30, 1942
Laboratory		
Ottis R. Causey, M.D.	August 4, 1939	June 30, 1942
Gustavo M. de Oliveira Castro, M.D.	April 1, 1939	September 30, 1939
Henrique Maia Penido, M.D.	December 27, 1939	October 3, 1941
Gladstone de Mello Deane, M.D.	June 14, 1939	October 16, 1939
Leonidas de Mello Deane, M.D.	June 14, 1939	June 30, 1942
Maria Paumgartten Deane, M.D.	June 16, 1939	June 30, 1942
Antonio Conserva Feitoza, M.D.	April 28, 1939	April 7, 1940
Epidemiology Section		
Richard G. Hahn, M.D.	September 8, 1939	December 4, 1940
Carlos Eugenio Porto, M.D.	January 20, 1940	July 15, 1941
Cartographic Section		
C. G. Inman	April 1, 1939	June 30, 1942
Division Directors		
Ceará		
Gastão Cesar de Andrade, M.D.	January 18, 1939	June 21, 1942
Frederico Acquer, M.D.	June 14, 1939	July 31, 1941
Octavio Pinto Severo, M.D.	September 30, 1939	February 9, 1941
Jefferson Carlos de Souza, M.D.	June 16, 1939	November 1, 1941
Miguel Scaff, M.D.	February 10, 1939	September 3, 1939

Medical Staff of the Malaria Service of the Northeast—*Cont.*

Name	Period of Service	
Division Directors—*Cont.*		
Ceará—*Cont.*		
Antonio da Silva Maltez Filho, M.D.	June 10, 1939	August 22, 1940
Luiz Ferreira Tavares Lessa, M.D.	January 18, 1939	August 31, 1939
Rio Grande do Norte		
Eleyson Cardoso, M.D.	January 22, 1939	November 19, 1940
Fernando Machado Busta-mante, M.D.	January 1, 1939	June 8, 1942
Abelardo Buarque Lima, M.D.	April 6, 1939	November 11, 1940
Assistants		
Plinio Teófilo de Aguiar, M.D.	January 10, 1939	June 21, 1942
Nisomar Pinheiro de Azevedo, M.D.	November 1, 1939	June 9, 1942
Arnobio Calheiros Bomfin, M.D.	June 22, 1939	June 21, 1942
Garibaldi Bezerra de Faria, M.D.	December 11, 1939	June 21, 1942
Eliezer Pará-Assú de Serra Freire, M.D.	September 20, 1939	June 21, 1942
Lauro Melloni, M.D.	May 24, 1940	May 31, 1942
Durval Bustorff Pinto, M.D.	February 11, 1939	June 21, 1942
Darcy da Rosa, M.D.	May 28, 1940	May 31, 1942
Mario Machado Sampaio, M.D.	December 13, 1939	June 30, 1942
Orlando José da Silva, M.D.	June 24, 1939	May 21, 1942
Vival Silva, M.D.	April 22, 1940	June 30, 1942
Antonio Mello de Siqueira, M.D.	November 3, 1939	June 6, 1942
Ruy Soares, M.D.	September 25, 1939	June 21, 1942
Vicente Zambrano, M.D.	October 1, 1940	June 30, 1942
José Pedro Bezerra, M.D.	January 1, 1939	September 5, 1940
Carlos Vinha, M.D.	January 1, 1939	February 29, 1940
João Damasceno da Costa, M.D.	April 14, 1939	August 31, 1939
Ivo Bugano, M.D	November 3, 1939	April 10, 1942
Gilberto de Freitas, M.D.	May 1, 1939	November 18, 1939
Oswaldo Novis, M.D.	March 4, 1939	June 23, 1939
Joaquim Gracindo Marques, M.D.	March 23, 1939	December 24, 1939
Irun Sant'Anna, M.D.	July 10, 1939	December 12, 1939
Germano Silval Faria, M.D.	March 9, 1939	December 24, 1939
Marcolino Gomes Candau, M.D.	June 14, 1939	January 4, 1940
Alcides de Albuquerque, M.D.	December 20, 1939	March 20, 1940
Mario Batinga de Araujo Lessa, M.D.	September 29, 1939	February 29, 1940
Nelson Camillo de Almeida, M.D.	November 1, 1939	March 31, 1940
Werther Leite de Castro, M.D.	December 8, 1939	April 3, 1940
Manoel A. F. C. Couto, M.D.	November 1, 1939	June 1, 1940

Medical Staff of the Malaria Service of the Northeast—*Cont.*

Name	Period of Service	
Assistants—*Cont.*		
Seraphim Paulo Werner, M.D.	March 13, 1939	June 5, 1940
Arnaldo Neves, M.D.	December 8, 1939	July 31, 1940
Lourival de Souza Neiva, M.D.	December 12, 1939	August 7, 1940
Luciano Moura Soares, M.D.	March 6, 1940	August 15, 1940
Eduardo de Souza, M.D.	April 3, 1940	September 9, 1940
Gentil Portugal do Brasil, M.D.	December 8, 1939	September 11, 1940
Edmundo Barros Leite, M.D.	December 8, 1939	September 23, 1940
Rubens Bezerra Valente, M.D.	November 1, 1939	October 3, 1940
Decio Guanabarino Freiria, M.D.	September 30, 1939	December 31, 1940
Nelson de Carvalho Teixeira, M.D.	December 5, 1939	January 7, 1941
Antonio Bernabé Martines, M.D.	September 23, 1939	May 31, 1941
Ramon Affonso Anhel, M.D.	December 11, 1939	June 30, 1941
Osorio Tenorio Lima, M.D.	April 15, 1939	August 8, 1941
Carlos Renato Grey, M.D.	December 19, 1940	December 31, 1941
Antonio Serpa, Jr., M.D.	September 22, 1939	February 29, 1940.
Elias Gerbatin, M.D.	February 10, 1939	July 31, 1939
Manoel R. T. Liborio, M.D.	September 22, 1939	January 16, 1941

INTRODUCTION

Few threats to the future health of the Americas have equaled that inherent in the invasion of Brazil, in 1930, by *Anopheles (Myzomyia) gambiae* Giles 1902. Only the undated arrival of another African mosquito, the vector of urban and maritime yellow fever, *Aëdes (Stegomyia) aegypti* Linnaeus, can be considered to have rivaled it in importance.

Warning voices emphasized the tragic import of the finding of gambiae in Brazil, but no sustained effort was made to eradicate the species until almost a decade had passed.

Although gambiae gave a small dress rehearsal of its future program in Natal and at several other points in the State of Rio Grande do Norte in 1930 and 1931, it went into its act proper only in 1938 after reaching the Assú and Apodí valleys in Rio Grande do Norte and the Jaguaribe Valley in the State of Ceará. The cataclysm of 1938 left nothing to the imagination and gave to the Brazilians a new concept of the possibilities of malaria as an epidemic disease: "What will be the future of Ceará and Brazil, invaded by *A. gambiae?* The continued presence of this invader amongst us throws a deep shadow on any optimistic prophecies regarding the destiny of our nation" (Belo da Mota, in translation).

And Dr. Barber, a veteran student of malaria in many parts of the world, after a 3-month survey (May to August 1939) of the gambiae-infested region of Brazil, was led to write:

There is no doubt that this invasion of gambiae threatens the Americas with a catastrophe in comparison with which ordinary pestilence, conflagration, or even war are but small and temporary calamities. Gambiae literally enters into the very veins of a country and may remain to plague it for centuries.

Even the penetration of yellow fever into the Orient might well be a lesser evil, because its vector is domestic and more easily controlled. When the medical history of this century is written the result of the contest of health agencies with this preventible invasion will form one of its most interesting chapters.

The present report will attempt to summarize the most important points in the history of gambiae in Brazil and to describe the organization of the control measures in 1939 which resulted in its eradication in less than 2 years. It is to be hoped that this "one of the most interesting chapters in the medical history of this century" will not have to be rewritten.

TOPOGRAPHY OF NORTHEAST BRAZIL

In considering the topography of upper Northeast Brazil as a whole, it will be seen that only a comparatively small part of the total surface of the three states included therein, Paraíba, Rio Grande do Norte, and Ceará, is suitable to the large-scale production of gambiae.

The term Northeast Brazil has been used to designate the extensive areas from Piauí to Baía between the 3rd and 13th degrees south latitude, with a climate, except along certain parts of the coastal plain, more arid than tropical. Northeast Brazil is, geologically, a degraded zone where the ancient plateau in large part has been worn down to the crystalline skeleton. The erosion of this plateau has been far from uniform, with the result that the three states forming the shoulder of Brazil, which are of especial interest in connection with the study of gambiae, Ceará, Rio Grande do Norte, and Paraíba, are almost completely blocked off from the rest of Northeast Brazil by plateaus and mountains, except where the coastal plain extends to the south into Pernambuco and to the west into Piauí. These states, lying between the 3rd and 8th degrees south latitude and covering approximately 257,000 square kilometers, make up the northeastern slopes of the great Brazilian plateau with a series of terraces facing north, northeast, and east, formed by the denudation of the ancient sandstone plateau which once covered this part of the continent.

Terrain

Three distinct zones may be pointed out in this region: the mountains, the lower plateaus of the interior, and the coastal plain.

MOUNTAINS. The mountains and tablelands, varying in altitude from 400 to 1100 meters, are the remnants of the ancient plateau which, through surface erosion, has been laid bare down to the Archean basement. There are, however, three main mountain ranges in the states under discussion which are still capped with complexes of sandstone alternating with thin layers of limestone. These are the Ibiapaba mountain range and the Araripe plateau, which bound Ceará on the west and south, and parts of the Apodí plateau, which is the watershed between the Jaguaribe and the Apodí river valleys in the boundary between Ceará and Rio Grande do Norte.

The soil of these three ranges absorbs much of the rainfall which they receive, but practically all the other mountains are dry and rocky and entirely unsuited to conserving water. Except for a thin layer of porous soil, resulting from the decomposition of the surface, water does not penetrate this terrain but rushes in torrents down the narrow rocky valleys during the rainy season. Even the thin layer of porous soil permits rapid evaporation and the little moisture retained quickly disappears.

LOWER PLATEAUS. The terrain of the major portion of the states of Ceará and Rio Grande do Norte slopes gently from the mountain masses to the coast. Much of it ranges from 100 to 300 meters above sea level, but it is broken in many places by hilly ranges or isolated hills, some with sharp, others with gently rounded profiles. Lying between these hilly ranges are broad shallow river valleys which carry the flood of water during the rainy season, drying up completely shortly thereafter. The main exceptions are the Jaguaribe River, which drains almost half of the area of the State of Ceará, and the Apodí and Assú rivers in Rio Grande do Norte, whose subsurface water sheet, even during the height of the dry season, allows of conditions which greatly favor gambiae production.

COASTAL PLAIN. The coastal plain, which is from 3 to 25 kilometers wide and rarely rises more than 100 meters above sea level, is composed of clays and soft low limestone cliffs, as well as sand dunes. All along this coastal plain seepage areas extremely favorable to gambiae breeding occur.

Drainage System

Except for a small section of western Ceará which drains into the Parnaíba Valley through the Boqueirão do Poti, the drainage of this region, following the slope of the terrain to the coast, is entirely independent of that of the rest of Brazil. Likewise, the drainage system of Ceará is completely independent of those of Rio Grande do Norte and Paraíba, which have some valleys in common.

In each of the states of Rio Grande do Norte and Ceará there are two main river valleys and a coastal section which is drained by small short rivers. In Rio Grande do Norte it is the eastern third which is drained by short coastal rivers rising in the easternmost mountains of the Borborema range and running eastward to the sea. These are all relatively unimportant, including the Potengí and the Ceará Mirím, which are somewhat larger than the others. The state's most important river, the Assú, draining its central section, rises beyond the southern border, in the State of Paraíba, and runs in a northeasterly direction to the northern coast. Parallel to the Assú, and separated from it by the João do Vale mountains, runs the Apodí River, which drains the western third of the state.

Across the Ceará boundary, on the other side of the Apodí range and paralleling the course of the Assú and Apodí rivers, lies the largest river of all the gambiae-infested area, the Jaguaribe, which, together with its tributaries, drains all the southern, central, and eastern sections of the state. The Acaraú River, the second largest in Ceará, drains the western section of the state at the foot of the Ibiapaba range, while small relatively unimportant rivers drain the central coastal area.

As has been mentioned above, most of the terrain is practically impermeable, with the exception of the sediment-covered mountain ranges (Ibiapaba, Araripe, and to a lesser extent Apodí), the sandy plains in the river valleys, and the coastal plain. Even the alluvial plains in the lower river valleys, away from the river banks, are of clay which does not permit much absorption, and water collecting here after floods and rains disappears only by evaporation.

As a result, although there is an average annual rainfall of about 960 millimeters, only a very small amount is taken up by the soil. The rest, from the moment of its first contact with the parched hot soil to the beginning of the subsequent rainy season, is subject to constant evaporation. Of the water which rushes down the steep mountainous slopes of the upper reaches of the rivers, flooding the wide shallow river beds and overflowing the banks, only a small amount ever reaches the sea. In the Jaguaribe, largest river system of the region, Pompeu Sobrinho calculated that of an average rainfall of 68,760 million cubic meters during the years 1912–1914, 4 per cent was taken up by the soil, 6.5 per cent was drained off to the sea, and almost 90 per cent was lost by evaporation.

In general, therefore, it can be said that the valleys of the rivers of this region are separated from each other by high dry plateaus or mountain ranges. Even the rivers of the coastal plain, which are short and parallel each other in a more or less direct course to the sea, are generally separated from each other by sandy or dry elevated areas, offering few opportunities for the formation of ground pools suitable for mosquito production.

DEVELOPMENT OF PROGRAM
Initial Difficulties

The Malaria Service of the Northeast (see Fig. 39) encountered many difficulties and made little apparent progress during the early months of its existence. The relatively large area would have been much easier to

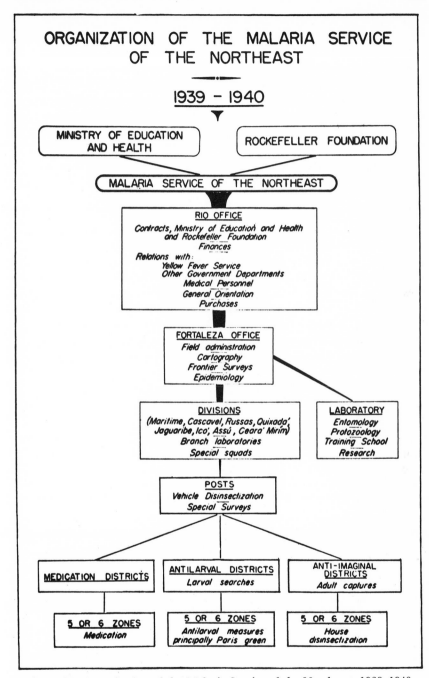

Figure 39. Organization of the Malaria Service of the Northeast, 1939–1940.

cover had it been an island, unable to expand daily as did the gambiae-infested area. Unduly rapid development of an administrative program is always uneconomical but the threat of farther spread of gambiae justified the attempt to cover the area as rapidly as possible.

While personnel was being selected and trained, gambiae was progressing in its march into previously clean areas. The 1938 surveys of gambiae distribution were dry season surveys and definite information was lacking regarding longevity of gambiae eggs, of possible estivation of adults, and the comparative extent of gambiae breeding in wet and dry seasons. These surveys had given a rough idea of the distribution of gambiae at the time they were made, but no one knew to what extent gambiae had been able to take advantage of later favorable opportunities to spread into contiguous regions.

The fact that the Malaria Service entered the field at the beginning of the rainy season was a great handicap. Malaria was epidemic once again, as in the previous year, and humanitarian considerations forced organization of a treatment campaign at a time when administrative energy should have been concentrated on developing and applying methods of gambiae control. Malaria also constituted a serious problem for the Service in its effect on the health of the personnel. Food was difficult to obtain in many areas, since malaria had reduced production during the preceding season. Transportation away from the main highways is always slow in the rainy season. Mapping was difficult and the assignment of definite areas to be worked by individual inspectors impossible. Checking of results was uncertain and there could be no assurance that all parts of a region were being worked. The great expanse of water during the rainy season caused a false impression of the necessity for drainage and led to the digging of useless ditches, later abandoned. The multiplication of potential foci during the rainy season also made it imperative to double the number of men employed for Paris green distribution and larval searches at a time when well-trained personnel was at a premium.

The personnel question was a serious one, and the absorption of the staff of the Antimalaria Service with its seven doctors and hundreds of employees, in the face of the transfer of many men from the Yellow Fever Service to key positions in the new organization, created certain problems which could have been avoided had the Malaria Service of the Northeast started from the ground up. The personnel from the Yellow Fever Service was well trained in the technique for eradication of aegypti but had had no experience in working with anopheles, whereas the personnel of the Antimalaria Service, trained as malariologists, was considering the gambiae program as a malaria, rather than as a species eradication campaign. The selection and training of the thousands of men needed was in itself no small task, and the fact that it was first necessary to instruct the doctors and chief inspectors before they in turn could train the subordinate personnel created serious delays. The legal requirement of a certificate of at least one year's military training for employment by any agency using federal funds could rarely be fulfilled by men in the back country and prevented the Service from rapidly acquiring the large number of workers needed until after special dispensation from this requirement was granted for certain types of workers.

The greatest handicap in the beginning, however, was the complete lack of a definite concrete technique which could be guaranteed to eradicate gambiae. Although it was known that the gambiae imago is highly susceptible to pyrethrum sprays and that Paris green is an effective larvicide for this species, no practical system had ever been worked out for the eradication of gambiae, and the new Service began operations without a definite preformulated plan. This rendered it inexpedient to order supplies at the beginning of the campaign before their utility had been demonstrated in the field. Under these circumstances the interval which elapsed before material could be received from Rio de Janeiro or from abroad was at times a serious factor in retarding the developing of the campaign.

First Six Months of 1939

In spite of the many difficulties, a great deal of important work was done during the first 6 months of 1939.

Surveys of gambiae distribution were made which showed the continued spread of this species in Ceará up the Jaguaribe and its tributaries and along the coast toward Fortaleza, while in Rio Grande do Norte the extent of infestation in the Apodí and Assú rivers was found to be greater than anticipated. Gambiae seemed to take advantage of the rainy season, spreading far and wide. In the Banabuiú River, an affluent of the Jaguaribe, gambiae was found in June 120 kilometers above the point which earlier in the year had been considered as the last outpost of infestation. Scores of such unexpected findings contributed to the uneasiness of mind felt by those responsible for the antigambiae campaign.

Antimalaria treatment was given to 114,000 persons, a field staff of 2500 men (May) was mobilized, rough maps of areas to be worked were prepared, vehicle disinsectization for prevention of the transportation of gambiae to clean areas was begun, and the Central Laboratory was installed at Aracatí. Administratively, the infested area of Ceará fell into three divisions, Russas, Quixadá, and Icó, and that of Rio Grande do Norte into two, Ceará Mirím and Assú.

Much was learned about the gambiae mosquito and the advantages and disadvantages of various antilarval measures in the campaign against this species. During the first 4 months of the year, 87 per cent of the antilarval work consisted of filling in and oiling, while Paris green accounted for only 5 per cent. By June, however, the advantages of the simplest methods of Paris green application had been demonstrated and from that month on, this larvicide became the mainstay of the antilarval work.

In spite of everything, however, no results of the general attack on gambiae, which could be given statistical presentation, were apparent at the end of June 1939. Those responsible for the orientation of the antigambiae program carefully nourished rays of hope originating from the apparent eradication of gambiae from the coastal village of Caiçara in May, from the labor camp at Lima Campos in the Iguatú area in June, and from a stretch of highway between Russas and Fortaleza, to bolster the decision to ask for additional resources with which to expand the Service to a point where all infested areas could be covered. During the first half of the year the Malaria Service of the Northeast had spent much more than the proportional part of the year's budget, without covering all the infested area with antimosquito measures. The central, heavily infested, lower Jaguaribe Valley was repeatedly sacrificed through the withdrawal of men for the protection of the frontiers where gambiae was still spreading. In June, before additional funds for the year were assured, some 250 men working in this lower valley were laid off to guaranty funds for the payment of salaries in the important frontier areas until the end of the year. An appeal was made for additional funds and before the end of June the Brazilian Government had agreed to increase its contribution by 2000 contos (about $100,000 U.S.) in spite of the fact that the only concrete result which could be claimed for the Service was the demonstrable reduction in mortality from malaria due largely to the treatment campaign. This was especially striking at Russas, where the antimosquito measures had not yet been adequately organized.

Second Six Months of 1939

During the second semester of 1939 gambiae made slight gains in territory in the Assú, Apodí, and Jaguaribe river valleys and a jump of 50 kilometers took place along the coast from the mouth of the Pirangí to Caponga in the direction of Fortaleza. As each new frontier focus was discovered, small armies of workers were sent in to cope with the situation.

In addition to the routine frontier surveys, special reconnaissance trips were made to many localities, well beyond the known infested area. These led as far afield as the states of Paraíba, Piauí, and Maranhão. Fortunately, although it was feared that gambiae might have been transported to some distant point and there established itself, no evidence of its spread beyond the states of Ceará and Rio Grande do Norte was ever found.

The three divisions into which the infested area in Ceará had originally been divided proved too large to be handled satisfactorily and in the second semester of 1939 two more divisions were organized, Cascavel and Jaguaribe. It was early in this semester that the Martime Division was installed.

An important development during this period was the inauguration of routine house disinsectization, at first in a few and later in all infested areas. Wholesale disinsectization was not instituted until December and so its full effect was not felt until the following year. Although antilarval measures alone had brought about the apparent complete elimination of gambiae in several of the most heavily infested districts, it was hoped that the introduction of anti-imaginal measures would speed up the process.

In the second semester of 1939 the Malaria Service continued to overspend its budget. It was felt that large amounts expended at the outset for encircling the known infested area and for a concerted effort to push gambiae back toward the lower Jaguaribe would, in the long run, be profitable by preventing extensions to well-watered areas which might render later eradication many times more difficult and expensive.

In addition, therefore, to the 2000-contos increase already agreed to by the government during the first semester, 3000 contos ($150,000 U.S.) more was requested. In asking for the additional appropriation, three facts were stressed: first, that the budget as originally planned had not included funds for medication and that up to August 1939 almost 800-contos' worth ($40,000 U.S.) of drugs had been bought and distributed in the infested areas; second, that although gambiae had made no long-distance hops it had nevertheless gotten within 25 kilometers of Fortaleza and was also traveling south, threatening the well-watered area around Crato from which extension to the São Francisco River Valley might be possible; and third, that in June 250 employees had been released, not because they were not urgently needed elsewhere, but because of the rapidly dwindling budget. The additional 3000 contos was granted, bringing the total sum appropriated for gambiae work by the Brazilian Federal Government in 1939 to 10,000 contos, or some $500,000 U.S.

By the end of 1939 the Malaria Service of the Northeast could begin to feel some real optimism (see Fig. 69). The places cleaned during the first 6 months had not become reinfested and before the end of the year, gambiae was no longer being found at Caponga, on the coast; at Forquilha, Bom Successo, and Cariús on the upper Jaguaribe (Ceará); and at Assú, Lake Piató, and São Gonçalo (Rio Grande do Norte). Before these gains could be considered definite, however, the disturbing question as to what extent the success of gambiae elimination from these areas was due to the effect of the dry season had still to be answered. Only after the rains of 1940 began would a satisfactory solution be forthcoming.

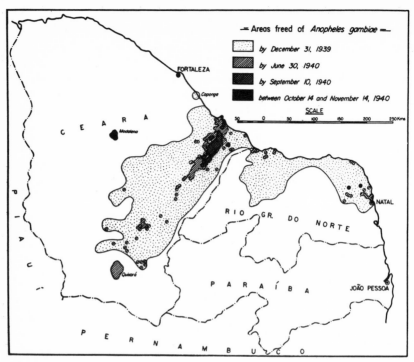

Figure 69. Areas freed of *Anopheles gambiae.*

First Six Months of 1940

Based not only on apparent results already obtained but also on the existence of a trained staff, the year began with some optimism of a proved technique and of what was confidently thought to be an adequate budget. The budget for the first 6 months of 1940 amounted to 12,500 contos ($625,000 U.S.): 10,000 contos ($500,000 U.S.) from Brazilian Government funds and 2500 contos ($125,000 U.S.) from The Rockefeller Foundation.

The rainy season set in earlier than usual in 1940, substantial rains having fallen in many places as early as the preceding December. In the first week of 1940 the special frontier squad discovered a gambiae focus near Quixará on the Cariús River. This represented a jump of about 50 kilometers from the focus at Cariús, which had been discovered and cleared up in the last half of the preceding year, and directly threatened Crato, less than 50 kilometers away on a passable highway. Large numbers of combat workers were at once dispatched and at the end of 4 weeks, gambiae had apparently been exterminated, as it did not reappear in this zone. No other new areas of infestation were found during the semester.

But in spite of this spearhead of invasion up the Jaguaribe valley, gambiae was giving way rapidly throughout the infested regions in the face of the onslaught with Paris green and insecticide. Reports from every division showed that gambiae-free areas were becoming more and more extensive, even during the rainy season. On the other hand, however, gambiae increased rapidly in Gracismões and Cumbe, the two districts where in order to permit the study of gambiae under natural conditions no control measures were being carried out.

In his paper (unpublished) before the IV Pan American Conference of National Directors of Health in Washington, D.C., in May 1940, Dr. Evandro Chagas, who directed the work of the Division for Studies on Endemic Diseases in Gracismões, said:

With the continuation of the dry season up to January 1940 the adult density (in the comparison area of Gracismões) went gradually down again, with a rise in October due to unexpected rains in this month. In January, February, and March, 1940, the adult density became very high so that in April, in the second half of the month we already had a very high index of adults. The rise appeared sooner this year than in 1939 and this fact coincides with the period of rainfall which was also earlier this year.

Concurrently with the reported decrease in the incidence of gambiae there was a greatly diminished demand for antimalaria treatment during the first half of 1940, and in many areas prophylactic administration of drugs to the personnel of the Malaria Service was suspended.

At the end of 1939 and in January 1940, respectively, Drs. G. K. Strode and L. W. Hackett visited the Malaria Service of the Northeast. In view of the apparent absence of gambiae in certain sections, each independently suggested that the validity of this disappearance be tested by abandoning all control measures and giving gambiae freedom to reappear.* However, it was not until mid-April 1940 that this challenge to gambiae was put into effect. The area chosen for the original test was a large part of the Salgado Valley in the Icó Division, at one time heavily infested but which had apparently been clean for some 3 months. Control measures were suspended and elaborate precautions were taken to guard against any unrecognized persistence of gambiae by instituting both larval searches and house captures of adults in the areas abandoned. The training of inspectors to recognize adult gambiae is fairly easy, but training to recognize larvae is more difficult. It was decided to trust entirely to microscopic examina-

* Dr. Hackett's experience in Durazzo, Albania, made him especially emphatic on this point. There, after a whole summer without a single *A. maculipennis* var. *elutus* in an area where the campaign against that mosquito was being waged through salinification of its only breeding place, intensive production of *elutus* followed when failure to keep open the saltwater intake made its former breeding place again suitable.

tion for the identification of larvae and therefore collections of larvae from all anopheles foci found were taken to the division laboratory for classification. No evidence of persistence of infestation or of reinfestation by gambiae in cleaned areas in which control measures had been suspended was found. The men released consequently from these areas were sent to the divisions on the lower Jaguaribe, which had never been adequately manned; the work of the Russas Division, the only one without a frontier, was especially affected by this measure.

With the decision to suspend gambiae control in Icó, orders were given simultaneously to inaugurate control measures in the study areas at Cumbe, near Aracatí, and at Gracismões, near Russas, for it was felt that gambiae now constituted a threat to the surrounding countryside there. That this danger did exist was confirmed by house captures which produced 2202 adult gambiae in 49 houses at Cumbe and 5825 gambiae in 47 of the 58 buildings in Gracismões. These figures are conclusive evidence that the season was a highly favorable one for the production of gambiae and that the reduction of density of this species at other points noted during the rainy season itself was due to control measures.

Gambiae's failure to reappear following the suspension of control activities was most heartening, and not less so was the demonstration that the Malaria Service of the Northeast now possessed a technique whereby gambiae could be pushed back and driven out even during the rainy season. By the end of the first semester of 1940 it was apparent to all that the final liquidation of gambiae in the known infested areas was but a matter of months, and the campaign became an exciting race between the personnel of different divisions to see who could finish with gambiae first.

Second Semester of 1940

The optimism of the first semester was reflected in a voluntary reduction of 20 per cent in the Service budget.

The retreat of gambiae continued rapidly during the second semester and the routine was followed of abandoning disinsectization in an area shortly after it failed to show either larvae or adults and of suspending the application of Paris green after a period of 3 months of freedom from gambiae. As the frontier areas became clean, more and more men were released and were then concentrated in the remaining dirty areas.

The monthly maps of gambiae distribution in 1940 (see Fig. 70) show clearly the way in which the cleaning of one section was followed rapidly by the cleaning of others. During the month of May, the Russas Division, the last of the known infested sections to be cleaned, had 226 dirty points; during June, 126; during July, 103; and during August, only 18, some of which were completely cleaned up before the end of the month. No gambiae was found in this division after September 9.

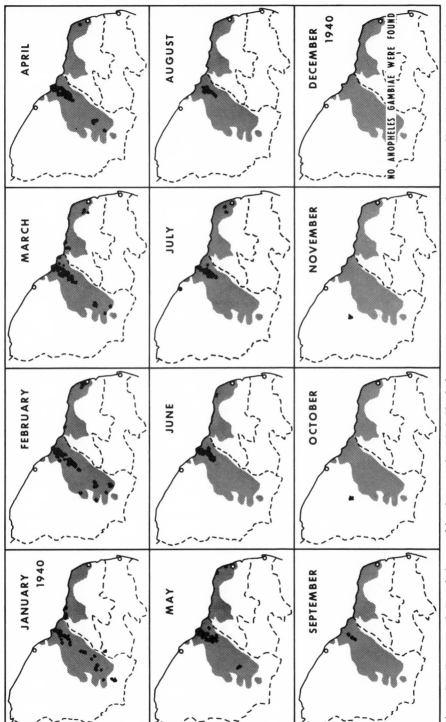

Figure 70. Retreat of *Anopheles gambiae*, by months, 1940. Shaded area represents greatest extent of gambiae dissemination; black dots indicate places where gambiae was found in 1940.

APRIL

AUGUST

DECEMBER 1940

NO ANOPHELES GAMBIAE WERE FOUND

MARCH

JULY

NOVEMBER

FEBRUARY

JUNE

OCTOBER

JANUARY 1940

MAY

SEPTEMBER

Once the Aracatí sector of the Russas Division was proved to be clean, the laboratory colony of gambiae in Aracatí was regarded as a potential source of reinfestation and was therefore killed off on August 31.

On September 7, Brazil's Independence Day, a luncheon was given to members of the staff of the Malaria Service in Fortaleza to celebrate the virtual extinction of gambiae in the Northeast. Some outside observers thought this premature but the staff knew from personal experience that control measures had been developed to the point where the trained personnel of the Malaria Service was capable of cleaning immediately any new area of infestation which might appear. The opportunity to test this optimistic attitude arose a few weeks later when a previously unknown pocket of gambiae infestation was uncovered in October at Madalena beyond the Quixadá Division, some 60 kilometers from Quixadá. The last autochthonous gambiae found in Brazil was collected November 9, the last larva November 14, 1940.

Another indication of the efficacy of the control measures was the decline in the number of individuals seeking treatment at the various posts. By September 1, 1940, there were not enough cases of malaria to justify keeping special employees to treat the few cases which did appear, and treatment was suspended throughout the whole area (see Figs. 72 and 73).

The year 1940 ended with all control measures against gambiae, including both Paris green and insecticide, suspended except in the small area at Madalena. Complete optimism existed regarding the absence of gambiae from the controlled areas, but considerable reservation was made as to complete species eradication because of the possibility of gambiae's having escaped to more distant regions.

Control Methods

Of all the measures devised for the control of mosquitoes only two, Paris green to kill larvae and pyrethrum spray insecticide to kill adults, were employed on a large scale by the Service.

Antilarval Measures

The so-called naturalistic methods of control were not attempted; the attack on gambiae was frontal and direct.

Drainage in general was of little use in the gambiae campaign and swamp drainage was found to be unnecessary.

Flooding land with seawater was used only on the lower Potengí River in Natal, in the area of original gambiae infestation.

Filling was used for the elimination of certain small collections of water which could be filled easily with nearby soil. New borrow pits, new water holes, and after the floods of the rainy season subsided, new marginal pools

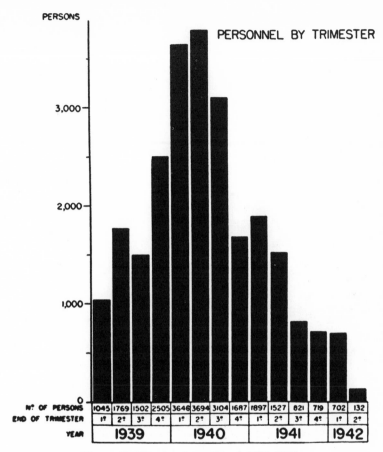

Figure 72. Personnel employed 1939–1942.

were constantly being formed, so that the number to be filled was always great.

Marginal filling and regulation were used at times to make all parts of pools and streams accessible to fish, but the artificial *distribution of fish* was not attempted.

Oil was used as an emergency larvicide, during the first 3 or 4 months of work, since supplies were at hand and some of the available workers were familiar with its use.

Paris green application to all foci was practically the only antilarval measure employed after the first few months. The method of application varied according to the season:

1. Wet method: a mixture of water and a stock emulsion of Paris green and kerosene, used during the rainy season when water was easily obtainable.

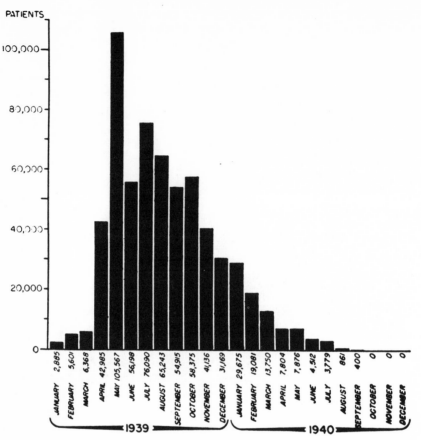

Figure 73. Number of patients under treatment for malaria, by months, 1939–1940.

2. Moist method: the stock emulsion mentioned above and moistened pebbles, wet sand, or even earth, used during the transition period between dry and wet season.

3. Dry method: dust, dry sand, or dry earth, used during the dry season when practically no water could be found.

OTHER MEASURES VERSUS PARIS GREEN. The failure to use many of the methods in the armamentarium of the modern malariologist was due to the urgency of the situation, to the peculiar local conditions which made some of them useless, and to the fact that measures designed for anopheles reduction may not be equally advantageous in eradication campaigns.

Drainage requires technical planning and supervision, is slow, expensive, and in regions subject to annual rainy season flooding must be renewed each year. Where the program is one of local malaria control for a limited population in a given area, drainage may often be used to advantage, but in a campaign for species eradication, there is no profit in moving water from one point to another, unless by so doing it can be eliminated as a possible source of breeding at the point of delivery.

The artificial distribution of fish was not employed in spite of the fact that the fish hatcheries of the Department of Agriculture offered unlimited supplies of local minnows which had proved very effective against aegypti larvae. The majority of gambiae foci during the rainy season were found away from the river beds and were too temporary to offer living conditions for minnows; dry season foci, on the contrary, were mostly in the river beds, where fish occurred naturally, it being necessary only to rectify the margins to permit their access to the entire water surface.

Oil has many disadvantages in a species-eradication campaign, among which may be cited its cost, the difficulty of distribution to workers in the field, and the rendering of essential water supplies unfit for use. After the application of Paris green was systematized, oil was used only as a disciplinary measure to force compliance with the protection of water holes against infestation.

One of the great advantages of Paris green, as used by the Malaria Service of the Northeast, is that at no season of the year is it necessary to spend money on the transportation of diluent for the larvicide. It is easy for the inspector to carry the necessary Paris green or stock emulsion and to find a suitable diluent at his place of work. The difference in distribution cost alone gives Paris green a tremendous advantage over oil as a larvicide for species eradication campaigns in which all the infested areas must be worked.

The application of Paris green presented some difficulties at first but soon came to be the only antilarval measure employed throughout the infested area. Both the low price of labor and the type of water collection preferred by gambiae made the hand application of Paris green the method of choice, although it may well be less effective against other anopheles which do not, as does gambiae, prefer open shallow pools without vegetation and only the margins of large collections of water.

PARIS GREEN AS USED BY THE MALARIA SERVICE OF THE NORTHEAST. Paris green as a larvicide has been known to Brazilian workers for many years, but it had never been used on a large scale and many minor but important details of technique had to be learned before its use was adapted to the conditions of Northeast Brazil. During the first months of 1939 there were no stocks of suitable Paris green available except a small order which had been placed by the Antimalaria Service, and no one in Brazil was familiar with the wet method of Paris green application. As the Malaria Service of the Northeast began to work during the rainy season when road dust was not obtainable, preliminary plans were made to use dust from one of the cement factories, but analysis of transportation costs showed this to be impracticable.

In the early months of the use of Paris green in the antigambiae campaign, the larvicide was applied on a weekly cycle, since gambiae may develop to the imago within 6 days after oviposition. Later, as peripheral areas were cleaned, freeing personnel for the final drive on the infested central areas, semiweekly treatment was adopted because, under field conditions, a given application of Paris green may fail to kill 100 per cent of the larvae present.

The first attempt to use the wet method of Paris green application gave unsatisfactory results, probably because distribution was by common garden sprinklers. When Excelsior horticultural pressure pumps equipped with mechanical agitator paddles became available, highly satisfactory results were obtained. Laboratory tests showed that constant agitation of the larvicide during spraying is imperative, but that the addition of egg albumen or castor oil to effect an even distribution of the Paris green is unnecessary. The addition of egg albumen did improve the suspension of Paris green in water, but it also rendered it less buoyant and therefore less effective, as large quantities immediately sank when spread upon water. It was also found that Paris green containing special floating agents is unsatisfactory, as it tends to froth and be blown to one side of pools being treated. Nine types of Paris green with particles varying in size from 2 to 25 microns were tested. Field and laboratory observations indicated that the 2 to 3-micron Airfloat Paris green was by far the best for antigambiae work.

The wet method finally adopted required the inspector to carry to the field a small amount of a stock emulsion in the proportion of 1 gram of Paris green to 2 cc of kerosene or diesel oil. At the site of application, 1 part of this emulsion was mixed with 100 parts of water taken from the foci to be treated and the resultant liquid was applied with knapsack pressure spray pumps. The only serious drawback to this method of application is that it necessitates carrying a pump, weighing some 20 pounds, from place to place.

The moist method proved its value during the transition from the dry to the wet season, when dry earth is not yet available and when pools with sufficient water to fill the knapsack pump are scarce. It is quite effective, especially for gambiae larvae which have been observed to feed at the bottom of pools as well as at the surface, but requires very careful application since the Paris green–kerosene–wet sand mixture, broadcast by hand, is not spread by the wind as is the Paris green–dust mixture.

The favorite method of the Malaria Service of the Northeast for the application of Paris green, however, was that in which the dry mixture was used. It was less messy and, aided by the wind, a given area could be covered more quickly than with the kerosene or oil mixture. Arrived at the place of application the inspector scooped up approximately 1 kilogram of dry earth, dust, or fine gravel and mixed this thoroughly with 10 grams of Paris green, repeating the operation until 5 kilograms had been mixed. For this work, the inspector only needed to carry around with him a small supply of Paris green, a standard measure for 10 grams, a pail with a mark indicating the approximate level reached by 5 kilograms of earth, and a grocer's scoop for collecting dust. In most divisions the mixture was dispersed by hand, but in others the scoop was also used, in which case the inspector needed some practice to acquire the proper knack of distributing the mixture evenly. But it was worth the effort as it diminished the risk to the operator of mild arsenic poisoning, which was uncomfortably frequent during the early months of the use of the larvicide by inexperienced men.

Such poisoning constituted the chief disadvantage of Paris green, as used in the antigambiae campaign. The most common manifestations were acneform dermatitis on the forearms and hands, vesicles on the upper lip and nasal alae, ulcers of the scrotum, with occasional secondary pyogenic infections, and epistaxis. Efforts to avoid this field hazard included insistence on frequent baths and clean fingernails. The men were trained to take every precaution in mixing and spreading the Paris green-dust mixture, but the veering gusty winds of the river beds made it difficult. Gradually the inspectors learned to work with minimal contact of skin and mucous membranes with the dust, with gratifying results; those who reacted severely and persistently were transferred from the antilarval to some other branch of the Service, when all signs of poisoning disappeared rapidly.

Official complaints were received from county authorities and private individuals in a score of localities to the effect that Paris green was killing cattle, goats, sheep, and chickens. Even abortions in domestic stock were attributed to the Paris green applied in the watering holes. A careful consideration of these complaints showed that some of the abortions were due to brucellosis, which had not hitherto been reported in Ceará. Agglutination tests on selected sera showed that brucella infection occurred in the human population, in dairy cows, and in goats.

Fortunately popular opinion did not attribute any human ailments to Paris green, and only six accidents were reported during the application of some 260 tons in Northeast Brazil. Paris green was the lethal agent for two suicides; it was swallowed by three children, two of whom recovered; and an overzealous inspector, who also eventually recovered, suffered severely from a public demonstration of the nontoxicity of Paris green in which he added a goodly portion of it to his beer.

Anti-imaginal Methods

Screening, which looms so large in some antimalaria campaigns, had no place in the program of the Malaria Service of the Northeast. The houses of the region worked could have been made mosquitoproof only with great difficulty; screening material was very expensive and, even had it been possible to screen on a large scale, this measure would not have had an appreciable influence in checking the spread of the species nor in eradicating it. As a matter of individual protection employees of the Malaria Service working in infested zones were supplied with special mosquito nets adapted to the hammocks in which they slept.

DESTRUCTION OF ADULT MOSQUITOES.

Historical. The attack on adult mosquitoes for the reduction of mosquito-borne disease is not new but dates from the first antimosquito campaigns organized after it was demonstrated that malaria and yellow fever are transmitted by mosquitoes. Fumigation was an integral part of the campaigns of Gorgas and Oswaldo Cruz for the eradication of yellow fever from Havana and Rio de Janeiro and, although he later abandoned the idea, Gorgas at first considered this measure to have been a major factor in his success at Havana.

Although Carlos Chagas (1906 and 1908) early advanced the theory that malaria is a domiciliary disease, acquired in the house and transmitted by house-frequenting mosquitoes, it is surprising that until recent years no large-scale attempts were made to control malaria through the destruction of adult mosquitoes, in contrast with the extensive and enthusiastic attempts to destroy adult mosquitoes in the control of yellow fever. But even in the case of yellow fever, adult destruction methods were aimed at the infected mosquito in an attempt to get rid of the disease and were not part of a program to eradicate the guilty species.

The first large-scale use of spray insecticide instead of fumigation for the destruction of infected mosquitoes is believed to have been made in the antiaegypti campaign during the 1928–1929 outbreak of yellow fever in Rio de Janeiro. Dr. Emygdio de Mattos found the spray insecticide very efficient, but its application by hand pumps impracticable in military barracks and other large buildings. An appeal for ideas was made to the local representative of the manufacturer of one of the more popular commercial spray insecticides, who suggested the use of the paint spray pistol operated by compressed air. This led to the development of equipment with which houses totaling 183,243 floors were disinsectized in Rio de Janeiro during the years 1928–1929.

In 1933–1934, the weekly spraying of houses and huts by hand pumps was introduced for the control of malaria in Natal, South Africa, where *A. gambiae* and *A. funestus* are the principal vectors. Park Ross reported that the systematic use of spray insecticide was invariably followed by a sharp reduction in the number of cases of malaria in huts and barracks and by the disappearance of epidemic conditions.

One of us (F.L.S.) had an opportunity to visit South Africa in 1935 and see at first hand the work done in Zululand, Natal Province, under the direction of Park Ross, and was duly impressed. Three years later Park Ross reported (Personal communication, 1938):

You will be interested to hear that we have prevented epidemic malaria in Natal and Zululand for five years now by hut spraying. We have seldom had such heavy breeding as during the past two years and had a sprinkling of cases all over the country; but only a sprinkling, and in every case we stamped it out by spraying before there was any semblance of even a minor outbreak.

The results in Africa led to the testing of adult destruction as a means of malaria control in other regions.

In India the use of spray insecticide apparently caused a great reduction in malaria transmission, without noticeably affecting the house density of the principal vector, *A. culicifacies*, which is not essentially a domestic species. In other words, the results were obtained by an attack on the parasite in the infected mosquito in the house rather than by an attack on the mosquito species itself.

TECHNIQUE OF SPRAY DISINSECTIZATION USED IN BRAZIL. The results obtained with spraying in South Africa were correlated with a great reduction in the number of gambiae in the huts, which suggested that spray insecticide might be useful in the campaign about to be undertaken in Brazil for the eradication of this highly domestic mosquito.

Spray insecticide was used by the Malaria Service of the Northeast

1. To reduce the density of adult gambiae and, as a result, the possibility of its spread from infested to clean areas by infiltration or by transportation.

2. To destroy adult gambiae being carried by train, car, truck, boat, and plane.

3. To shorten the period of continued egg laying, after larval control was begun, by killing off a large number of the adults which otherwise would have oviposited.

4. To reduce the incidence of malaria by preventing the mosquitoes which emerged, in spite of antilarval measures, from developing infectivity.

Various experiments were made before the insecticide mixture finally employed was evolved. Kerosene and various types of diesel oil were tested, and the diesel oil marketed under the trade name Combustol proved to be a more toxic vehicle than other oils and kerosene. Even when Combustol was applied alone in the routine way, many mosquitoes in cages placed in the houses sprayed were later found dead. With kerosene alone no mosquitoes were killed. Combustol had the disadvantage, however, of leaving a thin oily film on furniture and other household articles.

Since many of the houses sprayed had open kitchen fires, carbon tetrachloride was added to the insecticide to reduce inflammability. In the proportions used, the mixture would flare when sprayed into an open flame, but no accidents ever occurred from this source. The addition of more carbon tetrachloride would have greatly reduced the buoyancy of the atomized spray in the air. An attempt to use water as a vehicle for pyrethrum extract was unsuccessful, the atomized fog settling quickly to the floor.

The spray insecticide used was in most cases composed of 5 parts of a pyrethrum concentrate 1-20 (trade name Pyrocide 20), which contains 2.0 grams of pyrethrins in each 10 cc of the pyrethrum concentrate, 10 parts of carbon tetrachloride, added for its fire-preventing as well as insecticidal properties, and 85 parts of kerosene or diesel oil.

The equipment used consisted of a spray pistol of the DeVilbiss type requiring a tank for compressed air with at least 15 pounds pressure to the square inch for satisfactory operation. Most of the work throughout the rural areas was done with small portable hand-operated tanks, whereas gasoline-engine-powered tanks, capable of giving 35 to 40 pounds pressure for several spray pistols operating simultaneously, were used in the towns and at the larger disinsectization posts for vehicles.

In the rural areas the disinsectization squad, consisting of one inspector and three laborers, equipped with two hand-powered pressure pumps and two spray pistols, made the rounds weekly, spraying all buildings and outhouses in the zone assigned to it. All doors and windows were closed and, with two laborers manning the pumps and the inspector and one laborer each operating a pistol, the rooms were sprayed one at a time until a cloud of spray was visible from the roof to the floor. Instructions were left with the family to keep the house closed for 10 minutes after spraying. No attempt was made on routine disinsectization to count or collect the mosquitoes killed but a careful record was kept of the houses sprayed, the time spent in each house, and the amount of insecticide used. To facilitate checking the work of the squad the inspector noted the date of the spraying and the hour of his arrival and departure on a form which was posted in each house.

In the towns, mule-drawn carts were used to carry the gasoline-motor equipment with a number of spray pistols attached to the compressed air lines, from house to house. With such equipment, disinsectization of the larger houses and buildings of the towns is relatively easy.

No attempt was made to seal the houses before spraying. This would have been an impossible task in the thatch-roofed and mud-walled houses of the region worked. Spraying has an advantage over fumigation, in that the spray is a cloud of minute droplets which do not disappear by expansion and dilution as do gases such as sulfur dioxide. Rooms need not be hermetically sealed to force contact of disinfectant with mosquito, but simply closed for a few minutes.

After the decision was made to disinfect houses as a control measure, weekly spraying of all houses in infested areas was organized as rapidly as the necessary personnel and equipment became available. Preference was always given to the organization of disinsectization work in the peripheral and frontier areas, so that only relatively late in the campaign, after the periphery was clean, were the heavily infested central areas treated. After the adult capture and larval breeding indices of an area were both reported as zero, weekly disinsectization of houses was discontinued.

Disinsectization of trains, trucks, passenger cars, boats, and planes was regularly carried out at certain key points of departure from the infested areas or immediately after arrival in clean districts. Provision was made for 24-hour service at the more important points. The same pyrethrum extract mixture used for the disinsectization of houses was employed, except that for use in planes the proportions of pyrethrum and of carbon tetrachloride were both doubled.

DISCUSSION

Reality of Threat to the Other Americas

When the story of the 1938 gambiae-produced epidemic of malaria in Northeast Brazil became known in other countries of the Americas, many health officials grew alarmed over the future safety of their own provinces, whereas others adopted the philosophy "It can't happen here." Some of the first group, representing several different countries, gathered at the Xth Pan American Sanitary Conference at Bogotá in September 1938, went so far as to discuss unofficially the need for a common international war chest to finance the attempt to rid Brazil of gambiae. Others believed from the first that gambiae could not be eradicated and that it made little difference to their countries whether it was or not.

In the light of a careful analysis of gambiae's behavior in Africa and in Brazil, it is no exaggeration to say that vital interests of every country in the Americas, except Canada, were probably involved in the struggle with gambiae in Northeast Brazil. The gambiae threat was not limited to an increase in the malaria of regions already malarious, but included the introduction of the disease to many nonmalarious regions and the widespread dissemination of filariasis, of which gambiae is a vector. Probably 90 per cent of the gambiae-transmitted malaria in Brazil in 1938–1940 occurred among populations entirely unfamiliar with the disease.

Much of gambiae's success derives from the fact that it is most highly adapted to a simple, almost universal type of breeding place: shallow sunlit pools without vegetation. Gambiae's eventual distribution, then, would depend on simple climatic factors, of temperature and humidity, rather than on some of the more complex factors which determine the distribution of other species of anopheles. Although the hibernation of gambiae has not been recorded, nor have its eggs been kept alive more than a few weeks, the

possibility of gambiae-transmitted outbreaks due to annual spring importations of the species in areas where winters are severe and summers are
short must be taken into consideration since the transmission of malaria
may rapidly become intense following the introduction of gambiae.

An idea of the final range of gambiae in America may be obtained by
comparing the climatic conditions of those parts of Africa from which gambiae has been reported with those of different parts of the Americas.

From an analysis of the meteorological conditions under which gambiae
is found in Africa, it may be seen that conditions in the New World, from
the northern provinces of the Argentine Republic through all the South
and Central American countries and the West Indies and even to the
southern section of the United States along the Gulf of Mexico and the
Caribbean, are favorable for gambiae breeding.

There will, of course, be those who will argue that the apparent adaptation of gambiae to life in Brazil away from its normal habitat was always
precarious at best and that its disappearance following control measures
simply proves its failure to adapt itself and is an indication that its presence
in Brazil was of little importance to the rest of the continent. The same persons will be ready to insist that the disappearance of gambiae was mainly
because of biological factors rather than the result of control measures devised by man.

However, observers in Brazil are agreed that gambiae was thoroughly at
home in the new faunal region. The 8-month dry season in the invaded
region was a myth during 1939–1940, when a more than usual amount of
rain fell with a prolonged distribution throughout the year, especially in
1939. The occasional year-long droughts which occur in much of the area
infested with gambiae did not materialize even though the people of such
regions prayed for a drought year, or even two, rather than a repetition of
the 1938 outbreak of gambiae-transmitted malaria. But this could have
brought but temporary relief, gambiae having demonstrated its resistance
early in its Brazilian career by weathering the severe drought of 1932.

Those who had the opportunity to observe gambiae in Ceará and Rio
Grande do Norte from 1938 to 1940 have no doubt but that this species, unchecked, would have maintained itself indefinitely in Brazil and would
eventually have become a scourge throughout the Americas. They point
out that the biological factors responsible for the decline and disappearance of gambiae in Brazil, but not present previous to 1939, were Paris
green and pyrethrum.

Opinions on Species Eradication Before
Success of Campaign

Although in retrospect it is easy to say that gambiae could have been
rapidly eliminated from Brazil at a minimal cost had a well-oriented attack

been made on the species at the time of its discovery in 1930, at no time from 1930 to 1938, and even in 1939, was it possible to get serious encouragement on the possibility of species eradication from those experienced in antianopheles work. In 1930 those who argued that although gambiae had crossed the ocean and established itself in Brazil, it would not be able to survive indefinitely in this new faunal region, were the first to argue that if it did survive in America, there was no hope of chasing down the last of this or any other species, and eradicating it. When, early in 1931, gambiae was found in the interior of Rio Grande do Norte, the problem was regarded as hopeless from the standpoint of an eradication campaign, but in 1932 it was thought that the drought of that year might accomplish what man could never do. (N. C. Davis on receipt of Shannon's report, December 1930, that gambiae had spread since May over an area only some 6 square kilometers, replied under date of January 7, 1931: "Eradication would appear to be hopeless now." Seven months later E. R. Rickard on learning that gambiae had been found at São Bento, 182 kilometers from Natal, wrote, "This certainly looks serious and greatly diminishes any possibility of species extinction.") This hope was vain and in 1933 and 1934 when it was found that gambiae had weathered the drought successfully, no steps were taken to eradicate it.

The fact that gambiae was known to have spread 182 kilometers during its first year in Brazil led naturally to the suggestion that perhaps it had even gone much farther without its presence having been detected. The logical question raised was what hope there might be of erecting an efficient local barrier against the farther spread of a mosquito which had crossed successfully the 1680-mile saltwater barrier of the South Atlantic.

Recourse to the works of the masters failed utterly to provide inspiration for any attempt to eradicate gambiae from Brazil, as the following excerpts show:

No one has ever supposed it possible to exterminate mosquitoes from whole continents, or even from large rural areas. The operation must be confined principally to towns and suburbs. No one imagines that it will be possible to exterminate every mosquito even from towns—we aim only at reducing their numbers as much as possible (R. Ross, 1901).

The idea that vast tracts peopled only with natives, could be freed from any mosquito is too silly to require any disclaimer (—, 1923).

The work described in the first edition of this book recorded a new phase in antimalarial work, namely the control of malaria by anopheline reduction in rural areas.'. . . The radical method of mosquito reduction has everywhere given results superior to any other.

"Drainage and reduction of breeding areas is the all-important work in the antimalaria campaign" was the conclusion reached in Panama; and it confirmed my own views. Consequently, although *A. costalis* (*gambiae*) can be destroyed by open drainage, to eradicate malaria in Africa would require a more thorough drainage and upkeep than is necessary on the flat land of Malaya where mosquitoes like *A. kawari* and *A. umbrosus* are the carriers (Watson, 1921).

Only MacGregor, who made a survey of Mauritius in 1924, was found to be so bold as to advocate eradication of gambiae:

For this reason there is every likelihood of exterminating the species rapidly from the central parts of Mauritius down to an altitude of 600 feet if the comparatively small number of breeding places in the inland districts are destroyed. Below 600 feet the species can be successfully exterminated also in the course of time, I believe, once the efforts of the anti-malaria campaign in Mauritius are systematized so that the anti-malaria measures are carried out thoroughly, section by section, until at last the whole island has been dealt with.

In August 1938 a letter was written by one of us (F.L.S.) to Park Ross, whose work of controlling gambiae-produced malaria by disinsectization of houses had been visited in 1935:

We.... are beginning to consider the possibility of doing something about gambiae. This mosquito is apparently limited to regions where a great reduction in rainfall occurs during certain months of the year and where conditions enable us to dream of complete extinction of the mosquito from the continent. I say *dream* because I realize what many will think. I would appreciate very much getting your opinion as to whether with adequate funds and men you could clear gambiae entirely from a known limited area of infestation.

Under date of October 9, Park Ross replied:

It is not possible to give emphatic opinions because we do not know your terrain. We have no notion as to permanent rivers, perennial swamps, or whether your dry season is in cold weather as ours is, but seeing you know the terrain here, a few statements relating to it may be of service to you even if they may not be orthodox.

A. Winter control of breeding appears to us to be the key to the situation. In the Table Mountain area (Valley of a Thousand Hills) gambiae were not found for three years. There was no winter control. This year breeding again occurred in relatively small numbers. We did hut spraying only.

In the Mandini area of Zululand (which you know) we have now kept up winter control by spraying breeding places for some years. Funestus has now been absent for the same time. Until we had winter control, fever had never been absent from the area, at least not for 50 years. The summer incidence of gambiae used to average 200–300 adults per hut. It has now dropped to a summer average of two to three per hut and that mainly in the vicinity of uncontrollable streams. We are sure that had it not been for these streams we could have got 100% control by our winter measures plus summer adult work.

B. Our large perennial rivers, such as the Tugela, most certainly act as focal points. They provide good breeding places for gambiae during winter in seepages and laterals. In summer, owing to floods, they are not so difficult to handle. We cannot, with our staff, get 100 per cent winter control.

C. The fact that gambiae larvae are usually found in certain favoured situations does not mean that eggs are laid exclusively there. The hatch may be dependent on favourable conditions of water, environment, etc., and not on selective laying on the part of the mosquito. . . .

Around perennial swamps, as soon as temperature conditions become favourable and cattle create suitable breeding puddles, there is, with us, immediate breeding in these puddles. This makes one surmise that limited breeding is taking place in the more permanent water all the time, even if larvae may be almost impossible to find.

D. We have proved that adults are not only easily carried by cars but they readily reinfect an area. Unless you control car traffic from an infected area into a sprayed area, reinfestation is bound to occur. . . .

One hundred per cent success by spraying will depend on your terrain and men.

It is clear from a careful reading of the above paragraphs from Park Ross's letter that he believed the problem to be essentially an administrative one. In 1938, at the time plans were being made for the organization of the Malaria Service of the Northeast, the only persons who seriously considered the possibility of the eradication of gambiae from Brazil were those familiar with the work of the Yellow Fever Service in the eradication of aegypti from many parts of Brazil, beginning about 1932.

Previous to 1930 yellow fever campaigns were based on the reduction rather than the eradication of the urban mosquito vector, since it had been shown that a considerable density of aegypti is required to keep yellow fever virus in circulation and that the disease generally disappears long before the extinction of its vector. Such disappearance of recognized yellow fever occurred not only in the larger centers of population, where the density of the vector was reduced, but also throughout entire tributary areas. Under these circumstances, it was logical to organize temporary antimosquito services to eliminate yellow fever simultaneously from all the larger centers of the endemic regions and thus terminate the threat of yellow fever forever. Unfortunately this program was shown to be untenable when yellow fever blossomed out as a jungle disease not susceptible to control by antimosquito measures. The development of methods rendering possible the species eradication of aegypti went unnoted except by those working with the problem at a time when the discovery of jungle yellow fever and new methods of vaccination were attracting universal interest. Shannon who had made a detailed study of aegypti breeding in the city of Salvador, Baía, in 1929–1930, previous to the introduction of the modifications in method which made the local eradication of this species possible, revisited Salvador and personally verified the absence of aegypti breeding in 1936, becoming enthusiastic over the administrative work of the Yellow Fever Service. This enthusiasm was the basis for Shannon's opinion openly expressed in November 1938 that the eradication of gambiae from the State of Ceará was within the possibilities of the administrative technique of the Yellow Fever Service. .

In spite of this favorable opinion, it should be stated here that the Directors of the Yellow Fever Service themselves were far from convinced. While it was known that certain individual breeding areas could be cleaned of larvae and that adults could be killed in the houses with spray insecticide, it was by no means certain that the entire infested region could be cleared of gambiae with the funds which might become available before the infested area became so extensive that all thought of eradication would have to be abandoned. And so it was that the Yellow Fever Service undertook the solution of the problem of gambiae eradication rather as a moral obligation than as a reasonable program with fair chances of success. It was recognized that new administrative techniques would have to be developed and the principal incentive to faith in the possibility of such successful development was the foreknowledge of the dire results of failure to eradicate gambiae before the problem became further complicated by extension to other regions. Excerpts from the letter of November 28, 1938, in which the project was recommended to The Rockefeller Foundation for approval show this clearly:

> I am enclosing herewith Shannon's seven page report on conditions in Ceará as noted in his work up to the 17th of this month . . . I find it impossible to be as optimistic about final results at as early a date as is Shannon but cannot force myself to be entirely pessimistic as to final results if we are able to avoid the spread to the Parnaíba and São Francisco River valleys. The amount of work to be done in the areas already infested and threatened is enormous; whether final eradication is possible or not, I believe the effort will justify the expense in the actual reduction of malaria in the region during the time that operations are carried out. The most hopeful factor in the whole situation is the small proportion of the total infested area which is capable of year round breeding of any mosquito. . . .
>
> With the present extension of gambiae I feel that any failure to take immediate steps would be criminal if means can be made available for immediate action. . . .
>
> There can be no doubt that we are asking for an enormous headache for quite some time in offering to organize this program but I see no way to avoid the issue. And if work is going to be done it must be done on as large a scale as possible from the beginning. . . .

No one foresaw the relative ease and rapidity with which gambiae might be eradicated, estimates running as high as 10 years' time and $10 million.

Dr. Evandro Chagas stated, in 1938, that at present gambiae is still limited to an area from which eradication will not be impossible and where control is perfectly practicable; that it is a mosquito of extraordinary resistance and adaptability, breeding easily under the meteorological conditions of the Northeast, and that it will only with difficulty be eradicated from its new habitat; and that only years on end of unrelenting systematic campaigns, of vigilance and isolation of the infested region, will remove and annul the enemy.

Dr. Lessa Andrade, who had worked on the control of malaria at Natal and Macaíba, gave it as his opinion in November 1938 that under conditions existing in Rio Grande do Norte it should be possible to get rid of gambiae within 5 years, if the necessary men and money were provided and if the state could be *protected against reinfestation from Ceará* (personal communication).

It is interesting to note that the time and money spent in the eradication of the Mediterranean fruit fly in Florida, 1929–1930, were also far less than the original estimates: Congress, facing requests for appropriations of nearly $20,000,000, made $8,780,000 available, of which less than $6,000,000 were spent; eradication of the fly did not require several years as anticipated, but was accomplished in 16 months.

Only after several months' work and the expenditure of large sums of money did those in charge of the Malaria Service of the Northeast dare to believe that the eradication of gambiae was possible. Just at this time Corradetti was writing that malaria in the presence of gambiae could not be eliminated, but control might be attempted with screens, quinine prophylaxis, and treatment. Barber, who was in the infested region from May to August 1939, was hopeful regarding the temporary limitation of gambiae's range but frankly pessimistic as to species eradication. Barber believed the people would have to adapt themselves to living in a so highly malarious region and advised education as to methods for making the homes mosquitoproof through the use of homespun cotton netting: "We often demonstrated to them the cause of their trouble, showing them gambiae caught in their dwellings ... the beginning of an education which may take a generation or two to accomplish ... If it is no longer possible to extirpate gambiae in Brazil, its spread to large up-river and up-coast regions may be prevented or delayed for many years."

GROWTH OF FAITH IN SPECIES ERADICATION

In addition to the data on the speed of cleaning individual places, it is interesting to see in retrospect how those responsible for the work gained increasing confidence as the campaign progressed. This can best be done through quoting from the *President's Review, 1939,* of The Rockefeller Foundation, which gives the attitude as of the end of that year, and from correspondence between the field staff (F.L.S.) and the New York Office (W. A. Sawyer) of the Foundation throughout the year 1940.

The following cautious prophecy was made in the *President's Review* of the work of the Foundation for 1939:

If the mosquito can be held within its present limits during the wet season of 1940, we can begin to think of the possibility of its eventual eradication from the entire region. This, of course, would mean extermination of the last surviving pair. It must be admitted that eradication is a rash word in terms of prophecy.

On February 9, 1940, after a trip through the State of Rio Grande do Norte, the report (F.L.S.) to the New York office included:

I arrived at Mossoró, Rio Grande do Norte, on January 26th and spent the following days until the 31st with Doctors Hackett and Wilson looking over the gambiae situation in the State of Rio Grande do Norte and discussing the situation in Ceará as well . . . I was surprised to find Dr. Hackett somewhat more optimistic than I had ever permitted myself to become regarding the rapidity with which results can be obtained in much of the infested area. On the other hand, I found him more pessimistic regarding the final clean up of certain difficult areas. I have felt, and still do, that if it were possible to prevent the spread of gambiae to regions other than those already known to be infested, the final elimination would depend only on having adequate funds and efficient administration. . . .

The Service is now facing the first real test of its work with the onset of this year's rains. Both Wilson and I feel that the rains will disclose any defects in the organization which are not now apparent; but that, on the other hand, many places will fail to produce gambiae this year which had serious outbreaks of gambiae-transmitted malaria last year. We are even hoping that a mistake has been made and that the Malaria Service is greatly overstocked with drugs for treatment of malaria this year. . . .

On April 11, growing optimism was reflected in the report of another visit to the infested area:

Dr. Wilson and I arrived back in Fortaleza yesterday after a week in the Jaguaribe River valley during which we traveled a total of some six to seven hundred miles and visited the laboratory at Aracatí and the administrative centers at Russas, Jaguaribe, Icó, and Iguatú. . . .

The rains around Aracatí have been heavier this year than last and the region has also suffered more from the flood waters of the Jaguaribe River, since excess water has fallen throughout the valley. In spite of the extremely favorable breeding conditions, Aracatí itself, and much of the surrounding region, is free of gambiae . . . That this absence of gambiae from large areas is due to control measures is indicated by the way in which gambiae has increased rapidly during the past two months at Cumbe, the near-by study area where control measures are not being taken. The absence of gambiae is further attested to by the great reduction in malaria this year. . . .

At Russas, which is the headquarters for the lower Jaguaribe valley, I was truly surprised to find Dr. Gastão Cesar de Andrade so apologetic for the continued existence of a number of dirty spots in his division. We have all recognized this lower Jaguaribe as probably the most difficult problem to be solved with regard to gambiae in Brazil, and, when the heat was on us last year, we drained it of trained men repeatedly, feeling that the frontier had to be protected at all costs. And so it was that this division did not really have a chance to get organized until well toward the end of the year. Even so, some parts of the division are remarkably clean, and none of them are as they were last year, with the exception of Gracismões which is a study area under the direction of the group from the Oswaldo Cruz Institute working under the direction of Dr. Evandro Chagas. In checking over the results of house captures it was interesting to note that the dirtiest places in the entire division were those contiguous to the uncontrolled Grascismões area. Our Service has been fumigating all the houses in the contiguous areas since January, but even so the number of mosquitoes to be found is many times higher than in other parts of the division. (I sent a wire to Dr. Chagas yesterday requesting his acquiescence to the organization of antilarval and fumigation services throughout the Gracismões area) . . . .

In the Jaguaribe Division which extends from just above Limoeiro up the river to Bebedouro, we found Dr. Severo claiming complete lack of evidence of gambiae except for a distance of twelve kilometers along the river above the junction with the Russas Division not far from Limoeiro.

In the Icó Division we found Drs. Oswaldo Silva and Jefferson de Souza both quite optimistic regarding the future, with known foci of gambiae infestation at only a few points—viz., a small area just west of Lavras, two isolated points on the Riacho dos Bravos just south of Cariús, and a rather large area at Barroso on the Jaguaribe River, thirty-six kilometers down stream from Iguatú. Both of these men know from experience that once they have found a focus of gambiae infestation in this region they can get rid of it with present methods, and both have undertaken to have no gambiae in their division during the month of June 1940. [This promise was fulfilled in both cases.]

We did not visit either the Quixadá or Cascavel Divisions, both of which have failed to report gambiae for some time, now. It is entirely possible that these divisions are really clean at the present time. [Cascavel has not been again found infested, nor has the Quixadá Division itself, although frontier infestation was found at Madalena 6 months later.]

With all my optimism of the November and January visits, I did not expect to find things as satisfactory as they are at the present time. Gambiae has increased most markedly in Cumbe and Gracismões where no control measures have been applied, but elsewhere it has been held in check much better than was to have been foreseen. Except in certain very limited areas malaria is not a serious problem this year, and in most places our own personnel is not taking preventive treatment. No problems have been found which are considered insoluble by the men responsible for solving them. Difficulties there are, of course, and much remains to be done, but everyone is now satisfied that with present measures, adequate funds, and a little time, the problem of gambiae in Northeast Brazil can be solved.

By July 10 confidence in the antigambiae measures adopted had grown to such proportions that definite expectations of gambiae eradication were expressed:

The rapidity with which a place can be cleaned of gambiae in this part of the world with present technique is almost incredible. Cumbe, a rural area close to the laboratory, was reserved for many months for laboratory studies and no control measures were undertaken there until April 29, 1939. During the third week of April, laboratory workers caught with hand tubes 800 gambiae in the houses of Cumbe and, in the days just before control measures were applied, division capture squads, working with insecticide, caught over 2,200 gambiae. Control work consisted of Paris green and house fumigation twice a week. The last larvae were found on May 15 and the last adults during the last week of May!

I fully believe that all visible infestation with gambiae will be exhausted before the end of September, possibly before the end of August, and that by the end of the year we will be justified in reducing the Service to one of skeleton proportions to search for dirty spots and for unexpected reappearance both within the previously known infested region and outside the region.

I am authorizing reducing the Quixadá service to a sentinel service on a monthly cycle and having the cycle for Jaguaribe changed from 15 to 30 days.

By September 3, the situation was so favorable that the suggestion was made that the budget for the following year be reduced:

I have just returned from a two weeks' trip through the gambiae areas of Brazil and as result am wiring you,

"Request one hundred thousand gambiae budget 1941 Soper."

This reduction of $150,000 in the amount requested from The Rockefeller Foundation for 1940 is only a partial measure of my present optimism since I very much doubt that it will be necessary to spend all of this amount. However, there is so much at stake and so much already invested in this program that ample provision should be made for all possibilities of unexpected reaction on the part of the fast disappearing gambiae.

I left Fortaleza on the morning of August 19 in the military air-mapping plane which has been working with the gambiae service in mapping the lower Jaguaribe valley. We flew down close to Caponga, the closest point to Fortaleza at which gambiae has been found, and then went over Cascavel and followed the highway from Boqueirão to Russas. At Russas we came down to a few hundred meters and flew over the study area, one of the last points of gambiae resistance in this State. Then up the river to Limoeiro and a short distance up the Banabuiú River before turning back and covering the Jaguaribe River between Peixe Gordo and Aracatí. The flight was a most interesting one and gave me the proper background for an optimistic week in the region in which gambiae production has fallen so markedly during the past few months. As I got out of the plane at Aracatí I fully realized for the first time that the gambiae mosquito in Brazil is doomed to extermination, not at some shadowy time in the uncertain future, but here and now. The reduction which has occurred in the breeding in the lower Jaguaribe, as well as elsewhere throughout the region during the past few months, has taken place in spite of an exceptionally wet and prolonged rainy season!

I remained with Causey at the laboratory a couple of days but refused to get excited over the fact that he had recently shown that gambiae eggs can be kept in wet sand for 25 days and still produce larvae; careful checking of the Icó district where control of larval production was abandoned in April has failed to reveal any persistence of gambiae beyond the period routinely used before discontinuation of control measures.

On the 21st of August I went with Dr. Paulo Antunes to Assú in Rio Grande do Norte. Here we found Dr. Bustamante getting ready to drop control measures to give gambiae a chance to show its presence; no gambiae have been found in the Assú Division since March. The work in Rio Grande do Norte has not been organized in such a thorough way as it has been in Ceará, but even so it is quite probable that gambiae is already absent from the Assú Division. . . . [No further production of gambiae was found.]

While in Rio Grande do Norte we went to the Division of Ceará Mirím where we found much to criticize in the organization of the work in spite of which we came away willing to believe that gambiae is absent from the area or is continuing only in small areas of low production where eradication should follow discovery rapidly. [No further production of gambiae was found.] This entire region has given only a few scattered positive findings this year with less than 100 adults and less than 100 larvae found since the first of January. However, we are taking no chances on the area; it will be air-mapped this week and we are throwing a large number of trained men from Ceará into the division to find out if gambiae is still present or not and to get rid of it if found.

From Natal we returned to Russas . . . Here, to the surprise of many, only one adult gambiae was found during the month of August. From Russas we drove up to Jaguaribe and Icó where all control measures have been taken off and gambiae let breed at will. There is a monthly check on both adult and larval findings throughout the once infested areas now believed to be clean. In Icó the discontinuance of Paris green was followed by a great increase of Nyssorhynchus production. The field inspector is not expected to recognize the difference between gambiae and Nyssorhynchus larvae and is responsible only for collecting samples from all foci found and sending them in to the laboratory of the post. In the Icó laboratory seven microscopists are at work, each with his helper to prepare slides, whereas in Jaguaribe there are only four microscopists. Up to 35,000 larvae are examined daily in the two laboratories. After seeing this machine at work one cannot avoid a certain confidence in the negative reports from these areas.

On the way back from Jaguaribe we stopped once more at Russas and got the final results for the month of August. Only two of the four sectors of the Russas Division—viz., Russas and União, showed adults or larvae during the month, and the number of places infested was minimal in comparison with previous months. During May the Russas Division had 226 dirty points, during June 126, during July 103 and during August only 30. Also the density of infestation in the dirty spots was very low; of the places found with gambiae during the month, several which were dirty at the beginning of the month, were examined once more during the past week and are now clean.

The Aracatí sector was clean in August so Antunes and I drove to Aracatí and helped Causey eliminate the laboratory colony (August 31, 1940).

During the last days of the trip we were forced to realize that summer has at last begun and with clear skies and hot winds a standing order for the next four or five months, there would seem to be no reason for letting any gambiae infestation *which can be found*, be carried over into the next wet season. With the possibility of discontinuing antilarval measures in all areas well before the end of the dry season and giving gambiae a free hand to declare itself, there seems to be little chance for gambiae to exist in any suspected region without being found.

Please don't get the idea that I will be ready to declare gambiae absent from Brazil at any time in the near future. However, I do believe that we are entering now on the second phase of the campaign during which a great deal of watchful waiting must be done before vigilance can be relaxed (Icó, Quixadá, and Jaguaribe are already in this phase of the campaign).

I did not mention it above but instructions were given during the past 15 days to discontinue all treatment throughout the gambiae area. There are still some cases of malaria but not enough to justify keeping special employees to treat the few cases which do appear.

Of course I do not expect you to believe that the situation is as rosy as I have painted it above. . . .

But a month later (October 3) the report read:

During the early days of September some gambiae breeding was found but during the past three weeks no adults, or larvae, have been discovered by the Malaria Service of the Northeast. During the entire month of September, six foci of gambiae larvae were found: one in Araújos, one in Patos, one in Pedro Ribeiro, and three in Timbaúbas. Araújos and Timbaúbas are villages included in the Chagas study area where we took over control late, and Patos and Pedro Ribeiro are neighboring villages. During the month of September only one adult gambiae was found in Brazil: at Jurema, a village lying between Russas and União not very far from the points at which larval foci were found. . . .

On November 8 announcement was made that control measures had been suspended except in a very limited area and that the happy results obtained with gambiae in Brazil were stimulating visions of similar victories over both gambiae and other anopheles in other parts of the world:

In April 1940 at the height of the rainy season both antilarval and anti-adult measures were discontinued in a large part of the Icó Division which had been at one time heavily infested but had been apparently clean for some time. After a considerable period of time during which gambiae did not again appear in this area, the other areas believed to be free of gambiae were put to the test of discontinuing all control measures. To date no area has been found reinfested where work has been discontinued in this manner. I have officially authorized the discontinuation of all control measures throughout the Russas Division except in a very limited area where gambiae was found in August. All control measures have already been discontinued in all of the other divisions. (As you know, a small infested area has been found outside the previous limits of the Quixadá Division in an area which was never worked and never suspected. This area is cleaning up rapidly and in and of itself is of very little importance.)

I really believe that we have come to the point with gambiae in Brazil where it is now only a matter of "mopping up," that is, searching out all possible missed foci very few of which should be found outside of the area of operation and probably none inside this area. [None have been found.]

My attention has recently been called to Dr. Boyd's address of last year in which he suggests that malaria control should be based on long-term operations with gradual results rather than on blitzkrieg methods. I believe this attitude is becoming general among malariologists . . . In most cases this may well be the logical program, but I am wondering if there are not many special malaria problems which can be best attacked by methods similar to those used with gambiae in Brazil. For example, I am thinking of the malaria problem of the Pacific Coast of Peru. This area is separated from the Amazon valley by the high range of mountains over which anopheles probably pass very rarely so that reinfestation from this region would probably not occur. The Pacific Coast malaria problem is naturally linked with the river valleys but these river valleys are comparatively short and separated from each other by stretches of desert. I believe it would be entirely feasible to attempt the elimination of *Anopheles pseudopunctipennis* from these valleys one at a time with the expectation that only at rare intervals would reinfestation occur either over the Andes or from neighboring valleys. [The possibility of eradication of *A. pseudopunctipennis* in Peru had been previously suggested by R. C. Shannon.] In a comparatively few years it should be possible to get rid of all malaria on the coast of Peru through the complete elimination of the species. Once eliminated, an occasional survey at regular intervals should be made to discover any reinfestation and eliminate it before it becomes of any size. Once the original work is done the upkeep should be very low.

In the light of what has already been done in Brazil I believe that a total species elimination campaign would be highly efficient in that part of the Anglo-Egyptian Sudan about Khartoum where gambiae breeding is an important problem along the River Nile and in the irrigation system. . . .

In Africa there must be many places where gambiae has a precarious existence during at least part of each year and from which it would be relatively easy to exclude this species if it were once eliminated. Even in that part of South Africa where Park Ross has been working it would probably be good business to spend enough to get rid of gambiae and then work only a frontier zone next to the unworked infested area.

And of course, once one starts to let his imagination go he cannot avoid considering the many islands where malaria is a serious problem which are limited geographical units with a definite area to be cleaned and with some natural protection against reinfestation. Small islands such as Mauritius and Granada may lead one eventually to attack such problems as *A. culicifacies* in Ceylon. . . .

Has Gambiae Been Completely Eliminated from Brazil?

While admitting the inferiority of negative to positive findings, it must be recognized that negative findings for gambiae should be given a very high rating, because

1. The adult is prone to enter houses and its presence in the community is easily established by house captures.

2. The larva occurs predominantly in the most simple and accessible type of breeding place.

3. The presence of the species in an area for even short periods generally results in an explosion of malaria.*

The value of negative findings was probably somewhat increased by the offer in January 1941 of approximately 10 days' salary as a premium to any inspector finding gambiae; in July this premium was increased to 20 days' pay but without result.

It now seems reasonably safe to state that gambiae no longer exists in the previously known infested regions of Northeast Brazil, or in the neighboring districts of Ceará and Rio Grande do Norte, or in the states of Paraíba, Pernambuco, Alagôas, and Piauí.

This statement is based on the following evidence:

1. Continued search for the species in all previously infested areas for periods ranging from 1 to 2 years after the interruption of all control measures.

2. Since no measures of a permanent character were used in the campaign against gambiae, the infested region remained as suitable as ever for gambiae production so that the discontinuation of control was an open invitation to gambiae to resume breeding.

3. Repeated search for the species in the surrounding regions.

4. Anopheles surveys at more distant points.

5. Absence of malaria in regions which had severe malaria during the period of gambiae infestation, and failure to find gambiae in areas which have recently reported outbreaks of malaria.

SELECTIVE SPECIES ERADICATION

Although *Anopheles* of the *Nyssorhynchus* group found in the gambiae-infested areas are highly susceptible to both weapons used by the Malaria Service, Paris green and insecticide, this susceptibility becomes operative

---

* However this does not always occur and gambiae can remain for a considerable time in areas where there are no gametocyte carriers without causing an outbreak. At Madalena, the last point found infested in October 1940, there is reason to believe that gambiae had been present for 1 year or longer without anything happening to call attention to its presence. This can be attributed to the small number of carriers in this area, which is not favorable to malaria transmitted by local anopheles, and to the fact that one of the partners owning the property knew of the serious outbreaks of malaria in the Jaguaribe Valley and as a matter of precaution gave orders that everyone on the property coming down with fever should be removed immediately.

only in case of direct attack. While it is true that the measures taken greatly reduced the density of Nyssorhynchus in the areas worked, the results were never so complete as those observed with gambiae, and the production of Nyssorhynchus rapidly returned to normal once control measures were abandoned.

The very characteristics of gambiae's biology which made its spread in Brazil possible and made it so much more effective as a transmitter of malaria than are the native anopheles also made gambiae more vulnerable to Paris green and insecticide than are the latter. The preference of the gambiae larvae for shallow sunlit pools without vegetation makes it very susceptible to attack by Paris green; while gambiae's innate desire for shelter in human dwellings makes it easily discoverable and susceptible to attack with spray insecticide.

Various species of Nyssorhynchus, on the other hand, breed in a much greater variety of places: in much less exposed waters, in the midst of vegetation, in the shade, in the center of pools, in deep water, all of which are much less easily treated with Paris green. Furthermore, only a small percentage of Nyssorhynchus is to be found indoors, making these species much less accessible to insecticide than is gambiae.

Although Nyssorhynchus has just been discussed as a unit, as a matter of fact there are wide differences in the breeding habits and domesticity of different species of this subgenus. Any future attempts at eradication of anopheles in Brazil should be based on careful selection of the individual species to be attacked rather than on a general campaign against all anopheles. After it was reasonably certain that gambiae no longer existed in the region, an attempt was made to eradicate all anopheles from the test area at Cumbe. The results of this attempt indicate that, given the men, money, and necessary materials, there is nothing basically impossible about the eradication of various species of the Nyssorhynchus subgenus.

DANGER OF REINFESTATION FROM AFRICA

While there may be some hidden focus of gambiae infestation still present in Brazil, it seems much more probable that any future finding of gambiae in this country should be attributed to future air traffic between Africa and America. That there is great danger of reinfestation was shown by the finding of a female gambiae on a plane arriving in Natal on October 9, 1941; on January 8 and 10, on May 17 and 26, and on June 15 and 23, 1942, additional specimens of gambiae were found on planes arriving from Africa. Those found in January were somewhat damaged and had apparently been killed by disinsectization in flight, but those found in May had probably arrived in Natal alive. Permanent vigilance over all types of aircraft is necessary and, in addition, gambiae surveys should be made at frequent intervals in areas subject to reinfestation from Africa. Gambiae, rather than anopheles, surveys are suggested, since the native anopheles are only slightly domestic; gambiae surveys could be most easily and cheaply made by the Yellow Fever Service, which makes house searches for aegypti infestation as part of its routine work.

Should gambiae once more invade Brazil or should it be found to have already extended its range beyond the regions investigated by the Malaria Service of the Northeast, there now exist a technique and the personnel trained in that technique whereby a repetition of the tragedy of Northeast Brazil during the 1930s can be avoided.

PREVENTION OF TRANSFER OF DANGEROUS ARTHROPODS

The serious problem created in Brazil by the introduction of *Anopheles gambiae* in 1930, even though such introduction almost certainly occurred by boat rather than by plane, first called the attention of health officers to the serious problem of preventing the transfer of disease vectors from one region to another by the fast-developing air traffic of the world. Although, in the case of gambiae, the danger was due to the introduction of an efficient vector in an area where the disease already existed, it was recognized that the introduction of a disease itself in a region already well supplied with vectors but free of the disease in question might be brought about by the carrying of infected vectors by air traffic.

Especially was the question raised of the possibility of yellow fever being carried through the transfer of infected *Aëdes aegypti* to regions where the vector was present in large numbers, but where the disease was absent. The threat of summer epidemics hangs over such temperate zones as the southern United States, where aegypti is permitted to breed unrestrained, and the more terrible threat of permanent yellow fever endemicity casts a shadow over India and the Orient, should the virus of yellow fever ever reach those regions from Africa.

Considerable work has been done on the air transportation of arthropods and on methods of disinsectization of planes, but there has been no development of a universal consciousness of the threat that modern air transportation represents, especially in wartime when long-distance unannounced flights of large numbers of planes are the rule rather than the exception, through the transplantation of arthropods dangerous as vectors of human and animals disease and as agricultural pests. The problem of preventing the reinfestation of the American continent by gambiae imported from Africa is only one small phase of the more general problems of preventing the extension of the range of gambiae in any direction from its present habitat and of protecting every region of the world from the pests and diseases of every other region.

The experience of the Malaria Service of the Northeast in the disinsectization of planes arriving in Brazil from Africa has only served to emphasize the dangers of international air traffic and the difficulty of obviating this threat. As already stated, *Anopheles gambiae* has been recorded seven times, *Glossina palpalis* twice, and other arthropods whose possible importance has not been studied, many times.

Disinsectization of the large modern commercial and military planes is not easy and requires motorized equipment for its rapid execution. Great difficulty has been found in preventing the entrance of local insects into planes before disinsectization has been made upon arrival and after final disinsectization has been carried out on planes bound for Africa. (The Malaria Service of the Northeast has assumed the responsibility of attempting to prevent the infestation of Africa with American arthropods through disinsectization of planes before departure.) It is becoming increasingly clear, as experience accumulates, that disinsectization should be routine and should be carried out immediately before departure and repeated during flight. In the absence of compressed-air lines to different parts of the planes and to avoid carrying unnecessary weight, pyrethrum in much heavier concentrations than usual should be used in flight. Some efficient method of complete disinsectization in flight which will not involve carrying additional weighty equipment is urgently needed. Careful search of planes for living arthropods at the port of arrival, with adequate penalties if found, may be expected to secure satisfactory disinsectization before departure and during flight and eventually, the development of planes so constructed and equipped as to facilitate the prevention of arthropod transportation.

Under present conditions, however, it is probably more practical for the health officers of each region to assume the risk of possible debarkation of invading arthropods in the first minute or two after arrival of planes and limit their activities to routine disinsectization with motorized equipment immediately after the passengers and crew have left the plane but before baggage, mail, or anything else has been taken off. In Brazil, the Malaria Service of the Northeast insists on disinsectization of planes coming from Africa before either passengers or crew leave the plane.

The problem is one which merits the closest attention of health and military authorities in all parts of the world.

WILL BRAZILIAN ANTIGAMBIAE MEASURES SUCCEED IN AFRICA?

Now that gambiae has apparently been eliminated from Brazil, there are those who are willing to attribute its disappearance in large part to climatic and other factors rather than to Paris green and insecticide. While it is true that conditions in Northeast Brazil favor a program of eradication, it is just as true that any localized attempt to protect individual towns and villages from malaria transmitted by gambiae would have resulted in the permanence of the species in the region and its farther spread. It is also true that within the infested regions were various areas where conditions were highly favorable to gambiae throughout the year, as at Cumbe, but that the method of attack evolved cleaned it out rapidly.

On the other hand, it must be admitted that until the attempt is made to apply this eradication technique to gambiae in Africa, no one can predict with certainty the outcome of such application. It has been shown that the gambiae larva is very susceptible to Paris green and the adult to attack with insecticide. There exist large areas in Africa seriously handicapped by gambiae-transmitted malaria in which conditions for permanence of the species are no more favorable than are those in many parts of Northeast Brazil. In other areas gambiae exists only because irrigation water is available for breeding. Where unfavorable conditions exist throughout an area large enough to justify the expense of eradication and the permanent maintenance of a frontier barrier zone, eradication should, in spite of the original cost, prove to be a highly profitable investment. For example, Symes' exposition of the malaria problem at Nairobi, Kenya, and of the cost of malaria to the community there gives the impression that the gambiae mosquito in this area could be eradicated with methods used to good advantage in Brazil:

> There are, of course, great variations in seasonal and local densities of these species . . . *Anopheles gambiae* is the most notorious from this point of view. During the drier months it is absent, as far as can be ascertained, from all but a few permanent breeding places: the Nairobi River and irrigation canals in the swamp area, the Ngong River below the Prison and Infectious Diseases Hospital and a few of the more permanent murram pits or pools in other streams. But as soon as the early rains of February or March provide further areas of stagnant water it begins to spread until during June it occupies in great force almost every available pool, pit, and puddle in and around the township.
>
> Nairobi communities are losing in cash every year, nearly £4,000 through malaria. They are losing, in addition, from the same cause, some 35 to 40 people whose "cash" value cannot be ascertained, and another unknown amount through impairment of health and efficiency that so often results from malaria. Can we assume that these last two losses amount to at least another £4,000?
>
> Specific efforts to prevent these losses over some ten years have cost about £1,000 a year. It is now obvious that such efforts are inadequate.
>
> In order to put an end to this annual loss of £8,000, what ought the community to be prepared to expend on permanent control measures?

Workers contemplating gambiae control in Africa should not be too greatly influenced by the amount of money spent on gambiae eradication in Brazil. It should be remembered that the Malaria Service of the Northeast worked under emergency conditions, spent large sums on the treatment of malaria, and purchased much equipment and material which was never used. Also the Service never succeeded in making careful studies to determine how long control measures must be continued after the species can no longer be found in a community. It is known that the 3-month period adopted errs in being too conservative. The results in certain areas suggest that an intensive campaign of combined antilarval and anti-imaginal measures of 6 weeks will be sufficient to clean many places completely. The cost of gambiae eradication in future campaigns can definitely be greatly reduced far below that of the work in Northeast Brazil.

As time goes on it will almost certainly be found that an increasing number of areas can be cleaned of gambiae and freed of gambiae-transmitted malaria. The problem of eradication in Africa would, of course, be centrifugal rather than centripetal; in Brazil the thwarting of rapid expansion required the cleaning of the periphery first, together with protection of the frontier zones, but in Africa, where the species is already widely disseminated, it would seem logical to attempt eradication by beginning at the center of the area to be cleaned and working always outward. While it is true that cleaned areas in Africa will not enjoy the barrier of hundreds of miles of ocean against reinfestation of clean areas, there is no question in the minds of those who have worked on the problem in Brazil but that once a fairly large area has been cleaned, the maintenance cost of frontier services to prevent the reinfestation of those clean areas, and the elimination of such reinfestations as may occur before they become important problems, will be far less than any other possible means of controlling malaria in that area. It remains to be seen whether *Anopheles funestus*, another very efficient vector of malaria in Africa, will respond equally well to the same technique. This point is important since *A. gambiae* and *A. funestus* are active collaborators in many areas of Africa.

Feasibility of General Species-Eradication Measures

It has been demonstrated in Brazil that species eradication of *Aëdes aegypti* and *Anopheles gambiae* is feasible. The question naturally arises as to whether practical species-eradication methods can be worked out for other disease transmitters, other mosquitoes and insects. This will depend somewhat on the financial limits to be put on the term "practical." It will be argued by many that species eradication is an expensive luxury and that funds for this type of work could never be gotten in the districts in which they work. However, if species eradication is even remotely possible with available methods against a given species in a given region, it is well to consider the amount of money spent annually in partial control work and the loss attributed to the disease under consideration over a period of some decades, before deciding against species eradication on the basis of cost.

Before deciding on species eradication, the following points should be established:

1. That the insect to be eradicated produces enough disease in the community to justify the expenditure of the necessary funds.

2. That the insect is susceptible to attack in one or more, preferably all, stages of its life cycle.

3. That it is possible to eradicate the species from small areas.

4. That the area in which eradication is to be attempted possesses natural barriers against constant reinfestation or is large enough to make the cost of maintenance of a permanent clean frontier zone, an item of minor expense for the entire clean area.

5. That the necessary money, men, and authority to carry out the program will be available when needed.

6. That the insect in question can be easily found in at least one of the stages of its life cycle so that negative findings can be interpreted as definite indication of its absence from areas surveyed.

Before taking these preliminary requirements too seriously, it should be noted that many of them were not fulfilled before the development of the campaigns against aegypti and gambiae in Brazil, and against the Mediterranean fruit fly in Florida. The Yellow Fever Service developed its technique for the eradication of aegypti in the course of a mosquito-reduction program, and the Malaria Service of the Northeast undertook the eradication of gambiae under emergency conditions with a large infested area from which dissemination of the species was proceeding apace. Each additional extension of its range further complicated the problem of control, not only because of the increased area in which control measures had to be applied, but also by creating serious outbreaks of malaria which had to be taken care of by personnel sorely needed in the organization of antigambiae measures. Under these conditions it was not feasible to lose time in making careful surveys or extensive preliminary studies of possible control methods; it seemed rather more expedient to learn how to get rid of gambiae by actually getting rid of gambiae.

Ross (1910) called attention to the "learning by doing" technique as applied to the control of malaria:

Amateurs are fond of advising that all practical measures should be postponed pending carrying out detailed researches upon the habits of anophelines, the parasite rate of localities, the effect of minor works, and so on. In my opinion, this is a fundamental mistake. It implies the sacrifice of life and health on a large scale while researches which may have little real value and which may be continued indefinitely are being attempted. As a matter of fact, the campaigns of Havana, Panama, Ismailia, and the Federated Malay States were all commenced before the local carriers were definitely incriminated and their habits studied . . . In practical life we observe that the best practical discoveries are obtained during the execution of practical work and that long academical discussions are apt to lead to nothing but academical profit. Action and investigation together do more than either of these alone.

The campaign against gambiae differed from previous campaigns against malaria in that the objective was not simply the control of malaria in the local population but the eradication of the vector in the entire area, not only to protect the local population against malaria, but also to prevent its spread to other regions. When the declared purpose of a campaign is the eradication of a species rather than the reduction in the incidence of disease caused by that species, the entire viewpoint of the service changes almost automatically. As long as evidence for the existence of the species continues to appear, the campaign has been a failure. There is no such thing as partial success in species eradication; one either achieves glorious success or dismal failure. Estimates of progress based on the traditional method of the malariologist, such as spleen rates, blood parasite rates, clinical attack rates, infant infection rates, become invalid and subordinated to the simple question: Is the species under attack still present in the area being worked? This point of view is in direct disharmony with that of the modern malariologist, as is revealed by a perusal of the words of the Special Committee on Malaria, of the League of Nations:

As for the reluctance and criticism arising from a fear of incomplete success, we would like again to stress the point that in dealing with rural malaria, speed and perfection are costly out of all proportion to their worth. We believe in taking a *long-time view* [italics not in original] of the malaria problem and in having patience to prefer steady progress, slow and imperfect though it may be, to an indefinite postponement of any work whatever.

This may be good philosophy for the defeated, but results of work with both aegypti and gambiae indicate that it is much easier to evaluate perfect rather than partial results. If the time and money spent on evaluating partial results were spent on obtaining perfect results, greater progress might be made over a given period. It is when one takes the long-time view of the malaria problem that justification for attempting species eradication is found. By the creation of very large malaria control areas and pooling all resources for malaria work in both towns and rural districts, it should be possible in many areas to eradicate the responsible local vector at a great saving over a period of years. To quote once more: "The Committee desires to stress the fact that rural malaria, especially in the tropics, is one of the principal unsolved problems in the field of Public Health. . . ."

Those who have had an active part in the eradication of gambiae from Brazil hope that the work of the Malaria Service of the Northeast has done more than solve the local rural problem and that results of the attack on gambiae in Brazil may lead to the development of methods which will help solve for many rural areas, within and outside the tropics, their especial individual, malaria problems.

SUMMARY

The arrival of *Anopheles gambiae* in Brazil in 1930 was followed by serious outbreaks of malaria in 1930 and 1931. The first organized campaign in 1931 apparently resulted in the eradication of gambiae from Natal, its port of entry, but not until after it had found a footing in the relatively inhospitable interior of Rio Grande do Norte. From 1932 to 1937 it was more or less quiescent until it encountered more favorable conditions in the Assú and Apodí valleys of Rio Grande do Norte, and the larger and more favorable valley of the Jaguaribe, in Ceará. In 1938, terrific outbreaks of malaria with a high fatality rate occurred in the two states. To meet this emergency, the government organized the Antimalaria Service, which was fused in January 1939 with the Malaria Service of the Northeast, a cooperative service organized solely for the purpose of combating the gambiae mosquito and supported by the Ministry of Health of Brazil and the International Health Division of The Rockefeller Foundation. The Malaria Service of the Northeast, with the aid of the already existing Yellow Fever Service, undertook to organize a campaign of species eradication against gambiae, relegating the problem of malaria itself to a place of minor importance. After several disappointing months of intensive organization, the Malaria Service began a heavy attack with Paris green and pyrethrum spray insecticide on gambiae in both larval and adult forms, and initially concentrated its efforts on the peripheral and frontier zones. Gambiae was stopped in its career of invasion, was beaten back, and finally eradicated from the known infested area in less than 2 years. Observations covering a period of 1½ years, including two rainy seasons, after the suspension of all antigambiae measures, indicate that eradication has been complete. Precautions must be taken to prevent reinfestation by gambiae and the introduction of other vectors or diseases by modern facilities of rapid transportation.

APPENDIX I

Legal Decree No. 1042 (In Translation)

The President of the Republic, by reason of the powers conferred upon him by Article 180 of the Constitution, DECREES:

Article 1. The Malaria Service of the Northeast is hereby created in the Ministry of Education and Health.

Article 2. The Malaria Service of the Northeast shall be responsible for:

a. promoting the study and investigation of the transmission of malaria by the mosquito *Anopheles gambiae,* in the northeast of Brazil;

b. applying all measures necessary to fight the mosquito *Anopheles gambiae* in the northeast, as well as to prevent its spreading to other parts of the national territory;

c. applying all complementary measures relative to the fight against malaria in the northeast, such as treatment of the sick, and health education of the population, etc.

Article 3. The Malaria Service of the Northeast shall be headed by a specially appointed director with a Class O salary.

Paragraph 1. The technical and administrative personnel of the Malaria Service of the Northeast shall be appointed in accordance with provisions of the law.

Article 4. The Federal Government is empowered to entrust the direction and administration of the Malaria Service of the Northeast to The Rockefeller Foundation for the period of time deemed necessary.

Paragraph 1. The financial contribution of The Rockefeller Foundation as well as the administrative regulations under which the Malaria Service of the Northeast will operate according to the provisions of this article, will be specified in the contract to be signed with the Foundation by the Ministry of Education and Health.

Article 5. The necessary expenditures for the operation of the Malaria Service of the Northeast, in 1939, shall be charged to the funds of the special budget as established by Legal Decree No. 1007, of December 30, 1938.

Article 6. This law shall be in effect as from the date of its publication.

Article 7. Provisions to the contrary are hereby revoked.

Rio de Janeiro, January 11, 1939, 118th of the Independence and 51st of the Republic. [signed] Getulio Vargas

Gustavo Capanema

Appendix II

Terms of Contract Drawn up by the Ministry of Education and Health and the International Health Division of The Rockefeller Foundation for the Study and Combat of *Anopheles gambiae* throughout Brazil during the Year 1939 (In Translation)

On the twenty-sixth day of January, 1939, there being present in the Department of Financial Affairs of the Ministry of Education and Health, the respective Minister, Dr. Gustavo Capanema, representing the Federal Government, and Dr. Fred L. Soper, duly authorized representative of the International Health Division of The Rockefeller Foundation, the latter stated that the said Division would assume responsibility for the studies of and campaign against *Anopheles gambiae* during 1939 throughout Brazil, under the following conditions:

First. The International Health Division of The Rockefeller Foundation will assume entire responsibility for the combat and study of *Anopheles gambiae*

throughout the entire northeastern part of the country, from the first day of January to the thirty-first day of December, 1939. Should the existence of *Anopheles gambiae* be verified in other parts of the national territory, the International Health Division of The Rockefeller Foundation will extend its activities to those localities.

Second. The representative of the International Health Division of The Rockefeller Foundation shall be the director of the Malaria Service of the Northeast, and shall have the power to choose employees and stipulate the conditions under which they work with the approval of the Ministry of Education and Health.

Third. In selecting candidates for the technical staff, preference will be given to those who present proof of having satisfactorily completed a course of training in malariology or of having had long experience in antimosquito work.

Fourth. The two parties to this contract shall designate, in accord with available information as to the results of entomological surveys, the areas in which antilarval measures against *Anopheles gambiae* are to be carried out.

Fifth. In addition to the campaign against *Anopheles gambiae*, complementary measures for the control of malaria, such as treatment, chemical and mechanical prophylaxis, education of the public, etc., will be undertaken at the discretion of the Director of the Malaria Service of the Northeast.

Sixth. Since the International Health Division of The Rockefeller Foundation is cooperating with the Federal Government, it is understood that the legal entity, for all purposes, shall be the Malaria Service of the Northeast, of the Ministry of Education and Health.

Seventh. In combating and studying *Anopheles gambiae*, the personnel of the Malaria Service of the Northeast shall have authority to enforce such health measures as now exist or may later become effective, relating to the collection of blood samples, control of mosquitoes, notification of deaths, permits for burials, examination of bodies, the performing of autopsies or any other measures which may be of interest to the Malaria Service of the Northeast.

Eighth. When on duty the doctors and authorized employees of the Malaria Service of the Northeast shall be entitled to exemption from postal and telegraphic charges, to passes on government railroads and to discounts allowed public departments by ocean and river navigation and air transportation companies, all such concessions being extensible to employees in charge of posts where the Service does not maintain resident doctors. Authorized doctors and other employees shall requisition passes for subordinates and for transportation of necessary materials on government railroads as well as free telegraphic service on government lines.

I. Passes, transportation, and telegrams requisitioned from government lines shall be considered to be in the public interest and, therefore, not chargeable.

II. Expenses incurred through the requisition of passes, transportation, and telegrams on government lines shall be considered as part of the contribution of the Federal Government to the Malaria Service of the Northeast, in charge of The Rockefeller Foundation.

Ninth. The personnel and material of the Antimalaria Service of the Ministry of Education and Health, now operating in the Northeast, shall be incorporated in the Malaria Service of the Northeast.

Tenth. The Malaria Service of the Northeast may, whenever necessary, request the collaboration of other federal, state, and municipal departments directly or through their respective ministers, interventors, or mayors, in applying the necessary technical measures or in securing necessary supplies.

Eleventh. For the execution of the service herein contracted, the Federal Government will contribute 5,000 contos ($250,000 U.S.) and the International Health Division of The Rockefeller Foundation the sum of $100,000 (one hundred thousand dollars), including in this figure the value of material supplied by the Division.

For the execution of this clause, the following conditions are established:

I. The quota of the Foundation ($100,000) in milreis shall depend on the exchange rates in force at the time payments are being made by the Division;

II. The Federal Government shall deposit in advance, in the Bank of Brazil, its corresponding quota (5,000 contos) to the credit of the representative of the International Health Division of The Rockefeller Foundation in Brazil, after due registration of this contract, the interest accruing to revert in favor of the National Treasury;

III. The cost of the Malaria Service of the Northeast shall be debited to the contributions of the Federal Government and the International Health Division of The Rockefeller Foundation in the proportion of 70% (seventy per cent) to the former and 30% (thirty per cent) to the latter;

IV. Should the contribution of the Division become exhausted, due to modifications of the exchange rate, further expense shall be met exclusively by the quota of the Federal Government;

V. Financial statements of the total expenditures of the Malaria Service of the Northeast shall be submitted by the International Health Division of The Rockefeller Foundation showing that the stipulations of Item III are being carried out.

VI. The taxes and imposts already created or which may be created by law during the term of this contract, which financially affect the budget of the Malaria Service of the Northeast, shall be charged against the sum of 5,000 contos ($250,000 U.S.) herein established as the quota of the Government.

Twelfth. The salaries and traveling expenses of the doctors of the staff of the International Health Division of The Rockefeller Foundation, who may be brought to Brazil for work with the Malaria Service of the Northeast, shall be paid by the Division and, therefore, shall not be subject to the terms and conditions of the eleventh clause of the present contract and its subitems.

Thirteenth. The expenses up to 5,000 contos ($250,000 U.S.) entailed in carrying out the present contract which will be valid until December 31, 1939, shall be chargeable to the reserve set up by the special credit opened by Legal Decree No. 1007 of December 30, 1938.

Fourteenth. Reports on the work of the Malaria Service of the Northeast shall be sent monthly to the Ministry of Education and Health and to the Director of the National Health Department, in addition to any other information which may be requested from time to time.

Fifteenth. Personnel, equipment, and transportation facilities of the Malaria Service of the Northeast and of the Yellow Fever Service shall be interchangeable.

Sixteenth. The present contract shall only become effective after due legal registration, the Government not being liable for any indemnity should registration be refused.

Seventeenth. Under the terms of Art. 36, No. 72 of Decree No. 1137 of October 7, 1936, the present contract is exempt from the stamp tax. And since both parties are in agreement, the present contract has been drawn up, which on being read and found in order, will be signed by Dr. Gustavo Capanema, Minister of Education and Health, on behalf of the Federal Government, and by Dr. Fred L. Soper, representative of the International Health Division of The Rockefeller Foundation, by the witnesses below and by me, José Medeiros de Carvalho, administrative officer of class "J," who drew up this contract. Rio de Janeiro, January 26, 1939— [signed] Gustavo Capanema, Fred L. Soper, and the witnesses: J. A. Kerr, José Medeiros de Carvalho, and Jorge Modesto de Almeida.

| Paris Green in the Eradication
of *Anopheles gambiae*: Brazil, 1940;
Egypt, 1945*

In March 1930 *Anopheles gambiae,* probably the world's most efficient vector of malaria, was found at Natal, Brazil. Its arrival was associated with the development of rapid communications with Europe by way of Dakar. Although the breeding of gambiae when discovered was less than 1 square kilometer in extent, a serious outbreak of malaria occurred in the following month. The severity of this outbreak was such that the Health Department had to distribute "food as well as quinine."

Twelve years later, in March 1942, severe outbreaks of malaria in Upper Egypt signaled the invasion of Egypt by gambiae coming from the Sudan. This invasion was associated with greatly increased traffic into Egypt from the south, owing to wartime difficulties of shipping in the Mediterranean. In the fall of 1942 gambiae-transmitted malaria struck as far north as Asyut, some 320 kilometers from Cairo.

Gambiae was eradicated in Brazil in 1940 after a sojourn of 10½ years in the country; in Egypt eradication came in 1945, 3 years after the invasion occurred. The basic method used in each country was a straightforward chemical attack with Paris green. Victory in each country came only after unnecessary and costly delays. These delays can be attributed to lack of vision, lack of courage, lack of salesmanship, and lack of administrative experience.

Through a series of coincidences I participated in the delays in eradicating, and in the eradication of, gambiae in both Brazil and Egypt.

[The remainder of the discussion of the eradication of *Anopheles gambiae* from Brazil has been omitted. The campaign there terminated June 30, 1942. *Ed.*]

Anopheles gambiae IN EGYPT, 1942–1943

Six months later, on January 7, 1943, as a member of the United States of America Typhus Commission, I arrived in Cairo to learn that Egypt had been invaded by *Anopheles gambiae* the previous year. The fall months of

* Excerpt from a paper presented at Seminar on Mosquito-Borne Diseases—Past, Present, and Future, Communicable Disease Center, Atlanta, Georgia, March 10, 1966. The entire paper was originally published *(117)* in *Mosquito News 26:* 470–476, 1966. Dr. Soper was a Special Consultant, Office of International Health, Public Health Service.

1942 had been marked by a disastrous epidemic of malaria, paralleling in severity the gambiae-malaria outbreaks seen in Brazil but on a much larger scale.

On invitation of the Under Secretary of Health, I visited the infested epidemic area; my report emphasized the threat of continuing epidemic malaria if gambiae were not eradicated. I explained that the "same factors which make gambiae such a dangerous vector of malaria, namely, its tendency to breed in shallow sunlit pools without vegetation and its habit of resting and feeding in human habitations, make it highly vulnerable to simple frontal chemical attack." I stated that complete species eradication, although not easy, was "entirely possible with the careful meticulous application throughout the entire infested area of *measures already known and demonstrated.*"

I recommended that an emergency Anti-Gambiae Service be organized; that this Service be of temporary character, directly under the Minister of Health, and responsible only for "the prevention of the spread of gambiae to those parts of Egypt not already infested, and the complete eradication of gambiae from Upper Egypt . . . that this Service should have adequate funds and necessary liberty of action to carry out the administrative measures necessary for the rapid discharge of these responsibilities."

The Service should not be responsible in any way for the study and treatment of malaria.

I insisted the Director be given full autonomy in the choice, appointment, and discharge of all personnel; have full freedom to determine how and where work should be carried out; and be able to requisition needed items, including technical personnel, from other branches of the Health Department.

My report was also submitted to the diplomatic and military authorities of the United Kingdom and the United States since Egypt was at that time occupied as an active theater of war. I appeared before the Middle East Supply Center recommending the allocation of shipping tonnage for the importation of Paris green. This was approved.

I failed to convince interested British workers that eradication of gambiae was possible; I likewise failed to convince the Egyptian authorities that they should request The Rockefeller Foundation to participate in the attack on gambiae with experienced administrators from Brazil. Failing this, I gave the Egyptian workers the manuscript of the then unpublished book "Anopheles gambiae in Brazil, 1930 to 1940" and a manuscript copy of the detailed manual of instructions of the Brazilian operation. (This manual had been carefully prepared after *Anopheles gambiae* had already disappeared from Brazil, as an historical record of the procedures used and in the hope that it might be useful later in gambiae eradication programs in Africa south of the Sahara.)

Anopheles gambiae IN EGYPT, 1944–1945

I left Egypt in June 1943, and not until February 24, 1944 did I learn of Egypt's catastrophic epidemic of the fall of the previous year. Then I saw at Naples, in the U.S. Army newspaper *The Stars and Stripes,* a British denial of the Egyptian charge that the occupation forces had so depleted the country's food supply that thousands had died of starvation in Upper Egypt. The British claimed that foodstocks were adequate, that starvation had occurred because of paralysis of food distribution by an overwhelming epidemic of malaria. (Again emphasis on "food as well as quinine.")

On invitation of the Government of Egypt, I returned to Cairo early in May 1944 to make recommendations on malaria in the Nile Valley. The enormity of the 1943 catastrophe had made malaria a top political issue in which King Farouk himself became involved. The true measure of the 1943 epidemic will never be known; His Majesty told me a Royal Commission, after visiting the blighted areas, had estimated malaria deaths in 2 years at 130,000. Interest, finances, and authority would not be lacking for the attack on the invader.

After a week-long visit to the infested area, I rewrote for the Minister of Health the essential recommendations I had made 16 months before; I again offered the administrative assistance of The Rockefeller Foundation. These recommendations and offer were accepted, and in June 1944 a special Gambiae Eradication Service was created, independent of the Malaria Service, directly under the Minister of Health, and responsible only for the eradication of gambiae from Egypt.

Foundation participation began on July 15. Fortunately, the Egyptian Malaria Service had used the manual of instructions of the Malaria Service of Northeast Brazil in zoning the gambiae-infested area and had adequate personnel already in the field.

It had, however, failed to substitute Paris green for oil in the attack on gambiae; the logistics problem for using oil had not been solved.

Beginning in July, the shift from oil to Paris green was made as rapidly as possible, but the flood season was imminent and a great deal of malaria occurred in the fall of 1944.

In Egypt, as in Brazil, gambiae proved to be highly susceptible to Paris green larviciding. The last gambiae in Egypt was found on February 19, 1945, just 7 months after routine application of Paris green began.

COMMENTS

Thus the invasions of Brazil and Egypt by gambiae, together covering a decade and a half, terminated with the invader rejected. Although the two campaigns were administratively and technically very similar, the geographical and psychological problems were quite different.

In Brazil gambiae was actively spreading at the periphery with an entire continent in jeopardy. The technique of blocking this spread and of eradicating gambiae in the infested area was unknown. Not the certainty of winning but the cost of failure was the stimulus to action.

In Egypt gambiae had been successfully blocked at Asyut; the infested area was the narrow irrigated zone along the Nile surrounded by hostile desert; the limits of the problem were known as was its solution; no research was needed nor attempted; from the start the result could be foretold.

In Brazil work began with an inadequate budget; at a critical time during the first year there was considerable difficulty in financing operations. In Egypt instructions from the Minister of Health were from the beginning that gambiae must be driven out. He said, "Go on spending!"

It is now 36 years since gambiae invaded Brazil and 24 years since it came down the Nile into Egypt. Brazil and Egypt are just as vulnerable to invasion by gambiae today as they were decades ago; many other regions of the world are equally vulnerable. Also it seems certain that some areas now suffering from gambiae malaria could be more easily freed of this curse by eradication of gambiae than by other means. Malariologists should not fail to study the records of Brazil and Egypt as they face up to the challenge of African malaria. In Brazil, toward the end of the campaign, a small test area was cleared completely of gambiae in 3 weeks; in Egypt, gambiae was widespread in November but had disappeared before the end of February.

I have retold this story of long ago because it has lessons for each generation of conscientious public health administrators. I have told it in the first person because I have referred to killing and costly delays due to lack of vision, lack of courage, lack of salesmanship, and lack of administrative experience; even the casual reader may identify examples of each.

Part VIII | The Philosophy of Eradication

Species Eradication: A Practical Goal of Species Reduction in the Control of Mosquito-Borne Disease*

FRED L. SOPER AND D. BRUCE WILSON

The first application of antimosquito measures† for the control of malaria and yellow fever, following the demonstrations that these diseases are mosquito borne, was made by Gorgas in Havana, Cuba, in 1901. Since the measures applied were aimed at mosquitoes in general, all mosquito-borne disease was affected, but the striking reduction of the mortality from malaria was overshadowed by the dramatic disappearance of yellow fever. Similar comparative results were later observed for malaria and yellow fever, following general antimosquito measures in Panama and in Rio de Janeiro, Brazil. It is significant that the great American sanitarian Gorgas and the great Brazilian sanitarian Oswaldo Cruz both worked to control malaria as well as yellow fever, but that the fame of each is based on results obtained with yellow fever rather than with malaria.

These early general antimosquito campaigns for the control of malaria

* The work on which this paper is based was conducted with the support and under the auspices of the Ministry of Education and Public Health of Brazil and the International Health Division of The Rockefeller Foundation. The antiaegypti campaign has been carried on for many years by a large number of colleagues on the staff of the Yellow Fever Service. For all practical purposes, the antigambiae campaign has been carried out by many of the same group, although under a special service designated as the Malaria Service of the Northeast. More detailed reports of the organization and work of these two services are in preparation. Dr. Soper was the Representative in South America (Rio de Janeiro Office) of the International Health Division of The Rockefeller Foundation; Dr. Wilson was a staff member.

This article was originally published (*42*) in the *Journal of the National Malaria Society 1:* 5–24, 1942.

† The term "mosquito eradication" has been widely misused in the literature of mosquito campaigns where mosquito reduction is meant. "Species eradication" should be defined as the complete extermination of the species under consideration in all phases of its development; ovum, larva, pupa, and imago. When species eradication has been accomplished, the crucial test of discontinuation of all control measures, in the presence of suitable breeding places, is not followed, in the absence of reimportation, by reappearance of the species.

and yellow fever were very expensive. Once it became apparent that the control of yellow fever is easier than, and independent of, that of malaria, it became customary to organize special yellow fever services for the control of *Aëdes (Stegomyia) aegypti* breeding. Just as it was discovered that general antimosquito measures are not essential in the control of yellow fever, so also was it learned that malaria can often be controlled by attacking a single species of anopheline without consideration of other anophelines present in the community. Thus it came about that general antimosquito campaigns devoted to the solution of health problems have given way to special "species sanitation" campaigns: anti-aegypti campaigns for the control of yellow fever and special malaria campaigns taking as their objective the most dangerous local anopheline.

The program of such species sanitation campaigns has been one of reduction of the density of the individual species concerned below the critical threshold at which such species can continue to transmit disease under the existing local conditions. This report is based on such species sanitation campaigns against *Aëdes (Stegomyia) aegypti* and *Anopheles (Myzomyia) gambiae,* in which "species reduction" has been pushed to its logical conclusion—"species eradication." The eventual great economy and administrative simplicity of species eradication over species reduction justify a careful study of all mosquito-control projects to determine those in which the species-eradication technique may be practicable.

Species Eradication of *Aëdes aegypti*

Early campaigns for the control of mosquito-borne disease demonstrated that it is not necessary to eradicate vector species in order to curtail active transmission. Rather was it found that as the species density was lowered by control measures a "critical index" was eventually reached, after which transmission no longer occurred. This critical index is, of course, a variable function, depending on many factors other than the density of the vector, such as the incubation period of the etiological agent in the vector, the infective period of the human host, the development of lasting immunity, the number and distribution of susceptible hosts, and the number and distribution of sources of infection.

In dealing with aegypti-transmitted yellow fever, experience shows that generally the critical index has been reached when careful house-to-house inspection reveals the aquatic forms of the vector on not more than 5 per cent of the premises visited.*

* This house-breeding index is, of course, only a rough indirect measure of adult aegypti density, since it takes no account of the size or productivity of the larval foci found. However, no figures are available, based on imago surveys during outbreaks of yellow fever, to determine the corresponding critical index.

In practice it was found during many years of antiaegypti measures to be fairly easy to reduce aegypti breeding to the point where larval foci could be found in less than 5 per cent of the houses in the area worked, but that attempts to force the house-breeding index below 1 or 2 per cent were very costly and that final species elimination was never obtained. In the light of this experience, yellow fever work came to be based on a program for the reduction of the aegypti house index to well below 5 per cent, but no attempt was made to secure complete eradication.

It was also found that any relaxation in the antiaegypti measures resulted in a dangerous increase of aegypti production. The cost of the regular antiaegypti services is high, so that funds for adequate services of this type were generally available only during and for a limited period following outbreaks of yellow fever.

A surprising result of the early antimosquito campaigns in Havana, Panama, Santos, and Rio de Janeiro was that yellow fever disappeared not only from these cities but from surrounding areas as well. As long as yellow fever was believed to be only a human disease, transmitted by a single species of mosquito, it seemed logical to attempt the eradication of yellow fever from the American continent through temporary intensive campaigns in the principal cities of known endemic regions to reduce aegypti density below the critical index. No plans were made for permanent aegypti control measures since, once yellow fever disappeared from these principal cities, it would soon disappear also from the surrounding areas and not reappear unless imported from Africa.

This concept of the strategy of yellow fever control received a rude shock in 1928 when yellow fever appeared unexpectedly in Rio de Janeiro, the capital of Brazil, after an absence of 20 years. Although it was universally recognized that the modern development of Rio de Janeiro dated from the first notable campaign of Oswaldo Cruz, antiaegypti measures had been practically abandoned after a number of years of freedom from yellow fever. The disease reappeared at a time when no nearby foci of infection were known and it was not until the discovery, a few years later, that yellow fever is also a disease of wild animals in the tropical forests that a satisfactory explanation of the origin of the reinfection of Rio de Janeiro became available. Jungle yellow fever constitutes a permanent source of virus for the reinfection of aegypti-infested areas and makes the permanent eradication of yellow fever through a temporary reduction of the domestic vector, *Aëdes aegypti,* impossible.

The Rio de Janeiro epidemic of 1928–1929 forced a recognition of the danger of unchecked aegypti breeding in those centers of population within striking distance of infection. The development of air transportation of passengers has so shortened the travel time between distant points that practically the entire world is threatened by the possibility of infective cases arriving from the endemic regions of Africa and South America during the incubation period, which may be as long as 6 days. *While required vaccination of all air passengers may be of some value in protecting against this threat, the only guaranty of safety is elimination of the aegypti mosquito.*

Various solutions to the problem of the high cost of aegypti control have been suggested and tried in an effort to develop a program of permanent control. As early as 1927 the attempt was made to use monthly, instead of weekly, cycles of inspection in those cities in Northeast Brazil where a low house-breeding index had been maintained for several years. This lengthened cycle permitted a great reduction in personnel and in operating cost, but also permitted a dangerous increase in aegypti density and, eventually, yellow fever reappeared in some of the cities with such lengthened cycles.*

In 1928 a serious attempt was made to eradicate aegypti from João Pessôa, the capital of Paraíba State, at that time a city of some 35,000 people. This attempt failed, but produced the concept of the "mother," or "generating," focus as responsible for the perpetuation of the aegypti species in cities where antiaegypti measures were being carefully applied.

It was reasoned that, since the aegypti mosquito is relatively short-lived, any prolonged perpetuation of the species must be due to hidden production not subject to elimination at the time of the inspector's regular visit. This reasoning was based on the fact that when low house indices are obtained, practically all the foci found by the regular inspectors contain larvae only, the final aquatic or pupal stage being absent. When these larval foci were plotted on the map of the area worked, they were found to form clusters, each of which was the product of one or more nearby hidden primary foci. Searching out and destroying hidden foci in this way helped to reduce the already low index but did not alone lead to eradication.

Previous to the introduction of the search for adult aegypti to indicate the presence of this species, the officer in charge of yellow fever control had to rely on the larval index,† based on foci found and reported by the in-

---

* A given house-breeding index based on weekly inspections is correlated with a much lower density of adult aegypti than is a similar index based on longer inspection cycles. With a weekly cycle, the foci found are destroyed before they come to fruition, since the minimum cycle of reproduction of the aegypti mosquito is longer than the interval between inspections. With a monthly cycle, however, such foci may produce as many as three broods of mosquitoes between inspection. In the first case adult production is necessarily limited to such foci as are not found by the inspection, whereas in the second case there is added to this production of hidden foci, that which can occur during a month from observed foci. Thus a house index of 5 per cent on a weekly cycle may indicate the presence of relatively few adult mosquitoes at any one time, whereas the same index on a monthly cycle may correspond to a much higher adult density.

† Technically includes pupal foci as well, since most pupal foci also have larvae.

spectors who were themselves responsible for maintaining a low aegypti density. The inference is obvious.

In some tragic instances in which fatal yellow fever reappeared in controlled areas, it was found that the reported larval index utterly failed to represent the true breeding conditions. At times this discrepancy was due to careless work and often to failure to report conditions as found, but when well-trained chief inspectors and health officers repeated the inspection, even in areas worked by able and conscientious inspectors, an appreciable number of missed aegypti foci were generally found. Often, especially in areas where the total number of foci was low, the number found on reinspection equaled that reported initially. It eventually became apparent that the greater experience and imagination of those checking the work were often responsible for finding additional foci missed by the routine inspector.

On the other hand, it was found that when the regular inspector's visit occurred immediately after that of those checking his work, he sometimes uncovered foci missed by his superiors. In any case, the second inspection was merely a repetition of the first and both pitted human intelligence against aegypti instinct in the discovery of actual or potential hidden breeding places. In this struggle, instinct often won, the really difficult foci missed by the regular inspector being missed also by the checking inspector.

In order to get an independent estimate of aegypti density, a page was taken from the malariologists' handbook and the search for adult aegypti introduced toward the end of 1930. The adult capture method has proved to be the most sensitive indicator of the presence of aegypti in an area and is invaluable in locating the position of such hidden primary perpetuating foci as may remain after the gross infestation has been eliminated by routine antilarval measures.

At about the same time, effective measures were introduced to eliminate, as mosquito-producing foci, all water containers found with larvae, by destruction or by oiling with a mixture of three parts of fuel oil and one part of diesel oil.

It is believed that the use of adult captures for the localization of hidden primary or generating foci and the routine destruction or oiling of all foci found were responsible for the complete absence of aegypti breeding which has been reported from an ever-increasing number of Brazilian cities and towns over long periods since 1932 (see Table 1).

The first effect noted in the curves of mosquito indices following the introduction of adult captures for the location of hidden breeding was the gradual separation of the aegypti index from that of other mosquitoes. Previously, the indices of aegypti and other mosquitoes had fluctuated together throughout the year, according to the amount and distribution of rainfall and other climatic factors. Thereafter, however, the index of other

Table 1. Quarterly Summary of Houses Found with Aegypti Foci before and during Species Eradication Program

Brazilian ports	Approximate population	Approx. No. of houses	Year	Before species eradication[a] Quarter 1st	2nd	3rd	4th	During eradication program[a] 1938 quarter 1st	2nd	3rd	4th	1939 quarter 1st	2nd	3rd	4th	1940 quarter 1st	2nd	3rd	4th	1941 quarter 1st	2nd	3rd	4th
Manáos	63,574	13,753	1933	1182b	1218b	3068b	2458b	2	1	2	1	2	0	0	0	0	0	0	0	0	0	3	0
Belém	159,088	32,405	1932	1507b	886b	571b	394b	0	3	1	0	0	2	0	0	0	2	1	1	0	0	0	1
São Luiz	63,617	12,327	1931	2794b	2922b	3173b	1151b	0	0	0	0	0	0	0	0	0	0	0	0	1	0	1	0
Terezina	40,248	9,650	1932		3892b	816b	330b	0	0	0	0	0	0	0	0	0	0	0	0	0	0	0	0
Parnaíba	21,395	5,620	1933	512b	271b	126b	336b	0	0	0	0	0	0	0	0	0	0	0	0	0	0	0	0
Fortaleza	122,273	28,206	1931	4265b	4494b	1795b	532b	6	4	0	1	1	1	0	0	0	2	0	0	0	0	0	0
Natal	50,630	12,501	1931	7165b	8460b	4048b	1047b	0	0	0	0	1	0	0	0	0	0	0	0	0	0	0	0
Macáu	7,469	1,966	1931			892b	637b	0b	1b	0b	0b	0b	0c	0c	0c	0c	0c	0c	0c	0c	0c	0c	0c
João Pessôa (Paraíba)	74,134	12,645	1931	29	40	28	9	0c	0c	0c	0c	0c	0c	0c	0c	0c	0c	0c	0c	0c	0c	0c	0c
Cabedêlo	6,322	1,704	1932	140b	151b	92b	44b	0b	0	0	0	0	0	0	0	0	0	0	0	0	0	0	0
Recife	333,600	76,684	1931	5626b	7449b	5231b	1779b	0	0	0	0	0	0	0	0	0	0	0	0	0	0	0	0
Maceió	74,723	20,765	1931	4787b	4052b	3042b	3464b	0	0	0	0	0	0	0	0	0	0	0	0	0	0	0	0
Penedo	12,559	3,970	1931	437b	432b	276b	138b	0	0	0	0	0	0	0	0	1	0	0	0	0	0	0	0
Aracaju	51,561	13,274	1931	142b	130b	115b	55b	2	0	2	0	0	0	0	0	8	2	0	0	0	0	0	0
Salvador (Baía)	255,166	58,252	1931	3988b	3019b	2973b	2921b	2	0	0	2	1	1	0	1	0	1	0	0	0	1	0	0
Ilhéus	19,035	4,985	1931	2724b	4150b	1767b	957b	0	0	0	0	0	0	0	0	0	0	0	0	0	0	0	0
Vitória	61,635	13,586	1931		1864b	2455b	1677b	0	0	0	0	0	0	0	0	0	2	0	0	0	0	0	0
Niterói–S. Gonçalo	193,449	45,632	1932	3133b	4773b	2934b	2051b	0	0	0	0	0	0	0	0	0	0	0	0	0	0	0	0
Federal District	1,787,440	383,713	1932	451b	185b	71b	192b	1	0	0	0	0	0	0	0	0	0	0	0	1	0	1	0
Santos	143,351	27,612	1935		190	0b	7b	0c	0c	0c	0c	0c	0c	0c	0c	0c	0c	0c	0c	0c	0c	0c	0c
Florianópolis	33,680	5,257	1936		135b	10b	10b	2b	1	—	—	—	—	—	—	—	—	—	—	—	—	—	—
Total	**3,574,949**	**784,507**		**38,882**	**48,713**	**33,483**	**20,169**	**13**	**12**	**3**	**4**	**3**	**5**	**1**	**1**	**8**	**6**	**4**	**2**	**0**	**5**	**1**	**1**

Houses with foci of Aëdes (Stegomyia) aegypti

[a] In the period "Before species eradication" the number of foci found is appreciable in spite of weekly destruction; in period "During eradication program" the number of foci found remains low in the face of lengthened inspection cycles, generally 28 days.

[b] Weekly inspection.

[c] Regular inspection suspended; presence of aegypti checked by adult captures only. All others, lengthened cycle, generally 28 days.

mosquitoes continued to fluctuate, whereas that of aegypti tended to continue on a regular downward course, eventually reaching the base line. It became evident that species reduction of aegypti was being carried to the extreme of species eradication without greatly affecting the breeding of other species of mosquitoes.

The use of the capture method brought some unexpected results, one of which was the modification of the handling of the "unoccupied house" problem. Previously it was found that the empty house constituted a serious problem in the reduction of aegypti breeding in an area. Since the empty house was generally locked at the time of the inspector's regular visit, such foci as might be present were not found and destroyed. Eventually the problem was handled by special empty house squads which carried special equipment and were responsible for getting the keys to all unoccupied houses, entering them, and eradicating all potential aegypti foci so that further visits would not be required until the house was again inhabited. The work of these empty house squads was effective but expensive, and was in many cases devoted to aegypti-proofing houses which would not in any case have produced aegypti, either because of absence of potential foci or because of absence of aegypti in the immediate neighborhood to take advantage of such potential foci as did exist. With the introduction of the capture method it was found that examination of empty houses could be discontinued except when the presence of aegypti breeding in the neighborhood of such empty houses was revealed by the capture of adult aegypti in nearby houses where they had gone to feed.

The use of the capture method, followed by routine elimination of all foci found, revealed, as should have been self-apparent, that though the number of potential breeding places of aegypti may appear to be almost infinite in certain areas, actually the number of permanent producing foci on which the species depends for its continued existence is finite. Such casual breeding places as roof gutters and flower vases are not generally responsible for maintaining the species.* Roof-gutter breeding may be a very important factor in building up a high adult density during the rainy season in cities where an otherwise low index has been obtained by control measures, but only occasionally do roof gutters form permanent primary foci, and the presence of these will be revealed by the finding of adult mosquitoes in the houses; it is no longer necessary to maintain costly routine roof-gutter inspection.

* This concept of selective breeding is important in considering other species which may appear to present insoluble problems because of the wide variety of conditions under which they may occasionally be found to breed. On careful investigation it will often be found that the effective breeding of the species in question, that is, the breeding which is responsible for the year after year maintenance of the species, is limited to certain special types of containers or foci.

The first zero indices were obtained in 1932, and a sufficiently long period has now elapsed for sound conclusions to be drawn regarding the possibilities of aegypti eradication. In the early days of zero indices it was often found that a city which had apparently been free of aegypti for some time would be reported dirty again. Careful investigation showed that this reappearance of aegypti was often due to some householder putting water once more, sometimes after an interval of several months, in water jars on the walls of which were still viable eggs of aegypti. In contrast to this "internal" reinfestation, it was found in other cases that reinfestation had occurred from outside the clean areas by transportation of eggs or aquatic forms in the water containers of families moving from "dirty" areas, or through transportation of adult aegypti on trains or boats.

Experience showed that the internal reinfestation could be exhausted in time but that it was necessary to extend anti-aegypti measures to tributary communities to overcome the threat of "external" reinfestation. Such extension has been carried out on an ever-larger scale, without increased expenditure, by suspending routine inspection in clean areas and using personnel thus released for work in dirty tributary areas. The capture of adult aegypti has proved to be an adequate indicator of reinfestations, internal and external, when such occur, in clean areas where routine inspections have been suspended.

As this program continues, the areas free of aegypti become larger, the chances of reinfestation decrease, and the number of men available for work in remaining dirty areas increases in relation to the size of these dirty areas.

The search for adult aegypti is slow and expensive and is not used in the initial stages of a campaign while the adult aegypti density is high; its special purpose is the discovery of hidden breeding after the bulk of aegypti production has been eliminated by the routine antilarval measures.

Administratively there is a great psychological advantage in undertaking species eradication rather than species reduction, and classifying each area as "dirty" or "clean," rather than as with "safe index" or with "dangerous index." The demand for 100 per cent efficiency removes the last defense of the inspector who does sloppy work. The basic question, Is aegypti present? requires an answer of but one word and cuts short all argument.

The great reduction in staff possible in a given community once eradication has been accomplished, and the reduced contact of this staff with individual households are conducive to administrative simplicity.

Table 1 presents, in summary form,* quarterly reports of the actual num-

---

* More details of this work from 1935 to date have been published from time to time in the *Boletín de la Oficina Sanitaria Panamericana.*

ber of premises* found with foci of aegypti in various cities of Brazil before and after the adoption of the program of species eradication.

In attempting to eradicate aegypti, it was found that certain cities, after some months' work, were almost clean, only to continue with a small number of foci every trimester; that other cities were very slow in acquiring relative cleanliness; while others, after being clean for some time, suddenly showed an appreciable number of foci. The trickle of an occasional focus in a clean city generally resulted from reinfestation from nearby dirty areas or even from distant areas by river boats (Manáos, Belém); the failure of a city to become clean in a reasonable period generally was the result of lax administrative supervision at a time when more serious matters were demanding attention elsewhere; and the sudden increase in the number of foci in a city, followed by their early disappearance, often represented only an apparent increase, because of the inclusion in the control area of dirty suburbs not previously worked and which had been found to be dangerous sources of reinfestation.

The data presented in the table cover only a few of the more important centers worked among the hundreds, nay thousands, of cities and towns, villages, hamlets, and even rural districts in which antiaegypti measures have been applied in Brazil in recent years. Local species eradication of aegypti has been accomplished in many of the larger cities and even in entire states, and these have been protected against serious reinfestation for years at a time for but a fraction of the expense previously incurred in maintaining "safe" aegypti indices in a few of the larger cities. A large percentage of funds now charged to yellow fever control is devoted to the campaign against nuisance mosquitoes in cities where aegypti no longer exists. The development of a technique for the eradication of these nuisance species would permit further great economies.

With regard to the possibilities of aegypti eradication, it can be said that no insoluble problems have been found in Brazil and that with the present organization and orientation of the National Yellow Fever Service of the Brazilian Department of Health, a few more years should find Brazil practically free of this species.

In the officially adopted "Internal Regulations" (1942) of this Service, the Section of Stegomyia Control is given the responsibility for

* The house-breeding index or percentage of houses found with aegypti foci is useful in estimating the possibility of yellow fever transmission and in comparing the situation of one "dirty" city with another. Once eradication is undertaken in an area, the interest shifts to a comparison of local conditions at intervals in the same area over a period of time. For this purpose the actual number of premises found with foci is a much more stimulating figure than is the house-breeding index, which often masks the trend of small numbers behind a series of decimal places.

a. Preparing plans for the campaign against *Stegomyia* (=*Aëdes aegypti*) looking towards the complete elimination of this species. . . .

c. Supervising the work of eradicating the vector (*Aëdes aegypti*).

SPECIES ERADICATION OF *Anopheles gambiae*

In 1930, following the discovery at Natal, Rio Grande do Norte, Brazil, of *Anopheles gambiae,* the most notorious of the African vectors of malaria, there were some informal discussions of the possibility of attempting the eradication of this newly imported species while the infested area was still small. No serious attempt was made, however, and the demonstration in 1931 that the species had spread to several points in the interior of Rio Grande do Norte led to the conclusion that eradication was no longer possible through the application of control measures, and to the reliance on the empty hope that this dangerous species would not find conditions in Brazil suitable for permanent residence and further dissemination.

In March 1931* a local antigambiae service for Natal was organized and before the end of the year control measures were extended to various points in the interior of the state.

The initial campaign against gambiae was essentially an antimalaria campaign, and once the malaria problem of the state capital was solved, no further measures were taken. This abortive attempt to deal with gambiae was of great importance since it may well have been one of the deciding factors of gambiae's failure to spread southward along the coast from the city.

Paradoxically enough, the success of antigambiae measures in Natal, instead of stimulating a continued program for the eradication of gambiae from the relatively small area infested in the interior of the state of Rio Grande do Norte, actually resulted in the neglect of this infestation until after it had assumed gigantic proportions in 1938.

---

* At the request of the Director of the National Health Department of Brazil, the Cooperative Yellow Fever Service, maintained by the Ministry of Education and Health of Brazil and the International Health Division of The Rockefeller Foundation, undertook the organization of antigambiae measures in Natal to mitigate the effects of the second gambiae-transmitted outbreak of malaria in the New World, the first epidemic having occurred the previous year. In October 1931 the responsibility for the control of gambiae was taken over by the State Health Service of Rio Grande do Norte, under the direction of one of Brazil's best known malariologists, who had been especially appointed because of the gambiae situation. The special budget of 300 contos ($20,000 U.S.) made available by the federal government to meet this problem was exhausted within a few months and control measures abandoned in April 1932.

During the period 1932–1937 inclusive, gambiae was little in the public eye, although it was known to persist in the interior of Rio Grande do Norte. Apparently the Assú, Mossoró, and Jaguaribe valleys were invaded about the same time, either late in 1936 or early in 1937. The year 1938 witnessed, in this region, what may well have been the most severe epidemic of malaria ever occurring in the Americas; official estimates give over 100,000* cases and a minimum of 14,000 deaths during the first 6 months of the year. The demand that something be done about this African invader was insistent, and at the end of October, the Brazilian Government organized a control service with a budget for the rest of 1938 of 1000 contos ($50,000.00 U.S.) under the name of Service for Anti-Malaria Operations (SOCM). At the same time, the International Health Division of The Rockefeller Foundation undertook an independent survey of the extent of the infested region and those factors which might influence the success of a belated attempt to eradicate gambiae from the country.

On the basis of this survey and the experience of the Service for Anti-Malaria Operations, the Malaria Service of Northeast Brazil was created by presidential decree in January 1939, especially for the purpose of attacking the gambiae problem. The Malaria Service of the Northeast began the year's operations with a total budget of 7000 contos ($350,000 U.S.), of which 5000 contos ($250,000 U.S.) were contributed by the Ministry of Education and Health and 2000 contos ($100,000 U.S.) by the International Health Division of The Rockefeller Foundation.

The Malaria Service of the Northeast was, from the beginning, organized as an antigambiae service rather than as an antimalaria service, although sizable sums and much effort were devoted to the treatment of fever cases during 1939 and the first half of 1940, in a humanitarian effort to reduce the mortality from malaria during the period of continued gambiae transmission. The chief objects of the service were, first, to learn how to eradicate gambiae and, second, to eradicate gambiae. The urgency of the situation and the shortage of technical personnel precluded any careful study of malaria.

The reasons for undertaking the eradication of gambiae and gambling such large sums as were eventually used on this effort can be understood only by those who have witnessed the effects of true epidemic malaria, which are many times more severe than are those of annual "epidemics" in endemic areas. The realization that the 1938 outbreak would be repeated over and over again in the same river valleys until the survivors among the

---

* This estimate of cases is undoubtedly ultraconservative. In the following year the Malaria Service of the Northeast treated in the same region 176,000 persons, and probably failed to reach at least 25 per cent of the sick during the epidemic season.

local populations had become thoroughly malarialized and relatively immune, and that this tragic picture would be drawn in the same sombre tints in many parts of the Americas, as other suitable parts of the continent were invaded, one by one, left those who might no choice but to attempt to eradicate the species, no matter what might be the odds against success. Factors which influenced the decision to make the attempt were

1. The previous demonstration by the Yellow Fever Service that the eradication of *Aëdes aegypti* is a practicable public health measure.

2. The failure of gambiae to persist in Natal itself or to reinfest the original focus of 1930 following the initial 1931–1932 campaign.

3. The apparent limitation of gambiae to parts of the states of Rio Grande do Norte and Ceará where meteorological and topographical features might be expected to delay extension and favor eradication.

4. The existence of the large staff of well-trained men of the Yellow Fever Service, experienced in the species eradication technique as applied to aegypti, which could be drawn upon at will.

Among the many factors which suggested caution were

1. Absence of adequate experience with methods which might be successful in dealing with gambiae.

2. Almost complete lack of encouragement from malariologists and others having experience in attempts to control many species of anophelines, including gambiae.

3. Lack of knowledge of critical points in the biology of gambiae, such as duration of viability of ova and hibernation and estivation of imagoes.

4. Failure to find any record of species eradication of insects except that of the Mediterranean fruit fly in the United States, against which intensive combat was begun immediately after its discovery.

No previous estimates were made of the time and money which might be needed to explore the possibilities of eradication. It was fully realized that the effort might well end in failure; none could foretell the rapidity nor the direction of spread of gambiae which might occur before control measures became effective. Even though local eradication in known infested areas might be accomplished, it would always be reasonable to fear that a mosquito which had crossed the 1600-mile expanse of the South Atlantic might have spread during the 9 years it had been present in America many hundreds of miles to regions where it had not yet been recognized. Many would question the expenditure of large sums of money to eradicate gambiae from Brazil while inexhaustible supplies of the species in Africa constituted a permanent threat of reinfestation.*

* The reality of this threat was revealed by the capture on October 9, 1941, of a female gambiae on a flying boat at Natal at the end of a 21-hour flight from Lagos, Nigeria, West Africa, during the routine inspection and desinsectization which are carried out on all transatlantic planes on arrival in Brazil.

The Malaria Service of the Northeast began operations after the rainy season of 1939 had set in, without a definite plan as to how gambiae could be controlled, although it was known that Paris green had given good results as a larvicide for this species and that gambiae-transmitted malaria had been controlled in Zululand by the use of pyrethrum insecticide spray.

The first 6 months of work was very discouraging in spite of the fact that the funds allotted for this period were overspent. Malaria was rife on all sides and gambiae paid little heed to the ineffectual efforts of hundreds of untrained men but proceeded up the Jaguaribe and its tributaries apparently unrestrained. An appeal for additional funds brought a generous response from the Brazilian Government of an additional 5000 contos ($250,000.00 U.S.) for the year; simplified methods of applying Paris green, both wet and dry, were adopted; antilarval work was reinforced by pyrethrum spray desinsectization; the hand capture of adult gambiae as an independent check on the distribution of the species was replaced by the flit-umbrella method; the intensive training of carefully selected men eventually gave visible results; and before the end of the year gambiae had apparently been eradicated from certain districts and its dissemination successfully blocked at most points.

The first year's work ended on an optimistic note, quite different from that emitted at the end of the first half year; it was felt that the demonstration of local eradication with available materials and technique had been made and that the problems still to be solved were largely of an administrative character. Arrangements were made for adequate funds (12,500 contos or $625,000.00 U.S.) for the first 6 months of 1940, and a staff sufficient to cover the infested area was developed, eventually reaching a total of 4000 men.

Even under these favorable circumstances the most optimistic observers failed to foresee the rapidity of gambiae's retraction during the second year's campaign. To the surprise of everyone, the area in which gambiae infestation could be found continued to diminish right through the rainy season, an unusually heavy one, at a time when exceptionally high densities were registered in two uncontrolled areas reserved for unhampered study of the biology of the species. Early in April (1940) it was decided to make the crucial test of the significance of negative findings, and all control measures were suspended in a previously heavily infested section of the Salgado River Valley, where the species had not been found during the first 3 months of the year. With the failure of gambiae to reappear in this area, it became routine practice to discontinue all control measures in a district after 3 months of failure to find the species. Continued careful systematic observation of the Salgado Valley over a period of 18 months (April 1940 to October 1941) has failed to reveal any recurrence of gambiae, and in no case has this species reappeared in a district in which control measures were suspended on the basis of 3 months of negative findings.

Before the end of June it was apparent that gambiae would probably be eradicated within a few months and on September 7, Brazil's Independence Day, a staff luncheon of the Malaria Service of the Northeast, in Fortaleza, celebrated the new freedom of Brazil from the African invader. Some weeks after this celebration, an isolated pocket of gambiae infestation was found some 60 kilometers beyond the last previously known frontier. This pocket was intensively worked, with the result that the last evidence of infestation in Brazil to date was recorded on November 14, 1940, less than 2 years after the organization of the Malaria Service of the Northeast.

Since January 1941 all antigambiae measures in Brazil have been suspended, a cash reward has been offered for the finding of gambiae, and a large staff of trained men have been kept searching for the species in the previously infested areas and throughout contiguous regions, with negative results. Provision is being made for continuing these activities of the Malaria Service of the Northeast as a cooperative project financed by the Brazilian Government and The Rockefeller Foundation, at least until the end of the 1942 rainy season. After this it is hoped that the responsibility for future checking and vigilance will be turned back to the regular health authorities, thus obviating the necessity for the continuation of a special service.

DISCUSSION

Many workers in the control of mosquito-borne disease have been more than reluctant to accept the idea that man has it in his power to eradicate any mosquito anywhere, no matter what the effort made. Psychologically it is apparently much easier to visualize the geometric increase of a species from a single gravid female to the millions of gambiae existing at one time in northeast Brazil than it is to picture the reverse process, as all possible breeding places in a region are treated week after week with Paris green and the highly domestic and extremely susceptible adult is subjected at frequent intervals to pyrethrum insecticide spray in the buildings of infested districts. The traditional ingrained philosophy that species eradication is impossible, that a species is something sacred and eternal in spite of the example of the dodo, the passenger pigeon, and the dinosaur to the contrary, and that when species disappear they do so only in response to "cosmic" or "biological" rather than man-made factors, is most persistent.

It is still too early to claim, on the basis of negative findings, that the last infestation of gambiae has disappeared from Brazil, but there can be no doubt that the failure of hundreds of well-trained searchers to find any trace of this mosquito, which is especially easy to find because of its larval and adult habits, many months after all control measures have been sus-pended,* is at least indicative of local eradication in many areas. Likewise, although large areas of Brazil are still infested with aegypti, it is a fact that this mosquito cannot now be found under favorable conditions in many cities and towns and even in entire states where it previously abounded.

Those who have followed the work in aegypti and gambiae in Brazil are convinced that local species eradication has been adequately demonstrated for both species; that the present program of the National Yellow Fever Service may well lead to the eradication of aegypti from Brazil and that a technique is available for the rapid elimination of any future gambiae in-festation which may perchance be found in northeast Brazil.

In the face of these results, it is interesting to consider the possibility of extending species eradication of aegypti and of gambiae to other regions and of applying the same concept to other species of mosquitoes. The wide variety of difficult aegypti situations already solved in Brazil gives confi-dence regarding possibilities elsewhere, and it is believed that no insuper-able difficulties will be encountered in applying eradication to this species wherever it exists. Antiaegypti measures in Bolivia have already resulted in cleaning many previously infested areas. Going further afield, a most attrac-tive problem would be the organization of an eradication program for aegypti in Egypt, the country from which it takes its name.

With regard to gambiae, it may be argued that the Brazilian experience proves nothing, since the species was outside of its normal habitat.† Those who saw gambiae in action in 1938–1939 have no doubts but that this species, unchecked, would have spread to many parts of the Americas and succeeded in maintaining itself as successfully as has that other invader from the Old World, *Aëdes aegypti*.

The senior author visited Africa in 1935 and saw many regions, from Zululand in Natal Province, South Africa, to the Anglo-Egyptian Sudan to the north, where gambiae-transmitted malaria is a serious problem. On the basis of Brazilian results he believes that some of these can be cleared of

---

* Since both Paris green and pyrethrum, the essential elements in the anti-gambiae campaign in Brazil are ephemeral in action, the suspension of control measures left conditions as favorable for gambiae proliferation as before the cam-paign. Draining and filling, considered so important in many malaria control projects, took no essential part in the eradication of gambiae.

† A prominent European malariologist writes: "I learn with pleasure that the last larvae and adults of gambiae were seen in October of 1940 in northeastern Brazil. I believe that you will agree with me in holding that, if this be true, we must suppose that biological factors have intervened to cause this disappearance; this would not be surprising considering the fact that the anopheline is of recent immigration."

gambiae at a reasonable cost with the same methods and then protected against reinfestation with relative ease.

With regard to eradication of other species, no conclusions should be drawn previous to a careful study of all factors involved, followed by even more careful work and observation in the field. The U.S. Department of Agriculture, in spite of its success in the eradication of the Mediterranean fruit fly, has not undertaken the complete elimination of the Japanese beetle, and the Brazilian National Yellow Fever Service, which has embarked on a program of aegypti eradication, has not considered undertaking similar projects against those species responsible for the transmission of jungle yellow fever.

Among the factors which make species eradication feasible are

1. Ease in discovering both aquatic and adult forms.

2. Efficiency of methods of destroying or sterilizing, permanently or temporarily, all breeding places.

3. Opportunity to eradicate the species in a sufficiently large or isolated geographical area so that the periphery, subject to reinfestation from dirty unworked areas, represents but a small fraction of the area worked.

4. Demonstrated public health and economic importance of species to be eradicated. Men, money, time, and full authority are needed for carrying out species eradication and these are generally available in adequate quantity only for truly serious problems.

Using these criteria there are undoubtedly a great many problems which can be solved by species eradication at much lower cost, in the long run, than by any other method.

One reads, for example, of the loss of 100,000 lives and the expenditure of £350,000 in a single great epidemic of malaria in the island of Ceylon and wonders what the immediate cost and ultimate advantages might be of eradicating *Anopheles culicifacies* from the island and thereafter maintaining a sentinel service to prevent reinfestation from the mainland.

One sees the short narrow irrigated valleys of the Pacific slope of Peru, isolated from the rest of the world by the high Andes to the east and the Pacific Ocean to the west, and from each other by long stretches of absolute desert, under the heavy economic handicap of annual outbreaks of malaria coinciding with the busy harvest season, and realizes that here is an ideal physical setting in which to attempt the piecemeal eradication of *Anopheles pseudopunctipennis,* the only vector of the region, from one valley after another.

The advantages of attacking problems having definite limits are so great that attempts at species eradication in the immediate future may well be limited to such geographical areas as present important obstacles to reinfestation, both during the campaign and after eradication has been accomplished. In addition to the problems already cited, the many malarious islands of the world, including those in the Caribbean region, would seem to offer a challenge to the responsible public health authorities. On the other hand, it must be remembered that the species-eradication technique was developed in Brazil in the absence of any natural obstacles to widespread dissemination of aegypti.

It is not the purpose of this paper to give the impression that species eradication is easy and simple. Final results can be disappointingly slow with a species such as aegypti, the ova of which may be viable for a year or more and are not infrequently transported from place to place by travelers; or gratifyingly rapid, with a species like gambiae which has no such means of defense and is so highly domestic that it can be easily attacked in the adult as well as in the larval form. But in each instance, success is attained only on the basis of careful organization and meticulous administration. It is not sufficient to plan the program and give orders for its execution; it is essential that there be careful independent checking of results.

Each species will present different problems which must be met by altered methods. For example, eradication of aegypti has proceeded from the larger cities to the tributary areas but in the attempt to eradicate gambiae special emphasis was placed on its elimination first from the peripheral zone of the infested area, since it was here that expansion was occurring.

It must be remembered that failure to find a species during a short period should not be interpreted as an indication that eradication has been accomplished; only after all control measures have been suspended and free opportunity given for multiplication of the species do negative findings become significant. A case in point is the experience at Durazzo, Albania: In the third year after the salinification of the only breeding place of *Anopheles maculipennis* var. *elutus* (=*A. sacharovi*), which could be found for miles around, not one of this species was found in eight scattered catching stations visited weekly during an entire summer, but in the following year, the silting up of the outlet canal produced an area of relatively fresh water, with the result that by the middle of the summer heavy production of elutus was again apparent. Here negative findings did not stand the test of even temporary interruption of control measures.

SUMMARY

Species eradication has been successfully demonstrated as a practical method of handling the problems of *Aëdes aegypti* and *Anopheles gambiae* in Brazil. The suggestion is made that eradication may be equally feasible for these two species in other countries and even for some other species under certain conditions.

Hans Zinsser, in 1935, when louse-borne typhus was of no concern to health workers in the United States and DDT was still unknown as an insecticide, wrote:

> Typhus is not dead. It will live for centuries and it will continue to break into the open, whenever human stupidity and brutality give it a chance as, most likely, they occasionally will. But its freedom of action is being restricted and, more and more, it will be confined, like other savage creatures, in the zoological garden of controlled diseases.

I have taken the long-memoried elephant as the symbol of the savage communicable disease, whose activities are being more and more restricted but which have never lost their instinct and capacity for human destruction.

Within 5 years of Zinsser's prophecy, World War II, with its excess of "human stupidity and brutality," unleashed typhus in Poland, Russia, Iran, Egypt, North Africa, Italy; in the concentration camps of Germany and Australia; and in Japan. Over 300,000 cases occurred between 1942 and 1946 in countries occupied by U.S. troops, and only the timely development of the chemical attack on the louse avoided a widespread major catastrophe, with millions of cases such as had occurred after World War I.

While louse-borne typhus may possibly continue for centuries, the chemical attack on the louse, spearheaded by DDT, is so popular with infested populations, that there would seem to be a possibility of eventual eradication, in spite of delayed relapses of the type of Brill's disease, unless the recent disturbing report from Korea, of body lice resistant to DDT, be confirmed. Should a resistant strain of lice be spread to other regions of the world by soldiers of the United Nations returning from Korea, it might well be one of the most disastrous results of the Korean War.

Although typhus did not become a problem in the United States during World War II, this country would not necessarily escape, should the United States itself come under attack in some future war. The destruction of housing, followed by inevitable overcrowding, with shortages of water, fuel, and especially of soap and insecticides, might well cause a return of epidemic typhus in the United States.

Zinsser, in 1935, did not urge that the zoological garden of controlled

* Presidential address, American Academy of Tropical Medicine, Chicago, Illinois, November 16, 1951. Dr. Soper was the Director of the Pan American Sanitary Bureau and Regional Director for the Americas of the World Health Organization.

This article was first published (73) in the *American Journal of Tropical Medicine and Hygiene 1: 361–368, 1952.*

diseases be cleared through eradication of its savage creatures, as he surely would do were he alive today, with full knowledge of residual insecticides, antibiotics, chemotherapeutic substances, and proved examples of eradication. How Zinsser, who was at heart a public health worker, would have been thrilled by last year's Symposium in Savannah on "Nation-Wide Malaria Eradication Projects in the Americas"; and by the recent liquidation of malaria as a public health problem in the United States, which is dramatically signalized here in Chicago this week by the amalgamation of the National Malaria Society and the American Society of Tropical Medicine to form the new American Society of Tropical Medicine and Hygiene.

As responsible public health workers, we must not be misled by the inactive status of certain diseases, no matter how long such apparent inactivity may persist, so long as the conditions suitable for their recurrence are permitted to continue.

Before visiting the Bwamba forest of Uganda some years ago, I was told the story of an English hunter in Africa who, having paid his £50 fee, was out for elephant. The first tusker sighted was a beautiful specimen but was inactive—was, in fact, sitting down. Not only was this elephant sitting, but he failed to rise and become a proper target even after a gentle cough or two from the hunter. Of course, a sitting elephant could not be shot any more than a sitting bird, so the hunt for an active target went on. But the second tusker was also sitting down and likewise showed no inclination to rise. When, at last in desperation, the hunter poked him with the muzzle of his rifle, the elephane is reported to have said: "Oh, go away and leave us alone. Can't you see we're playing bookends?"

With this pacific tale fresh in mind, I was rudely brought back to reality late one night in the forests of Uganda by the sudden braking of the station wagon in which I was riding together with a number of mosquito catchers when, unexpectedly, the rear of an elephant as large, in the headlights, as a barn, loomed suddenly out of the darkness as the highway made a sudden bend. The car was stopped, the lights doused, and the party remained in complete silence for 4 or 5 minutes until the great beast had had time to amble off into the forest. Only then did the driver, who had never heard of elephants playing bookends, have the courage to proceed.

Each of the communicable diseases, which have come to mean so little to many of the health workers in the United States and certain other favored countries, is still a dangerous enemy of many millions in other lands.

Yellow fever, like typhus, is not dead in spite of all the conquests and conquerors of this disease, nor is it likely to die out as long as the tropical and subtropical forests maintain their mammalian hosts and insect vectors. Jungle yellow fever remains as a potential source of virus for undoing the conquest of urban yellow fever, wherever *Aëdes aegypti* is permitted to continue. as witness the 1928–1929 outbreak in Rio de Janeiro. the scene of

Oswaldo Cruz's signal triumph two decades earlier. All too many health authorities have thought of yellow fever as "playing bookends" as long as it occurs only as jungle yellow fever. It is in every way as serious to the laborer, infected in the forest, as aegypti-transmitted yellow fever is to the person infected in the city, and urban outbreaks, arising from the chance introduction of the jungle virus, are classical in symptoms and in severity.

Since November 1948, a small series of cases of jungle yellow fever have been diagnosed in the Republic of Panama. The first cases found occurred east of the Canal Zone, with each succeeding case further west, the last occurring close to Almirante, near the frontier with Costa Rica, in June 1951.

A study of the distribution of immunity to yellow fever in monkeys, begun shortly after the first cases were reported and working ahead of the apparent movement of the disease from east to west, indicated that animals in the forests of all parts of Panama had been previously infected. At Almirante, immune monkeys were shot over a year before a human case was found there.

With the monkey immunity survey results positive for almost all of Panama, plans were made for a similar survey of Mexico and Central America beginning in Mexico and continuing south and east, country by country, until immune animals were found. It would then be obvious that the forests intervening between this point and Panama were also subject to yellow fever. The first study made at Palenque and Cintalapa, in Chiapas, in March and April of this year, showed up immune animals at both points.* Before these results were available, cases of yellow fever began to be observed in Costa Rica in June, not far from the Panamanian frontier and on the Caribbean side of the Continental Divide.

The activity of yellow fever has been much more apparent in Costa Rica than in Panama and over 150 cases are known to have occurred during the past 5 months, with each new group of cases found progressively farther west and north, until quite recently, when cases have appeared south of the Divide on the Pacific slope. The Costa Rican outbreak has been accompanied by reports of an epizootic among monkeys and the finding of the lesions of yellow fever in the livers of animals found naturally infected in the forests.

The observations in Costa Rica give strong support to the suggestion, based on the scattered Panamanian cases, that yellow fever is working from east to west and northwest, in an epizootic wave, remaining in a given area

---

* *Editorial note:* At Palenque, in 1953, J. Boshell-Manrique and H. Groot [Encuesta inmunológica sobre fiebre amarilla en primates silvestres de América Central (1952–1957), *Boletín de la Oficina Sanitaria Panamericana 43:* 309–322, 1957] obtained serological evidence from howler monkeys that casts much doubt on the validity of the serological data.

only a matter of weeks or, at most, months, and burning itself out, apparently through exhaustion of the supply of susceptible animals.

Such an epizootic wave was observed from 1934 to 1940 in the Brazilian states of Mato Grosso, Goiáz, São Paulo, Minas Gerais, Paraná, Santa Catarina, Rio Grande do Sul, Rio de Janeiro, and Espírito Santo; in Paraguay; and in the Province of Misiones, Argentina.

On the other hand, certain areas may, apparently because of large numbers of short-lived highly reproductive susceptible mammals, maintain jungle yellow fever as a permanent enzootic, as in Ilhéos, Brazil, and in Muzo and San Vicente de Chucurí, Colombia. In Ilhéos, there is reason to believe that, in the small rain-forest cacao-producing zone comprising only two or three counties, the virus of yellow fever has been constantly present during the last 20 years. In the same way the county of Muzo, Colombia, which has had yellow fever reported intermittently since 1907, reacted to viscerotomy in the three years before systematic vaccination was introduced with human cases every year and, in one or another of the 3 years, in every month of the calendar. San Vicente de Chucurí, which first came under scrutiny with yellow fever deaths in 1933, has had fatal cases in 10 of the past 18 years and, in 1951, had deaths in January, May, July, August, and October.

It remains to be seen whether the present Panama-Costa Rica epizootic will be traced by the observation of human cases through Nicaragua, Honduras, and Guatemala into Mexico, or whether its movement may be blocked by some intervening zone of animal immunity, owing to a previous local enzootic.

The observance of jungle yellow fever in Panama and Costa Rica, and the finding of immune monkeys in Mexico, have not altered the basic picture of yellow fever in the Americas; rather do they complete the jigsaw mosaic pattern of jungle yellow fever in the Americas almost 20 years after the first isolation of the yellow fever virus, in the absence of *Aëdes aegypti,* in the Valle do Chanaán, Brazil, in 1932.

Looking at the 20 year map of the distribution of known yellow fever in the Americas, and noting how recently Central America and Mexico have fitted into the picture; how, in 1949, an outbreak of over 800 cases appeared in southern Bolivia in a valley where yellow fever had not occurred during the past 18 years, and how, in 1951, the first outbreak of jungle yellow fever ever to be registered west of the Andes occurred in Ecuador, in the coastal region where no yellow fever at all had been found since 1919, it would appear that the yellow fever elephant never permanently forgets.

Today we know that jungle yellow fever, an important public health problem in its own right and a permanent potential source of virus for the reinfection of towns harboring aegypti, occurs from time to time in all of the suitably inhabited tropical and subtropical forested areas of Mexico, Central America, Panama, and South America. In South America, only Chile and Uruguay are free of this disease. Jungle yellow fever has been known in Colombia and Venezuela for many years, within easy striking range of the United States and of the West Indies by air transportation; and the jungle infection in Panama, Central America, and Mexico does not significantly increase the threat, as long as the cities and towns of the infected countries remain free of infection. Fortunately, Panama City was practically free of aegypti when the infective cases came to the Santo Tomás Hospital in 1948, and the 1951 outbreaks in Ecuador and Costa Rica found the campaigns for the eradication of aegypti already under way, not only in these countries, but also in the other countries of Central America and in Mexico.

Following the discovery of yellow fever at Almirante, close to the Costa Rican frontier, the health authorities of Costa Rica began an intensive vaccination campaign among the rural residents in areas lying in the anticipated route of invasion. In the more isolated districts, where refrigeration for the preservation of vaccine often was not available, the Dakar neurotropic vaccine was used in the belief that it is more stable than the 17D vaccine.

A number of typical cases of yellow fever have been observed in vaccinated persons beginning as long as 4 and 5 weeks after vaccination. This is in contrast to the field experience with the 17D vaccine, which, used in epidemic areas, has apparently prevented infections after only a few days, leading to the conclusion that the vaccinated individual is fully protected by the end of a week. Likewise, recent studies with 17D virus show that this vaccine prevents the circulation of the Dakar virus if a period of only 4 days intervenes between the applications of the two viruses. It seems logical to conclude that the failure with the Dakar vaccine indicates that it had not survived exposure to field conditions, or had been applied ineptly.

A series of cases of encephalitis occurring in persons vaccinated with the Dakar vaccine in Costa Rica and, more recently, in Honduras, is now being studied to determine the nature of this encephalitis. Until further data become available, vaccination in Central America is being limited to the use of the 17D chick embryo vaccine by injection.

There is real need for greater comprehension of the tragedy of jungle yellow fever and of the necessity for the routine vaccination of the relatively inaccessible populations who live and work in contact with the tropical forests of the Americas.

A tragic occurrence early this year was an outbreak of jungle yellow fever with over 2000 cases and several hundreds of deaths, among the newly arrived settlers in the State of Goiaz, Brazil. This area had suffered an outbreak in 1945, at which time extensive vaccination was carried out in the then relatively small population. During the past 6 years, however, an important agricultural development has brought in large numbers of non-immunes from Northeast Brazil. Traveling overland, these newcomers passed through no place where routine vaccination would reach them. Ironically enough, these newcomers came from the previously highly endemic region of aegypti-transmitted yellow fever of Northeast Brazil, where there is no jungle yellow fever. It was here that The Rockefeller Foundation initiated its campaign in Brazil against aegypti-transmitted yellow fever in 1923, with the resultant development of this nonimmune susceptible population.

Much greater attention would be given to the vaccination of all exposed populations and more ready collaboration in the campaign for the eradication of aegypti would occur, if jungle yellow fever more regularly caused outbreaks of urban yellow fever. Health authorities have short memories and tend to forget the outbreaks in Rio de Janeiro, 1928–1929; in Guasipati and Tumeremo, Venezuela, 1929; in Socorro and Simacota, Colombia, 1929; in Santa Cruz de la Sierra, Bolivia, 1932; in Cambará, Paraná, Brazil, 1936; in Buena Vista, Colombia, 1937; and in Sena Madureira, Brazil, 1942, all of which are attributed to urbanization of the jungle virus.

As the years pass and jungle yellow fever continues to be jungle yellow fever, without invasion of the cities, the potential threat seems unimportant to many who do not realize the tremendous effort which has gone, and is going, into the eradication of aegypti in all the towns and cities in close contact with the infected forests. Years ago, the yellow fever workers in Brazil discovered that the only permanent friend of the Yellow Fever Service was yellow fever itself. The very success of the program for the eradication of aegypti in some areas in preventing urban yellow fever militates against the completion of the task in other regions.

My attention has recently been called to an address, by the Dean of the School of Public Health of Harvard University in which the following paragraph from the inaugural address of the President of the American Medical Association, June 1950, is quoted: "Dread diseases like typhoid, diphtheria and smallpox which, 50 years ago, took a heavy toll in sickness and death, virtually have been eliminated as national health problems and all the infectious diseases have been brought under effective methods of prevention, control and treatment." Dean Simmons challenges this as "a statement so obviously incorrect, that it deserves comment only because it comes from an official authorized to speak for the leading medical organization of the country." He then calls attention to (1) the occurrence of a group of diseases which have not been brought under effective methods of prevention, including poliomyelitis, measles, the common cold, and infections of the respiratory tract, and (2) the continued occurrence of another group of diseases for which adequate methods of prevention are now avail-

able, including intestinal infections, insect-borne infections, and the venereal diseases.

In other words, returning once more to Zinsser's figure, the distinction is
made between two groups of savage creatures, the first, as yet untamable;
the other already "confinable in the zoological garden of controlled diseases."

The statement is then made, referring of course only to the second group,
that "the American people are not yet deriving the full benefit of our pres-
ent-day knowledge about the prevention of disease and that we have a long
way to go before we dare announce that the infectious diseases are really
under control." But when we analyze the figures given by Dean Simmons
for these controllable diseases in relation to the population at risk, or in
relation to the number of practicing physicians, it is found that the control
is excellent and that what is being demanded is really the eradication of
these diseases.

The criticism of the statement of the President of the American Medical
Association becomes then a criticism of the members of the sister organization, the American Public Heath Association, who have not completed
the task of preventing the preventable diseases and possibly a criticism of
the Harvard School of Public Health which, together with similar faculties,
has not yet created a generation of health workers trained to distinguish
between eradicable and noneradicable diseases, and to push on to eradication when possible.

That the American Public Health Association is not fully alive to the
possibilities of eradication as was the National Malaria Society is evident
from the records of the recent 79th meeting of the APHA in San Francisco,
when, with registration of over 4000 members and with a multiplicity of
sections, only 30 papers were presented on all phases of communicable diseases and no general analysis of future possibilities was made.

Of these papers, 17 related to diseases for which more or less adequate
methods of control are available: Brill's disease, 1; brucellosis, 1; diphtheria, 2; infantile diarrhea, 1; pertussis, 1; rabies, 2; salmonella, 1; shigella, 1;
smallpox, 1; syphilis, 1; tuberculosis, 4; yaws, 1.

Lest the picture I paint may seem too somber, it should be pointed out
that bovine tuberculosis in humans, which was so common in the hospitals
of Chicago when I was an interne, has become a rarity here, and this city
has announced that, beginning January 1, 1954, all milk sold here must
come from brucellosis-free herds. At least there is the conviction here that
animal diseases can be eradicated. It should also be mentioned that some
workers in tuberculosis and venereal disease are seriously beginning to consider the possibility of what might be termed "area eradication" of these
diseases. But "area eradication" calls for permanent protection from reinfection or reinfestation from other areas or other countries. The alternative

is to undertake eradication as an ever-expanding program, as has occurred in the case of the program for the eradication of the aegypti mosquito during the past 18 years, on a regional and, possibly, eventually on a world basis.

Such expanding eradication requires a mechanism through which the affected countries can unite on common programs, approved and supported by all, with identical technical orientation and with no loss of sovereignty to any nation. Fortunately, there already exists such a mechanism, based on treaties ratified by practically all the countries of the Americas and of the world, ready to function in the coordination of such programs; I refer, of course, to the mechanism of the official international health agencies, the Pan American and the World Health Organizations.

| Eradication Versus Control in Communicable Disease Prevention*

The eradication concept of disease prevention requires, for its best application, continuing expansion at the periphery and across international frontiers. The Pan American Sanitary Bureau has long recognized the interdependence of human and veterinary preventive medicine; the Bureau organized the first official international veterinary public health activities in 1949, planned and created the Pan American Aftosa Center in Rio de Janeiro, Brazil, in 1951, and the Pan American Zoonoses Center in Azul, Argentina, in 1956.

In considering eradication versus control of communicable diseases, the principles involved are the same in dealing with human, animal, and plant diseases, and with the zoonoses which attack both animals and man (see Fig. 1).

By reversing the dictionary procedure and giving examples of usage before defining terms, the differentiation of eradication and control may be simplified. The first example is from the *Annual Report of The Rockefeller Foundation for 1915*: "The policy . . . of the International Health Commission (of The Rockefeller Foundation) has been that of demonstrating, in a limited area of each country, the feasibility of bringing disease . . . under control . . . By showing that it is possible to clean up a limited area, an object lesson is given, the benefit of which is capable of indefinite extension." The concept of cleaning up a limited area and extending it indefinitely is the concept of eradication.

Quoting again from the Foundation's 1915 Report: "Preliminary arrangements have been made for a survey to determine the feasibility of undertaking at this time the eradication of yellow fever, and for experiments to test the practicability of controlling malaria." Here is a clear-cut differential usage of the terms, the eradication of yellow fever, meaning the worldwide eradication of the virus of yellow fever, the local eradication of which had been demonstrated in Havana, Panama, Rio de Janeiro, New

* Presented before the Section on Public Health and Regulatory Veterinary Medicine at the Third Pan American Congress of Veterinary Medicine and 96th annual meeting of the American Veterinary Medical Association, Kansas City, Missouri, August 23–27, 1959. Dr. Soper was Director Emeritus of the Pan American Sanitary Bureau.

This article was originally published (*98*) in the *Journal of the American Veterinary Medical Association 137*: 234–238, 1960. (A small amount of text has been omitted.)

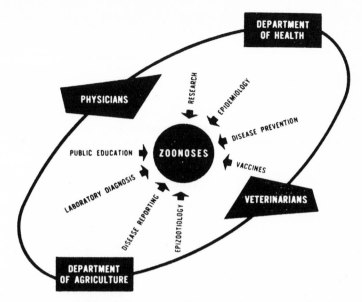

Figure 1. Physicians, Department of Health Workers, veterinarians, and Department of Agriculture employees work together against the zoonoses.

Orleans, and elsewhere; and the control of malaria, which was destined to be a frustrating problem in most rural areas of the world until the introduction of DDT, three decades later.

Another example of usage of the terms "eradication" and "control" is from a recent article by T. E. Jones: "Using methods that make medical health officers envious, veterinarians in several countries have completely stamped out such diseases as rinderpest, contagious bovine pleuropneumonia, glanders, dourine, hog cholera, foot-and-mouth disease, and others, and have brought under control such diseases as brucellosis and bovine tuberculosis, all by the short-cut of slaughtering affected animals." Here is a clear-cut distinction, in referring to past accomplishments, between eradicating and controlling disease, even though there are well-advanced eradication programs for both brucellosis and bovine tuberculosis. These eradication programs are not control programs, and they have done much more than bring brucellosis and bovine tuberculosis under control; they have resulted in establishing areas of local eradication as essential stepping stones to national eradication.

Just as the police officer considers crime to be under control when it is at such low level that it is of importance only to the victims, so the public health officer considers a given disease to be under control once its incidence has been so reduced that it is no longer a serious public health problem except to the few voiceless victims who still suffer. May I assume that in veterinary practice, control means the reduction of a disease until it is no longer a source of serious financial loss to the community as a whole, although it may be to those whose animals are affected?

Eradication, on the other hand, refers to the complete disappearance of all sources of infection of a given disease agent, so that no recurrence of that disease is possible, even in the absence of all preventive measures. Local eradication indicates the elimination of all sources of infection from a given area, so the disease does not recur unless reintroduced from outside the area.

ERADICATION PROGRAMS

Eradication programs must cover fairly large areas from the beginning to minimize the possibility of reintroductions of the infection into clean areas, and they must be able to expand at the periphery. Local eradication, to be successful, must provide for protection against reinfection. Such protection can be best obtained by increasing the eradication area. Eventually the limits of the eradication area will coincide with the national boundaries. At this point, the nation acquires a vested interest in eradication in neighboring countries. Eradication programs evolve naturally as local, state, national, international, regional, and world programs.

Fortunately for the ultimate development of health programs throughout the world, there is no convenient stopping point; eradication is not something one area can do for itself and maintain indefinitely with ease. It is obvious that clean areas can best be protected by sharing the burden of cleaning up less fortunate areas through pooling financial and technical resources. Only in recent years, with the development of the Pan American Health Organization, the World Health Organization, the Food and Agriculture Organization of the United Nations, the International Cooperation Administration of the U.S., and UNICEF, has there existed an adequate mechanism for coordinating and assisting regional and world eradication programs.

The first international and world eradication attempt antedates the effective development of these organizations by 30 years. The survey to determine the feasibility of undertaking eradication of yellow fever, mentioned in the quotation from The Rockefeller Foundation 1915 Annual Report, led to an attempt to eradicate yellow fever from the world. The Rockefeller Foundation, a private philanthropic organization, coordinated the antimosquito programs of affected countries, and gave the technical and financial assistance needed.

Wickliffe Rose, who, after consultation with William C. Gorgas, committed The Rockefeller Foundation to yellow fever eradication, was without training in medicine and public health administration. Rose had been a professor of philosophy and a college dean before entering the field of public health as executive secretary of the Rockefeller Sanitary Commission for the Eradication of Hookworm Disease in 1910 and continuing as director of the International Health Commission when the Foundation was chartered in 1913. Raymond Fosdick has said of Rose: "Always his thinking and his strategy were in planetary terms. Whether it was mathematics or chemistry or astronomy, he worked on a global scale. His effort was constantly to break over the boundaries of parochialism and lay his plans in accordance with world patterns."

The yellow fever eradication program is the most magnificent failure in public health history. When the Foundation withdrew from the program in 1949, after 34 years of effort, during which the lives of six staff members were sacrificed to accidental infections and some $14 million were spent on the control and study of the disease, yellow fever virus persisted widespread in the forest animals of Africa and South America. But the attempt to eradicate yellow fever led inevitably, as many decades of control might not have done, to studies which clarified the epidemiology and epizootiology of yellow fever and to the perfection of a live attenuated virus vaccine. (The techniques for handling viruses, developed during the studies of yellow fever virus, have been of inestimable value in the study of other virus diseases.)

With the discovery of jungle fever in 1932, it became obvious that the eradication of yellow fever virus had, from the beginning of Rose's dream in 1915, been impossible. But by 1934, the last endemic focus of human yellow fever in the Americas had been cleared of infection. Since 1935, yellow fever in the Western Hemisphere has behaved essentially as a zoonosis; few urban cases of yellow fever have occurred in the past 25 years, and those have come from transient invasions of cities and towns by the jungle virus brought in by persons infected in the forests. In the future, even this threat to urban communities should disappear; already it has largely disappeared with the progress of the campaign for the eradication of the *Aëdes aegypti* mosquito, the only urban vector of yellow fever in the Western Hemisphere.

A full quarter of a century before Rose, the philosopher, undertook the eradication of yellow fever, a young man destined to become one of America's great public health leaders, Charles V. Chapin, presented a philosophy of disease eradication as a natural corollary of the acceptance of the germ theory of communicable disease. In 1888, a few years after Koch's discovery of the tubercle bacillus, Chapin said:

In regard to the prevention of consumption, it must be admitted that the germ theory has done little except to emphasize the importance of hygienic measures. But it should have great influence . . . The germ theory—now no longer a theory in the case of tuberculous consumption—tells us what we have to do with a contagious disease. Now there is no theoretical reason why a purely contagious disease like tuberculosis cannot be exterminated. If we can prevent the spread of contagion at all, we can prevent it entirely.

This last sentence is a fitting slogan for all who are responsible for the prevention of communicable diseases. Once this principle is accepted, the problem becomes one of devising economically feasible administrative methods adapted to each situation. This "economically feasible" restriction is most important; methods chosen must be not only feasible, but economically so.

Eradication programs are based on a variety of measures: For *Aëdes aegypti,* on an attack on the aquatic stages of development; for smallpox, on herd vaccination; for yaws, on mass treatment of cases and contacts; and for malaria, on the destruction of infected mosquitoes.

Not every disease, or every disease vector, is presently eradicable; the campaign for the eradication of the urban vector of yellow fever is well advanced, but no one has yet proposed any eradication of the forest mosquito vectors of jungle yellow fever.

Chapin recognized the need of concomitant solution of the problem of bovine tuberculosis. To quote:

> But with the increasing prevalence of tuberculosis among domestic-animals something more is imperatively demanded. Active measures should be taken to free the country from animal tuberculosis. The proper authority for dealing with this, as with all other contagious diseases of animals, is the Bureau of Animal Industry of the Department of Agriculture. It is a wasteful method for states to act independently. The powers and expenditure of this Bureau should be greatly increased and it should take active measures against this disease.

The exact measures suggested are

1. The reporting of all cases of tuberculosis in domestic animals to the proper authority by both owners and veterinarians or other persons having a knowledge of the same.

2. The slaughter of all infected animals and the isolation and slaughter of all exposed to infection. The government should partially indemnify all owners of slaughtered cattle.

3. Thorough disinfection of all buildings occupied by diseased cattle.

4. The confiscation of the flesh and milk and milk products of all tuberculous animals.

Chapin had the vision and the voice of a prophet; he recognized instinctively that the rejection of spontaneous generation and the acceptance of the germ theory of disease implied the concept of contagious disease eradication. Were Chapin alive today he would be emphasizing that it is a wasteful method for nations to act independently, and he would be championing the cause of world eradication programs.

Only recently did I learn from Dr. H. C. King that the Bureau of Animal Industry, which Chapin called upon to eradicate bovine tuberculosis, had been created only 4 years previously, in 1884, specifically for the "suppression and extirpation of contagious disease among domestic animals." To quote Dr. King:

In 1843 . . . contagious pleuropneumonia gained entrance to the United States . . . For the next 40 years, this disease spread up and down the Atlantic Coast. Other diseases began to spread and become increasingly alarming. Boycotts by Great Britain against American livestock aggravated growing livestock disease problems, and added economic pressure to the desire by the people that Congress do something about the situation. As a result there was passed by Congress on May 29, 1884, "An Act for the establishment of a Bureau of Animal Industry to prevent the exportation of diseased cattle and to provide means for the suppression and extirpation of pleuropneumonia and other contagious diseases among domestic animals."

Five years later, contagious pleuropneumonia had been eradicated (from the U.S.) with the expenditure of $1.5 million.

The eradication of contagious pleuropneumonia was a dramatic illustration of what could be accomplished through unified activities in animal disease eradication. The principles involved have been applied successively to a number of zoonoses with gratifying results. Many benefits have accrued to the people of the United States through the suppression of diseases which are transmitted from animals to man. Animal husbandry, as we know it today, with its concentration of animal populations and efficient, rapid, long-distance transportation of livestock, would be practically impossible, had not these diseases been eradicated or effectively controlled. As new tools and methods for disease eradication became available more diseases were included in programs designed to wipe them out. Accomplishments in programs aimed toward the eradication of tuberculosis, brucellosis, cattle tick fever, vesicular exanthema, foot-and-mouth disease, scrapie, and screwworm, are worthy of review and comment.

It is not only the public health authorities who today are thinking in terms of world disease eradication. The *Food and Agriculture Organization/OIE Animal Yearbook for 1957* states:

It has often been said that diseases know no frontier; regional control of infectious diseases, therefore, is an objective which must receive full consideration and support . . . an example is rinderpest which, although its ravages have been widespread in the past, is now confined to a few areas, and even in them is gradually being eradicated . . . One of the main objectives of international organizations interested in livestock production is to encourage and participate in the regional control of epizootics leading to their final eradication, not only from the regions but from the world. This is a task fraught with many difficulties; progress, however, is gradually and surely being made.

In the control of diseases of animals, full consideration has to be given to that important group now termed zoonoses, in which both animals and human beings are involved . . . in such diseases the simplest and probably the most effective measures of control concern the eradication of the infection from the animal populations. There must, therefore, continue to exist close collaboration between veterinary and medical authorities, whose common objective should be to so interweave their activities that zoonotic diseases will eventually be well controlled and even eradicated. In this work veterinary authorities have an important part to play.

However, if they are to play this part, the leaders of the veterinary profession must recognize their responsibility in promoting and advancing the philosophy of communicable disease eradication; the schools of veterinary medicine must emphasize the teaching of the basic elements of epizootiology and of the prevention of communicable diseases; veterinary authorities must accept Chapin's dictum: "If we can prevent the spread of contagion at all, we can prevent it entirely." The veterinarian must join the physician in showing more concern over the gap between current incidence of a disease and the zero base line than in satisfaction in such reduction of disease incidence as may have occurred. In taking credit for such reduction, the public health officer and the animal health officer must accept blame for what remains. To the eradicationist, the demonstration of his ability to reduce the incidence of a disease constitutes proof of his culpability in not eradicating it. In determining eradication programs for certain diseases, especially the zoonoses, the veterinary health officer must be ready to substitute humanitarian consideration for financial consideration.

Finally, the veterinary health authorities of each country must get their respective governments to accept the responsibility, as members of the community of nations, to prevent their territories from becoming or remaining sources of infection for countries from which a disease has been eradicated, although the disease in question may be relatively unimportant in their countries.

Rehabilitation of the Eradication
Concept in Prevention of
Communicable Disease*

The eradication concept in the prevention of communicable diseases is quite modern; it had to await the discovery of effective methods of disease prevention, the rejection of the concept of spontaneous generation, and the identification of specific etiologic agents of individual diseases.

The introduction of vaccination as a preventive of smallpox led Thomas Jefferson to enunciate the eradication concept in the early years of the nineteenth century. Some decades later Pasteur said, "It is within the power of man to rid himself of every parasitic disease." ("Parasitic" for Pasteur was a general term including infectious diseases.)

In 1884 the U.S. Congress created the Bureau of Animal Industry to eradicate contagious bovine pleuropneumonia and to prevent the export of other animal diseases from this country.

In 1888 Charles V. Chapin declared that any disease which could be prevented in part could be prevented in its entirety and urged the eradication of tuberculosis.

In 1902, following the dramatic victory over yellow fever in Havana during the previous year, Gen. William Gorgas predicted its future eradication.

In the early years of this century, Ronald Ross worked out mathematical formulas for the disappearance of malaria, and Wickliffe Rose became the director of the Rockefeller Sanitary Commission for the Eradication of Hookworm Disease in the United States.

In 1915, the newly created Rockefeller Foundation established its Yellow Fever Commission, under the leadership of Gorgas, to undertake the eradication of yellow fever.

Of these early dreams of eradication, only that for the eradication of contagious bovine pleuropneumonia materialized; by 1930 the eradication

* This paper is based on the first Fred L. Soper Lecture given at the School of Hygiene and Public Health, Johns Hopkins University, October 27, 1959; it was first published *(112)* in *Public Health Reports 80:* 855–869, 1965, at which time Dr. Soper was a Special Consultant, Office of International Health, Public Health Service.

(There is much duplication in the content of this paper and Selection 38, which were presented within a year of each other, but to very different audiences. Both papers are included in extenso because this paper is primarily concerned with the principles of the eradication concept, while the other deals more with the practice of the concept as it affected the activities of the Pan American Sanitary Bureau.)

concept was thoroughly discredited in this country. Health workers accepted, and professors of public health administration taught, the philosophy of reduction of communicable disease to a reasonable level; a modicum of preventable disease became and, even today, remains respectable.

However justifiable the complacent acceptance of the persistence of preventable diseases may have appeared 30 years ago, it is no longer defensible. The success of local and national eradication efforts during the past three decades, the discovery of new methods of disease prevention, and the increasing participation of all nations in coordinated international health programs have led to rehabilitation of the eradication concept. Today the nations of the Americas are committed to the eradication of the *Aëdes aegypti* mosquito, malaria, smallpox, and yaws; the nations of the world have joined in the global eradication of malaria, and the demand for the eradication of other preventable diseases is inevitable.

ATTEMPT TO ERADICATE YELLOW FEVER

My introduction to eradication came, in November 1919, from Wickliffe Rose, director of the International Health Board of The Rockefeller Foundation. In outlining to me, a prospective staff member, the program of the board, Rose cited yellow fever as a scourge which could be and was, in fact, being eradicated by the nations of the Americas with the aid of the Foundation. Rose was confident that yellow fever would disappear within the next 5 years.

At Johns Hopkins in 1920, before my first visit to Brazil, I heard more of yellow fever eradication from General Gorgas, the hero of Havana and Panama. Gorgas cited the experience of two decades, during which campaigns against the aegypti mosquito in the large cities of endemic yellow fever regions had eradicated the disease in these regions and in the smaller communities in tributary areas.

Yellow fever was then being eradicated by the reduction of its mosquito vector in known endemic centers long enough to allow the virus to spontaneously disappear throughout the endemic zones. No consideration was given to attacking aegypti throughout its range or of eradicating it anywhere; eradication of yellow fever virus itself was the objective.

In Brazil I learned that the Government had organized its own eradication program (National Yellow Fever Commissions) in 1919, along the lines proposed by Gorgas in 1916. Yellow fever had receded as anticipated, and eradication seemed imminent. Soon after the disease had disappeared from the statistics of Brazil (1921–1922), the National Yellow Fever Commissions were transformed into the joint Federal-State Services for the Prevention of Rural Endemic Diseases (Profilaxia Rural). Shortly after this transformation, however, yellow fever reappeared, and the Brazilian Government in

1923 invited The Rockefeller Foundation to collaborate in its eradication campaign.

The reorganization of the eradication campaign by The Rockefeller Foundation was essentially a repetition of the preceding Brazilian effort; the failure of the national campaign was attributed to an inadequate coverage of the endemic centers for too short a period, rather than to any weakness in the plan itself.

Again, yellow fever receded rapidly with the attack on the aegypti in the capital cities of north Brazil; optimism about the imminence of eradication grew rapidly through 1925. However, a so-considered temporary setback occurred in 1926 when nonimmune troops moving through north Brazil became infected and seeded a number of widely scattered towns with yellow fever.

Antimosquito work was instituted in the infected towns in the interior. Yellow fever once more receded below the threshold of visibility, and during an 11-month period in 1927–1928, no case of yellow fever was recorded for the entire American continent. Optimism was such that in January 1928 the health workers of Brazil were assured that should another 3 months pass without cases of yellow fever, they could consider the disease eradicated. In March 1928, one case occurred in Sergipe and 2 months later Rio de Janeiro, Brazil's beautiful capital with almost 2 million people, became infected with yellow fever for the first time in 20 years.

This unexpected invasion of Rio, heavily infested with aegypti, provided yellow fever virus its most active center of distribution since 1910. During the next 3 years, the disease occurred in numerous towns in the interior of Brazil, on shipboard, in port cities from Buenos Aires on the south to Belém at the mouth of the Amazon, and even as far as Manáos, some 800 miles up the river.

During this period, yellow fever workers were shocked by the occurrence of the disease at Recife, Pernambuco, in 1929, after 5 years of uninterrupted antiaegypti work. Investigation revealed a much greater density of aegypti there than reported by the inspectors. This led many to believe that Rio de Janeiro had been reinfected from Northeast Brazil; that failure to eradicate yellow fever had again been the result of inadequate antiaegypti measures in the known key-centers of infection.

The contrast between the absence of reported yellow fever in the period immediately preceding its appearance in Rio and the widespread epidemicity which followed was a dramatic demonstration of the influence of the large city in the distribution of infection. This was indeed a confirmation of the key-center epidemiology on which eradication was based. On the other hand, at about the same time, outbreaks of yellow fever were occurring elsewhere, and these could not be explained by the key-center theory. In 1929, isolated outbreaks were reported in Socorro, Colombia, and Guasipati, Venezuela, both small centers far from all Brazilian foci of infection, inaccessible to each other, and isolated from all large cities.

ERADICATION CONCEPT DISCREDITED

The period between the late 1920s and the early 1930s was probably this century's low point in acceptance of the eradication concept in the prevention of communicable diseases. The 1928–1929 outbreak of yellow fever in Rio seemed to invalidate previous optimism about its eradication. Hookworm disease campaigns everywhere had failed to entirely eliminate hookworm infestation. The eradication concept was thoroughly discredited, and The Rockefeller Foundation suffered severe criticism because of its support of eradication programs.

ERADICATION OF *Aëdes aegypti*

In 1930 I became directly responsible for the administration of The Rockefeller Foundation's effort to eradicate yellow fever in South America. Before assuming direction of the Cooperative Yellow Fever Service (maintained by the Brazilian Government and The Rockefeller Foundation in north Brazil), I discussed the disease and its eradication with Dr. Wade Hampton Frost, professor of epidemiology, at Johns Hopkins. He asked me if I believed that yellow fever could be eradicated from Brazil. My answer was equivocal, "If the eradication of yellow fever was ever possible, it is definitely so at present because of the great interest aroused by the Rio outbreak and the infection of many smaller cities and towns."

Frost then inquired if I planned a blanket attack on aegypti throughout north Brazil, not to eradicate it but to get rid of unrecognized foci of infection. My protest that this would be very costly brought a reply worthy of the dean of American epidemiologists: "No matter how great the cost, the eradication of yellow fever is so important that none will question the expenditure once the job has been done." And he made it clear that getting the money was part and parcel of the job itself. (The point is too often missed by public health administrators that theirs is a selling as well as an administrative job.)

Following the meeting with Professor Frost, I returned to Brazil determined to find out if yellow fever could be eradicated. An analysis of the 1930 yellow fever situation indicated that (a) the epidemiology of yellow fever was not fully known, the disease could continue unobserved for months or years, (b) the aegypti mosquito could maintain itself indefinitely in hidden breeding places despite trustworthy inspectors who worked under close supervision, and (c) it is difficult to maintain an efficient antiaegypti service in the absence of yellow fever. Specifically, then, these problems had to be solved:

1. Silent endemic yellow fever: how to discover when and where cases occurred?

2. Hidden aegypti breeding: how to find residual breeding responsible for the continued existence of the species?

3. Supervision and checking of antiaegypti operation: how to maintain safe aegypti levels and guarantee accuracy of reported breeding indices?

Seeking the answers to these questions and applying them was to occupy the best efforts of Rockefeller Foundation and Brazilian workers, aided by workers of other South American countries, during the next decade.

Determining when and where yellow fever occurred proved most difficult. Although the clinical symptoms of classic fatal yellow fever are dramatic, experience had repeatedly shown that the disease could and did continue over long periods of time without reported cases. The then newly developed protection, or neutralization, test in monkeys was too expensive for routine surveys. The results of such surveys, when positive, indicated only that the disease had been present within the lifetime of persons with immune bodies, but did not establish the date of infection. This problem was solved through the routine collection of pathological material throughout possible yellow fever areas.

Yellow fever, when fatal, generally kills within 10 days after onset and produces a characteristic lesion in the liver. The practical difficulty of collecting postmortem material was greatly reduced by the development of a simple instrument, termed the "viscerotome," for the rapid removal of liver tissue without autopsy. Viscerotomy was not designed to substitute for autopsy when yellow fever was suspected; rather was it applied systematically to all persons who died after less than 11 days of febrile illness.

A field organization of local representatives was created to collect and forward liver tissue to the central laboratory for diagnosis. Although initial opposition to the desecration of bodies soon after death was encountered, all difficulties were eventually overcome. Viscerotomy has proved the most fertile source of information of the current distribution of yellow fever infection throughout South and Central America.

The discovery of hidden aegypti breeding places came to be based on the search for adult aegypti mosquitoes; once a house with hidden breeding had been identified, special squads were assigned the task of uncovering the concealed breeding. This relatively simple procedure, although costly in time and effort, proved unexpectedly productive.

Yellow fever workers had previously found the capture of aegypti of little value in control campaigns where the objective was to reduce breeding to less than 5 per cent of the houses. At levels of incidence below 2 per cent, however, the capture of adult mosquitoes proved the most sensitive index of the presence or absence of aegypti in an area.

The supervision and checking of antiaegypti work in Brazilian cities was greatly strengthened by careful mapping of all areas, definite delineation of individual responsibility for each area, detailed reporting of all work done, and continuous checking and cross-checking of work at all levels. (The declared objective was to make the reported aegypti breeding index as trustworthy and certifiable as were the bank account statements of the Yellow Fever Service.)

Viscerotomy indicated that Northeast Brazil maintained a silent but widespread endemic yellow fever, transmitted by the aegypti mosquito even in the rural areas. This endemic disease had been overlooked year after year by the Yellow Fever Service with its sentinel services in the coastal cities. The endemic was limited almost entirely to Brazilian children under 15 years of age. Since viscerotomy is applied only postmortem, the falsity of the belief long held in this area that yellow fever was a "febre patriótica" which slew only foreigners became obvious.

The unusual rural distribution of the aegypti mosquito, which permitted this endemic to be self-perpetuating as an infection transmitted from man to man, had not been foreseen in the development of the key-center plan of yellow fever eradication. But once this silent endemic was uncovered, it was a relatively simple and straightforward, if tedious and expensive, task to eradicate the disease by taking anti-aegypti measures in all the towns and villages and many rural areas.

By August 1934 this final endemic focus of yellow fever in the Americas was eliminated, and had the aegypti mosquito been the only culprit in the transmission of the disease, as Gorgas believed, that year would have marked the end of yellow fever in the Western Hemisphere.

An even more unexpected result came from viscerotomy: the demonstration that yellow fever is basically an animal disease in the forests of tropical and subtropical America. Following this revelation, previously described epidemics in various countries were identified as jungle yellow fever.

Between 1947 and 1959 jungle yellow fever was observed in all the countries of South America except Chile and Uruguay, and in all the countries of Central and North America except El Salvador, the United States, and Canada.

The observation of yellow fever in forested areas, involving mammals other than man and mosquitoes other than aegypti, led to recognition of jungle yellow fever as a permanent reservoir of virus for the reinfection of urban areas. Therefore, the dream of yellow fever eradication had been, from the beginning, impossible.

The introduction of the search for adult aegypti to reveal hidden breeding and the meticulous supervision of antiaegypti operations led unexpectedly to the disappearance of aegypti itself. In 1933 this mosquito had disappeared completely from many of the coastal cities of northeast Brazil. I wish I could say that we carefully planned to eradicate aegypti and then did so. In truth, this was a free ride, so to speak; some would call it serendipity. It was not planned, but came as a reward of careful administration and of lowering the visibility of aegypti breeding below the survival threshold.

Eradication of aegypti in certain Brazilian cities came only after more than three decades of antiaegypti campaigns, beginning with that of Gorgas in Havana in 1901. In 1928 Rockefeller Foundation workers had made a special effort in the town of Parahyba (now João Pessôa), with a population of some 35,000 people. Although a point was reached when inspectors no longer found pupal or producing foci, some aegypti larvae continued to be found week after week, far beyond the maximum lifespan of aegypti. The instinct of the mosquito had proved superior to the intelligence of the inspector in finding residual water containers suitable for breeding.

Failure to eradicate aegypti was explained on the basis of the sanctity of the species, the law of diminishing returns, and the irreducible minimum. But these explanations became untenable in the face of adult captures and meticulous administration. The decision to undertake such meticulous administration was based in part on the unhappy experience with false reports in Recife in 1929, mentioned previously, and in part on my experience in the field.

Before assuming the direction of the yellow fever program, I spent some weeks in the cities of north Brazil learning the details of antiaegypti work from the various inspectors. Beginning at Belém at the mouth of the Amazon River, I moved southward from city to city along the coast. In each city I worked with the man who actually inspected houses, not with the supervising inspector or with the service physician. I started with the inspector in the morning and performed the same tasks as he all day—examined the same water containers, climbed the same roofs, and kept the same records. The experience was exciting and highly educational.

The work was always excessive; each inspector knew he was working with the new chief of the Yellow Fever Service and, to make a good impression, he visited many more houses that day than usual. Since I worked with a different inspector each day, the routine was exhausting. Many days I would have been tempted to shirk and falsify the house visit records had I not been closely watched by the inspector.

Gorgas and Le Prince have said that to combat mosquitoes, one must think like a mosquito. After initiation in the hard school of the inspector, I felt it more important to think like the inspector—the man who, in the final analysis, alone determines whether the job is done or not. On his routine job, the inspector needs the stimulus of his supervisor's interest in the quality of his work. Nothing is so deadly to his interest and morale as visiting the same houses week after week without sympathetic, although rigid, supervision.

The "Manual of Operations" eventually prepared for the Yellow Fever Service provided detailed job descriptions, definitions of individual responsibility for carefully mapped zones, regular itineraries, immediate entries on special forms of all work done, routine checking of all reports, registers posted in all houses visited and countersigned on all visits, and bonuses to the inspector based on the efficiency of each month's work as determined by the supervisor. (The inspector came to have a special interest in having his work checked by the supervisor, since he was not eligible for a bonus in any month in which the supervisor failed to check a certain percentage of his work.)

Once organized, meticulous administration seemed logical and simple and it belied the difficulties suffered in its development. Unavoidably, such administration was criticized at times by some who overlooked the serious responsibility of the Yellow Fever Service. The press in Niterói once violently attacked the service for dismissing an inspector because he had not been killed the day before. The inspector's itinerary required him to spend much of the same morning each week in the arsenal across Guanabara Bay from Rio de Janeiro. On the morning of one scheduled visit, the arsenal was destroyed by an explosion and everyone on the premises perished. The press insisted that the Yellow Fever Service should have rejoiced over the inspector's escape rather than penalize him for dereliction in performance of his duty.

The observation of aegypti eradication came simultaneously with the discovery that jungle yellow fever was not a chance observation but a widespread phenomenon precluding the eradication of yellow fever virus. Eventually the eradication of the aegypti became the objective of the Yellow Fever Service, since the threat of reintroduction of virus from the forests was permanent.

Eradication of aegypti started in the large cities, but the cities could not be kept free of this mosquito without clearing up the suburbs; it was cheaper to clear the suburbs than to maintain the antiaegypti measures in the large cities. Of course, once the suburbs were cleared, reinfestation came occasionally from the interior. Again, it was always easier to clear the periphery than to maintain the costly central service year after year. Thus, gradually, the eradication of aegypti expanded in Brazil.

The initial proposal to undertake eradication of aegypti in Brazil was made in 1934. Eradication of this vector proved a much more identifiable goal than its reduction in endemic yellow fever centers. The campaign was waged on the basis of the existence or nonexistence of the aegypti rather than on the presence or absence of yellow fever itself.

(See Part II of this book for additional information about the eradication of aegypti.)

ERADICATION OF *Anopheles gambiae*

My return to Brazil in 1930 coincided with the discovery of *Anopheles gambiae,* Africa's most effective vector of malaria, in the Americas. This dangerous immigrant was found at Natal, Rio Grande do Norte, in March 1930. The invasion of Brazil by gambiae, while not directly related to the yellow fever problem, did in effect constitute a moral obligation for the Yellow Fever Service, since it was the only organized administrative health service in the region at the time capable of taking action against this new threat.

The invasion of the Western Hemisphere by gambiae posed a problem for tropical and subtropical America: how to eradicate this vector before it reenacted in North, Central, and South America and the West Indies the tragedy of malaria in Africa?

The solution to this problem was long delayed. In 1930 I failed to interest the Governor of Rio Grande do Norte, the Federal health authorities, and The Rockefeller Foundation in an attempt to eradicate this African invader. My presentation may have been half-hearted; aegypti had not yet been eradicated from any Brazilian city nor was there any definite plan to propose for the eradication of gambiae. In any case, proposals for an attempt to eradicate were rejected: a lack of salesmanship on the one hand and of vision on the other.

The eradication of gambiae was delayed by the very success of partial measures which should have hastened it. Early in 1931, during the second gambiae-transmitted outbreak of malaria in Natal, The Rockefeller Foundation was urged by the National Director of Health to organize an emergency malaria control program. This emergency effort, based on the use of Paris green as a larvicide, relieved the pressure and, as later observations were to show, eradicated gambiae from Natal.

The full importance of gambiae's disappearance from Natal was not recognized at the time, and the advantage gained was not followed up with a comprehensive eradication effort in the interior, where the infestation was in a relatively unfavorable area. Gambiae spread slowly during one of Brazil's cyclical droughts. However, in 1937 it reached the Assú and Jaguaribe river valleys, where in 1938 it caused catastrophic epidemic malaria such as, from time to time, used to decimate the Indian Punjab and Ceylon.

The seriousness of the situation in Rio Grande do Norte and Ceará was a preview of what was in store for a large part of Brazil and of tropical and subtropical America if gambiae was to continue its march unchecked. There had been little support for the proposal to eradicate gambiae when only a few square miles were infested; 8 years later there was a general demand for its eradication. Yet uninfested areas of Brazil and other countries of the Americas, alarmed by the 1937–1938 mortiferous epidemics of malaria in gambiae-infested areas, joined in demanding its eradication. There was no choice but to attempt eradication, although we knew not how to begin. The catastrophic nature of the problem outweighed all other considerations.

Whereas in 1930–1931 no obvious precedent existed for attempting eradication of gambiae, the intervening years showed a convincing example of the expanding eradication of aegypti from Brazilian cities and towns.

Although The Rockefeller Foundation refused, as a matter of policy, to commit itself to the eradication of gambiae, it joined late in 1938 in the organization and financing of the Malaria Service of Northeast Brazil, which undertook the feat. The Malaria Service was financially and administratively independent of the Yellow Fever Service. However, disciplined skeleton staff of all grades, experienced in the eradication of aegypti, and emergency equipment, supplies, and transportation units could be made freely available from the older organization.

The administrative methods used in the eradication of gambiae were adapted directly from those which led to the eradication of aegypti.

Fortunately, the threshold of visibility of gambiae in Brazil was low; the larva, when present, was readily found in gambiae's preferred breeding place—the shallow sunlit pool. The adult always rested indoors, and the invasion of any new area was soon declared by unwonted epidemic malaria. Fortunately, also, the method of attack on gambiae that proved successful in practice was quite simple—a direct chemical attack on all suitable breeding areas in the infested region.

Following the introduction of Paris green as a larvicide in the control of anopheles breeding in 1921, malariologists had developed highly refined methods of diluting it with specially prepared dusts to be applied with pumps, blowers, and airplanes. Such refinement was valuable where the malaria control operation was designed to limit anopheline breeding in a circumscribed area; it proved an insuperable logistic handicap in the gambiae eradication campaign which had to cover the entire infested area.

Gambiae was eradicated from Brazil by inspectors, each carrying an empty pail and a small container of Paris green, who routinely visited and dusted all potential gambiae breeding areas within a carefully delineated geographic area for which each was responsible. The Paris green was mixed with whatever diluent came to hand at the site of application—dust, dirt, sand, pebbles (in the rainy season, mud)—anything which could be thrown by hand over the surface to be treated. The dusting inspector did not search for aquatic forms of gambiae in his area; his responsibility was the routine dusting of all suitable breeding surfaces, while others made the entomological appraisal of results.

In less than 2 years gambiae was eradicated in the Western Hemisphere. As in the case of aegypti, the eradication of gambiae in Brazil did not necessitate a new method of attack against the mosquito, but depended rather on the simplification of existing techniques and the complete coverage of the infested area.

[Part VII for additional information regarding the eradication of gambiae. *Ed.*]

REHABILITATION OF ERADICATION CONCEPT

The eradication of gambiae in Brazil, belated by a full decade, was much more effective in rehabilitating the eradication concept, after the disastrous epidemics of 1937–1939, than it could have been immediately after the invasion from Africa. The high rate of mortality in these epidemics had been widely publicized among public health workers in many countries. The final eradication of gambiae was widely hailed as an important public health victory, and eradication became once more a respectable term. It was only after the eradication of gambiae was known and accepted that the eradication of aegypti from large areas of Brazil was freely published. Even then, after 7 years of observation, the eradication of aegypti was tied in with the eradication of gambiae in a paper on species eradication to make it palatable to public health administrators.

The renewed interest in the eradication concept in the prevention of communicable diseases has not been limited to insect-transmitted infections. An important contribution had been made in 1937 by Wade Hampton Frost, who reported that tuberculosis in man was being eradicated in the United States and certain other countries.

Following the reports on the eradication of aegypti and gambiae in Brazil, other eradication campaigns were organized. One of these was the campaign in the Nile Valley in 1943–1945 for the eradication of gambiae from Egypt. This invader from the upper reaches of the Nile, discovered in Egypt in 1942, caused epidemics of a violence unheard of in Egypt; a Royal Commission appointed to investigate the situation in 1944 estimated the number of deaths at more than 130,000 in 2 epidemic years.

The invasion of Egypt by gambiae led to another lamentable failure in salesmanship with disastrous results. Arriving in Cairo early in January 1943 with the United States of America Typhus Commission, I was invited by the Egyptian health authorities, who knew of the eradication of gambiae from Brazil, to visit the invaded area above Asyut. I did not find any breeding foci in Egypt which could not be readily cleared by the Paris green technique used so successfully in Brazil. Enthusiastically, I reported that with adequate authority, personnel, and Paris green, the eradication of gambiae could be accomplished in a single season. The participation of experienced leaders from the Brazil campaign was recommended, but this suggestion was not accepted. The 1943 campaign was therefore based on larviciding with oil, which failed to prevent the second tragic epidemic. This outbreak led to reorganization of the Malaria Service in the Nile Valley along the lines so successful in Brazil. The reorganization began in July 1944; the last gambiae was found 8 months later, on February 19, 1945.

The eradication of gambiae from Egypt is a striking example of the value of international pooling of information and experience. Other local and national eradication campaigns have been aimed at *Anopheles labranchiae* in Sardinia; *Anopheles elutus* in Cyprus; *Anopheles sergenti* in the Western Oases in Egypt; *Anopheles gambiae* and *Anopheles funestus* in Mauritius; *Anopheles pseudopunctipennis* in the coastal region of Peru; bovine tuberculosis in Costa Rica; yaws in Haiti; foot-and-mouth disease and smallpox in Mexico; vesicular exanthema of swine, bovine tuberculosis, brucellosis, the Mediterranean fruit fly, and the screwworm in the United States; and malaria in Argentina, Greece, Italy, the United States, and Venezuela.

Eradication as a Regional Objective

Some of these campaigns have succeeded, some have failed, and some are still in progress; but all were local or at the best national efforts which, when successful, would require eternal vigilance to prevent reinfestation or reinfection. On the other hand, The Rockefeller Foundation had undertaken eradication of yellow fever from the Western Hemisphere, cooperating with each infected country to attain the common objective.

With the discovery of the jungle infection, it became obvious that yellow fever was not eradicable; only by the eradication of aegypti could the safety of urban populations be guaranteed. The observation in 1933 that aegypti had been eradicated in a number of Brazilian cities did not lead to a foundation-sponsored effort to eradicate aegypti from the Americas. Health officers of Bolivia, Colombia, Cuba, Ecuador, Paraguay, Peru, the United States, and Venezuela were trained in the eradication techniques, but Foundation support of eradication efforts was limited to Brazil, Bolivia, and Paraguay. Attempts to obtain The Rockefeller Foundation's support for continental eradication failed, as did a later attempt in 1942 to interest the newly created Institute of Inter-American Affairs.

The Rockefeller Foundation's withdrawal from antiaegypti work in Brazil in January 1940 left this program fully staffed by Brazilians. This withdrawal did not handicap the national effort but did, however, destroy the mechanism through which experienced Brazilian workers could be made available for eradication projects in other countries as they had been in Bolivia and Paraguay. This withdrawal was to delay for 8 years the development of the continental program of aegypti eradication. But it was not a lost issue; it came to life eventually as a result of the continued expansion of the aegypti eradication program in Brazil.

At the time of the Rockefeller Foundation's withdrawal, aegypti could no longer be found in Brazil's capital, Rio de Janeiro, or in 6 of its 20 states. The Yellow Fever Service, after its reincorporation into the National Health Department, boldly declared its objective to be the complete eradication of aegypti from the rest of Brazil. The continuing progress in eradication of this vector was such that by 1946 Brazil was suffering reinfestation from neighboring countries across national frontiers.

In that year, the Brazilian Yellow Fever Service suggested to the Rockefeller Foundation that it negotiate with the Government of Paraguay for the cooperation of the Foundation and the Government of Brazil in the eradication of aegypti in Paraguay. The Foundation demurred, pointing out that although Paraguay might be willing to sacrifice its mosquitoes, eradication there would only move the line Brazil had to defend against aegypti to Paraguay's frontiers with Argentina. Analyzing the situation in the light of its 10 frontiers with neighboring countries, the Brazilian Yellow Fever Service concluded that the defense of Brazil from reinfestation with aegypti required nothing less than the eradication of this ancient and well-established African invader from the Americas.

In 1947, Brazil proposed, and the Directing Council of the Pan American Health Organization approved, a program for the eradication of the aegypti mosquito from the Americas. This action is an important landmark in international health policy; for the first time the governments of an entire region committed themselves to the continental solution of a common health problem.

Fortunately, the introduction of DDT made the eradication of aegypti much less onerous than it had been when oil had been the insecticide of choice. Before the end of 1947, the Pan American Sanitary Bureau was collaborating with the Government of Paraguay in a truly international effort to eradicate aegypti. The Pan American Sanitary Bureau was supplying the framework of collaboration; Brazil, the technical leadership and essential technical supplies; Argentina, the motor transportation; and Paraguay, the necessary manpower.

Progress in the continental eradication of aegypti was slower than anticipated, but nevertheless gratifying. In 12 years (1947–1959), during which only three cases of aegypti-transmitted yellow fever were reported from the entire continent, the following countries were certified as free of aegypti by the Pan American Health Organization: Bolivia, Brazil, Ecuador, Guatemala, Honduras, Nicaragua, Panama, Paraguay, Peru, Uruguay, and British Honduras. (Additional countries certified by 1964 included Argentina, Bermuda, Costa Rica, Chile, El Salvador, the Canal Zone of Panama, and Mexico. The United States initiated, in 1963, its program for the eradication of aegypti in nine infested states, Puerto Rico, and the Virgin Islands.)

The international public health worker of 1959, accustomed to official group action of nations through the World Health Assembly, the Pan American Sanitary Conference, and the Executive Board of the United Nations Children's Fund (UNICEF), found it difficult to imagine the vacuum in which the International Health Board of The Rockefeller Foundation operated in 1920. The Pan American Sanitary Conference, established in 1902, had held no meetings between 1912 and 1920. The Office International d'Hygiène Publique, established in 1907, was limited by its charter to an exchange of information between countries on the incidence of epidemic diseases. The Health Section of the League of Nations was still to be created.

When The Rockefeller Foundation was chartered in 1913, there was no effective international framework through which countries could consider and act on common health problems. The Foundation quite naturally operated through direct negotiation with each country concerned, whether the problem was one of internal interest only, such as hookworm disease, nursing education, and health centers, or one of truly regional international concern as was the eradication of yellow fever.

The stimulus for The Rockefeller Foundation interest in yellow fever eradication came from the fear of invasion of Asia through the Panama Canal, newly opened in 1914. The decision to undertake the eradication of yellow fever was made by The Rockefeller Foundation on the advice of consultants without the calling of an international conference, or even an expert committee as, would be done today. There was no previous agreement among the countries of the Americas to eradicate yellow fever or a willingness to collaborate in such a project.

The creation of the Pan American Health Organization in 1947, through which the Pan American Sanitary Bureau previously limited to the 21 American Republics operates throughout the Western Hemisphere, and its alliance with the World Health Organization, created in 1948, has resulted in a permanent framework through which all countries of the Americas can work together for the solution of common problems. The development of this framework has been especially significant at a time when the eradication concept is being rehabilitated, and when the introduction of residual insecticides, specific drugs, antibiotics, biological techniques, and new and improved vaccines make the eradication of certain communicable diseases feasible.

In 1947 a bus passenger from the Mexican border was found to be infected with smallpox on arrival in New York City. This caused great agitation and the emergency vaccination of millions of persons in the metropolitan area. This incident emphasized the difficulty of maintaining efficient barriers against the entry of communicable disease and the difficulty of keeping populations immunized against diseases which are not a constant threat.

Although smallpox has long been an eradicable disease, a 1948 study led to the conclusion that eradication throughout the tropics would be greatly eased by perfection of a desiccated heat-resistant vaccine. As a preliminary to this eradication effort, the Pan American Sanitary Bureau requested the U.S. Public Health Service to review methods for preparation of a dry smallpox vaccine. In collaboration with the Michigan Public Health Laboratory, the Public Health Service developed a method of producing a "thermostable" vaccine for use in the tropics.

In 1950 the XIIIth Pan American Sanitary Conference approved a continental program of smallpox eradication, and established a special fund for promoting the production of desiccated vaccine and for technical assistance in the organization of national eradication campaigns. Meanwhile, Mexico had taken the lead in organizing a successful national eradication campaign with glycerinated vaccine. The disappearance of smallpox from Mexico in 1951 was followed by the absence of reported cases in North America, Central America, and the islands of the Caribbean since 1954. Considerable progress has been made in reducing the incidence of smallpox in South America.

In 1949 Haiti, stimulated by the surprising results obtained in field trials of the treatment of yaws with penicillin, requested the assistance of the Pan American Sanitary Bureau in a campaign for the eradication of this infection. The countrywide campaign, based on the mass treatment of the rural population, began with the collaboration of WHO and UNICEF in 1950. Mass treatment was justified on the basis of the high incidence of yaws in Haiti and on the necessity of treating infected contacts during the incubation period.

The yaws eradication request from Haiti led to widespread interest in the disease and to treatment campaigns in many parts of the tropics. The 1950 Pan American Sanitary Conference approved the eradication of yaws as a Pan American Sanitary Bureau-sponsored program for the Americas. To date, the standards for international certification or eradication of yaws have not been established. In any case, the incidence of yaws in Haiti is low, and eradication efforts are being carried out in many tropical areas of the world.

Reports in the late 1940s of the dramatic reduction of malaria in the United States, Brazil, Venezuela, British Guiana, and Argentina, after the introduction of DDT, led the Pan American Sanitary Bureau, in 1950, to make a reconnaissance of malaria control in the Western Hemisphere. This was followed by a recommendation of the 1950 Conference that the Pan American Sanitary Bureau collaborate with the malarious nations of the Americas in national malaria eradication programs.

The action of the conference on malaria eradication proved to be ahead of its time; the Pan American Sanitary Bureau itself was not sufficiently developed to give adequate leadership nor were the chiefs of malaria control programs in many countries willing to admit the inadequacy of their efforts.

The finding of Anopheles resistance to residual insecticide, the recurrence of malaria in areas believed to have been freed from all danger, and another reconnaissance of the malaria situation in 1954 which showed little advance over the position in 1950, led the XIVth Conference to declare malaria eradication an emergency need and demand that the Pan American Sanitary Bureau carry out its 1950 resolution. The Conference established an emergency fund of $100,000 available immediately for administrative expenses and provided for additional voluntary financing. Developments since this October 1954 action of the Conference have been startling.

Eradication as a Global Objective

In January 1955, the President of Mexico authorized the Minister of Health to arrange the financing of a national malaria eradication program. In March 1955 the Executive Board of UNICEF, looking with favor on Mexico's appeal for aid, asked for a meeting of the UNICEF/WHO Joint Committee on Program to consider malaria eradication as a suitable program for UNICEF support. The favorable action of the UNICEF/WHO Joint Committee in May was followed almost immediately by action of the Eighth World Health Assembly sponsoring a program for world malaria eradication.

The response of the nations of the world has been almost universal, and the program has developed faster than could have been foreseen. A most important factor in this development was the decision of the U.S. Government, in 1956, to sponsor the programs of the Pan American and World Health Organizations. U.S. contributions to the Malaria Eradication Special Accounts of these organizations have been greatly increased in value by the decision to transform control projects supported by the International Cooperation Administration (AID) to eradication campaigns.

History tends to repeat itself. In the eradication of malaria, some of the same difficulties are being encountered as with yellow fever eradication in 1930. With efficient tools available, despite difficulty in some areas with anopheline resistance to residual insecticide, the problems are (a) how to get meticulous administration and complete coverage of all human habitations in malarious areas, and (b) how to identify the residual foci of transmission once the incidence of malaria is below the threshold of easy visibility. These are the problems which are preoccupying malaria workers in the Americas, Europe, the Middle East, and Asia.

The malaria problem in Africa is particularly difficult because of the high efficiency of the principal vectors, *A. gambiae and A. funestus,* the lack of trained personnel, the difficulties of transportation, and the poverty of the region. However, the factors which make the African vectors so efficient, among which is their high domesticity, should in the long run prove to be their undoing. Available evidence strongly suggests that there are no insuperable obstacles to the eradication of malaria in Africa.

The Pan American and World Health Organizations, UNICEF, and the Agency for International Development are all committed to malaria eradication: each recognizes that the task is too great for one organization and welcomes the full collaboration of the others. This attitude augurs well, not only for malaria eradication, but also for the future solution of other important health problems.

Just as the Pan American action sponsoring the eradication of the aegypti mosquito marked a milestone in international collaboration in the regional solution of a common problem, so did the action of UNICEF and the World Health Organization, in 1955, establish the precedent for global collaboration in the solution of a world problem.

At the end of the sixth decade of the twentieth century, disease eradication and vector eradication, where feasible, offer great advantages in this shrinking world. Improved methods of prevention in national programs coordinated by international health organizations make certain eradication programs feasible; the rapidity of travel makes eradication in endemic foci the most logical defense against the spread of communicable diseases. With the eradication programs already organized and with continued improvement in methods of disease prevention, the public health administrator is sure to hear much of the eradication concept in the future.

SUMMARY

The eradication concept in the prevention of communicable diseases was formulated almost as soon as modern methods of disease prevention appeared.

The first serious attempt at regional eradication was The Rockefeller Foundation's effort to eradicate yellow fever from the Americas. This effort failed because of the unrecognized existence of jungle yellow fever, a permanent source of virus for the reinfection of cities and towns. However, this failure led to a program for the eradication of yellow fever's urban vector, the *Aëdes aegypti* mosquito.

The progress of this program in the Western Hemisphere and the eradication of *Anopheles gambiae,* first in Brazil and later in Egypt, began the rehabilitation of the eradication concept which had been discredited by public health workers.

Improved methods of disease prevention, both technical and administrative, and the coordination of national efforts in regional and global programs by the Pan American and World Health Organizations make certain regional and even world eradication programs feasible.

Part IX | The Control of Epidemic (Louse-Borne)
Typhus Fever by Insecticide Powders

Selection 34 | Louse-Powder Studies in North
Africa (1943)*

F. L. SOPER, W. A. DAVIS, F. S. MARKHAM,
L. A. RIEHL, AND PAUL BUCK

Severe and extensive outbreaks of typhus fever occurred in both Algiers and Morocco during the winters of 1941–1942 and 1942–1943. A survey visit to this area by Richard Allen of the American Red Cross and Dr. George K. Strode of the International Health Division of The Rockefeller Foundation in January 1943 led to negotiations with Dr. Edmond Sergent, Director of the Pasteur Institute of Algiers, with Dr. Grenoilleau, Director of Health for Algeria, and Dr. Gaud, Director of Health for Morocco, for collaboration in studying methods of typhus control, based on the use of insecticidal powders. The American Red Cross sponsored the studies, which were undertaken with the approval of the State Department.

The Rockefeller Foundation Health Commission assigned Drs. Fred L. Soper, William A. Davis, Floyd S. Markham, and Louis A. Riehl to the project. (The services of Dr. Paul Buck were contributed by the Pasteur Institute.) Through transportation facilities provided by the War Department and the Surgeon General's Office this group came to North Africa late in June 1943 and established contact with the Pasteur Institute of Algiers, the Health Department of Algeria, and the Medical Section of NATOUSA (North African Theater of Operations, U.S. Army).

Plans were made for the initial testing of materials and methods in collaboration with the Pasteur Institute of Algiers. Demonstrations of epidemic control measures were planned in both Morocco and Algeria, if epidemic typhus again became a serious problem during the ensuing winter season.

The initial activities were devoted to (1) evaluating the effectiveness of different louse powders on natural infestations, (2) studying locally available excipients for the preparation of louse powder, (3) testing the feasibility of mixing DDT powder in the field, (4) determining the duration of effect of insecticides in the face of constant reinfestation, (5) developing methods for the rapid application of powder to the individual, and (6) developing administrative methods for rapidly and economically delousing communities for the purpose of blocking the spread of epidemic typhus.

Considerable difficulty was encountered in securing adequate supplies,

* This article was originally published (*49*) in *Archives de l'Institut Pasteur d'Algérie 23:* 183–223, 1945. (The 11 tables that accompanied the original article have been omitted from this excerpt.)

357

transportation, and personnel for the field studies, and the program proceeded more slowly than had been anticipated. However, during the following months the initial testing of materials and methods in a civilian prison was completed, and field demonstrations of delousing without the removal of the clothing had been made in prisoner of war camps and in the county of L'Arba, Algeria. The anticipated epidemic conditions required for field control demonstrations had not developed in North Africa when the rapid increase of typhus in Naples, Italy, led to a transfer of this part of the program to that city on December 8, 1943, under the auspices of the Allied Military Government. This epidemic in a nonimmune population, well seeded with typhus at the beginning of winter, afforded an unexcelled opportunity for the rapid and dramatic demonstration of the practical value of the method of delousing without removal of clothing developed in Algeria.

The present report covers (1) intensive studies carried out at the Maison-Carrée Prison near Algiers on the relative efficacy of factory-prepared MYL powder and powders containing DDT prepared with local excipients and applied by various methods, (2) the extensive field application of insecticide to the general population of the town and county of L'Arba in Algeria, and (3) a rapid field test in a prisoner of war camp of the new factory-prepared U.S. Army 10 per cent DDT–pyrophyllite powder.

The most important developments of the work in North Africa were (1) the demonstration, on naturally acquired infestations, that both MYL and DDT are highly efficient pediculicides; (2) the development of the air-blown application of louse powder without removal of clothing from the body of the person being deloused; (3) the demonstration that lousy people will take the trouble to come to accessible delousing stations to get relief; and (4) the development of administrative methods for the rapid disinsectization of both military and civilian populations.

Personnel Engaged in Studies

In Algiers, Dr. Edmond Sergent, Director of the Pasteur Institute, took a personal interest in the program from the beginning and assigned Dr. Béguet as the representative of the Pasteur Institute to follow the scientific aspects of the work. Dr. Paul Buck was assigned from the staff of the Pasteur Institute to work with the Foundation group in the actual application of insecticide and in ascertaining the degree of louse infestation before and after treatment.

Col. W. S. Stone of the Medical Section of NATOUSA was kept informed of the plans of these studies and was of great assistance in making available needed materials with which to work. Col. Stone was also instrumental in assigning a number of officers from Malaria Units to work in the field application of insecticide at L'Arba. Several of these officers later took an active part in the Naples campaign.

Dr. Sergent was responsible for making arrangement with M. le Directeur de la Sécurité Générale du Gouvernement Général for the studies at the Maison-Carrée Prison and with M. le Préfet du Département d'Alger and the Président de la Délégation speciale of L'Arba for the work in that county.

All details of the work and the observations herewith reported are the direct responsibility of the Rockefeller Foundation Health Commission Typhus Team and Dr. Paul Buck.

Materials

Insecticides

Initial plans called for the study in North Africa of various newly synthesized insecticides in an attempt to develop a formula better than the MYL of the U.S. Army. By the time the work began in North Africa, however, the laboratory tests of the new insecticide, DDT, had proceeded far enough to warrant concentrating efforts on field studies of MYL and DDT preparations.

MYL INSECTICIDAL POWDER OF THE U.S. ARMY. The MYL powder tested in the Maison-Carrée Prison was part of a shipment of powder manufactured by the McCormick Company of Baltimore which had arrived in Algeria in April 1943. This material was packed in 2-ounce shaker tins. The MYL powder used in the field at L'Arba was material ordered early in 1943 from the McCormick Company and packed in specially designed 2-ounce envelopes. The shipment arrived in Algeria in July of the same year.

DDT (2,2-BIS (P-CHLOROPHENYL)-1,1,1-TRICHLOROETHANE). When the North African studies began there was available a small lot of 5 pounds of DDT which had been received for field tests from Mr. Knipling at the Orlando Laboratory of the U.S. Department of Agriculture. An additional 30 pounds of DDT (probably of the grade now designated "technical") was received later from the Medical Section NATOUSA, which also furnished the 10 per cent DDT–pyrophyllite powder used in the prisoner of war camps.

CRESYLACETATE-2,4. 2,4-Dinitrocresylacetate was tested in combination with DDT in a single experiment at Maison-Carrée.

HAIR LOTION. The hair lotion used at L'Arba was a modification of that described by Davis. An emulsion of the active ingredient, phenyl Cellosolve, was made in water by the use of a sodium alkyl sulfate, Tergitol 07, at a concentration of 0.1 per cent. Since phenyl Cellosolve and Tergitol 07 are miscible liquids, a stock emulsion may be prepared and used as required.

The emulsion was easily and simply prepared. Five per cent by volume of the stock solution of phenyl Cellosolve and Tergitol 07 was placed in a container of convenient size, such as a 1-liter wine bottle. After the proper volume of water had been added and the bottle corked, the mixture was shaken vigorously before application. The suspension separates on standing for several hours but can be quickly reestablished by shaking.

Diluents for Insecticides

BARYTES (BARIUM SULFATE, Ba_2SO_4). Barytes is mined at Maison-Carrée, only a short distance from the prison where tests were carried out. Two samples of this material were received from the Cie. Produits Barytiques Nordafricains. The sample Blanc Extra Fin was found to be sticky but the Extra Blanc proved to be a suitably fine smooth white powder with little or no tendency to stickiness. It passed a 200-per-inch mesh screen easily and had a pH of 6.8 but was very heavy, being over three times the weight of pyrophyllite used in the preparation of MYL.

CEMENT DUST. The Société Lafarge, at Point Pescade, a suburb of Algiers, furnished a finely ground limestone which is used in the manufacture of cement. Chemical analysis showed this limestone to consist mostly of calcium carbonate with some magnesium carbonate and oxides of silica, aluminum, and iron. This limestone powder was a dirty gray-brown in color, was gritty to the touch, and had a pH of 9.0. It was, however, much lighter than the barytes, weighing approximately the same as pyrophyllite.

Preparation of Insecticides

SOLVENT METHOD. Suitable quantities of DDT "technical" and the excipient were weighed out. The DDT was then completely dissolved in a volume of acetone sufficient to yield a workably wet paste when the solution was added to the excipient. The resulting paste mixture was stirred thoroughly and continuously until the bulk of the acetone had evaporated, leaving the active ingredient evenly distributed on the excipient. The slight amount of acetone remaining evaporated when the mixture was spread in a thin layer on a paper-covered surface for final drying.

MECHANICAL METHODS. *Hand Mixer.* Weighed amounts of the active ingredients and excipients were placed in the baffle chamber of a small hand-operated mixer and rotated for specified time intervals. The mixing chamber was fitted with baffle plates and eccentrically placed on the surface of a revolving disc so that maximum distribution and mixing of the components could be obtained. When more than one sample was prepared for use in the same experiment the batches were mixed for equal periods of time.

Bread Mixer. Two batches of 10 per cent DDT powder were prepared in a bakery-type bread mixer. The machine consisted of a large cast-iron tub which rotated freely in the horizontal axis and an eccentrically placed set of mixing paddles which caused the tub to revolve slowly as the paddles moved through the contents of mixing chamber. From time to time during the mixing period the paddle action was augmented by manual redistribution of the materials in the tub. DDT concentrate becomes hard and lumpy on standing and must be milled shortly before mixing. Since the melting point of DDT is relatively low, the heat generated at the grinding surfaces of the mill produces a slight stickiness which prevents a smooth blend with the excipient in a bread mixer. This can be avoided if a certain amount of excipient be added to the DDT concentrate at the time of milling.

HOT TABLE. When clothing is examined to determine the incidence and degree of lousiness, searching the seams becomes a laborious task, and any simple means of driving out the lice greatly facilitates their discovery. The louse has a limited adaptation to temperature, and a slight increase of heat causes it to move about and leave the seams. The louse generally crawls upward and, even though negatively phototropic, will expose itself to light to escape heat applied beneath it. The heat applied must be moderate to avoid stupefaction or even death of the insect.

During the early work at the Maison-Carrée Prison it was found that effective use could be made of sunlight to heat a black metal surface which served as a "hot table" on which clothing was examined. Lice present in the clothes emerged from the seams and crawled about the exposed surface of the garments. As the season advanced a kerosene stove was placed below the metal surface with fair results. Later, a cylindrical barrel frame with a superimposed rack for suspending clothing at an angle in the warm current of air rising in the barrel was placed around the kerosene stove. This arrangement was not entirely satisfactory but proved useful in the final examination of clothing not obviously infested.

Applicators of Insecticide

SHAKER TINS. Previous experience led to the use of a special type of shaker tin for the application of MYL, which is too moist and sticky to sift well from the tin in which it is packed. The shaker tins used in North Africa were made by drilling one or two rows of holes in the side wall about the base of a cylindrical tin can having a diameter of $3\frac{1}{2}$ inches. With the perforations in the side wall (not in the bottom of the tin) it is possible to keep the powder flowing continuously by rotating the tin slightly with each shake.

AGRICULTURAL DUSTERS. The agricultural dusters used were of two types (trade names Toxine and Corona), both used by the wine growers in North Africa for dusting their vineyards.

The Toxine duster is a bellows-type knapsack duster in which the dust is picked up by an air stream directed downward on the surface of the powder and carried out through an aperture placed near the top of the chamber.

The Corona duster is a bellows-type knapsack duster in which the powder drops from the hopper into a tube below. The air stream picks up the dust as it passes through the tube.

Attempts were made to adapt the Hudson Rotary Powder Duster No. 608 for the application of MYL powder to clothed individuals, but the physical properties of this powder as well as the mechanical design of the duster rendered its use impractical.

HAND DUSTERS: HUDSON, CADET-MAJOR, PLUNGER TYPE. The powder chamber is immediately in front of the compression chamber, forming with it a continuous tube with an air valve located in center of partition separating the two chambers. The outlet aperture for dust consists of an axial tube, beginning about one third of the length of the chamber from its distal end. Powder tends to pack around the outlet tube and discharge as "slugs." The axial inlet and outlet tubes, together with its small capacity cause this duster to be relatively inefficient. However, it can be used in an emergency to good advantage, as was demonstrated later in the Naples epidemic.

DOBBINS SUPERBUILT No. 133, PLUNGER TYPE. Air passes from the compression chamber through a tube placed at the circumference of the powder chamber and enters the powder chamber at the distal end. Outlet consists of a series of apertures well back of the distal end opening into a delivery tube placed diametrically opposite the inlet tube. When the duster is held so that the outlet tube is on the upper side, the air, en route from the inlet to the outlet, must pass upward through the powder carrying some of it into the air space of the powder chamber and thence out through the delivery outlet. This (together with the similar Hudson Admiral Duster No. 765) proved to be a highly satisfactory tool for applying louse powder.

DEVILBISS HAND POWER SPRAYER OUTFIT AND MODIFIED DUST GUNS. (For use with portable power-compressor units). The DeVilbiss sprayer outfit No. TZ-601 is a hand-operated unit consisting of a compressor to which is attached a spray gun fitted with a glass or metal container for liquids. The gun was modified to use positive rather than negative pressure but was found to be unsatisfactory because of the continued demand for high pressure required for its operation.

The modified DeVilbiss sprayer gun and several others built through the cooperation of the Surgeon's Office NATOUSA and the U.S. Army Air Corps shops were used with varying degrees of success when attached to gasoline-driven air-compressor units. In general, the limitations of this type of equipment are (1) the ability of the compressor unit to maintain sufficient pressure to operate two or more guns continuously, (2) the ability of the powder chamber to withstand the abrasive action of the excipient dust, (3) the facility with which the powder chamber can be refilled, and (4) the need for mechanically trained operators to care for the equipment.

Methods

Determination of Louse Infestation

The degree of louse infestation was determined with varying degrees of thoroughness. In work at the Maison-Carrée Prison the degree of lousiness of each individual was determined by removing all the clothing and carefully examining the inner surfaces and seams for lice. In preliminary survey work, when an incomplete search revealed the presence of 10 or more lice, the individual was registered as 10 plus. (Previous experience in community surveys had shown that populations can be roughly divided into two groups: those having not over 9 lice and those having 10 or more. Most of the persons falling in the first group will be found to have not more than 5 lice.) In posttreatment examinations all garments were examined and complete counts made.

The examinations were generally made in bright sunlight and negative garments were often subjected to hot-table treatment to aid in the discovery in insects.

The classification of posttreatment lice as to stage of development was found to be very useful in evaluating the insecticide tested. Each insect was recorded as newly hatched, immature, or adult. The posttreatment finding of only newly hatched lice indicates that the insecticide, although not ovicidal, has a persistent action which destroys the instars before they reach the nymphal or adult stages. The finding of immature forms on treated garments is not necessarily an indication for repeated treatment.

At L'Arba the subjects were not disrobed to determine the degree of louse infestation. A louse-index based on a rapid examination of the clothing about the collar and over the shoulders was considered sufficient for the purpose of this study.

At Maison-Carrée Prison all examinations were carried out by members of the Rockefeller Foundation Typhus Team or Dr. Buck, with a few specially trained prisoners working under their direct supervision.

Application of Powder

SHAKER TIN. If bedding is to be treated the blankets are first spread out flat on the floor or table top and lightly dusted with powder from the shaker tin. The blanket is then folded over once. Next, the upper garments after having been turned inside out are laid one by one in the center of the folded blanket and dusted individually. Particular care is taken to ensure thorough powdering of the neckband, and the seams about the shoulders, arms, and waist. Coats, shirts, and undershirts are treated alike. The lower garments after being turned inside out are treated in the same fashion. The side seams of the trousers and the seams about the waistband, seat, and crotch of both the trousers and underwear are heavily powdered. A certain amount of powder can be worked under the overlapping seams of the trousers by a brisk back and forth brushing movement over the surface of the garment. The inside of the hat or cap is then powdered and added to the pile in the center of the blanket.

Finally the corners of the blanket are folded over the dusted clothing so as to form a closed bundle which is given several smart blows at the sides and top in order to fluff the powder throughout the treated garments and blanket. If blankets are not being treated, the overcoat or waistcoat may be used as the covering of the bundle of clothing in the final step.

MECHANICAL DUST PUMPS. Essentially the same technique is employed in applying powder with both the hand-operated and the power driven compressed-air dust pumps.

The following paragraphs are quoted from the directions for powdering prepared November 2, 1943:

Powdering Technique

In using the duster, the operator should remember that powder should be distributed on the inner surfaces of the inner garments and on the skin itself. Those doing the work for the first time should have the clothing removed from the first persons powdered to observe the results obtained. If properly done, the entire inner garments should be more or less completely covered with powder and there should be visible powder on the body hairs of the chest, back, thighs, armpits and of the pubic and perineal regions. Since body lice are most often found in the seams of the clothes about the neck, armpits, waist, shirt-tail and crotch of the pants, these areas are particularly important ones to be powdered.

The dusting of individuals should follow a certain routine to avoid missing some parts of the clothing as must occur at times where each person is handled differently. The following routine has been found useful:

1. Dust inside of hat and replace hat on head.

2. With arms extended at shoulder height at the sides (not in front of the body) insert delivery tube up first the right and then the left sleeve and pump powder in between the skin and the innermost garment. Powder should reach well into the armpit and the position of the gun should be shifted to get powder all about the shoulder.

In case the subject is wearing more than one layer of clothing, dust should be applied between his underwear and shirt as well as between the underwear and the skin.

3. The delivery tube is next inserted at the back of the neck and a liberal charge of powder shot down the back, care being taken to dust the neckband itself.

4. The tube is next inserted inside the clothing from in front and powder sprayed first on one side, then on the chest and lastly on the other side, special care being taken to again reach the armpits.

5. The tube is next inserted, after the trousers are loosened, inside the innermost garment and a good dose of powder delivered to the crotch and pubic area. With the tube still in contact with the skin, the underclothing is powdered, special attention being paid to the waist and side seams.

6. With the trousers still loose, the tube is inserted down the rear of the pants next to the skin and powder is shot down over the buttocks and rear of the crotch.

Note: If more than one layer of clothing is being worn, steps 3, 4, 5, and 6 above are repeated for the second layer from the skin.

SECTION I: Studies at the Maison-Carrée Prison

The Maison-Carrée Prison had, at the time of these studies, approximately 1000 prisoners, accommodated in three wards, two for males, one for females. Only small demonstrations were attempted in the ward for females and no further reference will be made to the work there. The male prisoners, most of whom were Arabs, differed in prison status, clothing, and living conditions.

A considerable number of prisoners were employed as trusties in handling others. These trusties received better food, clothing, and quarters than did the other prisoners. Special concessions were made also for mechanics, cooks, and other specialized workers.

Some prisoners, especially those serving short sentences, had friends or relatives with sufficient funds to supply them with extra food, soap, and clothing. These were considerably better off than were prisoners depending entirely on prison issues. The latter were obviously undernourished and had little or no soap for washing the trousers, jacket, and blanket which comprised their entire wardrobe.

The prison routine calls for the use of woolen clothing in winter and heavy cotton in summer. Owing to the war and scarcity of materials, summer clothing had not been issued to many of the prisoners and numbers of them continued to wear winter woolens throughout the summer.

The work of the prisoners at Maison-Carrée varied according to the length of sentence imposed. Thus the prisoners in Ward I were of two groups, those condemned for life and those confined for minor offenses. The minor offenders were hired out in gangs to do agricultural work outside the prison grounds, whereas the lifers worked in the open courtyard of the ward at relatively light labor weaving mats and baskets for which they received a small stipend. The lifers in Ward I had not been issued summer clothing, whereas most of the short termers wore cottons.

The majority of prisoners in Ward II had been sentenced to forced labor. These men worked at hard physical labor preparing fiber for basket and mat weaving. This work was done under guards in a large room where the prisoners were crowded together on the floor.

Prisoners in both Wards I and II were provided with fiber mats and blankets and slept in groups of 80 in large dormitories where they were confined from 5:30 in the afternoon until 7 A.M.

Because of the intimate contact and crowding, particularly in Ward II, the opportunity for a daily interchange of parasites was excellent. Under these conditions only the most industrious of the prisonsers were able to keep themselves relatively free of lice. The steam-sterilization plant at the prison was little used, because of shortage of fuel and mechanical break-downs.

The first visit to Maison-Carrée was made on July 23 with Dr. Béguet, at which time arrangements were made with the Director of the prison for beginning work. Work began with a preliminary prepowdering louse survey, July 26 to 29. This survey revealed 153 lousy prisoners among 158 examined, 116 of whom had more than 10 lice each. Further surveys of unpowdered individuals were made from this time on through the end of October with the finding of even higher degrees of infestation. From these results it is clear that any reduction from the July level noted in the louse burden of test groups must be attributed to the insecticide used.

Experiment I

The initial test at Maison-Carrée was to compare the action of repeated doses of 5 per cent DDT in barytes and of MYL on natural infestations in an environment where exposure to reinfestation from untreated persons could be almost entirely prevented.

Ward I was chosen for the first test with observations in Ward II to serve as a check against the possibility of a seasonal reduction of louse incidence being attributed to the use of insecticide.

The prisoners were called by number and checked off as the clothing of each man was dusted by hand (shaker tins).

The 108 men examined in Ward I were divided into three groups of 36 men each, and hand dusted (shaker tins) as follows:

The clothing and blankets of the men in group 1 were treated with 5 per cent DDT in barytes (barium sulfate) and redusted with the same material 17 days later; those of the men in group 2 were dusted twice at a 7-day interval, and those of group 3 twice at a 14-day interval with MYL.

All other inmates of Ward I were treated with MYL twice with an interval of 14 days to prevent them from grossly reinfesting the study groups.

Insecticide MYL was applied also to the garments of all new prisoners coming to Ward I and to those returning to the ward after a stay in the prison infirmary.

As far as is known, the only prisoners in Ward I to escape the initial dusting were 3 who assisted the guards in the administration of the ward and 15 who worked in the bakery. These assistant guards were dusted 3 days and the bakers 13 days after the rest of the prisoners. This failure to dust all simultaneously is probably of little importance, since these 18 men all enjoyed special privileges, had separate quarters, and were much cleaner than the common run of prisoners.

The clothing and blankets of groups 1, 2, and 3 were examined at intervals after both first and second treatments. In pretreatment examinations, counts were discontinued on any given individual when 10 lice had been found, but posttreatment examinations covered the entire inner surface of all clothing worn and both sides of blankets.

The first posttreatment counts on groups 1, 2, and 3 showed that both DDT and MYL had been very effective in reducing the louse burden of the treated prisoners. The 2- to 4-day counts indicated that the immediate effect of DDT had been somewhat less than that of MYL, but the 7-, 10-, and 14-day counts definitely favored DDT. The DDT-treated group showed a steady decline in numbers of lice up to the day 17, when it was retreated. The hatching of young had apparently ceased by day 10 or 11. In the MYL-treated groups, 2- to 4-day counts were lower than 7-day counts and in the group not re-treated until day 14, there was a decline in the louse infestation between days 7 and 14 with hatching of young forms practically nil between days 10 and 14. The striking reduction in adult forms in all three groups is most significant, since the egg-laying function on which the species depends for continued existance is a function of adult life.

The second treatment of group I with DDT 17 days after the first was followed by examinations at 7, 13, 25, and 39 days after this second treatment, with practically no lice being found.

The last examination of this group, made 67 days after the second treatment (83 days after the first treatment), showed that about one third of the group was again lightly infested. This infestation was so slight that the prisoners still considered themselves louse-free.

Examinations of the MYL-treated groups (2 and 3) failed in both cases to reveal the presence of an appreciable number of lice for some weeks. As was to be expected, evidence of reinfestation was found earlier, in group 2, re-treated after 7 days, than in group 3, which was re-treated at an interval of 14 days.

In all three groups, negligible infestations were found at the end of 56 days after first treatment. The difference in the degree of infestation of groups 1 and 3, re-treated after 17 days and 14 days, and of group 2, re-treated after only 7 days is probably significant.

DISCUSSION. A study of the behavior of the louse population on groups 1 and 3 before re-treatment suggests that for the maximum result with the minimum amount of insecticide, the period between treatments may well be longer than 17 and 14 days.

Theoretically an insecticide which is fully effective immediately against all forms present except the ova, but which has no delayed residual action, should be repeated at about 14 days to catch the early posttreatment-hatched lice before they come into active egg laying. With the demonstration of continued activity of the insecticide this period may be lengthened accordingly.

From the epidemiological standpoint, it should be emphasized that the posttreatment counts are complete counts based on a thorough search in the seams of the clothing and an examination of blankets. The degree of lousiness found 83 days after treatment began was not such as to have permitted the rapid dissemination of typhus in the ward, had it been introduced. It seems reasonable to suggest on the basis of these counts that a population which has been thoroughly powdered twice may be considered safe from important outbreaks of typhus for at least a 3-month period.

The results in Ward I suggest that the complete eradication of lice in an institution or even in a community may be feasible with the proper application of either MYL or DDT.

Experiment II

Experiments II and III carried out in Ward II were designed to test, under conditions favoring reinfestation, the action of single doses of 5 per cent DDT, of 10 per cent DDT, prepared in various ways, and of factory-prepared MYL, applied in various ways. An additional accidental variable was introduced in Experiment II through the failure of mechanical equipment used to apply the same amount of insecticide as was applied by hand.

Whereas in Experiment I the possibility of reinfestation was reduced to a minimum, reinfestation was favored in Experiments II and III. Only the clothing of the prisoners in these experiments was powdered; their infested blankets were ignored. The remaining prisoners of Ward II, where conditions were more favorable to reinfestation than in Ward I, were not powdered. Intimate contact continued between treated and untreated individuals both day and night.

In Experiment II eight groups of 10 men each were treated with varying combinations of DDT, barytes, and cement dust, some by hand-shaker application and others by agricultural mechanical duster (Toxine) without removal of the clothing. This was the first attempt to dust mechanically any considerable group of people. Unfortunately, owing to an unrecognized defect in the duster used, only about one half as much insecticide was used on the machine-dusted groups as on the shaker-dusted groups.

The results of Experiment II are not as clear cut as one might wish, owing in part to the large number of variables present. It is apparent, however, that even in the face of constant exposure to reinfestation, six of the eight test groups treated with the variously prepared and applied insecticides, had greatly reduced louse burdens 1 month after a single application. Only in groups 5 and 7, in which about one half of the usual amount of 5 per cent DDT per person was used, were the results poor. That these poor results were to be attributed to the small amount of DDT actually applied rather than to the method of application is suggested by the fact that the same amount of 10 per cent DDT applied in the same way (groups 9 and 11) gave satisfactory results.

The data suggest that good results can be gotten when an adequate amount of 5 per cent DDT is used, but that 10 per cent powder affords a better margin of safety.

Epidemiologically, these results indicate that monthly powdering with DDT of persons subject to constant reinfestation will prevent them from becoming an important source of typhus dissemination.

No significant evidence was found for the superiority of solvent mixed over mechanically mixed powder. There is some suggestion that barytes may be a better diluent than is cement dust.

Experiment III

Although the results with cement dust in Experiment II were not quite so favorable as those with barytes it was felt that the great advantage in weight justified further tests of DDT in cement dust. Experiment III was set up in Ward II, under conditions favoring heavy reinfestation to test:

1. 10 per cent DDT in cement dust, to which had been added 2 per cent cresyl acetate, applied by agricultural duster (Corona) by hand.

2. 10 per cent DDT in cement dust without cresyl acetate applied by agricultural duster (Corona) and by hand.

3. MYL applied by Dobbins No. 133 duster and by hand.

4. Repeated hand picking and removal of lice from clothing.

The results of Experiment III suggest the following conclusions:

1. DDT is slow to act but continues to exercise an influence on the louse population for several weeks.

2. The addition of 2 per cent cresyl acetate to 10 per cent DDT powder is without apparent advantage.

3. MYL is more rapidly effective than is DDT but has a more limited residual action.

4. The mechanical application of insecticide without removal of the clothing gives results comparable with those observed after hand applica-

tion. There is some suggestion in the results that the insecticide blown forcibly into the texture of the clothing may have a more prolonged effect than has insecticide which is just shaken on the cloth.

5. Weekly hand picking of lice from the clothing does not appreciably reduce the total louse population where reinfestation with adult egg-laying forms occurs constantly.

Observations on Lousiness Made During the Course of Experiments I, II, and III

It is apparent under the conditions of life at the Maison-Carrée Prison that the great majority of viable ova hatch before day 10 or 11 after egg laying ceases. The fact that this period is so short may be in part explained by the fact that the prisoners wore their clothing day and night and that the warm weather persisted during the first two experiments.

The number of lice found on a given individual often varied from week to week in the absence of treatment. This was sometimes due to changing clothes, to washing clothes, and to very recent hand picking of lice.

Very few head lice were seen, possibly because the heads of the prisoners are close-clipped periodically.

Surprising numbers of lice and some ova were found on the blankets, which were used only at night. The blanket undoubtedly served as an important source of reinfestation in Ward II, where blankets were not powdered.

Lice were found to show a distinct preference for certain regions of the body. The seams at the armpit, the neck, the waist, and the crotch were particularly favored. When only a few lice were present, they were generally confined to these areas. On the other hand, when a prisoner was heavily infested, lice were found widely distributed all over the clothing and bedding.

A very noticeable preference was noted for certain types of cloth. Cases were observed in which several hundred lice were present on the shirt with practically none on the trousers. In other cases large numbers of lice were counted on the trousers with few or none on the shirt. In these cases the distribution was correlated with the material and weave of the cloth in the garment. Those making the observations in the prison came to know which types of cloth were favored by lice and could predict the distribution on a given individual before examination.

The average louse count increased rapidly after the cool weather began. The weather during July, August, and September was hot and clear but a sudden change to colder and rainy weather came early in October. The louse count rose rapidly at this time. This may be attributed to the fact that without adequate changes of clothing the men ceased to remove their clothing for washing, tended to huddle together indoors, and often wore their blankets both day and night.

SECTION II. FIELD PROGRAM IN L'ARBA COMMUNE, ALGERIA

The work at the prison had established the efficacy of MYL and DDT on people naturally infested with lice but confined within narrow limits and subject to prison discipline. Before undertaking epidemic control with the methods used in the prison, it seemed desirable to get experience in de-lousing a civilian population in which individuals were free to come and go as they pleased. Discussions with Dr. Edmond Sergent and Dr. Béguet of the Institut Pasteur, Algiers, and Dr. Grenoilleau, Director of Health for Algeria, led to the selection of L'Arba, which lies some 30 kilometers south of Algiers, as the site for such a study. Late in August, the commune of L'Arba was visited and the approval of the Mayor and the Caid obtained for a delousing program, to begin in October, after the end of Ramadan.

Typhus had been present in L'Arba during the seasons 1941–1942 and 1942–1943. Within the town proper live approximately 1500 Europeans, mostly French, and 3500 Arabs. That lice were present in the community was demonstrated on the first visit. Rapid examination of the collars and shoulder yokes of the upper garments of several boys at the school showed all to have lice.

It was hoped that information could be gained from the work in L'Arba on (1) means of establishing contact with and handling the people to be treated, (2) methods of applying delousing powder to free civilians, (3) type of records to be kept, and (4) availability of labor for the delousing of Arab populations.

It was decided that the delousing work at L'Arba would be based on the use of two applications of MYL powder per individual with an interval of 14 days between applications.

Preliminary Trial in Lotissement Bugeaud

It was agreed with local officials of L'Arba that a demonstration of de-lousing methods would be conducted in Lotissement Bugeaud, part of a ward-like subdivision near the town hall with some 600 inhabitants, mostly Arab.

The initial demonstration followed the general plan used in Mexico. The streets in the section were not named, and the houses did not have numbers. The first step, therefore, was the drafting of a map to orient teams of field workers.

The actual work of delousing began on October 11, 1943 Workers were organized into three teams of three members each—one person having had experience in the work at Maison-Carrée plus one male and one female assistant. Two of the women were French public health nurses. The third was an Arab girl, about 15 years old; permission had been obtained from her family for participation in the work, and it was hoped that her example would encourage other Arab women to accept employment. It was anticipated that the experience gained here would qualify these women for later supervisory work.

The population of the lotissement was divided into 3 approximately equal portions and a section assigned to each team. The team carried a basket containing the following equipment: a map of the lotissement, a clipboard with 2 sets of forms, one for recording census, louse incidence and powdered individuals and the other a daily team summary, a piece of chalk for marking the house numbers, a flashlight, a supply of MYL powder in 2-ounce paper envelopes, a Dobbins Superbuilt hand duster, a 1-liter bottle containing a 5 per cent emulsion of phenyl Cellosolve lotion for treatment of heads, and a supply of absorbent tissues to protect the eyes of the subject during the treatment of his head.

Each team began work at a different designated point on the map. Arab houses are built around a central uncovered court and because the light was usually better and the space greater than in the rooms, most of the treatments were given in the courtyards. The number of the families in the court was determined; names and ages of the members of each family were listed on the individual record form under the father's name. The name of the wife followed that of the husband; the children were listed in order of their age. If there was more than one wife, children were listed under the mother's name. After completion of the family census the treatment of individuals began.

Usually in each household a child of 8 to 12 years was selected as the first individual to be deloused. The children regarded it as a game and were perfectly willing to submit to powdering. The response of these children generally removed the hesitancy of older and younger members of the family.

Before application of powder, the collar, shoulder yoke, and armpits of the upper garments were examined for lice. The presence of either lice or viable eggs was used as an index of lousiness. Lousiness was recorded as zero, slight, or heavy.

Treatment of the subject began with the application of powder to the clothing. With the exception of the treatment of the head, the procedure used in applying powder to the clothing was that outlined previously.

When powdering of the clothing had been completed the person was seated, and the hair treated with phenyl Cellosolve lotion. The individual was given a piece of absorbent tissue and instructed to hold it in place against the forehead and over the eyes. Lotion was shaken from the bottle into the hair and rubbed in by hand until the hair was thoroughly wetted. The piece of absorbent tissue was then used to wipe the forehead and hair to prevent lotion from reaching the eyes. When treatment of all residents present in the house had been finished, the team moved to the adjoining house and so on until their section of the lotissement had been finished.

First treatments in lotissement Bugeaud were completed in October 14. The second application started on October 18 and was carried out by a single team consisting of one doctor, a French nurse, and the Arab girl. This second series of treatments was finished on October 25.

The work in L'Arba was interrupted by the invitation of the Surgeon's Office NATOUSA to conduct a delousing demonstration in prisoner of war camps. As personnel again became available to continue the program in L'Arba, a survey of the initial experience in Lotissement Bugeaud showed that (1) Arab men are not able to enter houses other than those of their immediate families and are of little use in house-to-house work; (2) treatment of Arab women and female children would have to be done entirely by doctors, nurses, or women workers; (3) Arabs were willing to accept treatment (only 1.7 per cent of the inhabitants of Lotissement Bugeaud refused to be treated); and (4) Arabs expressed their appreciation at being freed of lice, fleas, and other body-infesting insects. While the difficulty of obtaining employees for delousing Arab women remained a problem of considerable importance, the willingness of the Arabs to accept delousing measures and their desire for additional work in the community encouraged the consideration of a larger program in the area.

Expansion of Program in L'Arba Commune

On November 2 the Mayor of L'Arba and Monsieur Mohieddine, grandson of the Caid, were consulted regarding the expansion of the delousing program. Since the men from the douars (mountain districts) came in to L'Arba at least once a week to trade, they would be a constant source of reinfestation for the villagers if they and their families were unpowdered. This would mean the treatment of approximately 10,000 additional persons, but it offered an opportunity to gain valuable experience. Moreover, lousiness in the douars was universal, and typhus frequently made its first appearance in these areas.

If delousing measures were to be undertaken in the douars, the people living on the farms should also be included. It was decided, therefore, to accept the limits of the commune of L'Arba as the boundaries for the delousing program. This area encompassed the town of L'Arba, with a population of some 1500 Europeans and 3500 Arabs; the six mountain douars, with roughly 8000 inhabitants; and approximately 100 Europeans and 1900 Arabs living on the various farms on the plain north of the town.

LIBRARY
HOLY CROSS JUNIOR COLLEGE
NOTRE DAME, INDIANA

The primary obstacle to the execution of the enlarged program was the nonavailability of female assistants. For a variety of reasons connected with the war; full employment of the menfolk; local, social, and racial prejudices; inability to transport and feed imported personnel; etc., the bulk of the work would have to be done with a very limited amount of assistance. The entire project was ultimately carried out by two staff supervisors, two public health nurses, and a 15-year-old Arab girl to powder the Arab women. They were aided from time to time by the leader of the local Girl Scout organization, two of her friends and some of their young charges working on a voluntary basis.

A central base of operations was established in a combination garage-stable located in the ground floor of a dwelling house. This was the most suitable site available and it served as headquarters, powdering station, and supply depot. Three of the staff found living accommodations with the family occupying the house.

In spite of these unimpressive facilities and the nature of the problem being attacked, as well as the doubts expressed by early advisors, the project was well received and won the active cooperation of the local religious, educational, political, and medical leadership.

VILLAGE HOUSE-TO-HOUSE DUSTING. It was decided to start the delousing work in L'Arba in the section of the town known as Lotissement Eglise. The Mayor and the representative of the Caid felt that the Arabs would be more receptive to the program if house-to-house work was used in the beginning as had been done in Lotissement Bugeaud. In accordance with their wishes the work in Lotissement Eglise was planned on this basis.

In general the sections of the town in which the Arabs live do not have named streets and numbered houses. Since it was desired to have a record of the location of treated and untreated families and individuals, the first step was the drafting of a map. A rough sketch map was considered sufficient for the purpose of locating individual families and for assigning work to the census and delousing teams. The limits of the lotissements of L'Arba are quite definite and are generally known by the residents of the town; this greatly facilitated mapping. Several copies of the map were then made so that one could be supplied to each of the powdering teams.

The lotissement was divided into three approximately equal areas. The work assignment for a given delousing team was indicated on the map supplied it. Teams were directed to begin at the lowest number and work the families in order.

The powdering teams for Lotissement Eglise were made up of three females each; one recorded the census of the family while the two others applied the insecticide.

MYL was used on both the head and clothing in treating Lotissement Eglise, since the liquid pediculicide for the head required extra equipment and material. The women offered no objection to having their heads powdered.

TEMPORARY POWDERING STATIONS IN L'ARBA VILLAGE. House-to-house work as conducted in the Lotissement Eglise gave a relatively high percentage of coverage (91.8 per cent), but the number of treatments per man-hour of work was low. Inquiries showed that a fair proportion of the inhabitants of Lotissement Djipoulou were willing to come to the djama (community house) to be dusted. The area was therefore mapped and censused and the people notified when to present themselves at the djama for powdering. As they appeared and were treated they were checked off on the census lists. This system resulted in an increase in the number of persons treated per man-hour of work.

A further modification in the plan of operations was made in Lotissement Medjabri because it had been found in Djipoulou that valuable working time was lost in checking the census lists to locate the names of applicants for treatment. To overcome this difficulty when the census of Lotissement Medjabri was made each family was given a numbered ticket which was to be presented when it appeared at the powdering station. This proved to be satisfactory and effected a further saving in time per treatment.

In those lotissements which had no djama, the cooperation of influential residents of the area was enlisted and temporary powdering stations were set up in the courtyards or others convenient places in the residences of private citizens. Sometimes only the women and girls were dusted at these stations while the men and boys were asked to go to the central powdering station to be treated.

These various schemes of operation at temporary powdering stations in the lotissements were combined with a program of "cleanup" work so as to reach those who had failed for one reason or another to present themselves at the temporary treatment centers. A small squad armed with the census list called at the home of each family that had been missed according to the checked census record. As a rule the girls and women were reached in their homes during the daytime by the follow-up squad. The men and boys were accommodated at a temporary station which operated at a set time after working hours in the early evening. This type of follow-up dusting helped greatly to maintain the relatively high percentage of coverage obtained in the L'Arba lotissements.

Temporary Powdering Stations in the Commune Outside the Village of L'Arba

The delousing program in the douars (mountain districts) outside the village of L'Arba was arranged through the cooperation of the Mayor and the Chefs de Fractions, or district leaders. Mapping and census of these outlying regions was not practical, owing to the scattered nature of the population and the difficulties of communication. The Chef de Fraction therefore assumed the responsibility of having the inhabitants of his districts at a convenient and suitable point in the douar for powdering at a designated time. Names were listed as the people were dusted and separate facilities were provided for the treatment of males and females. Estimates of the coverage in the douars were made by checking the lists of persons treated against the number of ration cards issued for the district.

The farms in the L'Arba plain were handled as individual units. Arrangements were made with the owner as to a suitable time and place for the dusting. He prepared lists of his employees and their families for use by the powdering squads. The men were usually treated at a central point on the farm while the women and children were dusted at the gourbis (family dwelling places).

Permanent Central Powdering Station

The name, age, sex, and address of those coming to the permanent powdering station were recorded. Checking these lists presented many difficulties, but insofar as possible the individuals who came to the station were credited to the lotissements, douars, or other subdivisions where they resided. This detail was somewhat simplified after the introduction of numbered tickets. The station was kept open until 7 P.M. every day and the bulk of its patrons were older men, youths, and children; women seldom came.

In addition to the central powdering station a certain amount of dusting was done in the market place on Wednesdays and Sundays, the local market days. Records of this work were kept and treated in the same manner as those at the central station.

Institutional Delousing

Early in the L'Arba program arrangements were made with the local school authorities for the delousing of the school children in their classrooms. The effectiveness of the treatment would thus be demonstrated in homes throughout the community and it was hoped that this would facilitate the general acceptance of the program by the adults.

With the assistance of the directors and teachers the work was carried out in both the boys' and girls' schools, the only difference in handling of the two groups being the application of the hair lotion to the hair of the girls. Most of the boys wore their hair very short and it was easier to treat them with powder than with lotion.

Records were kept of the names and addresses and the incidence of lousiness among the pupils.

Discussion of Results

During the course of the delousing project in L'Arba 9376, or 66.8 per cent, of the 14,030 Arab inhabitants of the commune were powdered. There were 4241, or 30.2 per cent, dusted twice; and 4671, or 33.2 per cent, were not treated.

Personnel

The primary problem of the L'Arba program was the shortage of female assistants to work with Arab women. It is impractical to attempt large scale delousing in the region relying only on professional personnel such as doctors and nurses to powder the Arab women. With the greatly inflated family incomes of wartime, Arab women are not willing to work outside their homes. With the return of peace and the easing of transportation and food problems it may be practical to import female assistants from the urban centers where some Europeans and less orthodox Arab women are to be found. On the other hand, if a community were actually confronted with epidemic typhus, local leadership would probably become more effective in solving this problem.

Problems of Community Delousing

The favorable reception of the delousing treatment by the citizens of L'Arba is better indicated by the low percentage of refusals (1.7 per cent) than by the percentage of overall coverage in the community as a whole. The obvious effectiveness of the antilouse powder and the personal convenience and ease of applying it without removal of the clothing were primarily responsible for the results attained.

Racial discrimination, a question which was raised during the formative phase of the program, never became a problem because the Europeans, both at school and in the home, accepted the treatment without protest.

Aside from the personnel difficulties already mentioned, the major problem of the project was administrative: What practical method would reach the greatest number of people? The treatment was acceptable, but experience showed that it was not as actively sought for as might be expected in such a generally infested population. The character of the response may perhaps be explained in large part by two factors: the almost Oriental indifference of the Arabs born of long association to the discomfort and danger connected with blood-sucking ectoparasites, freedom from which the majority of the people have seldom or never known, and the multitude of proscriptions that so completely hedge and limit the activities of Arab women.

By far the simplest administrative procedure is to set up a central powdering station and invite the people to come to it for treatment. But during the month of its operation the central powdering station in L'Arba was utilized by only 10 per cent of the village inhabitants as compared to 8.7 per cent of the farm dwellers and 3.9 per cent of those living in the douars. Moreover, 92.7 per cent of the patrons at the central station and 95.8 per cent of those treated at the market place in L'Arba were males. It is very probable that had other delousing work been going on simultaneously in the lotissements the response at the central station would have been much greater. Nevertheless, it is evident that this system would fail to reach most of the females and very young males. It appears, therefore, that the treatment must be made more convenient by bringing the facilities closer to the home and establishing rather direct contact with the people, as was done by the house-to-house work and the use of temporary powdering stations in the lotissements, farms, and douars.

Considering the distance involved and the difficulties of communication the response in the douars is worthy of comment. Many of the people in these mountain districts traveled on foot for several hours to reach the wayside powdering station in the hills. In two of the six douars all the inhabitants came in for the first treatment while in two others between 65 and 75 per cent of the residents were dusted. In the remaining two, Khodja and Bakir, which were the largest and the ones therefore where travel and communication was most difficult, the response was poor. They brought the overall percentage for all the douars down to 46.3. This figure is to be compared with 87.1 per cent coverage in the lotissements of L'Arba village, where precensus and house-to-house cleanup work established direct contact with the greater part of the population. In the douars, explanation of the program and notification of the time and place of the dusting was the sole responsibiliy of the Chefs de Fractions and the success of the work there was determined by the extent of their cooperation. Unlike the people in the village, those in the douars did not have the benefit of a convincing preliminary demonstration such as that in Lotissement Bugeaud, which greatly facilitated the work in the other lotissements of L'Arba.

In the village of L'Arba itself, where 87.1 per cent of the population was dusted, 72.2 per cent of the untreated group were males over 16 years of age. Of the adult males only 65.5 per cent were dusted, whereas 94 per cent of the rest of the population were powdered. Most of the adult males were employed, many of them on night shifts, in the military installations and depots in the area and it is believed that absence from home and personal inconvenience rather than a reluctance to be treated accounts for the high proportion of untreated males over 16 years of age. This interpretation is supported by the fact that in the douars where the men were engaged in the fields the proportion of treated and untreated adult males was about the same as that observed in the other population categories.

While the reaction to different administrative methods varied from one part of the community to another it is believed that in normal times a sustained delousing program would meet with a very favorable response in a population familiar with its benefits.

Second Treatments

A single treatment gave prompt relief from the discomforts of being lousy, which persisted beyond the date set for retreatment. The result was that the people could not be convinced of the need of exerting themselves to seek a second treatment so soon. In the douars where the most effort was required to get treatment, only 10.3 per cent of the inhabitants presented themselves for the second powdering. In the village of L'Arba where relatively little effort was involved, only 52.3 per cent were treated a second time. The smallest percentage of second treatments was among adult males, again the group that would have to exert itself the most to be re-treated.

Costs of the L'Arba Delousing Project

The figures listed are based only on necessary expenditures for insecticides, payroll, transportation, and storage; staff salaries are not included:

Total expenditures	U.S. $1580.10	
Total people treated (once)		9,406
Cost per person	16.8¢	
Total number treatments given		13,708
Cost per treatment	11.5¢	
Cost of insecticide per treatment	6.5¢	
Cost of labor per treatment	1.6¢	
Cost of transportation per treatment	2.5¢	

The high cost of the insecticide was largely due to the fact that it was packaged in specially designed shaker envelopes which had to be filled by hand. The use of the hand dust pump made the special envelopes unnecessary but the production costs were included in the purchase price of the insecticide. Bulk powder is preferable for use in dust pumps and much less expensive.

Transport charges were inordinately high, owing to the scarcity of vehicles and the market price of fuel. Much of the work in the douars and farms was done with a truck hired at the rate of $20 per day.

In normal peacetime the cost per treatment would probably be reduced to about one third that of the experimental program.

Treatments per Man-Hour

Man-hours are calculated on the basis of the total number of hours for which the workers were paid, not the actual time spent in dusting, census taking, etc. The time spent going to and from a given place of work is included in the man-hours charged against each farm, douar, or lotissement. In the lotissements of the village the time spent in travel was slight, whereas it represents a very considerable part of the man-hours charged against the work in the douars. In small units such as lotissements Lamartine, Carnot, and Blandan, the women and girls were done by a single worker going from house to house while the men and boys were done at the central station. The result in these small units has an appearance of great efficiency when compared with the larger units where several crews were at work.

Control of Lice

Among the working class people and farmers of the L'Arba commune lousiness was almost universal. Indirect qualitative evidence of the success of the work was not lacking. Those who came for a second treatment frequently expressed their delight at being able to sleep undisturbed by lice, many of them for the first time since they could remember. Often workers were offered 2 to 4 eggs, worth 25 to 30 cents each, in exchange for a packet of powder. One or two enterprising young workers had to be discharged when it was discovered that they had stolen envelopes of powder and sold them at stiff black market prices as high as 70 cents each. Since there is little conceivable misuse to which the powder could be put, these incidents indicate that the value of the insecticide was thoroughly appreciated and suggest that were it possible to market the powder through normal commercial channels the community might do much for itself in suppressing lousiness.

Control of Typhus

There was no opportunity to determine the effectiveness of the delousing at L'Arba in the control of typhus. While typhus had been present in the area during the two previous winters, no cases were reported during the time the work was in progress nor were cases of typhus reported in neighboring communes. The opportunity of collecting data on the prevalence of typhus was lost by the transfer of Rockefeller Foundation personnel to Italy to organize the campaign against typhus in Naples early in December 1943.

SECTION III: Prisoner of War Camp Demonstrations

The experiments in the Maison-Carrée prison and the preliminary field test at L'Arba amply showed the practical nature of the method of applying insecticide to infested individuals without removing their clothing. Recognishing the advantage of this technique in the handling of prisoners of war, the Surgeon's Office NATOUSA invited the Rockefeller Foundation Typhus Team to stage a series of demonstrations in the Mediterranean area. The invitation was accepted and arrangements were made for demonstrations in Algeria, Morocco, Tunis, and Sicily during October and November.

A small stock of the U.S. Army's recently adopted 10 per cent DDT–pyrophyllite louse powder was available and it was decided to field test this new preparation in one of the prisoner of war (POW) camps where demonstrations were to be held. The following is a brief summary of the conditions under which the test was carried out and the results observed. The work was done with the full cooperation of the Base Section Surgeon, the commanding officer of the POW camp, and with the assistance of U.S. Army Sanitary Corps Malaria Control Units in the area.

A stockade made to hold approximately 1500 prisoners at one of the Algerian POW camps was selected and work was started on October 18, 1943. The commanding officer agreed not to add new prisoners to the stockade after the powdering had been done but did make some withdrawals during the period of observation.

The prisoners lived in pyramidal tents which were numbered individually and by row. Tents in various parts of the stockade were chosen at random and their occupants thoroughly searched for lice. Using the technique previously described, the examinations were made under the supervision of the Typhus Team by 12 enlisted men of the Sanitary Corps under the command of Lt. J. F. Stallworth. Records were kept of the name and location of each man examined and of the number and developmental stages of the lice discovered. The clothing of 252 prisoners was examined and 193 (77 per cent) were found to be infested. Of the 193 men 75 (30 per cent) had 10 or more lice.

The application of powder with Dobbins Superbuilt No. 133 hand dusters began on October 19 and was completed the following morning. It is of interest to note that although the enlisted men of the Sanitary Corps started the dusting of the prisoners, within a short time they had the prisoners themselves doing the dusting under their supervision. All the garments worn by the prisoners together with extra clothing and blankets were powdered. Between 1300 and 1400 prisoners were dusted.

On November 4, after a lapse of 16 days, two of the Typhus Team returned to the POW camp to supervise the follow-up examination and to observe the effectiveness of this first field test of 10 per cent DDT louse powder. The examinations were made by the same personnel as before. Of the 252 prisoners whose garments had been searched previously, 152 were still in the stockade. The examination of the clothing of 151 of these men failed to disclose lice. On the 152nd man 8 nymphal and 2 adult lice were found. Upon questioning, this man said that he had been admitted to the hospital on the evening of the preliminary examination and that he had returned to the stockade after the dusting crews had finished on October 21 and thus had escaped being dusted. His statements were confirmed by an inspection of the infirmary records.

It was concluded from these observations that (1) the technique of applying insecticidal powder without removal of the clothing was a thoroughly practical procedure, even when carried out by unskilled personnel, and (2) the 10 per cent DDT–pyrophyllite powder is a highly effective preparation.

Other demonstrations were held in Morocco on October 22, in Tunis on November 12, and in Sicily on November 16.

SUMMARY

Field work to test the efficiency of louse powders on naturally infested population groups and to develop methods for the rapid application of louse powders was carried out in North Africa during the second half of 1943. The powders tested were MYL and various combinations of DDT. Observations were carried out in a civilian prison, in a rural county with both European and Arab populations, and in prisoner of war camps. Administrative techniques tested included (1) house-to-house block dusting, (2) delousing stations, (3) local temporary delousing stations open only for a day at a previously notified time and place, (4) farm-to-farm delousing, and (5) institutional delousing. In the early tests in North Africa, the powder was dusted by hand from shaker tins to the inner surfaces of garments which had been removed from the wearers. In August, the first demonstration was made of the possibility of satisfactorily powdering the clothing without removal from the body. This was followed by tests of various types of hand- and power-operated dusting equipment.

CONCLUSIONS

1. In a closed population group where everyone is treated and the group protected from reinfestation from untreated groups, two treatments of either MYL or DDT at an interval of a fortnight may be expected to reduce lousiness immediately and prevent a dangerous degree of infestation during a 3-month period. Louse eradication in such a closed population should be possible with a few additional treatments.

2. Individuals living, working, and sleeping in close contact with heavily infested population groups show a very low infestation 1 month after a single treatment with DDT powder. Monthly powdering of native labor groups should almost eliminate all risk of such groups spreading typhus to the people with whom they come in contact.

3. MYL is more rapidly effective than DDT but has a more limited residual action. DDT continues to influence the degree of lousiness for several weeks.

4. The mechanical application of insecticide without removal of the clothing gives results comparable with those observed after careful hand application. There is some suggestion in the results that the insecticide blown forcibly into the texture of the clothing may have a more prolonged effect than has insecticide shaken on the cloth.

5. Vermin-infested populations welcome the application of insecticidal powders and will make some effort to be treated. The choice of administrative technique used will depend on the distribution of the population to be treated, the existence of transportation facilities, and the personnel available to do the work.

Selection 35 | Typhus Fever in Italy, 1943–1945, and Its Control with Louse Powder*

F. L. SOPER, W. A. DAVIS, F. S. MARKHAM,
AND L. A. RIEHL

A suggestion from the Office of The Surgeon General of the United States Army to the National Research Council led, in 1942, to the development of an effective pyrethrum-containing louse powder, MYL, by a U.S. Department of Agriculture group working in Orlando, Fla. Field tests of this powder in artificial louse infestations during the summer of 1942 gave such promising results that similar studies on natural infestations were planned for Mexico and the Middle East. Early in 1943 it was demonstrated in Egypt by the United States of America Typhus Commission that two applications of MYL powder with a 14-day interval between treatments would reduce the louse infestation of an individual to a low level, and that with an adequate staff large numbers of persons could be deloused at central powder stations in spite of the time consumed in removing the clothing of each individual for dusting. Furthermore, in a village where typhus was epidemic, the spread of the disease ceased following the delousing treatment.

Later in 1943, in Algeria, a technique was evolved for blowing louse powder on the inner surfaces of garments, especially those next the skin, without undressing the person treated. Tests of MYL and the then new DDT powders, carried out in the absence of typhus infection but controlled by louse counts before and for a considerable period after hand or mechanical application of the powders, indicated that either should be efficacious in arresting transmission of epidemic typhus.

Since a résumé of the Naples epidemic with an account of the measures instituted for its arrest has appeared, the present report will not attempt to relate the particular activity of each of the organizations which collaborated in the fight against typhus in Naples. Rather, it will describe the evolution of the epidemic and the persons affected thereby, it will discuss the measures instituted for the control of the outbreak and evaluate their merits, and it will describe in some detail the techniques and procedures

* The authors were all members of the Typhus Team of the Rockefeller Foundation Health Commission.

This article was originally published (52) in the *American Journal of Hygiene* 45: 305–334, 1947. (Eight figures have been omitted.)

recommended for applying louse powder in the event of subsequent typhus outbreaks.

The typhus team of the Rockefeller Foundation Health Commission organized and administered the delousing service in Naples under Col. W. H. Crichton (British), Public Health Officer, Allied Military Government (AMG), Region III, 15th Army Group, from December 9, 1943, to January 2, 1944; continued in charge of the mass delousing section of the typhus control service under Brig. Gen. Leon A. Fox and Col. Harry A. Bishop, United States of America Typhus Commission, January 3 to February 19, 1944; and resumed full responsibility for all delousing under Brig. G. S. Parkinson and Lt. Cols. W. C. Williams and Gordon Frizelle, director and deputy directors of the Public Health Sub-Commission for Italy, from February 20, 1944, to July 31, 1945.

Administrative personnel were drawn from both military and civilian sources, including Allied Military Government agencies; the Municipal Health Service, Naples; the Public Health Sub-Commission of the Allied Control Commission for Italy; the Peninsular Base Section, United States Army; the North African Theater of Operations of the United States Army (NATOUSA); malaria control units from North Africa, Iran, and Iraq; the Royal Army Medical Corps (British); the United States of America Typhus Commission; the United States Navy; and the Italian Red Cross and civilian medical profession.

EVOLUTION OF THE EPIDEMIC

The earliest incursion of typhus in the mainland of Italy during World War II apparently occurred in late February 1943 when a hospital train bringing soldiers from the Russian front arrived at Foggia, where 281 soldiers and officers were hospitalized. The train then proceeded to Bari, where 226 others were discharged to hospitals. On March 12 and 13, 80 cases of typhus appeared among these repatriated soldiers. Two additional cases were reported from the crew of the hospital train, a third in the staff of the Red Cross Hospital in Foggia, and another in a soldier who had gone to Messina on leave from one of the military hospitals.

The first cases of typhus in Naples were reported in March among patients in the military hospital, one in a soldier returned by train from the Russian front and three others in men brought by hospital ship from North Africa. The initial case of typhus in civilians was reported at Aversa, some 12 miles from Naples, where the first of eight cases, all in the same family, had its onset on April 24. The diagnosis was confirmed serologically at the Cotugno San Giorgio municipal contagious disease hospital in Naples. This patient had traveled to Foggia province twice during the week preceding onset, making portions of the trip in military vehicles operating to and from the military hospital. The commandant of this hospital at Aversa claimed that there was no typhus among his patients; however, his records of wounded and sick included several typhus convalescents who were brought from North Africa directly to Aversa.

In July two cases were reported among patrons of a bathing establishment in Naples and a third case (Giuseppe Grassi) with onset on July 16, occurred at the Poggioreale prison, a large provincial institution located in the industrial area of Naples. Grassi was released on July 21. On July 28 he was taken to the Cotugno Hospital, where a diagnosis of typhus was confirmed serologically.

Poggioreale prison, the most important in the area, was surrounded by military barracks, airplane and locomotive works, and soap and textile plants. Several direct hits during the Allied air raids of 1943 rendered some of its pavilions uninhabitable. The bathing plant was demolished, and hygiene in the prison sank accordingly. There were no shelters, and while raids were in progress the prisoners were herded together in the basement. The inmates were almost all louse-infested, so that conditions for the transmission of typhus were ideal once the causal agent had been introduced.

There were many opportunities for the introduction of typhus into Poggioreale during the winter and spring of 1942–1943. The disease was unusually prevalent in North Africa at this time, and there are records of large numbers of prisoners, both French and Italian, who were evacuated from Tunisian prisons, some by way of Sicily and others directly to Naples. Dr. Saporito, Medical Inspector General for Italian prisons, admitted that there was typhus among the prisoners in Sicily* and that louse control there consisted of burning and replacing clothing because there were neither chemicals nor equipment for delousing. Large numbers of Yugoslav prisoners also passed through Poggioreale as late as April 1943, and the names of some of these appear in the infirmary reports.

The records at Poggioreale are restricted largely to the infirmary registers which escaped destruction when the rioting prisoners burned the personnel records in the late summer of 1943, but a number of the inmates were traced through transfer records at branch prisons. Following the case of Grassi, mentioned above, Vincenzo Petriccione, who apparently contracted the disease in the prison infirmary, became ill on July 19. On July 23 he went to Cotugno Hospital, where the diagnosis of typhus was made. De

---

* The first outbreak was at Milazzo, Sicily, where 37 cases with 9 deaths occurred among Libyan prisoners between January and April 1943. Twenty cases occurred among 130 Libyans at Nicosia in July 1943, just before the Allied invasion. No civilian cases had been registered up to the prison break which came in August during the invasion, but escaping prisoners may have been responsible for scattering the infection in Sicily.

Luca, a clerk in the prison, became ill with the disease on August 13 and Guerrino, one of the carabinieri, contracted it on August 15. How many other cases occurred among the prisoners and staff between this time and December, when the first cases were actually reported from the prison, is not known, but inspection of the infirmary records reveals a long list of suspicious diagnoses, and one is impressed by the frequency with which acutely ill prisoners were liberated or transferred to branch prisons.

Typhus appeared in men transferred from Poggioreale in at least four branch institutions. One prisoner with a fully developed infection was transferred to Casoria on July 17. In July and August the Poggioreale infirmary was filled to capacity, so patients from the prisons at Gragnano, Casoria, and Aversa, in whom typhus was diagnosed serologically, were refused admission. Some of these patients returned to branch prisons while others were liberated.

The Pozzuoli prison, a reformatory for boys and mental delinquents which was evacuated in July to receive the overflow from Poggioreale, is the most interesting of the four branch prisons where typhus occurred during the summer of 1943. Large numbers of prisoners were transferred to Pozzuoli on July 12, 26, and 27, and shortly after their arrival some 25 cases of typhus developed. One patient died only 6 days after admission, and onsets among the others began on August 5. When the disease was finally diagnosed the prison was quarantined, and the patients were sent to Cotugno Hospital. Of no little significance is the fact that during August, when at least 25 typhus patients were present, no less than 100 prisoners were liberated, 40 or more were transferred to other institutions, and some 25 escaped. In the mounting confusion of August and September in Naples these potential carriers of the disease were lost to sight. Many probably sought refuge in the air-raid shelters, locally called *ricoveros,* which were as admirably designed to protect runaway prisoners from the law as honest citizens from bombs. The ricovero in "Tunnel 9th of May," a main traffic artery between Naples and Pozzuoli, began to yield cases of typhus in August and September.

Although Naples is a city of nearly a million inhabitants, it is relatively small and compact. The tenement districts about the port and industrial areas suffered extensive damage during the Allied raids in the spring and summer of 1943, so that large numbers of families were forced to reside in air-raid shelters. These were large underground chambers, most of them old quarries for tufa, the chief building material of the region. Many of the ricoveros were equipped with lights, some had water and toilet facilities, and a few afforded some measure of privacy in cubicles built of wood or stone, but in general the shelters were draughty, damp, and almost always dirty. Most of their permanent dwellers came from the poorest sections of Naples.

There are no official or reliable estimates of the usual population of the air-raid shelters in the summer of 1943, but their estimated capacity of 220,000 must have been severely taxed during the heavy raids of July, August, and September.

On September 23 the Germans ordered the evacuation of a zone 300 meters deep about the port and coastal area, and some 300,000 persons were obliged to leave their dwellings on that day, which resulted in further crowding of the air-raid shelters. Among the evacuees were thousands who lived in the "Tunnel 9th of May." Typhus had been incubating in this shelter for weeks, and its occupants were now dispersed to the shelters beyond the 300-meter zone. With characteristic thoroughness the Germans, before leaving Naples on September 30, opened the doors of Poggioreale and Pozzuoli prisons and emptied their infested occupants into the already overcrowded shelters of the city. Owing to the disorganization caused by the German evacuation and the Allied occupation of Naples, this serious situation went unchallenged. Transportation and communication facilities were inadequate for the needs of the civilian health authorities, with the result that the investigation of reported cases, isolation of known cases and even the preparation of reports were all delayed.

Persons Affected by the Epidemic

The final record of cases of typhus in Naples and the vicinity from July 1, 1943 to June 1, 1944, may be classified as follows:

	Cases	Deaths
Civilian cases in Naples	1403	318
Civilian cases outside Naples	511	82
Italian military personnel	23	3
Italian civilian prisoners	37	11
Unverified civilian cases	46	15
	2020	429

The unverified cases were those not hospitalized or seen by the control service staff, and the diagnoses were not confirmed by laboratory tests.

These data and the data presented in Table 1 differ from those reported during the epidemic, when lists of cases were being received from various sources. Duplications have been eliminated by careful checking of the names and identifying information regarding cases reported in municipal and provincial health department lists, death certificates, hospital admission records and laboratory reports, and the daily reports of the case-finding section.

Only the 1914 civilian cases in and outside Naples are included in the analyses in Table 1, since soldiers and prisoners constitute specially se-

Table 1. Distribution of Typhus Cases among Civilians in Naples
and Vicinity, by Weeks, July 1943 through May 1944

Week ending	Naples		Outside Naples		Total	
	Onset	Report	Onset	Report	Onset	Report
July 4	0	0	0	0	0	0
11	1	0	0	0	1	0
18	2	0	0	0	2	0
25	1	3	1	0	2	3
Aug. 1	0	1	0	1	0	2
8	2	0	2	0	4	0
15	3	2	1	1	4	3
22	1	3	0	2	1	5
29	4	1	0	0	4	1
Sept. 5	5	3	0	0	5	3
12	6	8	1	0	7	8
19	8	4	1	0	9	4
26	11	7	0	2	11	9
Oct. 3	8	11	1	0	9	11
10	3	8	0	1	3	9
17	8	3	2	0	10	3
24	6	6	1	2	7	8
31	1	6	0	1	1	7
Nov. 7	9	5	2	0	11	5
14	12	5	3	2	15	7
21	32	12	5	3	37	15
28	46	26	6	3	52	29
Dec. 5	40	42	11	7	51	49
12	64	42	7	9	71	51
19	129	48	8	11	137	59
26	224	115	21	4	245	119
Jan. 2	189	199	18	11	207	210
9	137	237	23	24	160	261
16	143	153	35	18	178	171
23	117	116	57	25	174	141
30	64	130	31	63	95	193
Feb. 6	43	75	37	32	80	107
13	33	38	35	34	68	72
20	16	38	28	37	44	75
27	9	20	26	24	35	44
Mar. 5	10	12	38	22	48	34
12	5	9	17	42	22	51
19	1	3	17	32	18	35
26	3	2	13	18	16	20
Apr. 2	4	3	16	21	20	24
9	2	4	9	2	11	6

Table 1—Continued

Week ending	Naples		Outside Naples		Total	
	Onset	Report	Onset	Report	Onset	Report
16	0	1	10	21	10	22
23	1	0	10	3	11	3
30	0	2	4	5	4	7
May 7	0	0	2	11	2	11
14	0	0	0	3	0	3
21	0	0	1	0	1	0
28	0	0	0	3	0	3
	1403	1403	500	500	1903	1903
Before July			8	8	8	8
Uncertain			3	3	3	3
Total	1403	1403	511	511	1914	1914

lected groups. Of the 1914 patients, 91 per cent were hospitalized; and serological confirmation of diagnosis, based on Weil-Felix, Castenada, or complement-fixation test, was recorded for 61 per cent. Eighteen of the patients were nurses or hospital attendants and two were physicians.

Table 1 contains the distribution of these 1914 cases by week of onset and of report, for Naples and outlying communities from July 1, 1943, through May 28, 1944. Between July 1 and September 26 (13 weeks), 32 cases were reported in Naples and only 6 outside. During the next 5 weeks the corresponding figures were 34 and 4. In the following 5 weeks (to December 5), 90 cases were reported in Naples and 15 outside, bringing the totals of *reported* cases to that date up to 156 for Naples and 25 outside. During this interval, however, 209 cases had their *onset* in Naples and 37 outside.

The date of onset was that given by the patient or his family, and there was a tendency for these dates to cluster about days readily recalled, for example, 45 cases with onset on New Years Day. Likewise, the date of report is not always epidemiologically significant, since it did not necessarily coincide with the date of hospitalization or of dusting with insecticide.

Although one or more cases occurred in Naples each week after the middle of August, the epidemic rise did not actually begin until the week ending November 7, when there were 9 cases. It reached its peak with 224 cases in the week ending December 26. The recession was not quite so rapid, but by March 5, 1944, the number of cases in Naples by date of onset had dropped to 10.

Figure 1 shows the gradual rise of the epidemic in November, a sharp skyrocketing in December, followed by a reversal in the form of the curve in late December and a rapid decline in the following months. When inci-

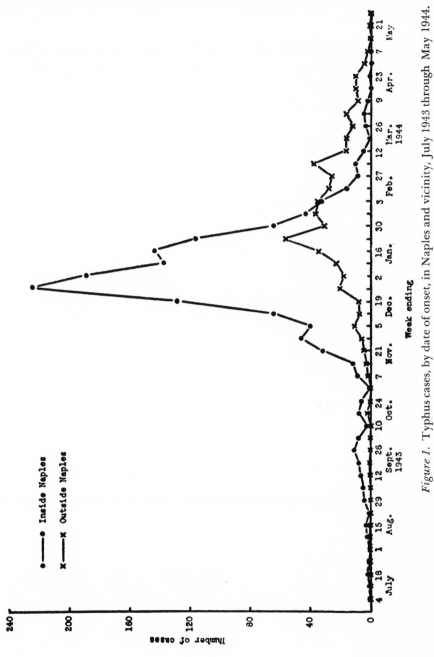

Figure 1. Typhus cases, by date of onset, in Naples and vicinity, July 1943 through May 1944.

dence in Naples is compared with that outside the city it is apparent that both acceleration and deceleration of the epidemic were more rapid in the city than outside. The median date of onset for the 1403 cases in Naples was December 29 and that of reporting January 6, giving an average lag of about 8 days.

The distribution of families or households with two or more cases is as follows:

Cases in Families

No. of cases	No. of families
2	130
3	49
4	42
5	28
6	16
7	9
8	8
9	6
10	2
11, 12, 16, 18, 20	1 each

Although louse-borne typhus is essentially a contact disease, only 1089 of the 1914 patients came from households having more than one case. The breaking up of families due to conditions prevailing in the city may have been partially responsible for this, but it is also probable that many cases were never reported. The application of louse powder to persons in the incubation period may also have prevented the spread of the disease within the family.

The distribution of typhus cases and deaths by age and sex are contained in Table 2, and in Fig. 2 the histograms showing the age distributions of cases among males and females are compared. The large number of persons between the ages of 10 and 24 years in each sex group is a conspicuous feature of figure 2 and may be a reflection of the breakdown of the normal discipline and order of family life in this wartorn area. Young people, when homeless, probably frequented the shelters, where the risk of exposure was greatest. Thus 9 of 14 cases recorded for one of the shelters were in boys from 13 to 20 years of age.

No less interesting is the greater number of cases in females between the ages of 35 and 44 years. Greater exposure may have been a factor here, and since women at these ages are usually mothers with numerous children, their illness disrupts the life of the family and they are more likely to receive medical aid and to be reported.

It is probable that cases of typhus were less well reported among young children in whom the disease may be mistaken for a childhood exanthema.

Table 2. Age and Sex Distribution of Typhus Cases and
Deaths, Naples and Vicinity, 1943–1944 ·

Age (years)	Cases			Deaths		
	Male	Female	Total	Male	Female	Total
0– 4	40	33	73	5	5	10
5– 9	70	64	134	2	3	5
10–14	124	112	236	2	3	5
15–19	175	134	309	16	13	29
20–24	94	121	215	6	11	17
25–29	57	75	132	9	6	15
30–34	55	77	132	16	13	29
35–39	50	109	159	22	19	41
40–44	51	97	148	24	27	51
45–49	59	70	129	31	21	52
50–54	35	64	99	20	27	47
55–59	24	35	59	14	18	32
60–64	15	24	39	9	15	24
65–69	12	11	23	11	9	20
70–74	4	9	13	4	9	13
75–79	2	2	4	2	2	4
80–84	3	2	5	3	2	5
85	0	1	1	0	1	1
Unknown	1	3	4	0	0	0
Total	871	1043	1914	196	204	400

The low frequency of cases among men of middle age may have been due partially to their employment on night shifts, which reduced their risk of exposure in the shelters, and to a large number of missed cases.

Owing to the uncertainty regarding the completeness of these data, attack or fatality rates derived from them would have little significance.

For practical purposes an assumption of universal susceptibility is believed justified. The only recent account of typhus in Naples was that of a group of 42 cases described in a bulletin of the Commune of Naples in 1927, originating in the winter of 1925–1926 from two small ships from North Africa, which entered the port without the formality of quarantine inspection. Vigorous measures appear to have suppressed the spread of the disease at this time. Prior to the epidemic, murine typhus was not reported from Italy. It is now known to be present in the area, but it seems unlikely that the disease is sufficiently widespread to affect appreciably the susceptibility of the population as a whole.

Although exposure to infection was by no means universal, the distribution of cases shown in Fig. 3 indicates that typhus permeated most of the 24 alphabetically designated districts of the city. Districts T, U, and W to

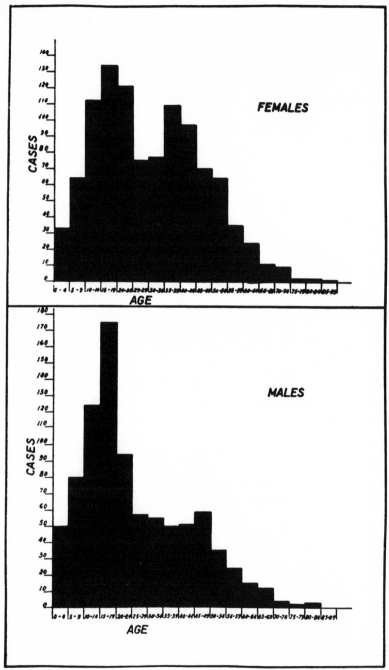

Figure 2. Typhus cases by age and sex, Naples and vicinity, 1943–1944.

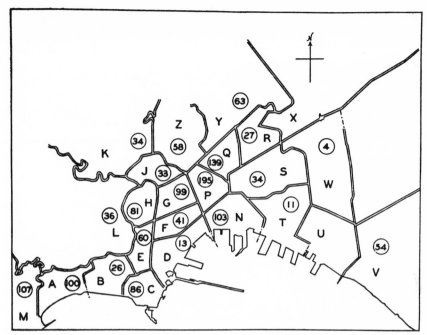

Figure 3. Distribution of typhus cases in Naples by administrative district, November 1, 1943, to April 30, 1944.

the east were industrial areas with few habitations, and few cases were reported from them. The evolution of the epidemic also varied within the districts. In area A, for example, half the cases occurred by mid-December, while in area V this stage was not reached until January 8. Areas A, C, G, M, N, P, and Q accounted for more than 50 per cent of the cases.

Outside the city 511 civilian cases were reported from 60 different communities of which 495 occurred within 25 miles of Naples (Fig. 4). This limited dispersion was probably due to difficulties in civilian travel as well as to less complete reporting of cases. The most remote point reached was Lecce and the greatest number in any one locality was 46 cases in Torre del Greco, a small, but busy, port at the foot of Vesuvius. This town like many others is really an extension of the city of Naples.

Epidemic Potential

The question of when a typhus patient becomes a menace to the community is not easy to answer. A person harboring a single infected louse is not a likely focus of disease spread during the period of survival of that particular louse. The individual and his own lice may remain well for 10 or 12 days or until the febrile period begins. The febrile period may last

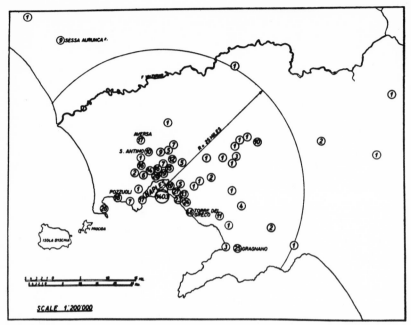

Figure 4. Distribution of typhus cases in and around Naples, July 1, 1943,
to May 31, 1944.

from 16 to 18 days, during which time the patient's lice may become infected and remain so until their death some 10 to 15 days after their first
infective meal. During this period the risk of transmission of typhus or-
ganisms from the patient to his associates will be greatest. Later in the attack when fewer rickettsiae are present in the bloodstream, the lice develop
their infections more slowly and the risk of transmission will lessen. In
view of the intermediate character of the period of potential transmission,
it was necessary to make an arbitrary assumption regarding its length, and
it was decided to define this period as one of 18 days following onset unless
in the meantime the patient had died, or had been dusted or isolated.

For each case reported in Naples, therefore, with onset between November 1, 1943, and April 30, 1944, the number of days (up to 18) elapsing between onset and isolation, dusting or death was counted. These periods of
infectiousness, when accumulated on a chronological basis, may be said to
constitute the *epidemic potential* of typhus with respect to the uninfected
population of Naples. Figure 5 shows the trend of these data when plotted
on a semilogarithmic scale, compared with the trends of persons treated
daily by the contact and station dusting services. The dramatic evolution,
progress and decline of the epidemic and the relation of the control measures to its various phases are clearly depicted here.

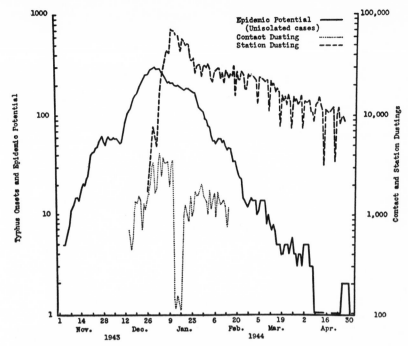

Figure 5. Typhus epidemic potential compared with the dusting activities, Naples, November 1, 1943, to April 30, 1944.

ORGANIZATION AND ACCOMPLISHMENTS OF DELOUSING ACTIVITIES

Headquarters for typhus control activities were established at the Provincial Laboratory on December 14, and delousing with insecticidal powder began on December 15 with the compulsory dusting of 700 passengers leaving Naples on the first passenger train to depart after Allied occupation. The first dusting crews were composed of nurses and inspectors from the Municipal Health Department. These proved to be intelligent, faithful workers and formed the nucleus around which the greatly expanded service developed later. Subsequently, recourse was had to personnel hired through the AMG Labor Office.

The delousing activities fell naturally into the following categories for administrative purposes and were initiated on the date indicated:

1. Contact delousing (December 16, 1943).

2. Air-raid-shelter delousing (December 27, 1943).

3. Mass delousing: (a) station (December 28, 1943); (b) block (February 6, 1944).

4. Flying squadron for work outside Naples (January 8, 1944).

5. Institutional delousing (January 9, 1944).

6. Military and military labor delousing (December 1943).

7. Refugee delousing (December 1943).

There will be no discussion of institutional, military, or refugee delousing, and no account of the isolation and treatment of the sick. Casual reference only will be made to vaccination as a method of combating the disease.

Insecticide and Dusting Equipment

The Surgeon's Office of the Peninsular Base Section made 20,000 2-ounce tins of MYL available immediately. The Surgeon's Office, NATOUSA, sent 400 pounds of DDT concentrate by air and authorized the use of such amounts of MYL powder, up to 500,000 2-ounce tins, as were required until the Allied Control Commission stocks began to arrive in January. The relative amounts of MYL and DDT used in Naples cannot be accurately determined, but since most of the early work was done with MYL, to this insecticide must go the credit for the early results of the delousing campaign.

Hand dust guns were used in the application of the powder and the workers were trained to follow a definite procedure in dusting each person, for which written instructions (reproduced below) were issued, so that the chance of omitting certain points might be lessened when dusters were working under pressure. Most of the work in Naples had to be done with the small Cadet type of Hudson duster, which is the least satisfactory of the three pumps eventually used because it requires refilling after each two or three dustings, and its delivery of powder tends to be in masses rather than in clouds of dust. There were a few Dobbins Superbuilt No. 133 guns on hand, and later the Hudson Admiral No. 765 gun became available, both of which were found to be equally satisfactory and far superior to the Cadet duster.

Contact or Spot Delousing

The names and addresses of all typhus patients reported after November 1 were assembled on December 12 so that the homes could be visited and the contacts of the patients discovered and deloused. An immediate result of this work was the finding of additional cases hitherto unreported, and, subsequently, this discovery of new cases became an important function of the contact-delousing squads.

The careful records of names and addresses of families dusted and new patients found, which were kept by the squads, provided the data for grouping the cases by families. They also facilitated the preparation of block histories for certain areas, so that what families had been dusted and when, in relation to primary and subsequent typhus cases, could be determined. Such information has aided materially in evaluating the spot-dusting measures, which were those first employed.

In practice, all members of a patient's family were dusted at the time of the squad's visit but absent members were not sought out. The family was urged to see that such persons attended the nearest mass-delousing station. The squad also powdered those other persons wishing to be dusted who lived in the same or contiguous buildings. Thus the term "spot dusting" more adequately describes its work. The crew usually worked in the court-yard or street in front of the building in which the patient lived.

On January 12 this spot delousing by persons accompanying the case-finding units was reduced to the immediate family and household contacts. Later in the month, however, the units reverted to a more extensive cover-age and shortly afterward collaborated with the mass-delousing service in dusting residents of certain blocks in areas where typhus persisted or where surveys revealed an appreciable amount of louse infestation.

Air-Raid-Shelter Delousing

The importance of the air-raid shelter as a focus of typhus transmission was recognized at once, but the organization and conduct of delousing ac-tivities there presented certain problems since the work had to be done between 6 P.M. and midnight, when the shelter held its maximum popula-tion. The service was organized to care for the dusting of approximately 10,000 persons weekly. Six teams, each consisting of a physician and 12 dust-ers, made the rounds of some 80 to 90 shelters, at first every 7 days and later once in 2 weeks, as the number of cases reported from the shelters declined.

Mass Delousing

STATION. When contact delousing was operating satisfactorily and ade-quate transportation and stocks of insecticide became available, plans were ready for opening 50 public delousing stations with an estimated capacity of 100,000 persons daily. Sites in hospitals, schools, churches, railway and streetcar waiting rooms, and similar places were chosen with consideration for population density and the known distribution of typhus. Each station was under the direction of a foreman and an assistant, who were responsible for the conduct of the work and the keeping of the daily records.

The first two stations opened on December 28. The one at the Ascalesi Hospital began by bringing children in from the street to be dusted. Its record jumped from 107 persons dusted the first day to 577 on the third and 1625 persons on the seventh day. The other station at the Anguilli School had the advantage of a large pediatric dispensary in the same build-ing and its clientele was sent to be dusted. This station deloused 837 per-sons on the first day, 2200 on the third, and 3585 on the seventh day. The delousing stations became popular overnight, so that soon the sight of persons on the street with powdered hair and clothing was too common to cause comment.

The supervision of the stations was carried out by Italian civilian inspectors, most of them physicians, who had a varying number of stations to visit twice daily. They issued powder and pumps, checked the work of the stations and collected the daily reports of operating personnel, supplies received and used, and the number of persons powdered. When received at headquarters these reports were summarized each day to provide the supervisors and administrators with current data on the operation of every station. In a summary of the work of 33 stations operating in Naples on January 15, 1944, there were, on the average, 13 persons working in each station, and an average of 1611 persons were dusted per station. Some 2500 pounds of powder were used in the 33 stations, with an average of 21 persons dusted per pound. It was only by daily checking of the activity of the stations that a proper level of efficiency could be maintained.

A problem involved in the operation of the stations was the hourly variation in the volume of work to be done. Visiting hours at hospitals, arrival and departure of trains and the opening and closing of business affected attendance at the stations. The staff provided had to be sufficient to deal with persons coming to be dusted at rush hours, which meant an over-staffing in slack hours.

BLOCK. As the work of the stations progressed it became evident that a certain portion of the population was not being reached, since typhus continued to occur in certain blocks within walking distance of busy dusting stations. It was decided, therefore, to survey different sections of the city with a view to answering the following questions: (a) were persons living near the stations being dusted repeatedly while those at a distance were missed; (b) was the dusting of men, women and children of equal proportion; and (c) what proportion of those dusted still had lice?

For this survey, groups of blocks representing different sections of a given district were chosen and detailed maps and census forms prepared. By the middle of February the canvass had covered over 100,000 persons, of whom 77 per cent claimed to have been dusted one or more times. The percentage varied from 65 around the Poggioreale prison to 93 in Fuorigrotta. Approximately 20 per cent had been dusted once, 28 per cent twice, and 29 per cent more frequently. Of some 13,000 children who had been powdered, 11.6 per cent were found to be louse infested, as compared with 20 per cent of 2500 undusted children.

As a result of these surveys, squads were organized on February 6 to work blocks having more than 5 per cent of louse infestation, less than 70 per cent of persons with a record of previous dusting, or both. Where typhus was being reported dusting was carried out if less than 90 per cent had been previously dusted. Block dusting was begun when the epidemic in Naples was definitely on the decline, so that the crews were augmented by persons released from the contact-delousing section. After February 14 the residents of each block where a case was reported were dusted, as well as residents of blocks contiguous to the one containing the infected house.

Block-dusting crews always started at the same point in each block, say the northeast corner, and proceeded to the right, calling at every door, entrance or courtyard, moving from floor to floor in the same manner, until they returned to their starting point ready to begin the next block. The squad kept a record of the dusted and undusted persons living in each household and those who were away from home were reached at school or at their place of employment.

Flying Squadron Delousing Outside Naples

The flying squadron began work on January 8, 1944, investigating typhus suspects outside Naples and operating in much the same manner as did the contact delousing squads in the city. Household and neighborhood contacts of infected persons were dusted, and a search was made for new cases. The squadron also vaccinated contacts as well as others in infected areas. Although 97 per cent of the cases of typhus outside Naples occurred within a 25-mile radius (Fig. 4), investigations had to be carried out at greater distances, at times even in the zone of military operations.

Some of the infected suburbs of Naples were heavily populated areas, and for these a special mobile unit was organized to carry on more extensive house-to-house delousing than could be done by the squadron. A report of delousing and vaccination activities performed by the flying squadron is given, by weeks, in Table 3 with reference to the probable cases of typhus seen from January 1 through May 28, 1944. Approximately 630 persons were dusted per case seen.

It is difficult to appraise the work of the flying squadron because of the likelihood of reinfection from Naples, and because many persons residing in these areas may have been dusted in the city. In 7 of the 60 places outside Naples where cases occurred no delousing was undertaken and in 26 places where measures were taken no subsequent cases occurred during a 12- to 14-day posttreatment period, so the typhus potential in these communities must be regarded as minimal.

Summary of Delousing Activities

From the middle of December, when dusting operations began, until the epidemic subsided, over 3,000,000 applications of powder were made in Naples and the surrounding towns. Table 4 contains a day-by-day report

Table 3. Weekly Block Dusting and Vaccination of Contacts Performed
by the Flying Squadron outside Naples, January to May 1944

Week ending	Probable cases seen	Persons dusted	Persons vaccinated
Jan. 9	1	13	13
16	6	402	44
23	17	8,484	16
30	48	13,430	226
Feb. 6	24	12,150	193
13	21	11,075	77
20	32	20,457	130
27	27	13,758	26
Mar. 5	17	11,720	38
12	37	20,336	63
19	26	12,023	139
26	17	10,066	47
Apr. 2	20	9,636	65
9	4	9,967	28
16	22	7,675	9
23	5	11,284	21
30	8	11,143	5
May 7	8	6,640	17
14	5	7,697	7
21	0	6,888	8
28	3	6,360	18
Total	348	211,204	1,190

of dustings by the services in Naples between December 15, 1943, and January 15, 1944, while the work was being organized and developed. Table 5 contains the weekly report of all dustings through May 31, 1944. From the standpoint of economy of effort and material, it is now important to decide whether contact or spot dusting alone is sufficient for typhus control or whether this method plus station delousing should be employed in future programs.

Appraisal of Typhus Control by Louse Powder

For evaluating the effect of dusting with louse powder upon the spread of typhus, the outbreak in Fuorigrotta, which was epidemiologically a part of Naples, has been chosen for consideration. This community, with its 11,000 inhabitants, is the area designated "M" in Fig. 3. Various tunnels through a narrow, high land barrier connect it with western Naples, but for the most part epidemiological factors appear to have operated locally. The eastern half of Fuorigrotta, lying west of the Naples tunnels, is characterized by narrow streets, bad sanitation and housing conditions like those

Table 4. Daily Dusting Totals, Naples,
December 15, 1943, to January 15, 1944

			Service		
Date	Mass dusting	Contact dusting	Ricovero dusting	Institution dusting, etc.	Total
Dec. 15		700			700
16		435			435
17		576			576
18		1,060			1,060
19		1,387			1,387
20		1,311			1,311
21		1,569			1,569
22		1,391			1,391
23		713			713
24		1,345			1,345
25		1,131			1,131
26		1,404			1,404
27		1,767	600		2,367
28	944	2,042	600		3,586
29	1,765	3,078	180		5,023
30	3,683	3,386	500		7,569
31	4,041	1,675	447		6,163
Jan. 1	2,568	1,808	446		4,822
2	5,158	3,311	492		8,961
3	11,495	4,231	488		16,214
4	19,581	2,463	1,055		23,099
5	22,935	3,838	1,761		28,534
6	28,658	3,344	1,041		33,043
7	37,960	3,360	1,275		42,595
8	38,971	3,405	1,224		43,600
9	37,750	1,911	1,228	200	41,089
10	66,126	2,994	2,092	1,410	72,622
11	63,210	3,533	2,321	—	69,064
12	66,476	147	1,588	1,215	69,426
13	60,862	112	954	667	62,595
14	59,995	149	1,414	1,304	62,862
15	53,153	71	1,648	1,966	56,838
Total	585,331	59,647	21,354	6,762	673,094

of Naples. The western half contains two municipal housing projects, one of which consists of a collection of four-family cottages, each with a garden plot, and the other of a group of large five-story apartment buildings.

The town suffered relatively slight damage during the Allied air raids of

Table 5. Weekly Dusting Totals, Naples,
December 15, 1943, to May 31, 1944

Week ending	Station[a]	Other	Total
Dec. 19	—	4,158	4,158
26	—	8,864	8,864
Jan. 2	18,159	20,332	38,491
9	197,350	30,824	228,174
16	408,163	27,558	435,721
23	334,785	19,085	353,870
30	188,346	29,052	217,398
Feb. 6	174,000	24,829	198,829
13	165,493	18,815	184,308
20	147,701	16,742	164,443
27	144,200	20,534	164,734
Mar. 5	139,355	20,664	160,019
12	130,829	18,046	148,875
19	102,421	20,986	123,407
26	83,564	11,931	95,495
Apr. 2	80,902	13,197	94,099
9	66,887	8,914	75,801
16	61,883	16,954	78,837
23	64,442	7,675	72,117
30	52,455	5,933	58,388
May 7	29,732	15,606	45,338
14	24,281	11,215	35,496
21	6,403	3,206	9,609
28	4,550	3,367	7,917
29–31	2,307	1,762	4,069
Total	2,628,208	380,249	3,008,457

[a]Includes mass delousing in out-of-town stations.

1943 so that its two shelters did not have a large resident population, but the German air attacks in the late fall and winter caused many people to resort to shelters at night. Since the combined capacity of the two shelters did not exceed 5000, they were extremely crowded during the raids.

The first typhus case in east Fuorigrotta had its onset on December 1, 1943, but was not reported until January 6. The second case in this section occurred December 10 and was reported on the 18th. This patient had slept in the shelter and was the probable source of many of the subsequent cases there and in the Via Grotta Vecchia. At the other end of the town two cases of typhus had their onset in the municipal housing developments on December 2. The people in this section used the shelter in Rione Duca d'Aosta.

Contact and spot dusting with louse powder began in Fuorigrotta on December 20, and, as elsewhere, disinfestation was welcomed by the people.

In the western end of the community more persons per case were dusted, owing to the greater density of population, with the result that here only one case had its onset more than 15 days after spot dusting began. In the eastern section of the community where the population was more scattered and nearer to Naples the final case had its onset on January 29, which was 6 weeks after contact dusting was started in Fuorigrotta.

Because of the alarm created by the discovery of 59 cases during the first week of January, a mass-delousing station was opened on January 7 and nearly 20,000 dustings were done in the first 5 days. Beginning with January 24th, applicants were refused dusting if they had been powdered during the previous 2 weeks. In the subsequent survey of Fuorigrotta 93 per cent of the people said they had been dusted, 15 per cent once, 32 per cent twice, and 46 per cent more than twice. When the station was closed at the end of April over 58,000 dustings had been done, representing an expenditure of 1.5 tons of louse powder in addition to the cost of labor and supervision. Could the job in Fuorigrotta have been accomplished with less money and material?

A criterion for determining the effectiveness of dusting operations must now be considered. Obviously delousing an individual during the incubation stage of typhus will not prevent infection from developing, so that cases may be expected to appear over a period of from 10 to 12 days after dusting begins, but when such persons are thoroughly dusted before onset the chances will be materially lessened that they will infect lice and so be likely to transmit the disease to others. Hence if cases decline in number or cease to appear after an interval of from 12 to 15 days, the presumption is that the treatment has reduced transmission of the disease. It is also obvious that with an average lag of from 8 to 10 days between onset and report, the effectiveness of control measures will be reduced. For maximum efficiency, therefore, the dusting service must be accompanied by an adequate and skilled case-finding service.

Figure 6 shows the individual cases in Fuorigrotta plotted in order of onset above the horizontal line and the same cases plotted below the line when reported. On December 20 when spot dusting began in Fuorigrotta, only 18 of the 106 onsets had occurred and of these only 5 had been reported. Twelve days later, on January 1, 87 cases had had their onset with the probability that none could have been prevented by the dusting. During the next 3 days 6 more cases occurred, but by January 5 the epidemic was virtually over although 13 cases had their onset between that date and January 29.

Figure 7 shows the rise and fall of the epidemic potential curve in Fuorigrotta plotted to a semilogarithmic scale. Between December 10 and 30, that is, 10 days prior and subsequent to the begining of contact dusting, the number of undeclared cases in the area rose steadily. The straight line

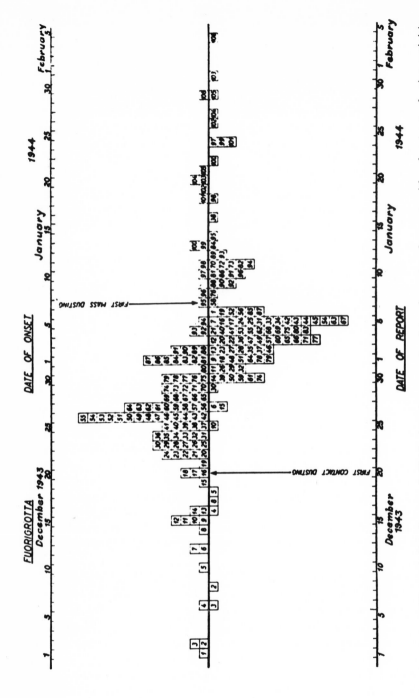

Figure 6. Fuorigrotta: individual typhus cases by date of onset and report, with reference to dusting activities.

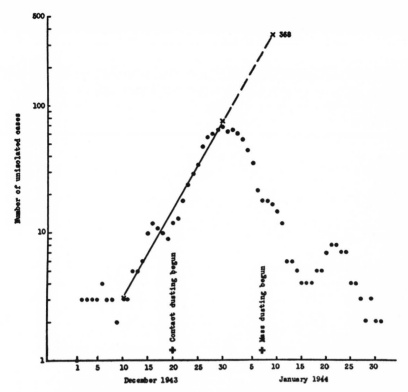

Figure 7. Fuorigrotta: rise and fall of the typhus epidemic potential with reference to dusting activities, December 1, 1943, to January 31, 1944.

fitted to the logarithms of the numbers of cases indicates a rate of increase of 17.2 per cent daily. If the curve had continued to rise at this rate during another 10 days, on January 9 there would have been some 368 undeclared cases in the community. Actually there were only 17. While one cannot prove that dusting was wholly responsible for the subsidence of the outbreak, one can confidently assert that it was an important contributing factor, particularly in view of the fact that no vaccinations were done. Figure 7 also reveals that the fall of the epidemic potential was not accelerated by the mass dusting activities begun on January 7.

A study of individual block histories in the city of Naples further strengthens the impression that prompt coverage by the contact-dusting and case-finding services resulted in early suppression of transmission. A single block in area P, for example, had 43 of the 195 cases occurring in this district. Twenty of these had onset after spot dusting began, but 13 of them occurred within 12 days of the first dusting. Of the remaining 7, 4 had been dusted before onset. How many patients in the Naples epidemic were actually dusted before onset is unknown, for the case histories are commonly incomplete on this point. From information available, however, it was ascertained that at least 10 per cent of the patients or their families were dusted prior to the onset of illness.

For Naples as a whole (Fig. 5) the peak of the epidemic potential curve was attained approximately 15 days after contact and spot delousing began. On December 10 there were fewer than 60 undeclared cases in the city, and by the end of the month there were over 300. With the exception of the work at the railway station, dusting in Naples between December 15 and 28 was done around typhus cases in homes, hospitals, and shelters, yet within 15 days after dusting was initiated the upward trend of the potential curve was arrested and reversed.

Thus spot dusting by itself was apparently an effective method of controlling transmission of the disease. The dusting stations probably also rendered certain infected persons innocuous by destroying the potential vectors, and the reduction in the lousiness of the population unquestionably decreased the likelihood of transmission by persons unfortunate enough to contract the disease.

STATION VERSUS BLOCK DELOUSING

The mass-delousing station probably offers the most practicable method of reaching great numbers of people in a large metropolitan area quickly, but for smaller populations block dusting is preferable because it affords more uniform and extensive coverage.

The relative efficiency of the two methods was tested in two small communities in the metropolitan area: Arzano, with a population of about 8500, and Casoria with one of about 10,000. Relatively little dusting had been done in either community before the beginning of the experiment. A mass-delousing station was established in Arzano after the town had been surveyed and each family given a ticket admitting its members to the station for dusting. Of more than 800 children examined before the station was opened, 33 per cent were found to be louse infested. A similar degree of infestation was revealed in Casoria. Squads with carefully prepared maps and family records then dusted all blocks in Casoria between April 3 and 12, with an expenditure of 107 man-days of labor. The station in Arzano operated from April 2 to 29, requiring 228 man-days of labor. Both communities were immediately resurveyed. Block dusting in Casoria had reached 86.6 per cent of the inhabitants and the residual louse infestation in approximately 3000 children was 5.4 per cent, while in Arzano only 53.9 per cent of the population had been dusted and 9 per cent of 2537 children were found infested.

Block dusting was, therefore, more extensive and effective and became the method of choice for most of the work outside Naples. Its effectiveness, however, depends on the availability of trained personnel and adequate transport, while the stations are more easily supervised and better suited to the training of new personnel for an expanding project. Finally, had an epidemic been present in Arzano, a greater proportion of its population would doubtless have applied for dusting.

Residual Lousiness

A survey in late April at 4 delousing stations in Naples revealed the distribution of residual louse infestation by age and sex of the applicants. Of approximately 9000 persons, 9.7 per cent were lousy and 66 per cent of those infested were males. There was less lousiness among both males and females between the ages of 10 and 44 years than among persons over 45. In the latter group, infestation increased with age, especially among females.

In July 1944 new surveys were made in those districts of Naples where the greatest number of typhus cases had occurred and the most intensive powdering had been done. The results indicated that the epidemic and dusting had not inspired any "louse-consciousness." Some 35,000 persons, including more than 9000 children, were examined. Of the latter, 641 (7 per cent) had never been powdered and had an infestation rate of 28 per cent, while 34 per cent of those who had been powdered were found to be infested at the time of the survey. In the Pallonetto Santa Lucia district, one of those most affected by typhus, 53 per cent of the children were louse infested at a time when practically everyone lived within a 10- or 15-minute walk from a free delousing station open 8 hours a day.

In late April and early May 1944, 14,584 persons were examined in 81 shelters, where among 5300 children, 8.5 per cent were infested. Routine dusting in the shelters stopped in June and another survey in late August revealed about 5000 still living there, with almost 50 per cent of the children infested.

It should not be inferred from the results of these surveys that DDT is not all that its champions claim it to be, an almost perfect insecticide. Mass dusting in Naples was not a louse eradication project; it was a typhus control measure for reducing the louse population to a point where typhus transmission would cease. Unless all the clothing possessed by all the people is dusted at about the same time, no more than a temporary reduction in lousiness can be achieved in crowded metropolitan districts.

Vaccination

Vaccination was not a part of the initial program in Naples and was used on a small scale for only a few weeks following the peak of the epidemic. From January through March 1944, some 26,000 persons were vaccinated by a three-dose technique and another 10,000 by a one-dose method, but nothing can be deduced regarding the effect of this measure upon the course of the epidemic. The 1190 vaccinations administered by the flying squadron outside Naples are reported in Table 3.

POSTEPIDEMIC ORGANIZATION OF TYPHUS CONTROL TEAMS

The civilian doctors who were released when the dusting stations in Naples were discontinued were employed to keep the public health officials and practicing physicians in the area alert to the possibility that typhus might remain undetected during the summer and reappear in epidemic form with the return of cold weather. The towns within a radius of 20 miles were repeatedly visited, with special attention paid to those communities where cases had occurred. The contagious disease hospital, as well as the infirmary of the Poggioreale prison, which had been one of the primary points of dissemination during the previous winter, was kept under observation.

During the fall of 1944 arrangements were made through the Ministry of the Interior for a series of meetings with the provincial health officers and their representatives throughout liberated Italy. At these gatherings the epidemiological and clinical features of both louse-borne and murine typhus were discussed, the importance of early diagnosis and reporting was emphasized and the technique of dusting demonstrated. Each provincial representative was required to dust at least 15 or 20 individuals under expert supervision. An emergency supply of powder and of dust guns was left in each province so that the local officers could do immediate spot dusting should typhus or suspected typhus patients appear within their jurisdiction.

These meetings began in October 1944 and extended to all but two of the southern provinces, both in Sicily. In December a similar instruction tour was undertaken in the liberated provinces to the north. Delegates from the three Sardinian provinces met in Cagliari. Also in December, the typhus control service, in cooperation with the Office of Hygiene of the Commune of Rome, supplied and supervised a dusting squad at the Prenestina railway station, where large numbers of refugees from the north were being discharged. This work was discontinued in June 1945 after dusting operations in the northern camps had been adequately organized.

POSTEPIDEMIC TYPHUS

Between June 1, 1944, and March 31, 1945, when the Naples headquarters were closed, 24 cases of typhus with two deaths were investigated; only one of these cases occurred in Naples. The patient, a baker, had arrived from Sicily only 10 days before onset, and his serum gave a positive comple-

ment-fixation reaction for murine typhus. The epidemiological and serological evidence is strongly suggestive that 17 of the 24 cases were of the
murine type. All were either food handlers or closely associated with ration
dumps where rats were numerous. In addition to the one case in Naples, 10
of the 24 cases were in the vicinity of that city, 6 were in Brindisi, 3 in Sardinia, 2 in Calabria, and 1 each in Sicily and Leghorn. During the months
of April through July, 1945, scattered cases were observed in northern Italy
in connection with the movement of displaced persons from Germany,
Austria and Yugoslavia. Spot dusting about these imported cases was done
by the local authorities who had previously been provided with powder
and guns.

At Cappizi, Sicily, a series of 39 cases with 9 deaths occurred between
March 12 and May 11, but typhus was not suspected until 26 cases had occurred, when the local authorities initiated contact delousing. As usual,
much powder was used after the epidemic was over. At Palermo typhus
was recognized in May after 10 or 12 cases had occurred and, in spite of the
local activities, some 25 cases and 3 deaths had occurred before the outbreak
ended. Figure 8 shows the distribution of cases during this period.

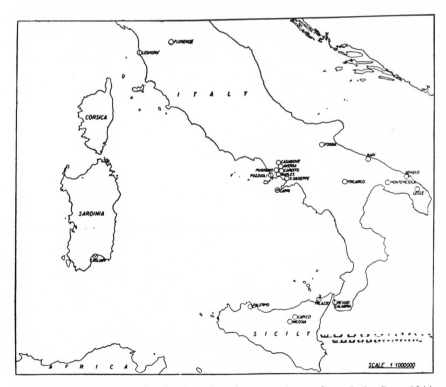

Figure 8. Postepidemic distribution of typhus cases in southern Italy, June 1944,
to July 1945.

RECOMMENDATIONS

Materials Required for Dusting

A motor compressed-air unit with multiple guns is a valuable apparatus for dusting large groups of people quickly, such as those in institutions, travel centers, demobilization points, ports, and hospitals, as well as in labor, refugee, and prison camps, where such an apparatus may be installed. With this implement the worker can dust more people with greater efficiency, since he is not fatigued by the operation of the gun. The simple hand-operated gun, however, is inexpensive, portable, and enables many workers to operate in a limited space. Dusting units with hand guns can be of any size, and additional dusters can be trained in a few moments from among the persons to be deloused. One person can easily carry a hand gun and enough powder to dust from 200 to 300 persons, and a pack mule can transport guns and powder sufficient for several thousand dustings. The most satisfactory hand pump used is one with eccentric entry and discharge air tubes to and from the dust chamber, exemplified by the Dobbins Super-built No. 133 and the Hudson Admiral No. 765.

The 10 per cent DDT louse powder can be readily blown from the dust guns. It does not kill nits but remains active and kills lice as they hatch for a considerable period, varying with the amount of insecticide used and the thoroughness of its application. In the Naples campaign 1 pound of powder was sufficient for dusting 20 persons, but in colder countries where more clothing is worn, a conservative estimate would be 1 pound for 15 persons. No evidence of sensitization or intoxication due to the DDT louse powder was observed during the Naples control activities.

Instructions for Dusting

Members of dusting squads should be trained to follow a definite routine in dusting so as to reduce the likelihood of missing one or more important points. The operator should bear in mind that the powder should be distributed on the inner surfaces of the inner garments and on the skin itself. Clothing should be removed from the first persons dusted so that the distribution may be observed. If properly done, the inner surface of garments should be covered and powder should be visible on the hairs of the chest, back, thighs, armpits, and of the pubic and perineal regions. Since body lice are most often found in the seams of the clothes, those about the neck, armpits, waist, shirt tail, and crotch of the pants should receive particular attention. A definite routine for dusting is as follows:

1. Dust inside the hat.

2. Dust the head, pumping the powder against the scalp, especially above the back part of the ears.

3. With the arms of the treated person extended at shoulder height at the side (not in front) of the body, insert delivery tube first up the right and then up the left sleeve and pump powder in between the skin and the innermost garment. Powder should reach the armpit and the gun should be shifted to eject the powder about the shoulder.

4. The delivery tube is next inserted at the back of the neck and a liberal charge of powder shot down the back, care being taken to dust the neckband.

5. The tube is next inserted inside the clothing from in front and powder sprayed first on the right side, then on the chest and finally on the left side, special care being taken to reach the armpits again.

6. (a) For men: The trousers are loosened and the tube inserted in front next the skin and a good dose of powder delivered to the crotch and pubic area. With the tube still in contact with the skin, the underclothing is powdered, with special attention to the waist and side seams. (b) For women: The skirt is lifted in front and the body and the inside of the underclothing are powdered as with men.

7. (a) For men: With the trousers still loose, the tube is inserted at the rear of the garment next the skin and the powder distributed over the buttocks and rear of the crotch. (b) For women: The skirt is lifted behind and the body and underwear are powdered. (If more than one layer of clothing is worn, steps 3 to 7 must be repeated for the second layer from the skin.)

Administrative Procedures

Contact or spot delousing is of primary importance in the event of a typhus outbreak. By the time a case is discovered, which may be several days after onset, infection may have been transmitted to the contacts, and these, when dusted during the incubation period, may be rendered innocuous at onset. Dusting only the immediate family contacts may not be sufficient to arrest the spread of the disease; hence all persons in the building where the patient's onset occurred as well as others in the neighborhood should be dusted by the spot-delousing squads.

Station delousing can be organized on a large scale with a minimum of trained personnel. Persons missed by the mobile units can be referred to a station for treatment. Also, the large-scale dusting reduces the louse burden of the community and for the time being protects those treated both from infestation by infected lice and from uninfected lice. Long continued work at a given station, however, is not economical because it is difficult to avoid redusting applicants, while an appreciable proportion of persons never applies for treatment. When trained workers are available more efficient work can be done by block-dusting squads, which follow a systematic plan that insures more uniform distribution and coverage.

Institutional Delousing

A minimum of trained personnel is required for this work since persons in the institution can be instructed and pressed into service as dusters.

Quarantine

It is virtually impossible to enforce quarantine in circumstances under which typhus flourishes, since infected persons can always find ways of avoiding barriers on fixed travel routes. On the other hand, infested and panicky citizens welcome dusting and when treated are relatively innocuous as travelers. All wearing apparel carried out of the epidemic area should, however, be dusted.

Isolation

Adequate care and hospitalization of the sick is practically impossible during a large typhus epidemic, and the public aversion to isolation hospitals is the chief cause of the concealment of cases. A thorough application of 10 per cent DDT louse powder to the patient, his clothing and bedding, and to the members of his household will greatly reduce the spread of typhus in the community. The patient should be hospitalized only if he requires and can obtain better care there than he would receive at home.

Vaccination

In the presence of an epidemic, mass vaccination should be undertaken only if personnel and transportation required cannot be used more profitably for case finding and contact or mass delousing operations. Vaccination should be available to doctors, nurses, assistants, dusters, and others who may be exposed by reason of their occupation to serious risk of infection.

SUMMARY

A well-seeded epidemic of typhus fever was revealed in Naples in November 1943, following the German evacuation and the Allied occupation of that city. The peak of the outbreak was reached in December and the trend reversed in January 1944. In Naples 1403 civilian cases were reported with an additional 511 cases from 60 points outside the city. Final cases in Naples occurred in April 1944, while those in outlying towns ceased in May 1944. None of the sporadic cases or small outbreaks observed in other parts of Italy in the following year could be traced to the Naples epidemic.

Delousing services were established in December 1943, so that an opportunity was afforded to test the efficacy of large-scale dusting with louse powders (MYL and DDT), applied with hand dust guns without the removal of clothing. Delousing was welcomed by the people and more than 3,000,000 applications of powder were made during the outbreak.

Examination of results revealed that the epidemic potential, that is, the number of undeclared cases in the population each day, reached its peak 15 days after contact or spot delousing began and before the effect of mass dusting at stations could have become operative. This was true of Naples as a whole and of the community of Fuorigrotta, where a more exact appraisal of the efficacy of dusting was possible.

Spot dusting of the patient's family and of persons otherwise associated with him is believed to have been an important factor in arresting and reversing the trend of the epidemic. Delousing in fixed stations and air-raid shelters and the systematic dusting in areas block by block, through reducing the louse burden of the community, supplemented the work of the spot-dusting squads.

During the winter of 1944 provincial health officers and their representatives were equipped with powder and dust guns to be used should cases of typhus appear in their jurisdictions.

Instructions for dusting with hand guns are given with recommendations as to dusting procedures in the event of an epidemic of louse-borne typhus.

Part X | International Health Administration

| Remarks Espousing Early
Regional Organizations of the
World Health Organization at
the First World Health Assembly*

My following remarks refer to the Provisional Agenda.

An examination of the provisional agenda of the Committee on Programme, the Committee on Administration and Finance, and the Committee on Headquarters and Regional Organization shows that no provision has been made for regional programs, for regional budgets, or for regional organizations prior to the end of 1949. Nor is there any proposal regarding the functions of regional organizations in the future. The failure to make provision for regional operations comes as a disappointment to the American republics, which during the past 2 years have given so much evidence of their interest in the regional program of the World Health Organization.

The XIIth Pan American Sanitary Conference, meeting in Caracas in January 1947, broadened the program of the Pan American Sanitary Bureau to correspond to that of the World Health Organization, and created a Directing Council with representatives of all Member States to correspond to a regional committee of the World Health Organization, as established by Chapter XI of the Constitution.

The Conference also acted to facilitate the participation of Canada and the non-self-governing political units of the Western Hemisphere. These measures were all taken for the purpose of making the Pan American Sanitary Bureau an organization which could function as a regional organization for the World Health Organization.

The American republics are greatly interested in the World Health Organization, but are most anxious that its activities be decentralized insofar as possible on a regional basis. One of the provisions of the draft agreement with the World Health Organization, approved by the last meeting of the Directing Council in Buenos Aires, stipulates that "an adequate proportion of the budget of the World Health Organization shall be allocated for regional work." But the Pan American Sanitary Bureau is not interested in regionalization for the Western Hemisphere only; it is obvious that it

* The First World Health Assembly was held in Geneva, Switzerland, June 24–July 24, 1948. Dr. Soper attended as an Observer from the Pan American Sanitary Bureau, which had not yet become a regional office of the World Health Organization.

These remarks (60) were published in *Official Records of the W.H.O. No. 13*, pp. 69–274 passim, 1948.

would be very difficult to establish satisfactory working relationships between a single regional organization in the Western Hemisphere and a centralized World Health Organization geared to handling matters for the rest of the world on the basis of direct arrangements between the Secretariat and individual governments.

American international health workers realize that success in the ultimate control of communicable disease must be based on a program of searching out and cleaning up endemic-disease centers, wherever they exist. Even perfect regional health work in the Western Hemisphere will not be sufficient to give protection from threats originating in other parts of the world. The unexpected appearance of cholera in Egypt in 1947 constituted a potential threat to Brazil and other American countries. Concerted action by health authorities of other regions must be taken if the American continent is to avoid exotic diseases and is to remain free of reimportations of *Anopheles gambiae* and *Aëdes aegypti* and is to avoid the importation of tsetse fly and other dangerous insects. Quite apart from the direct and indirect interest of the American republics in regionalization, attention should be called to certain very definite advantages inherent in a regional organization for an area.

Experience in the Americas has shown that general international conventions are not, in and of themselves, sufficient to establish satisfactory coordination of the activities of governments having common problems and common boundaries. Only through a regional organization with a trusted international staff, is it possible to develop a free interchange of information and harmonious action in attacking common problems. Regional collaboration is required for many problems in which the individual state is unable to act efficiently. As satisfactory eradication techniques become available for the solution of an increasing number of problems, the importance of regional action must increase rather than diminish.

In addition to the technical and administrative advantages of a regional organization, there is at this time a very pertinent financial argument in its favor. It is quite apparent from the budgets proposed that the funds of the World Health Organization are inadequate to solve the important health problems of the world. Eventually a considerable part of the international health program must be financed through the contributions of governments to budgets for the solution of regional problems in which they have a direct interest, as provided for in Article 50 of the Constitution of the World Health Organization. This development can come only after regional organizations are operating and after a demonstration of their value. This is the logical way open to increase the funds available for the program of the World Health Organization.

[Dr. Soper's participation in the discussion of regionalization of WHO is summarized as follows.]

Dr. Soper considered that the very first item on the agenda should be the organization and functions of regional offices. It was the experience of the Americas that one of the most important functions of the regional offices was the improvement of statistical information. Statistics would be the basis for the distribution of WHO activities and the yardstick for measuring results. The statistics which were at present being collected in the Western Hemisphere and furnished to WHO were very deficient. Field workers in statistics were needed to work with individual governments under a regional program.

The basic function of WHO was to create an administrative organization throughout the world, through which international health operations could be carried out. He cited the case of UNICEF: $4,000,000 was available for work on BCG, of which $2,000,000 had been allocated to Europe, leaving $2,000,000 for the rest of the world. The expenditure of that money should be made through WHO and its regional offices, but the administration of programs from a single center dealing with individual governments was extremely difficult. The items with regard to sanitary legislation, epidemiological studies, and health statistics, for instance, were essentially regional services. There should be, at the center, a system for the coordination of the work done in those fields in the regional offices. On the other hand, international standards, therapeutic, prophylactic, and diagnostic agents, and the development of an international pharmacopoeia were essentially central WHO matters.

With regard to publications, the Pan American Sanitary Bureau already had an important service of publications, particularly in the Spanish language. Provision would have to be made for reference and library services in the regional offices.

Dr. Soper thought that, as a question had been raised as to why the Pan American Sanitary Bureau still existed as an organization, apart from WHO, he should put before the committee certain facts which had not been properly appreciated by many delegates living in parts of the world other than the Americas.

The Pan American Sanitary Bureau existed on the basis of a treaty signed in Havana in 1924, which had been ratified by all 21 American republics and was the only one of the Pan American treaties so ratified. The treaty contained certain articles which, referring to the organization, functions, and duties of the PASB, permitted that organization to do in the Americas many things which the Constitution of WHO did not permit WHO to do throughout the world. It contained a clause providing that the Convention should become effective in each of the signatory states on the date of ratification thereof by the said state, and should remain in force without limitation of time, each one of the signatory states reserving the right to withdraw from the Convention by giving a year's notice in advance to the Government of the Republic of Cuba. None of the 21 republics had given such notice.

The functions which that treaty permitted in the Western Hemisphere were contained in Articles 54 to 59 of the Pan American Sanitary Code, and Dr. Soper said he would like those articles to be put on record.

Article 54 read:

The organization, functions and duties of the Pan American Sanitary Bureau shall include those heretofore determined for the International Sanitary Bureau by the various international sanitary and other conferences of American Republics, and such additional administrative functions and duties as may be hereafter determined by Pan American sanitary conferences.

Dr. Soper pointed out that under this article the Pan American Conference, which met every four years, had the full authority of the 21 countries to give additional administrative functions and duties to the PASB. It was under this article that the XIIth Pan American Sanitary Conference had met in Caracas in January 1947, 6 months after the meeting in New York of the International Health Conference, which had created the World Health Organization. At the Caracas conference, action had been taken to broaden the program of the PASB to coincide with that of WHO, taking in matters of medical care and the medical and sanitary aspects of social welfare. At that time also, the organization of the PASB had been changed, to conform to the type of regional organization laid out in the WHO Constitution, so that it would be possible to conform in every way to the administrative organization of WHO. At the same time, action had been taken to remove any political bars which had been thought to exist, and to make it possible for Canada and the non-self-governing political units in the Western Hemisphere to join the Pan American organization.

Article 55 read:

The Pan American Sanitary Bureau shall be the central co-ordinating sanitary agency of the various member Republics of the Pan American Union and the general collection and distribution centre of sanitary information to and from said Republics. For this purpose it shall, from time to time, designate representatives to visit and confer with the sanitary authorities of the various signatory Governments on public-health matters, and such representatives shall be given all available sanitary information in the countries visited by them in the course of their official visits and conferences.

Dr. Soper said that was a broad power in the Western Hemisphere, which was not provided for in the Constitution of WHO.

Article 56:

In addition, the Pan American Sanitary Bureau shall perform the following specific functions:

To supply to the sanitary authorities of the signatory Governments through its publications, or in other appropriate manner, all available information relative to the actual status of the communicable diseases of man, new invasions of such diseases, the sanitary measures undertaken, and the progress effected in the control or eradication of such diseases; new methods for combating disease; morbidity and mortality statistics; public-health organization and administration; progress in any of the branches of preventive medicine; and other pertinent information relative to sanitation and public health in any of its phases, including a bibliography of books and periodicals on public hygiene.

In order more efficiently to discharge its functions it may undertake co-operative epidemiological and other studies; may employ at headquarters and elsewhere experts for this purpose; may stimulate and facilitate scientific researches and the practical application of the results therefrom; and may accept gifts, benefactions, and bequests, which shall be accounted for in the manner now provided for the maintenance funds of the Bureau.

Under that article, the PASB was actually administering an antimosquito service in 1948 and 1949 in one of its member republics. PASB was working directly in that country; the service was under the direct administrative control of a representative of PASB, who was a health officer of another of the Pan American members.

Articles 57 and 58:

The Pan American Sanitary Bureau shall advise and consult with the sanitary authorities of the various signatory Governments relative to public health problems and the manner of interpreting and applying the provisions of this code.

Officials of the national health services may be designated as representatives, *ex officio,* of the Pan American Sanitary Bureau, in addition to their regular duties, and when so designated they may be empowered to act as sanitary representatives of one or more of the signatory Governments when properly designated and accredited so to serve.

Dr. Soper emphasized the importance of Article 58, under which it was possible for the Director of PASB to designate a health officer from any one of the 21 American republics to act as representative of the Bureau or of any one or all of the 21 governments without that individual having to resign or abandon his position with his own government, and in that capacity he was able to act for the Bureau anywhere in the 21 American Republics.

Finally, Article 59:

Upon request of the sanitary authorities of any of the signatory Governments, the Pan American Sanitary Bureau is authorized to take the necessary preparatory steps to bring about an exchange of professors, medical and health officers, experts or advisers in public health of any of the sanitary sciences, for the purpose of mutual aid and advancement in the protection of the public health of the signatory Governments.

Dr. Soper thought the committee would readily understand the reluctance with which the American republics would give up the possibility of close collaboration on the technical level which at present existed in the Western Hemisphere. The question had been raised as to the continued existence of PASB as an independent regional organization. When he had attended the third session of the WHO Interim Commission at Geneva in April 1947, as the newly elected Director of PASB, he had found that WHO had no plans for financing or organizing regional work, and he was very much disturbed to find that in the report of the Interim Commission no provision had been made for regionalization.

At the third session of the WHO Interim Commission, he had called attention to the fact that the discussion between the American republics and WHO was not a political one but essentially a question of whether WHO would have a large central organization or whether it would establish regional health organizations, which would make the influence of WHO felt by the people in the various countries. The PASB was not a political organization; it was not subject in any way to any international political organization. The treaty was entirely independent of any other treaty.

With reference to financing, he called atention to the fact that the United States had contributed only 11 per cent of the budget for 1948. At the meeting in Buenos Aires during the previous year, other countries had made voluntary supplementary contributions and had approved a budget of $1,300,000 for 1948, knowing that only $145,000 of that amount would be paid by the United States.

The PASB and the Pan American countries were much more interested in the development of a real world health organization than in maintaining independence for themselves. They realized that they could not protect the Western Hemisphere against the introduction of disease, unless regional organizations were functioning elsewhere.

Dr. Soper said he expressed the sentiments of the majority of the American republics in stating that they were very much interested in WHO, but, until such time as WHO was in a position to take over and finance the responsibilities of the Bureau, he did not believe the Pan American countries would be willing to abandon the organization which at present existed. He wished to call attention to the fact that, up to the present time, the Health Assembly had not discussed regional programs. The Bureau was continuing its work and could only indicate the broad field of activities in which it was working and ask WHO what it wished to take over as regional work.

He concluded by saying that the PASB was not asking for any special favors; it was asking for a regional organization and for adequate funds to be assigned to regional programs.

Dr. Soper feared that the resolution suggested by the working party had been agreed upon without full cognizance of the contents of a telegram which had been read out, but not circulated, at the meeting. That telegram contained the legal opinion of the United Nations that the interpretation of Article 9 of the proposed Agreement between PASO and WHO should be settled by the Health Assembly under Article 75 of its Constitution. Article 9 was the only article under discussion, and provided for the revision or annulment of the Agreement (by either of the parties) on a year's notice.

He pointed out that the Agreement had been approved by the Directing Council of PASO, and approval by the Health Assembly would make possible a final working agreement between the two organizations without further delay. Authorization had been given by the Directing Council (this action had been taken before any of the American states had become members of WHO) enabling him, as Director of PASO, to make the final arrangements with WHO on the basis of that Agreement. It was important that careful consideration should be given to the question before any changes were made, which might delay such agreement and might make it necessary to establish a temporary working agreement between the two organizations. He felt strongly that action should not be taken merely on the basis of the rapid consideration of the point by the working party.

Dr. Soper said he was glad the question had been raised, because he wished to emphasize again the fact that the Agreement which had come under discussion had been approved by the Directing Council of the PASB. But it had made a proviso that the Agreement should enter into force upon its approval by the Health Assembly. He thought it was essential to have some action by the Health Assembly confirming the final Agreement. The Directing Council was meeting in October, and, if the entire document were accepted as it stood, the final Agreement could be very rapidly concluded. Since there had been a question regarding Article 9, there should be a definite authorization on that particular item, so that it could be laid before the Directing Council. If a suitable wording agreeable to both parties was found, it would be possible to complete the arrangements between WHO and the PASB, so that the Bureau could begin to function as a full regional organization in 1949, without going through the preliminary stage of a working arrangement before the agreement had been reached.

Dr. Soper said he had been somewhat surprised at the discussion, because he thought the question was basically an administrative rather than a financial one. He outlined the development of the PASB from its beginning in 1902, with a budget of $5000 a year, to the present year, for which there was an approved budget of $1,300,000.

If WHO did not have regions, it would have to set up in Geneva special organizations for each type of work and attempt to deal with 60 different countries all over the world.

Dr. Soper said he wished to correct the impression that might be conveyed by a remark of the delegate of China, appearing in the minutes of the fourth meeting: "As Dr. Soper had pointed out, regionalization should be all or nothing." He stated that, although it would require a double system of administration to carry on activities in one part of the world through regional organization and in other parts through direct action by the central Secretariat and individual governments, he had not at any time considered the possibility of getting along without some regional organizations.

[The First World Health Assembly delimited the geographical areas of the WHO Regional Organizations. The Agreement, whereby the Pan American Health Organization has functioned also as the Regional Organization of WHO for the Americas since July 1, 1949, was signed on May 24, 1949. Brock Chisholm signed for the World Health Organization and Fred L. Soper for the Pan American Sanitary Conference.]

| Notes on the Progress of the Pan American Health Organization 1947–1950*

The developments during the past 4 years in the life of the Pan American Sanitary Bureau, summarized in this report, have been possible only because of many years of effort of a few individuals. Two preeminent figures in the life of the Bureau during the past generation have disappeared between the XIIth and XIIIth Conferences. I refer specifically to Dr. Hugh S. Cumming and Dr. John D. Long.

Dr. Cumming was the Director of the Bureau from 1920 to 1947 and continued devoted to its welfare as Director Emeritus until his death on December 20, 1948. Dr. Cumming was an outstanding leader in international health organizations; his memory is especially cherished by Pan American health workers, among whom he had a host of friends and admirers.

Dr. Long came into contact with Pan American health problems at the Vth Pan American Conference, Santiago, Chile, 1923, and from that time to his death in Guayaquil on September 18, 1949, never lost interest in their solution. Dr. Long was for many years Traveling Representative of the Bureau and at the time of his death was preparing to attend the Directing Council meeting in Lima as a consultant to the delegation from Ecuador. Dr. Long was the most important element in the transformation of the Pan American Sanitary Bureau from an information center to an active organization with numerous representatives in the field.

Dr. Long's patient work under great difficulties and with limited financial resources for the eradication of plague from the port cities of South America is an outstanding example of determination and resolution. Among Dr. Long's important contributions was his collaboration in the drafting of the Pan American Sanitary Code, 1924, which established for the Americas a liberal basis of international collaboration unequaled in the charter of any other international health organization.

Another whose passing must be noted here is Dr. Luis Gaitán, a wholehearted friend of the Bureau and an honorary member since the Pan American Sanitary Conference held in 1938, who died on July 21, 1949.

* This was Dr. Soper's first Director's report to a Pan American Sanitary Conference; it was read at the Inaugural Session on October 1, 1950, Ciudad Trujillo, Dominican Republic. The original Spanish text (*69*) was published in the *Actas* de la Décimotercera Conferencia Sanitaria Panamericana, Comité Regional, Organización Mundial de la Salud, published by the Pan American Sanitary Bureau as Publication No. 261, Vol. 1, pp. 37–44, 1952.

The period between the XIIth and XIIIth Pan American Sanitary Conferences has been one of gradual metamorphosis and expansion; Member States have been kept informed of developments through reports of the Director to the Executive Committee and to the Directing Council at intervals of about 6 months. A report covering the full 4-year period, January 1, 1947, to December 31, 1950, is now in preparation and should be ready for publication early in 1951. A preliminary provisional draft has been prepared for the information of Delegates to the XIIIth Conference. This draft carries much informational material which will be eliminated from the final report.

The XIIth Pan American Sanitary Conference (Caracas, 1947) was a hard-working body facing several difficult and complicated problems. The success of the reorganization and expansion of the activities of the Bureau have depended in large measure on the wisdom of the recommendations of that Conference.

The XIIth Conference entrusted to the Directing Council the consideration of proposed modifications of the Pan American Sanitary Code. The Directing Council at its First Meeting in Buenos Aires, 1947, after taking into consideration the fact that universal international regulations were to be prepared under the auspices of the World Health Organization, postponed consideration of the matter. A provision was written into the Constitution for suggested revisions of the Code to be submitted from time to time by the Director of the Bureau. It is anticipated that international sanitary regulations prepared by the World Health Organization will be submitted to the Fourth World Health Assembly in May 1951 and to the Directing Council of the Pan American Sanitary Organization later in the same year.

The XIIth Pan American Sanitary Conference established the bases for the present Constitution of the Pan American Sanitary Organization, which was approved in final form by the First Meeting of the Directing Council in Buenos Aires, 1947. Its provisions for the formation and regular meetings of the Directing Council and Executive Committee have been carried out.

The Conference also established the general terms of an agreement to be written between the Pan American Sanitary Organization and the World Health Organization. This agreement was formally signed on May 24, 1949, and became operative on July 1 of the same year. Through this agreement the Pan American Sanitary Bureau serves as Regional Office of the World Health Organization for the Americas. It is the first whereby a Specialized Pan American Organization has entered into direct working relationship with a corresponding Specialized Organization of the United Nations.

The Bureau has been regularly represented at the first three World Health Assemblies and at some of the meetings of the Executive Board of the World Health Organization. Likewise, the World Health Organization has been represented at each meeting of the Directing Council and some meetings of the Executive Committee. Although the finances and personnel of the two organizations are separate, considerable progress has been made in the development of a single operating unit in international health in the Americas. The collaboration of the World Health Organization has been devoted mostly to fellowships, maternal and child health, tuberculosis, venereal diseases, public information, and certain administrative functions.

There has also been success in the signing of another agreement. The Charter of the Organization of American States authorizes the signing of formal agreements between the Council of the Organization and Specialized Organizations. Thorough discussion by members of this Council and of the Council of the Pan American Sanitary Organization resulted in an agreement between the Councils of the two organizations signed May 23, 1950. This agreement fulfills the requirements of the Pan American system while at the same time it recognizes, but does not interfere with, the functions of the Bureau as the Regional Office of the World Health Organization.

In 1949, the Bureau drew up projects for the expenditure of UNICEF funds on health programs in Latin America. Later the Bureau became involved in the technical orientation of these same programs and in the preparation of other projects for UNICEF as the Regional Office of the World Health Organization. The handling of matters relating to these programs has required a considerable amount of extra work on an already overworked professional staff.

The XIIth Pan American Sanitary Conference determined that the professional staff of the Pan American Bureau should be inter-American in character and drawn from different geographical areas. In 1947 and previously, the professional staff of the Bureau had been largely composed of officers of the U.S. Public Health Service on loan to the Bureau and of special officers from other countries paid from special U.S. Government grants. Following the increases in the budget of the Bureau in 1948 and 1949, the U.S. Public Health Service withdrew its staff members, with the exception of a very few to whom leave without pay was granted. The XIIIth Pan American Sanitary Conference is the first to receive a report from the Director of the Bureau based on the work of its own professional staff drawn from a large number of Member States. With very few exceptions, professional staff members of the Bureau hold public health degrees.

The further development of the work of the Bureau's international staff is contingent on the provision of an adequate headquarters for the Bureau and increased financing. The XIIth Pan American Sanitary Conference stated in its Final Act: "The Conference also believes that the Personnel of the Bureau must be increased in proportion to the additional functions that it will assume, and points out the necessity for new quarters and an enlarged budget."

Through a misunderstanding of the actual financial situation of the Bureau, the XIIth Conference failed to take action to increase the quota payments of Member States. This failure forced the Director to take extraordinary measures. The Executive Committee at its First Meeting, May 1947, authorized the Director to approach Member Governments for supplementary contributions. Thanks to the timely generosity of certain governments, the Bureau was able to avoid bankruptcy in 1948 and even begin the expansion which has continued to the present time. Supplementary contributions have been received from Brazil, Chile, El Salvador, the Dominican Republic, Mexico, and Venezuela. (A 1,500,000-peso contribution pledged by Argentina in 1947 was received in 1954.)

The expansion referred to has been possible because of increased quotas beginning with the calendar year 1948. The 1948 quota was $1.00 per thousand population of Member States, in comparison with $0.40 per thousand during the previous 10 years. In 1949 the per capita quota system was abandoned, each country being assessed a certain percentage of the budget voted on the same basis as is used in assessment of the Organization of American States. The first budget (1948) approved under the new Constitution was for $1,300,000, but only some $300,000 of this was on the basis of assessed quota payments. Owing to inevitable delays in payment by Member Governments, expenditure at the rate of $320,000 for the year was possible only because of supplementary contributions as referred to above. (Although the budget expenditures of 1948 were considerably greater than those of 1947 which amounted to $176,000, actually there was a considerable decrease in the funds available for maintaining the activities of the Bureau, since during the year 1946 some $600,000, most of it contributed indirectly through agencies of the U.S. Government, had been expended.)

The increased appropriations of $1,700,000 for 1949 and $1,742,035 for 1950 have not been fully reflected in the rates of expenditure. In 1949 the Bureau spent only $786,000 and the expenditure for 1950 will not exceed $1,400,000. This delay in the increase of expenditures following the voting of budgets is due to delays in payment by Member Governments and to the fact that the Bureau must have a reserve at the beginning of each year sufficient to cover 9 months of operation.

Experience has shown conclusively that present budget levels are inadequate to meet the desires of Member States for technical services of the Bureau.

The inclusion of health projects among those of the Technical Assistance Program to be financed with funds contributed by governments is an official admission of this inadequacy. The development of such health projects with funds channeled through the United Nations and the Organization of American States has put a considerable extra workload on the already understaffed Bureau.

The need for adequate headquarters for the Bureau has been emphasized at each meeting of the Conference and in other meetings beginning in 1938. The Bureau moved away from the Pan American Union building in September 1947 but has completely outgrown its present home and has spread out to two small neighboring buildings. The available space is inadequate and some provision must be made looking toward the immediate solution of the problem as well as to the acquisition of suitable permanent headquarters through purchase or construction.

The presentation of this problem to the Directing Council in 1949 led to a discussion of the permanent site for the headquarters of the Bureau. The Directing Council concluded that this matter was of sufficient importance to be referred to this XIIIth Conference. The delay of 12 months has been most unfortunate but will have been eminently worthwhile if the decision as to the permanent site of the Bureau can be accompanied by the authorization of this Conference for the purchase or construction of suitable headquarters, in case these cannot be furnished by the government of the country chosen.

The recommendations of the XIIth Pan American Sanitary Conference with respect to specific programs included the following items: malaria, health education, brucellosis, rabies, typhus, plague, salmonellosis, trypanosomiasis, tuberculosis, venereal disease, rheumatic fever, and food and drugs.

Many of the detailed suggestions made by the XIIth Conference have not been carried out, owing to lack of funds or personnel, but some action has been taken on all the above items. Additional activities of the Bureau during this period have been related to the following subjects: the collection and exchange of statistical and epidemiological information, maternal and child health, nutrition, public health nursing and nursing education, hospital administration, garbage disposal, supply service, fellowships, training programs, hydatidosis, yellow fever, *Aëdes aegypti* eradication, smallpox, onchocerciasis, yaws, pertussis, diphtheria, and general insecticidal work.

In addition to the special relationship with the World Health Organization and with the programs of UNICEF, almost every program of the Bureau involves collaboration with one or more governments and in many cases with other agencies. During the period in question, the Bureau has had the collaboration of the National Yellow Fever Service of Brazil, the National Institutes of Health of the United States, the Institute of Inter-American Affairs, the Food and Agriculture Organization, The Rockefeller Foundation, the Kellogg Foundation, and certain commercial houses.

Special mention should be made of the Institute of Nutrition of Central America and Panama in which the countries in this region, the Kellogg Foundation, the Massachusetts Institute of Technology, and the Pan American Sanitary Bureau are collaborating. Agreements entered into by the Bureau with the governments of Brazil and Colombia make the services of the yellow fever laboratories of the Oswaldo Cruz Institute and the Carlos Finlay Institute, including the production of yellow fever vaccine, available to other American nations.

The basic proposition that long-term development of adequate health programs depends on the proper training of a full-time technical staff has been an important factor in planning the work of the Bureau and in determining the nature of the Bureau's aid to Member Governments through fellowships and other provisions for training.

Almost the first step taken by the Director of the Bureau in the development of staff and program was the appointment of a consultant in nursing education whose salary and travel funds were provided during the first year by The Rockefeller Foundation. Since generalized public health programs depend upon a good nursing service for much of their success, it was considered essential to begin immediately the long-term project of studying and assisting the schools which prepare the public health nurse. The educational field will for a long time continue to absorb much of the attention of the Nursing Section, but promotion of improved public health nursing programs in the Americas is the ultimate objective of the Bureau's efforts.

Although the Bureau subscribes to the tenet that general health services built around the family as a unit offer the best long-term program for the health of the community, it is not blind to the opportunity and need for special unilateral programs for attacking certain important problems for which there is a known solution, which can be carried out with relatively untrained nonprofessional personnel engaged in systematic routine operations.

Many examples of the opportunity for such unilateral programs might be cited as that for typhus control, in which the Bureau has been collaborating with the Government of Guatemala for several years, but one of the most interesting examples is that at present under way for the eradication of *Aëdes aegypti* from the American continent.

An important milestone in the orientation of public health programs in the Americas was reached in 1947 by the Directing Council, when the proposal made by the Delegate of Brazil that the continental eradication of aegypti be carried out was approved by the Council. The project for the eradication of aegypti from the Americas involves securing the collaboration of the governments in the organization of antimosquito measures in all countries and territories in the Americas between Canada and Patagonia. To be successful the campaign must bring about the local elimination of the mosquito species and must do that in every country in the region. Approval of this project was made by the Directing Council at a time when very little money was available for the activities of the Bureau and in place of a budget, the Bureau was authorized to take the necessary measures, in agreement with the interested countries, "to solve such problems as may emerge in the campaign against yellow fever, whether they be sanitary, economic or legal."

The success of this project which is receiving the support of the majority of governments in the Americas and is now well advanced in many countries is bound to have a far-reaching effect on the solution of other health problems which may be suitable to the eradication technique. It is setting a pattern for the coordination of technical programs of all countries in a given region through a specialized international organization.

During the past 4 years smallpox, the first disease for which an effective control method was developed, has been widespread from the northern border of the United States to Argentina and Chile. Experience has shown repeatedly that even highly developed areas with adequate general services are susceptible to the introduction of this disease, the eradication of which should be undertaken on a continental basis. The problem of its eradication in the Western Hemisphere is a challenge to the health workers of the Americas and to the Bureau as the agency responsible for the coordination of their activities.

But in the consideration of special unilateral projects for the control of individual diseases, the attempt should be made to develop such projects on as wide a basis as possible. Thus the campaign for the eradication of aegypti is combined, wherever finances permit, with programs for the control of other diseases transmitted by domestic insects, all under one section of the health department; in other campaigns, specialized personnel is to be utilized for more than one similar function, as in simultaneous vaccination against smallpox and yellow fever with desiccated vaccines.

In considering the emphasis which should be placed on eradication programs by the Bureau, it must be remembered that the Bureau has a special responsibility for aiding in the control of epidemic disease and for the prevention of the movement of epidemic disease from one country to another. This responsibility may move the Bureau at times to propose collaboration with individual countries in the solution of regional problems in which these countries are not greatly interested, but in which their collaboration is needed for the benefit of their neighbors. Great interest has been shown during the past 4 years in the development of local frontier health agreements between neighboring countries and groups of countries which can become fully effective only as the Bureau is able to develop its field staff to the point where active coordination based on these agreements can be carried out. All of the frontiers in South America excepting those with the Guianas are now covered by such agreements.

The introduction of DDT and other residual insecticides has greatly simplified the eradication of diseases transmitted by domestic insects. In the same way, the introduction of penicillin and other antibiotics has so greatly facilitated the treatment of yaws and of venereal diseases that optimism regarding the eventual eradication of these diseases is justified. The full impact of these insecticides and antibiotics has not yet become manifest, but with the relatively easy control of such important groups of diseases, it would appear that many of the regions of the Americas now suffering under a heavy handicap of ill health are on the eve of an important upsurge in health, population, production, and wealth.

From the foregoing it is apparent that the work of the XIIth Pan American Sanitary Conference, in paving the way for the development of a truly international health organization in the Americas having also the responsibility of the regional activities of the World Health Organization, has been highly fruitful.

International Health in the Americas, 1954–1957: Director's Review*

GROWTH OF A PATTERN
Triple-Anchored Hemispheric Structure

During the four years between the XIVth (1954) and the XVth (1958) Pan American Sanitary Conferences, the expansion of inter-American health activities envisioned by the XIIth Conference (1947) proceeded at an accelerated rate. In this period stress has continued to be put on the strengthening of national health services, the training of health personnel, and on communicable-disease control with special attention to the development of regional eradication campaigns. The stage for this rapidly developing international health program was set in the period preceding 1947.

Previous to World War II the example and the tradition of international collaboration in the development of national health services was built up over many years by The Rockefeller Foundation and by the Pan American Sanitary Bureau (PASB). These two agencies also set the pattern for collaboration in attempts to eradicate communicable diseases, the Foundation participating in the campaign for the eradication of yellow fever from the Western Hemisphere, and the Bureau in the effort to wipe out bubonic plague in the ports of America.

During World War II the United States, through its Institute of Inter-American Affairs (IIAA), developed cooperative health programs in 18 of the American republics. These programs were more extensive and more adequately financed than previous efforts had been. During the war period the United States also supplied funds to the PASB for field projects and training programs.

On the world scene the United Nations Relief and Rehabilitation Administration (UNRRA), created to serve populations of countries impoverished by World War II, expended many millions of dollars for health work in Europe, Africa, and Asia.

And so it was that at the end of World War II the nations of the Americas had had considerable experience with, and many nations of other parts

* Dr. Soper was the Director of the Pan American Sanitary Bureau and Regional Director for the Americas of the World Health Organization. This report *(91)* was published in *P.A.S.B. Official Documents No. 25,* pp. 1–20, 1958.

For several years after the creation of the World Health Organization the Pan American Health Organization was officially designated as the Pan American Sanitary Organization.

of the world had had a taste of, the benefits of international collaboration in health. The World Health Organization was created (1946–1948) as a technical agency of the United Nations system with broad functions and responsibilities, and in the Americas the Pan American Sanitary Organization expanded its field of operation from the American republics to cover the Western Hemisphere (1947) and prepared to serve also as the Regional Organization for the WHO for the Americas.

Historically it has taken a long time to bring about an effective alliance between the various international health agencies and to get a semblance of coordination of national health programs in regional and global efforts. The Pan American Sanitary Bureau, which dates from 1902, was followed by the Office Internationale d'Hygiene Publique in 1907, the Health Section of the League of Nations in 1923, and UNRRA during World War II. All too often each of these organizations went its own way, with unavoidable duplication of effort and confusion. The framers of the Charter of WHO were determined to correct this situation and create a single international health organization. The American Republics recognized the need for a World Health Organization and wished to participate but were unwilling to see the Pan American Sanitary Organization disappear. The Office Internationale, the health activities of UNRRA, and the postwar remnants of the Health Section of the League were absorbed by WHO; the refusal of the Americas to abandon the PASO led to the compromise under which the PASO continues to exist as a Pan American Organization and also serves as the Regional Organization of WHO for the Western Hemisphere. This adaptation was relatively easy since the Constitution of the World Health Organization (1946) provides for Regional Health Organizations in different geographical areas, and the Constitution (1947) of the Pan American Sanitary Organization was especially designed to permit the PASO to serve also as the Regional Health Organization of the WHO. The formal agreement between WHO and PASO establishing this relationship dates from 1949.

The PASO Constitution commits the Organization to the coordination of efforts to combat disease, lengthen life, and promote the physical and mental health of the people of the countries of the entire Western Hemisphere. For the first time, an inter-American health agency acknowledges its technical responsibility for the needs of the whole Region without regard to the political affiliation of the national and territorial governments of the Region. France, the Netherlands, and the United Kingdom, representing their interests in the Western Hemisphere, are active participants in the Pan American Sanitary Organization and are fully committed to the eradication and other health programs of the Americas. The PASO/WHO has complete double coverage of the Americas except for Canada, which does not participate in the PASO, and Colombia, which has not yet joined the WHO.

The final consolidation of the position of the Pan American Sanitary Organization as the responsible official international health agency of the Western Hemisphere came when an agreement (1950) with the Organization of American States recognized the PASO as a Specialized Organization under the OAS Charter of 1948. Only in the field of health has a united front been developed by the specialized technical agencies of the United Nations and the Pan American systems.

Providentially, health is a noncontroversial subject; everyone agrees that good health is desirable. No one argues that sickness is a benefit to the human race. The public health field is then an excellent proving ground for the initial trial of international working procedures.

The Pan American Sanitary Organization is completing a 10-year period of development and of adjustment, as a technical organization with its own Governing Bodies, while serving also as the Regional Organization of the WHO, and recognized as a Specialized Agency of the Organization of American States. The present structure and relationships with governments and with other organizations is believed to be suitable for application in other fields of activity to unite the interests and programs of agencies of the United Nations and of the Organization of American States.

The coordination of national communicable disease programs in regional and global eradication campaigns is setting a pattern for international cooperation, which should stimulate the development of many future programs for the solution not only of other health problems, but problems in agriculture and in other technical fields. There are few insoluble problems once the nations of the world come to unite their efforts in a common program under the auspices of technical nonpolitical organizations in which they have confidence.

The 10th Anniversary of the Constitution of the Pan American Sanitary Organization was commemorated in September 1957 by a special session of its Directing Council in the Hall of the Americas at the Pan American Union in Washington. The Secretary-General of the Organization of American States and the Director-General of the World Health Organization joined the Director of the Pan American Sanitary Bureau at this Commemorative Session in emphasizing the importance of the unification of international health activities covering all the Americas in a single program.

The Constitution of 1947 gives the Pan American Sanitary Organization a new status, without undermining the treaty status of the Conference and of the Bureau determined by the Pan American Sanitary Code (Havana, 1924). The PASO, in confirming the Conference as the Supreme Governing

Body and the Bureau as its executive agency, took pains to anchor itself firmly in the more than 40 years of inter-American public health tradition. Today American nations fully committed to the financial contributions needed for the global responsibilities of the WHO gladly pay double tribute to retain in active operation the agency, peculiarly their own, which they have known for so long and which they have supported in its own right since 1902. Only in the Americas do the nations of a Region financially support a regional health program in addition to that which can be financed from WHO funds.

The PASO, in becoming part of the worldwide organization, retained the experience, continuity, and regional orientation acquired over the years, and placed itself in position to profit as time goes on from the experience of the larger organization on a global scale.

By becoming also the Regional Organization for the Americas of WHO, the PASO, after 1949, maintains closer ties with what is happening in public health elsewhere in the world. By this affiliation the PASO takes on an even wider internationality than it had before. By anchoring PASO activities firmly in the worldwide health activities of WHO all attitudes of isolation become outmoded. Henceforth, what the Americas do in public health is of direct interest to world health and vice versa.

Just as the position of the PASO is immeasurably strengthened in the health field by its relationship with WHO, so also is its position as the Specialized Agency of the Organization of American States highly significant.

The OAS is not limited to the political field but sponsors cooperation between the nations of the New World in many fields, including agriculture, statistics, housing, geography and history, Indian affairs, child welfare, and the status of women. The PASO has many areas of interest in all of these fields.

As the sphere of cooperation widens, the bond of humanity is paramount; disease is the common enemy of all mankind. In the fight against disease, it is essential that nations, as well as individuals, be brought to stand shoulder to shoulder. It is only by putting health above national and organizational rivalries that the full benefits of international cooperation can be got.

The triple anchorage of the PASO structure permits the development of truly regional health programs in which all governments and peoples of the Americas participate.

Structure and Function

Structure and function are correlates. Because the purpose of the eye is to see, it has a corresponding structure built around a lens. Since the function of the heart is to force blood through the blood vessels, it has a structure roughly resembling a pump. In the same way the PASO, as it has now emerged, has a structure which corresponds with surprising aptness to the function of disease eradication—not just control but true regional eradication. Adequate plans for continental eradication campaigns could not be made as long as Canada, the Caribbean area, and certain parts of South America were excluded from its field of operation. No country can by itself banish a disease from the whole continent or permanently protect itself from reinfection. Every country and every area must cooperate. Eradication is inconceivable without an all-inclusive mechanism for international collaboration. Eradication cannot be operated on a small scale; it cannot be limited in extent, nor can any country, rich and great though it be, keep the benefits of eradication to itself alone. Theoretically and practically, eradication must continually expand until it covers first the Region and eventually the whole world. When malaria began to disappear from certain countries following the introduction of DDT, the eradication of malaria, first from the Western Hemisphere and eventually from the entire world, became a legitimate goal.

The PASO is now organized to operate on a hemispheral basis, covering the 21 American republics, Canada, and the interests of the United Kingdom, France, and the Netherlands, with a practical working relationship with all political units. Infectious disease cannot be eradicated on a limited political or geographical basis. The countries of the Americas have, for the first time, in the PASO, a convenient framework through which the effective teamwork so vital to eradication campaigns can be carried out, and they are now in a strategic position to declare a war of extermination on certain diseases, those diseases for which adequate control methods exist. Every country, colony, department, province, and island is within range of the coordinating action of the PASO, and there can no longer be an American refuge for any disease or disease vector from which it might later burst forth anew.

The present ideal structure of the PASO has come about after a long period of slow progress over a period of 45 years before the breakthrough of 1947, which made the present period of expanding activity possible.

Between the founding of the Pan American Sanitary Bureau, the first of the international health agencies, in 1902, and the adoption in 1954 by the XIVth Sanitary Conference of malaria eradication in the Americas as a high-priority emergency program, lies a long period of slow but essential development in the concept of international health.

In its earliest years the prime role of the Bureau was to prevent the movement of epidemic disease from country to country with minimal interruption to the movement of ships by quarantine.

The Bureau was to receive reports of occurrence of pestilential diseases, was to have every opportunity for careful scientific study of pestilential outbreaks in any of the American republics, and was to "lend its best aid and experience toward the widest possible protection of the public health of each of the said Republics in order that disease may be eliminated and that commerce between said Republics may be facilitated." (Many years were to pass before the function of facilitating commerce was to disappear as a justification for national interest in international health work.)

Once nations began to meet to discuss disease problems related to quarantine, it was inevitable that the scope of the health problems discussed should be increased. At the IVth Conference (1909–1910) much attention was devoted to such basic problems as compulsory vaccination for smallpox, antimalaria, and antituberculosis campaigns, centralization of national health legislation, promotion of research on tropical diseases, and establishment of laboratories at ports for purposes of diagnosis and research in tropical medicine and general pathology.

After another decade, in 1920, the Bureau was reorganized and authorized to prepare a sanitary code for the American republics. New functions required a fulltime professional staff for the permanent headquarters established in Washington, D.C.

The Pan American Sanitary Code (1924) enacted as a treaty, establishes the Bureau as the central coordinating health agency of the American Republics with a wide range of functions and duties, which may be modified from time to time by Sanitary Conferences. Under the Code the Bureau appoints representatives to confer with the health authorities of the various signatory governments; receives, publishes, and distributes information on vital statistics, public health organization, and preventive medicine; undertakes cooperative epidemiological studies; stimulates and facilitates scientific research; fosters the exchange of professors, health officers, experts, and advisers in public health; and provides technical information relative to the status of communicable diseases, progress made in control or eradication of such diseases, and new methods of combating them.

Specifically the Bureau began the regular publication of its *Boletín* to carry information in all fields of public health throughout the Americas, and appointed a traveling representative as a consultant in the eradication of plague from the ports of America. Later additional technical staff, including doctors, engineers, and nurses, were sent to the field by the Bureau for the stimulation of interest in both general and special health programs. During World War II the field staff of the Bureau was the nucleus for the development of certain programs of special interest because of the war situation.

The Constitution of PASO (1947) provides for a coordinated program to combat disease, lengthen life, and promote physical and mental health. The approach to this program has been through the strengthening of national health services rather than to the development of identifiable projects outside such services, and to the improvement of training facilities and to the training of health workers in all fields. A primary point of contact with national health services for the Bureau has naturally been the control of communicable diseases which has inevitably led to national and regional programs for the eradication of individual diseases. When the structural and financial breakthrough for the PASO came the program for the eradication of the *Aëdes aegypti* mosquito, the vector of yellow fever, was literally waiting on the doorstep.

At the first annual meeting of the Directing Council (1947), the countries of the Americas, at the suggestion of Brazil, where the final stage of the national campaign for the eradication of the aegypti mosquito was being hampered by the reintroduction of this mosquito from neighboring countries, committed themselves and the PASO to the eradication of aegypti from the Region. This action may well have set the pattern for the definitive solution of communicable disease problems by simultaneous national eradication programs coordinated by the international health agency.

Although the Bureau has maintained a balanced program devoted to technical aid to central health services, to education and training of national health service personnel, and to pilot projects in public health administration, as well as to the control of communicable diseases, by 1957 great emphasis was being placed on the eradication concept and concerted efforts are now directed toward the hemispheral eradication of the yellow fever mosquito, *A. aegypti,* yaws, smallpox, and malaria.

The increasing emphasis on eradication came because more and more health authorities are becoming convinced of the feasibility of such eradication; particularly are they impressed with the possibility of rapidly training the personnel needed for the specific tasks of eradication in any one campaign. Thus individual eradication campaigns can be carried out on a national scale long before the highly trained staff required for general health programs can be prepared. The eradication campaign can solve the specific problem without sacrificing in any way the development of the integrated health program.

In 1947, when the Directing Council of the PASO, at the suggestion of Brazil, solemnly entrusted "to the Pan American Sanitary Bureau, the solution of the continental problem of urban yellow fever, based fundamentally on the eradication of *Aëdes aegypti,*" relatively few public health workers were ready to accept the concept of eradication as a practical administrative objective. The public health administrator, responsible only for the health program in a single city, county, or state, found eradication of the causative organism or insect vector of disease impracticable because of constant or occasional reinfection or reinfestation from other areas; he came to believe that disease control depends not only on specific measures directed against the etiological agent but even more importantly on the correction of the accessory factors which favor disease incidence once it is in the community.

[There is much duplication in the content of this paper and Selection 33, which were presented within a year of each other but to very different audiences. Both papers are included in extenso for the reason that this paper is more concerned with the practice of the eradication concept as it affected the activities of the Pan American Sanitary Bureau, while Selection 33 deals mainly with the principles of the concept itself. *Ed.*]

Eradication—Early Dreams and Difficulties

By definition, the term "disease control" implies continuing effort to meet a permanent or recurring problem. Eradication, by contrast, means a concentrated, coordinated, all-out attack to end the problem permanently. It means the complete elimination of all sources of infection so that, even in the absence of specific preventive measures, the disease does not reappear. Eradication presupposes a recognized procedure by which a disease, or disease vector, is attacked with the intent of completely destroying it. All eradication techniques are alike in being committed to the goal of complete elimination. Every eradication campaign must have in it the element of thoroughness with no stopping point until the disease has disappeared. In the early parts of the campaign even that is not the end. Steps must be taken to maintain vigilance so that reintroduction of the disease into the cleaned area does not occur as the campaign expands peripherally until all infected or infested areas have been cleaned.

How did all the concern about eradication start? In a sense it can be said that when the germ theory of disease was established, the attempt at disease eradication had to follow. When Pasteur destroyed the concept of spontaneous generation of infectious disease, the concept of eradication of the causative agents of communicable diseases became inevitable. Charles V. Chapin, recognized pioneer and early professor of public health, commenting in 1888 on Koch's discovery of the tubercle bacillus, boldly declared, "There is no theoretical reason why a purely contagious disease like tuberculosis cannot be exterminated. If we can prevent the spread of contagion at all, we can prevent it entirely." Similar visions of liberating the human race from malaria, yellow fever, hookworm, and other diseases arose as the mechanisms of transmission of these diseases were found and methods of treatment and prevention devised.

Ronald Ross showed mathematically that malaria could be eradicated under certain conditions; General Gorgas believed that yellow fever could be "eradicated from the face of the earth within a reasonable time and at a reasonable cost;" and the first hookworm campaign was organized by the

Rockefeller Sanitary Commission for the Eradication of Hookworm Disease.

The early attempts at disease eradication were too limited in scope and too temporary, were based on inadequate information of the ways in which the diseases concerned are maintained in nature, and were undertaken with tools far less efficient and much more costly than those now available. Only in the case of the program for the eradication of yellow fever which began in 1915 was there the persistent, continent-wide effort, stimulated and supported by The Rockefeller Foundation, which led (1934) to success in eliminating urban yellow fever; failure to remove the threat of reinfection of urban areas was due to factors unrecognized for many years after the campaign began.

Disappointment and frustration were the lot of the early enthusiasts who dreamed of disease eradication as something that could happen overnight; tuberculosis receded slowly in some countries, not at all in others; the prevention of malaria proved too costly for rural areas; the campaign for the eradication of yellow fever appeared promising for some years but was doomed from its inception because of the unrecognized reservoir of infection in forest animals; and, although hookworm disease declined in many countries, hookworm infestation remained widespread.

The difficulties and delays in eradication led a whole generation of health workers to abandon the concept of eradication of communicable diseases and to undertake the gradual concomitant reduction of the incidence of all preventable disease through the activities of general health programs.

Rehabilitation of Eradication Concept

The rehabilitation of the eradication concept in public health has been gradual over the past 25 years. Various factors have contributed to this rehabilitation: (1) the success of eradication campaigns in the agricultural field, the campaigns for the eradication of the Mediterranean fruit fly in the United States and for the eradication of foot-and-mouth disease from Mexico and Canada; (2) the extreme reduction, and even local eradication of certain communicable diseases, brought about by carefully administered general health services; (3) the spectacular success of certain large scale campaigns for the eradication of vector species of mosquitoes; and (4) the discovery of new insecticides and therapeutic substances of greatly increased efficiency and ease of application.

Half a century after Chapin's youthful enthusiasm for the eradication of tuberculosis, Wade Hampton Frost, reviewing data on this disease in the United States, concluded (1936) that, "under present conditions of human resistance and environment, the tubercle bacillus is losing ground and the eventual eradication of tuberculosis requires only that the present balance against it be maintained." More recently the introduction of modern therapeutic measures has, during the past decade, caused such a remarkable drop, first in death rates and now in incidence, that Chapin's dream of eradication is shaping into reality.

In 1934, 19 years after The Rockefeller Foundation embarked on the eradication of yellow fever, the endemic human disease, maintained by the aegypti mosquito, the only form of yellow fever known when the campaign began, was cleared from its last American stronghold in Northeast Brazil. But true eradication had not been achieved; the discovery of jungle yellow fever in 1932 had revealed the previously unrecognized reservoir of infection among forest animals, which makes the eradication of yellow fever virus impracticable since it constitutes a permanent dangerous source of reinfection of aegypti-infested towns and cities. Fortunately, in the meantime, administrative methods had been (1932–1933) perfected for the eradication of the urban vector of yellow fever, the *Aëdes aegypti* mosquito. Thus it became possible to eliminate all threat of urban yellow fever, not through the eradication of yellow fever itself but through the eradication of the only species of mosquito causing urban outbreaks in the Americas.

The demonstration that aegypti can be eradicated led to successful campaigns for the eradication of *Anopheles gambiae,* Central Africa's most dreaded carrier of malaria, from Brazil (1939–1940) and from Egypt (1943–1945), which had been invaded with disastrous results by this highly adaptable mosquito. Inevitably these campaigns led to other anopheles eradication projects in the Western Oases in Egypt and on the islands of Cyprus, Sardinia, and Mauritius.

The discovery of the persistent insecticidal action of DDT, when sprayed on the inner walls of human habitations, led to the observation that malaria itself dies out in human populations if new infections are prevented during a period of only 3 or 4 years. For the first time malariologists had a method of malaria prevention applicable at reasonable cost to rural areas, and plans for national malaria eradication began to take shape in many countries. Inevitably the success of national eradication schemes led to the demand for international expanding eradication at the periphery.

The Pan American Sanitary Organization's involvement in eradication programs began with the Brazilian proposal to the Directing Council (1947) for a program of eradication of the aegypti mosquito from the Americas. This proposal came after most of Brazil had been freed of the yellow fever mosquito and reinfestation with aegypti from neighboring countries had become a major problem. Brazil recognized that the eradication of aegypti only from those countries bordering her territory would be but a temporary solution of her problem since these countries would be readily reinfested from their neighbors and thus in turn reinfest Brazil; hence the proposal for the regional eradication of aegypti.

The approval of the proposal for the eradication of aegypti is an important landmark in international health, constituting, as it does, a first pledge by the countries of the Americas of united and simultaneous action in the solution of a common problem. It marks the introduction into international health of the eradication concept as a common responsibility of the nations of a region and constitutes the first official recognition of the obligation of infested and infected territories to free themselves, not only to benefit their own people, but also to protect the peoples of other countries. The eradicationist, previously prone to dream of programs on defensible islands or areas isolated by mountains, deserts, or other natural barriers, can now plan boldly for all encompassing programs.

The Brazilian experience with aegypti had revealed the inexorable need for expansion inherent in the eradication concept; from the port cities of endemic yellow fever regions to the suburbs, then to towns and villages of the interior, to infested rural areas, to the seed beds of reinfestation in the cities and towns of nonendemic regions, and finally beyond national frontiers to all infested countries of the hemisphere.

The second proposal that the PASO become involved in an eradication program came in 1949 from the delegate of Haiti to the United Nations. Preliminary field trials of penicillin in the treatment of yaws, a disfiguring tropical disease widespread in Haiti, had shown that infectious cases could be made noninfectious by a single injection of penicillin. Previous campaigns using other drugs had always stopped short of eradication and had been followed by rapid recurrence of widespread infection of the rural population. Although Haiti's request referred only to the solution of the yaws problem in that island republic, it was obvious that yaws eradication to be successful would have to encompass other islands of the Caribbean and all foci of the disease in Central and South America.

The third official continent-wide eradication program, that against smallpox, long overdue, was proposed by Costa Rica in 1950, after the Bureau had been stimulating studies on the production of improved dried smallpox vaccine for use in tropical climates.

The most recent eradication program, and by far the most important in its implications for the welfare of the nations of the Western Hemisphere and of the world, is that for the eradication of malaria. The acceptance by the nations of the Americas, and later by those of the world, of the need for a supreme effort to eradicate malaria is largely due to three factors: (1) partial malaria control with residual insecticides entails unending annual expenditures which constitute a serious drain on public health budgets, (2) the success of several countries in limited and even national eradication, and (3) the observation that eventually certain species of anopheles become resistant to the residual insecticides. Wherever this occurs there is the threat that rural populations will be left once more, as they were before the advent of DDT, without any economically feasible measure of defense against malaria.

In 1950 the PASB surveyed the malaria control activities in the Americas and called the attention of the XIIIth Sanitary Conference to the possibility and desirability of eradicating this greatest of all tropical scourges. The Conference approved the concept of eradication and resolved:

> To recommend to the Pan American Sanitary Bureau to include henceforth in its operating programs the development of such activities as are necessary to provide for greatest intensification and coordination of anti-malaria work in the Hemisphere, stimulating existing programs, facilitating interchange of information and furnishing technical and, whenever possible, economic assistance to the various countries with a view to achieving the eradication of malaria from the Western Hemisphere.

In 1954 the Bureau again surveyed the malaria situation and was forced to report to the XIVth Conference that little or no progress had been made during the quadrennium, that the American nations were spending some $11 million annually for incomplete and partial control of malaria, whereas the expenditure of two and a half or three times this amount for a few years could conceivably lead to a permanent solution of the problem, and that disturbing observations of anopheline resistance to DDT after prolonged use of this insecticide in various countries of the world threatened the very basis of modern malaria control. The XIVth Conference passed the following resolution:

> 1. To declare that it is the utmost urgency to carry out the terms of Resolution XVIII of the XIII Pan American Sanitary Conference, which recommends that the Pan American Sanitary Bureau promote the intensification and coordination of anti-malaria work, with a view to achieving the eradication of this disease in the Western Hemisphere; and that the Member Governments should convert all control programs into eradication campaigns within the shortest possible time, so as to achieve eradication before the appearance of anopheline resistance to insecticides.
>
> 2. To instruct the Pan American Sanitary Bureau to take steps to implement the aforesaid resolution and to study international measures to ensure the protection of those countries or territories that have achieved eradication of the disease.
>
> 3. To authorize the Director of the Pan American Sanitary Bureau to secure the financial participation of public or private organizations, national or international, in order to further the aims set forth in this resolution.

It is indeed gratifying to note the worldwide interest which has developed since 1954 in malaria eradication and the support given by the World

Health Assembly (1955), by other international agencies, by the Executive Board of UNICEF, by the International Cooperation Administration of the United States, and, most essentially, by the governments of practically every malaria infected country in the Americas, in Europe, in the Near East, and in Asia. Even in Africa talk of malaria eradication is in the air.

ERADICATION IN PRACTICE
Administrative Problems

The following observations are based on administrative experience during various eradication campaigns extending over many years. The progress of the various eradication programs of the PASO is given elsewhere in this combined report. Here attention is directed to the experimental, executive, and general aspects of the eradication problem as exemplified in experience with several diseases. Disease eradication is still a new field in which much new ground is still to be broken. Mistakes and false starts are bound to be made, but errors tend to be self-corrective since progress is measured against absolute nonoccurrence.

Eradication methods vary with each disease and even with the conditions under which a given disease occurs in a given area. It cannot be overemphasized that the complete prevention of the occurrence of disease does not necessarily constitute nor lead to eradication, which implies the removal of the roots of infection or the correction of the conditions which permit the disease to exist. The continued prevention of congenital syphilis, for example, through the routine antibiotic treatment of all expectant mothers, can have little influence on the sources of infection. Today one does not speak of the eradication of yellow fever, but of the eradication of the aegypti mosquito for the protection of urban populations, and of the individual protection by vaccination of persons exposed in infected forests.

The general proposal for the eradication of malaria is based on a specific attack on the malaria parasite in those mosquitoes which have fed in human habitations, but in certain areas where habitations are not suitable for residual insecticidal action or where the habits of vector mosquitoes let it avoid such action, eradication must be predicated on other methods, as for example, the attack on anopheline-breeding areas with insecticides or on the malaria parasites with antimalarial drugs.

Yaws eradication campaigns are based on a direct attack on the causative spirochaetal organism by simultaneous mass antibiotic therapy of all apparently infected persons and all contacts living in the immediate population group.

Whatever the method of attack, direct against the organism or indirect against the vector, the administration of eradication programs requires a dedicated mental approach and a degree of efficiency, thoroughness, and prolonged persistence not common to health work. The change of objective from control, the reduction of disease incidence, to eradication, the removal of all threat of disease occurrence, forces a reconsideration of immediate and long-term objectives, procedures, and budgets. The basic nature and range of this reconsideration is shown in Table 1 for malaria, illustrating how methods differ at every point in the long process of dominating a disease when the end is eradication.

Financially and budgetwise, eradication requires a large initial expenditure sufficient to cover the entire infected or infested area, and a continuation of this expenditure until eradication has been accomplished. Eradication cannot be half done or two thirds done and then interrupted to be continued later without loss of the initial effort. Pains should be taken to ensure needed funds throughout the period required for eradication. Once eradication has been achieved, most of the personnel and funds, ex-

Table 1. Malaria Eradication versus Control

Item	Control	Eradication
1. Objective	Reduce the disease	Eliminate the disease
2. Area of operation	Start where the disease is worst	Every place is important
3. Standards of work	Good work acceptable	Perfection required
4. Duration of work	No end in sight	Definite terminus, perhaps 3 years
5. Residual malaria	Of little interest	Of prime importance
6. Economic aspect	Spray within budget	Pay extra, but spray
7. Other insects	May be considered	Not to be considered
8. Notification of malaria cases	Of secondary value	Of prime importance
9. Participation other health services	Not really necessary	Fundamentally necessary
10. Other professional assistance	No special interest	Needed for notification of cases
11. Suspicious cases	Not important	Of prime importance
12. Imported cases	Academic interest	Crucial after spraying is over
13. Epidemiological survey	Expensive and useless	Indispensable to knowledge of progress of eradication
14. Administrative evaluation of progress	Measurement of what has been done	Measurement of what remains to be done
15. Epidemiological evaluation	Reduction of parasites	Disappearance of all cases

cept those needed for vigilance against reintroduction from noneradicated countries, can be released for other health promotion programs.

The personnel needs of eradication programs are in general more readily met than are those of the more general health programs. The necessity of careful training of public health workers is universally recognized. The physicians, nurses, engineers, and sanitarians who direct public health work constitute a highly trained professional staff who, before assuming their posts, have received a diverse, lengthy, and costly preparation. This is because the positions of responsibility that these professionals occupy require from the occupant both versatility and judgment. On the other hand, once the eradication technique has been broken down into its component parts, the individual operation can be carried out by intelligent laymen with a common school education with special on-the-job training. These men are taught how conscientiously to carry out and record routine operations, the systematic and repeated performance of which are the backbone of eradication work. Almost any one thing that a professional does routinely as part of his many duties can be done as well or better by a person who has been taught to do just that one thing and nothing else.

Eradication campaigns are generally staffed with personnel trained for each particular disease. However, a corps of specially trained lay workers can, after one eradication campaign, be more easily trained for another eradication campaign.

Eradication campaigns require first-class staff work, strict discipline, detailed records, and continuous supervision and checking of all operations. Such staff work and supervision can be gotten only with a professional staff with a single responsibility. The eradication staff should not be expected to take on additional duties. To make the general health service responsible for an eradication program in an offhand way or without a great deal of supplementation does not lead to good results. Personnel with responsibility for multiple duties cannot be expected to concentrate on any single problem with the intensity and devotion needed for eradication. In eradication, singleness of purpose is essential.

The attempt to fuse aegypti eradication and malaria-control programs, while theoretically feasible, has proved unsound in practice. Although the house is the unit in both types of work, the house infested by aegypti tends to be urban, that in which malaria transmission occurs, rural. The application of insecticide is different when applied to the control of malaria. Also, malaria is generally an active disease causing illness in the community, whereas aegypti is only a vague threat of possible yellow fever in the future. Under these circumstances it is inevitable, since the administrative chiefs of the services are generally malariologists, that the malaria programs receive the greatest benefit of funds and staff and that comparatively little attention is given to the eradication of aegypti.

Eradication should not be lightly undertaken, but once begun must be pushed rigorously until achieved. Among the criteria for consideration in the decision for or against an eradication effort are

1. The public health importance of the disease.
2. The economic importance of the disease.
3. Ease of detection and diagnosis.
4. Existence of known methods of combat.
5. Ease of preventing reinfection.
6. Sufficient interest to guaranty financing and proper staffing of campaign to its conclusions.

The experience with each eradication effort has been instructive; the highlights of some of the lessons learned in each follow.

Aëdes aegypti

In the eradication of yellow fever the policy now followed is one of the containment of the virus in the infected forests. The yellow fever campaigns of the first 15 years after the incrimination of the aegypti mosquito, as the transmitting agent, were strikingly successful.

The disappearance of yellow fever from the Panama Canal, and from the principal seaports of South America, of the Caribbean, and of the Mexican Gulf is a fact of the greatest importance in the economic development of the Gulf ports of the United States, the Panama Canal, and the American tropics.

In 1915 The Rockefeller Foundation undertook to consolidate the victory over yellow fever through a coordinated attack in collaboration with the national health authorities wherever the disease might be found. The declared objective was the eradication of yellow fever from the face of the earth. This program for the eradication of yellow fever was the first serious proposal to solve completely a communicable disease problem through the eradication of the infectious agent. It was soundly conceived, adequately financed, and received the support of the infected countries. Just when victory appeared imminent over the human, aegypti-transmitted yellow fever, came the discovery of an almost untouchable reservoir of yellow fever in the jungle, kept there by a cycle of transmission involving monkeys and mosquitoes, other than aegypti. These forests where yellow fever virus hides, as a disease of monkeys, are virtually inaccessible to the application of eradication techniques and there can be for the present no thought of interrupting this forest cycle of yellow fever. Hence the policy of containing the threat of yellow fever within this "jungle" prison.

Obviously the best way to do this is to keep the areas outside of the jungle, where people live, free of aegypti, the only efficient urban vector. Otherwise a man infected in the jungle might come to a nearby town or even by airplane, to distant cities, where the aegypti mosquito could immediately take over again the task of spreading his infection to others. Repeatedly, in the past 25 years, since the final persistent foci of aegypti-transmitted yellow fever were suppressed in Northeast Brazil, yellow fever has been introduced from jungle to urban areas, lighting up aegypti-transmitted outbreaks anew. Fortunately, such outbreaks have been smothered before spreading to other urban areas. It is to safeguard the Americas once and for all from such dread recurrence that aegypti eradication must be pushed to completion.

The real difficulty today in dealing with aegypti, the urban carrier of yellow fever, is that yellow fever has long been absent from the cities of America. One has to deal with the threat of a disease rather than with the disease itself. It is more difficult to take measures looking to the future than to act when confronted by a present danger. Memories of the devastations caused by former onslaughts of yellow fever are now growing dim.

The big hurdle has been to convince health authorities, in the absence of urban outbreaks of yellow fever, that action should nevertheless be taken against the ever present menace of this disease, and that these authorities themselves have a responsibility not only to protect their own populations against possible mishap, but also to safeguard neighboring countries against reinfestation with aegypti once these countries have eradicated this mosquito. The fact that the battle must be waged indirectly against a forgotten enemy who has not been seen for many years in previously infected and still susceptible areas makes the aegypti campaign uphill work.

Thus it is that although the PASB began to organize the aegypti eradication campaign on a regional basis in 1948, the work is not yet finished in spite of the absence of insuperable obstacles. Eradication programs were projected and begun in the Caribbean area as early as 1948, but the 1954 outbreak of yellow fever in Venezuela and in Trinidad found both capital cities, Caracas and Port-of-Spain, dangerously infested with aegypti. On the other hand, gratifying successes were the eradication of aegypti from Ecuador before the invasion of Esmeraldas by jungle yellow fever in 1951, and the organization of aegypti-eradication programs in Panama and the countries of Central America ahead of the wave of jungle yellow fever which moved from eastern Panama to the border of Guatemala with Mexico between 1948 and 1957.

Aegypti is no longer found in many of the countries of the Americas, although final surveys for declaration of eradication have not been completed in a number of countries. The following areas are probably clean: Bolivia, Brazil, British Guiana, Chile, Costa Rica, Dutch Guiana, El Salvador, Ecuador, Guatemala, Honduras, Nicaragua, Panama, Paraguay, Peru, and Uruguay. The difficulty of eradication of aegypti in Trinidad and Venezuela has been greatly increased because of aegypti's resistance to

DDT in these countries. The situation in Colombia, where the program is well advanced, has been complicated by invasion of resistant aegypti from Venezuela. Argentina now has an active eradication program and no special difficulties are anticipated.

In the United States, preparation for eventual aegypti eradication has begun. A survey of aegypti distribution was made in 1957 and there is to be in 1958 a pilot eradication program in Pensacola, Florida, to provide a basis for estimating the technical and financial requirements of eradication under U.S. conditions. In Mexico aegypti-eradication work has been suspended, but the widepread use of insecticides by the Malaria Eradication Service is undoubtedly reducing the size of the task which lies ahead. The approximate status of aegypti campaigns is shown in the Quadrennial Report.

The decision has been taken to give the aegypti-eradication program both administrative and financial priority over many other programs in the infested countries beginning in 1958. This decision has been forced by the observation of the development of resistance to residual insecticides of aegypti in Trinidad and in Venezuela and the transportation of the resistant aegypti from Venezuela to Cúcuta, in northeastern Colombia, where aegypti had been practically eradicated.

There is considerable cause for alarm over the DDT resistant strains of aegypti which are developing. If these strains should invade the countries which have already been cleaned, the problem of aegypti eradication would suffer a setback and be rendered immeasurably more difficult. It is essential that the entire job of eradicating aegypti in the Americas be promptly finished.

Yaws

Yaws is a disfiguring and disabling disease still found in parts of the Western Hemisphere, and formerly worst in Haiti, where the disease held in its grip a large percentage of the rural population. Yaws was widespread also in other parts of the Caribbean area and is a problem in nine other countries: Bolivia, Brazil, Colombia, Costa Rica, Ecuador, Guatemala, Panama, Peru, and Venezuela.

This disease ran wild until arsenicals were introduced in the early 1900s. Then, about 10 years ago, came the miracle of treatment with penicillin. Penicillin is cheap and easily administered. A single dose is effective. An eradication campaign, begun in 1950 and now in its very final stages, is believed to be effectively eradicating yaws from Haiti. Any eradication campaign depending on the sterilization of infectious cases by individual treatment by hypodermic injection is bound to be difficult, especially in a country where seasonal nomadism is the rule. The program in Haiti is based on house-to-house visits by treatment teams to all parts of the Republic and the treatment of all obvious or suspect cases and, in a lesser dosage, all contacts, who may be incubating the infection. Practically everyone living in the rural areas of Haiti has been treated.

In the final search for remaining yaws in Haiti the field staff have been trained for and are carrying out a mass smallpox vaccination campaign. In this way it is possible to obtain on the arms of the populations an approximate record of the degree of coverage of the population in the final search for yaws, and at the same time, achieve the task of protecting the population against smallpox.

Now that the campaign in Haiti is coming to a close, increasing attention must be given to the problem in other countries, where the disfiguring and crippling effects of yaws are not so immediately apparent as they were in Haiti.

Smallpox

A cursory inspection 10 years ago of the reports of smallpox in the Americas revealed a disappointing picture of widespread infection and frequent movement of the disease across international boundaries. Considering that smallpox is the first communicable disease for which effective prophylaxis was developed, well over a century and a half ago, and that smallpox is one of the primary concerns of international sanitary regulations and of international health organizations, it was obvious that the Pan American Sanitary Bureau could not neglect this problem.

The Bureau did not have the funds nor the appetite for joining in the intensive vaccination campaigns that have so often given temporary relief, but became interested rather in improving the tools and methods through which permanent eradication might be brought about. At the suggestion of the Bureau the U.S. Public Health Service and the State Health Laboratory of Michigan joined in the development of a procedure for the manufacture of dried vaccine, adapted to transportation and use in tropical regions. Once this procedure was ready, the Bureau began to collaborate in the training of national staff in the preparation and use of the dried vaccine and has in many instances supplied the special equipment needed for its preparation. Although the Bureau's program for the eradication of smallpox in the Americas has been based on the belief that little was to be gained by additional demonstrations of smallpox eradication through high-pressure crash vaccination programs, the Bureau in some countries has collaborated in the organization of permanent immunization services, once adequate production of dried vaccine was available.

A seminar on smallpox vaccine was held in 1956 at Lima, Peru. Here professionals in charge of smallpox vaccine production in Argentina, Brazil,

Colombia, Cuba, Ecuador, El Salvador, Mexico, Peru, Uruguay, and Venezuela met together with representatives from the Lister Institute in England, the State Serum Institute at Copenhagen, and the laboratories of the State Health Departments of Texas and Michigan. These experts recommended that only dried vaccine be used in areas where no refrigeration exists, and that techniques for the production and testing of dried vaccine be standardized.

The PASB prepared in 1956 a detailed illustrated guide with organization hints, sample forms, and full technical information for the general guidance of smallpox vaccination campaigns and the training of workers.

Considerable progress in the eradication of smallpox in the Americas has been made; the records of North and Central America and of the West Indies are free of smallpox since 1954 and those of only five countries in South America show an appreciable number of cases in 1957.

The difficulties of smallpox eradication in South America are epitomized in Colombia, lying wholly in the tropics, with especially difficult travel from place to place because of topographical irregularities. Vaccination programs, as well as all other health activities, have been interrupted for long periods since 1948 in many areas because of disturbed political conditions. In 1955 with a high incidence of smallpox, fortunately of the mild "alastrim" type, it was estimated that 10,000,000 susceptible Colombians, two thirds living in rural areas, needed vaccination, since for many years smallpox vaccination had been largely limited to school children and travelers. In 1955, vaccination was made compulsory for everyone over 3 months of age. Colombia's national eradication campaign began on October 12, 1955. By the end of 1957 over 2,500,000 persons had been vaccinated and plans formulated to complete the job in 5 years, in time to begin another countrywide cycle.

Malaria

Almost half a century after the incrimination of the Anopheles mosquito as the vector of malaria, the malariologists of the world, armed with quinine, atebrin, ditching, filling, larviciding (with oil and Paris green), insecticides of various kinds, and biological control methods, still had no economically feasible solution to rural malaria, which constitutes the bulk of the world's malaria problem. The discovery of the residual insecticidal properties of DDT changed the picture amost overnight. The properties of DDT sounded to malariologists like a fairy tale when first announced 15 years ago.

The three eradication campaigns already mentioned each has its different method: The urban yellow fever campaign is dedicated to the eradication of the vector species of mosquito *A. aegypti;* the yaws campaign depends on a direct chemotherapeutic attack on the disease organism in each individual case; and the smallpox campaign is based on mass immunization of the susceptible population to break the chain of infectious cases on which the smallpox virus depends for its continued existence.

Theoretically, at least, malaria eradication may be based on the eradication of the mosquito vectors, on the treatment of individual cases, or on breaking the chain of transmission from person to person. Although species eradication of some anopheles has been demonstrated for limited areas, the variety and range of vector species in the world make this solution impossible; the treatment to a cure of individual cases has also been found administratively too onerous and expensive, and breaking the chain of transmission has to be based on some method other than immunization since there is no vaccine for malaria prevention. Previous to the introduction of DDT, attempts to break the chain of transmission through general reduction of anopheles mosquitoes were not economically feasible in many rural areas. DDT and other residual insecticides which maintain their toxicity for months after being sprayed on the walls are used to build a chemical barrier between the infected and the noninfected person living in the same home and even in the same room.

The female anopheles, the only one that bites, is in deadly peril if after a twilight flight in search of blood, which it needs for hatching its eggs, the wall on which it stops to rest has been sprayed with DDT. The anopheles is not a strong flyer. It is inclined to rest again when gorged with blood. Even though the anopheles escapes contact with DDT on its initial visit to the human habitation, it is in danger on each visit it makes for a blood meal during the 12 to 15 days before it becomes infectious.

The chemical barrier established between the infected and noninfected persons is effective in breaking the chain of malaria transmission by destroying the female anopheles in the home, either before it becomes infected or by destroying the infected anopheles before it is able to transmit. The cost of establishing the chemical barrier for the rural home is no greater than for the suburban or village home except for the added transportation costs of rural work. At long last the malariologist has an effective economical tool through which rural as well as suburban and village transmission can be blocked and malaria ended.

Instead of taking full advantage of the new tool, and undertaking the early eradication of malaria, the workers in many countries used it only for partial control, year after year, in the most malarious areas or in the most economically important ones.

Nature's children often find ways of circumventing obstacles and eventually various species of anopheles mosquitoes were found to be resistant to

DDT and other insecticides. To the other advantages of malaria eradication was added the necessity of using the sharp tool of residual insecticides before it becomes dull and useless because of anopheles resistance.

This is not the place to relate the many fascinating details of malaria eradication strategy. Something of what is being done is told later in this report and in the reports for 1954, 1955, and 1956. But it is important to stress the dependence of the program of malaria eradication on the continued susceptibility of vector species of anopheles to DDT and other residual insecticides. Thus far only a few anopheles in limited areas have lost this susceptibility. The threat is not only that this may occur in other cases but equally or more important is the danger of the spread of resistant anopheles from their original habitat to other areas. Once the barrier of the DDT-sprayed wall can be hurdled by a few DDT-resistant anopheles, the new resistant strain may multiply in geometric progression and gradually repossess the full faunal range of that anopheles species.

Quite apart from the development of resistance it is already apparent that the residual insecticides cannot be expected to solve alone all the world's complex malaria problems. Malaria occurs under such widely varying climatic and cultural conditions, with such a variety of anopheles vectors, with their different breeding and feeding habits, that considerable flexibility in methods of attack must be maintained until the final eradication of malaria has been achieved.

Medicine in a New Dimension
Medicine Revolutionized

The worldwide malaria eradication campaign marks a slowly developing revolution in medicine, as inevitable and as significant as other great revolutions of the present century—the revolution in physics—the more fundamental one in logic—and the even more dramatic revolution in transportation, with its assault on outer space! Truly this is a century of upheaval. In 1905 Einstein launched the atomic age with the theory of relativity; with his innocent-looking formula $E = mc^2$, he freed the world of the atom and the light-year ranges of stellar space, from the shackles of the Newtonian laws of gravity and motion. These laws, universally accepted during 300 years, while applicable to the usual range of human experience, are inadequate to an understanding of the infinitely small and the infinitely large in the universe.

"In the history of ideas, the past century is one marked by an extraordinary development of logic," says Morris Raphael Cohen, himself an eminent logician. "A discipline which had remained for more than 20 centuries in approximately the state to which the mind of Aristotle reduced it, suddenly entered upon a period of rapid growth and systematic development."

While the essential elements of the Aristotelian logic remain unshaken, modern logicians have produced a new logic in which Aristotelian logic occupies "only a tiny corner."

The field of transportation has been marked through the ages by a series of revolutions; the introduction of the sailing vessel and the wheeled vehicle, the steamship, and the steam engine for railroads have been overshadowed in this century by the automobile, paved highways, airplanes, jet planes, missiles, and satellites.

In the health field, the older pre-germ medicine with its sound advances in anatomy and physiology, such as Harvey's discovery of the circulation of the blood, and with exclusive emphasis on the treatment of the individual patient, has not been overthrown, but now occupies only a tiny corner in the greater sphere of modern curative and preventive medicine.

A century ago a few nations were groping in international conferences for agreements through which the movement of communicable disease from country to country might be prevented through quarantine; today, through the international health organizations the nations of the world are helping each other to build sound health programs everywhere and to attack and eliminate the seedbeds of disease wherever they occur.

The age of Pasteur, with its negation of spontaneous generation and the identification of the causes of certain communicable diseases, initiated a revolution in curative medicine and sowed the seeds of the modern public health movement. Pushing disease prevention to finality—eradication—must lead to even greater future changes in medicine and in basic public health practice.

Expanding Concept of Eradication

The very definition of the term "disease eradication" must be adapted to the present age. *Webster's New International Dictionary* had defined the verb eradicate, since before the age of Pasteur, as "to pluck up by the roots; to root up or out; hence to extirpate; as, to eradicate a disease." That this reference to disease eradication refers to the eradication of disease from the individual patient is shown by the accompanying definition of eradicative as "a medicine that effects a radical cure."

The term "disease eradication," then, is not new, but the modern concept of eradication, while not abolishing that of a century ago, no longer limits eradication to the individual, or even to the community, but expands its application to mankind. Penicillin is truly an "eradicative" for yaws, but in eradication campaigns the individual is treated not only for his own benefit but also for the elimination of yaws from the human race. Eradication forces the community to take an interest in every case of infectious disease and forces the world community to take an interest in foci of communicable disease wherever they exist.

The concept of eradication, which has just recently come on the horizon of many health workers, engrossed in the multiple problems of city and state health services, has had a considerable period of development. The first attempt to coordinate the efforts of many countries in a regional eradication program dates from 1915, when The Rockefeller Foundation began its long struggle with yellow fever in the Americas. This in turn led to the demonstration that the aegypti mosquito, the urban vector of yellow fever, can be eradicated (1933) and to the declaration of a war of eradication against aegypti by the National Yellow Fever Service of Brazil in 1940. Brazil's success on the national scale in turn led to the regional campaign for the eradication of aegypti from the Western Hemisphere (1947). In the meantime the eradication concept had become widely known through the eradication of *Anopheles gambiae* from Brazil in 1939–1940 and from Egypt in 1944–1945, in each instance under highly dramatic circumstances.

A World Movement

But these programs, as well as the campaigns for the eradication of yaws (1950), have been but steps toward the obvious ultimate objective of world eradication. The move of the Eighth World Health Assembly in 1955 in extending the program for malaria eradication previously approved for the Western Hemisphere by the XIVth Pan American Sanitary Conference (1954) is the first official declaration by mankind of total war against any disease. Planning the extirpation of even a single disease right out to the periphery of its distribution in the human race is a truly historic event.

In his message of the State of the Union, January 9, 1958, the President of the United States made the following statement:

We now have it within our power to eradicate from the face of the earth that age-old scourge of mankind: malaria. We are embarking with other nations in an all-out five-year campaign to blot out this curse forever. We invite the Soviets to join with us in this great work of humanity.

Here we have the concept of malaria eradication emerging at the highest of international levels. It is ranked among the great works of peace and is held before the attention of the entire world as one of the modern methods of waging the peace. Eradication of malaria is listed as constructive "cooperation on human welfare," and Mr. Eisenhower goes on to say: "Indeed, we would be willing to pool our efforts with the Soviets in other campaigns against the diseases that are the common enemy of all mortals—such as cancer and heart disease."

As if in reply, the Government of the Union of Soviet Socialist Republics is presenting to the Eleventh World Health Assembly (Minneapolis, May–June 1958) recommendations for the world-wide eradication of smallpox. The wording is as follows:

The Government of the USSR
RECOMMENDS
   (a) that during 1959–1960 the population be vaccinated in countries in which principal endemic foci of smallpox exist . . . and
   (b) that during 1961–1962 the eradication of smallpox be completed by means of the additional vaccination of the population in foci where the disease persists, that subsequently revaccinations be given to the extent it becomes necessary in accordance with the experience acquired in each country.
RECOMMENDS
   that all countries in which smallpox vaccination is compulsory continue to give smallpox vaccinations during the eradication of this disease throughout the world.

In the draft resolution on the eradication of smallpox, the USSR notes that, "with the eradication of smallpox, vaccination and all expenditures involved in its application will be redundant."

World eradication of such diseases as malaria and smallpox is no longer the dream of the idealist but the most practical approach to prevention. Truly a revolution is under way; in 1902 the PASB was founded to regulate quarantine and to convoke international health conferences; in 1958 the nations of the world, although still busy devising the means for mutual destruction, are ready to join in eradicating disease and making quarantine unnecessary.

Prosperous countries cannot afford to limit their participation in eradication programs to the clearing of their own territory but must be ready to aid less fortunate countries in the attack on the common enemy. During 1957 the PASB Special Malaria Eradication Fund received $1,899,600 in voluntary contributions from three countries: the Dominican Republic ($100,000); the United States ($1,500,000); and Venezuela ($299,600). For 1958 the United States has contributed $2,000,000 to the Fund. As each country becomes free of malaria it has a real financial stake in the eradication of malaria in countries from which it might be reinfected and must in self-interest be ready to support the continuing global effort until success comes.

Ramifications of Eradication

Eradication of malaria will mean more to the economic, social, cultural, and health conditions of the world than any other single health program. Malaria, when it does not kill, enslaves its victims by keeping them only half alive. Sick children cannot go to school. Impoverished populations cannot pay for education, and a truly successful malaria eradication campaign should repay within a few years all the money that governments put into it. Eradication should set off a chain reaction with the financial gains from malaria control, as the source of funds for investment in turn in the eradication of other diseases.

The PASO program is dedicated to many diseases other than the four on which specific eradication programs have been authorized. In this report occur chapters on rabies, leprosy, typhus, plague, influenza, with some comments on brucellosis, hydatidosis, and poliomyelitis. At whatever stage the work on these important communicable diseases may now be, the point is bound to be reached someday when eradication can be undertaken. In none of these diseases is it reasonable to aim only at alleviation. The whole communicable disease program is one in which eradication features will, as time goes on, become more general. Eradication of communicable diseases is a logical objective of modern public health practice, now that the international health organizations are setting the pattern for the coordination of national efforts in an overall international campaign. Once the eradication concept becomes firmly established, the public health attitude toward communicable diseases should come to parallel that of the fireman, who does not look at fire as something which must be reduced to a low level but kept burning just a little. Once the knowledge of how to prevent a given disease is available, the health conscience of the world should no longer permit that disease to continue as a regrettable but inevitable affliction of mankind. Eradication programs are not to be considered as something apart from the regular health services. Rather must the eradication concept come to permeate the integrated health services and must become part of public health training.

Extending the Work

The international health organizations cannot limit their collaboration with governments to a few major programs but are under constant pressure to undertake new efforts in practically all health fields. The presently neglected or largely undeveloped fields include such important ones as radiation, cancer, mental health, occupational health, heart disease, diarrheal diseases, basic sanitation (water supplies and sewage disposal), and pharmaceutical and biological products.

The PASO is engaged in what may be termed an experimental administrative adventure in long-term supervision of intercountry cooperation in specific fields beyond the reach of individual nations. The Institute of Nutrition of Central America and Panama, based in Guatemala, is financed and governed by a group of six neighboring countries for research in and the practical solution of their problems of tropical nutrition; the

Pan American Aftosa Center in Brazil is an inter-American center for research, and for training and for consultation, on the diagnosis, prevention, and eventual eradication of this destructive affliction of cattle, with its terrific effect on human nutrition; and the Pan American Zoonoses Center in Argentina, for field research and the training of experts in the control of diseases common to man and animals are examples of PASO assumption of direct administrative responsibility for internationally financed projects.

The PASO cooperates without direct administrative function with the Oswaldo Cruz Institute in Brazil and with the Carlos Finlay Institute in Colombia in providing technical laboratory services for the diagnosis of yellow fever and in producing and distributing yellow fever vaccine to the nations of America without charge.

As the eradication concept develops and as pressure develops to force the treatment and control of communicable diseases into the mold of disease eradication, inevitably there must be increasing emphasis on research, not limited laboratory research, but combined laboratory and field research. Only as the results of laboratory studies are taken to the field does the need for additional research appear, and only as the field work is checked by the laboratory can full confidence be placed in field results.

The experience in yellow fever has been most illuminating. In 1915 it was firmly believed that available knowledge was adequate for the planning of an eradication program to eliminate yellow fever forever. No provision was made for adequate laboratory studies, and not until a field laboratory in Africa succeeded in infecting monkeys with yellow fever and in transmitting the disease from animal to animal with mosquitoes other than aegypti did clues become available which later led to the discovery of jungle yellow fever in the Americas.

The PASO has had an important part in long-range studies in Brazil in the use of molluscocides developed by the U.S. Public Health Service for the campaign against the snail, the intermediate host of schistosomiasis. The results suggest that, under certain conditions, some host species of snails may be eradicable. The field testing of new products and methods is a natural field for coordination by the PASO/WHO, often bringing the worker with the product or method from one country to the country where needed conditions for field testing exist. An increasingly effective coordination of laboratory research and field experience looms up as a major desideratum in the development of new control and eradication techniques.

In the special case of the diarrheal diseases, today a leading cause of death, especially among infants, simple methods of treatment of early dehydration are often sufficient to prevent a fatal outcome. How can mothers be taught to take the elementary measures needed? The answer is being sought in field experimentation on domiciliary training, with careful observations and records of achievement. It may seem almost undignified to class these uncomplicated procedures as research, but the concept of field research must be broadened to include the development of new techniques for teaching and preparing the public and the standardization of mechanical operations such as the spraying of insecticides. There is here a growing science of practical application still in its early stages of development. In preparing the public health manuals of the future, great emphasis should be placed on the results of practical field research.

The emphasis placed on eradication in this introduction does not mean there has been any lessening of interest in all phases of health work, nor does it indicate that the PASO is ready to suggest embarking on additional eradication campaigns at the present time. Rather it is a call to arms to push to completion those programs to which the nations of the Americas are already committed, while intelligently developing and testing methods applicable eventually to other diseases.

Part XI | The Eradication of Malaria: Local,
Continental, Global

Selection 39 | Reduction of Anopheles Density
Effected by the Preseason
Spraying of Building Interiors
with DDT in Kerosene, at Castel
Volturno, Italy in 1944–1945 and
in the Tiber Delta in 1945*

FRED L. SOPER, F. W. KNIPE, G. CASINI,
LOUIS A. RIEHL, AND A. RUBINO

In the spring of 1944 the Surgeon of the Mediterranean Theater of
Operations of the United States Army (MTOUSA) requested that the members of the Rockefeller Foundation Health Commission who were working
in Italy undertake studies of the use of DDT for the control of house-infest-
ing anopheles of the Italian malaria-vector species *Anopheles labranchiae*.
At the time, the area facing the Allied Armies had been extensively flooded
and mined by the retreating German Army so that the customary application of larvicides for malaria control was hazardous if not impossible.
Later, the Allied Control Commission (ACC) for Italy issued a formal invitation to the members of the Health Commission to organize a Malaria
Control Demonstration Unit under the auspices of its Public Health Sub-
Commission.

One object of the investigation was to determine the effect upon anopheles of treating the interiors of all buildings with DDT in the absence of

* The studies and observations on which this report is based were made at the
request of the Surgeon's Office of the Mediterranean Theater of Operations of
the U.S. Army by members of the Rockefeller Foundation Health Commission
functioning as the Malaria Control Demonstration Unit of the Malaria Section
of the Public Health Sub-Commission, Allied Control Commission for Italy. Essential contributions were made by the Istituto Superiore di Sanità, Rome, by the
Health Department of the Commune of Rome and by the malaria control groups
of the British and U.S. Armies. Dr. Soper, Mr. Knipe, and Dr. Riehl were members
of the Rockefeller Foundation Health Commission; the services of Drs. Casini and
Rubino were provided by the Allied Control Commission.

This excerpt is reprinted by permission from the *American Journal of Tropical
Medicine 27:* 177–200, 1947. Copyright © 1947, The Williams & Wilkins Company,
Baltimore, Maryland. [The text of the original article *(51)* is complete, but 5 tables
and 6 figures have been omitted.]

other measures for their control. The area chosen for the initial studies was a part of the Bonifica di Castel Volturno extending along the southwestern coast of Italy between the Volturno River and the Lago di Patria. Later, similar but more extensive investigations were carried out in the Tiber Delta. In this paper the activities in the Castel Volturno region in 1944 and 1945 will be summarized briefly, and the work in the Tiber Delta will be discussed at greater length.

CASTEL VOLTURNO, 1944

A permanent river, the Regi Lagni, formed by the junction of the Aprano and Lagni streams flows from east to west, bisecting the 1944 experimental area at Castel Volturno in such a way that the southern of the two sections was approximately twice the size of the northern one. Prior to the outbreak of the war this previously swampy area had been drained and partially settled. In September 1943 the Germans destroyed the pumping stations, thus flooding the region along the Lagni, particularly that south of the river.

The test area was arbitrarily divided into six sections, as shown in the accompanying map (Fig. 1). Sections A and B lay between the Lagni and Volturno rivers, C and D were south of the Lagni, and E and F lay between C and D and the Lago di Patria. It was decided that the interiors of all buildings of sections B and D should be sprayed with a 5 per cent solution of DDT in kerosene, that those of sections E and F should be dusted with 10 per cent DDT in pyrophyllite and that the buildings in sections A and C should remain untreated, for observation purposes.

During the week beginning May 17, DDT spray or dust was applied to the walls and ceilings of all rooms (that is, bedroom, kitchen, stairway, stairwell, stable, pigsty, chicken run, toilet, cartshed, and oven) of all buildings in sections B, D, E, and F. The DDT solution was applied with an ordinary hand-operated knapsack sprayer with a disc-type nozzle giving a conical spray. Approximately a quart of liquid was used per 1000 square feet, giving an estimated dosage of 60 milligrams of DDT per square foot of sprayed surface.

The DDT powder was applied with a plunger-type hand dust gun, the Hudson Admiral. More powder adhered to the wall when the gun was held nearly parallel to it with the stream of powder directed toward the ceiling. A deposit of not more than 20 milligrams per square foot was thus obtained.

The buildings of sections E and F were redusted during the week beginning July 9; and between August 7 and 27 one team of four men sprayed the buildings on all the 216 farms in the four sections, applying approximately 80 milligrams per square foot of treated surface.

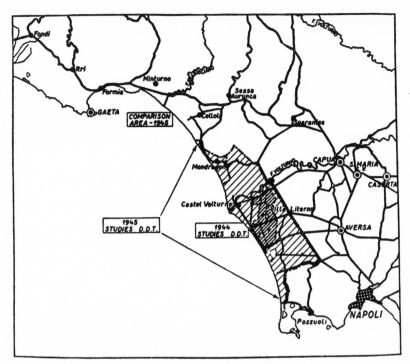

Figure 1. Castel Volturno areas covered in residual DDT studies, Italy, 1944 and 1945.

Certain premises in each section were selected for weekly captures of adult anopheles. Two inspections were made before the insecticide was applied, and subsequent captures were made routinely through July 8 and from August 10 through October 14. Captures were limited to a designated strip of bedroom ceiling 1 meter wide and 4.3 meters long and to an area of 1 square meter at each of the four corners of the stable roof.

Since captures prior to treatment in sections E and F were 10 times as high as those in section B and D, the superior effect of the 5 per cent DDT in kerosene was not clearly demonstrated until after all buildings had been sprayed in August. That even the powder is effective is shown by a comparison of the trends in anopheles density in sections E and F with those in the untreated sections A and C.

When captures were resumed in September, density in all sprayed sections had dropped to less than one anopheles per premises. For comparison, captures from two districts outside the study area were studied. In both districts the postseasonal decrease in anopheles density had set in but the levels were well above those in the treated sections.

Surveys made in June, August, and October to determine the species of anopheles present revealed *A. labranchiae, A. sacharovi, A. melanoon,* and *A. messeae.* While labranchiae was dominant early in the season, sacharovi became more prevalent later.

Spleen and parasite surveys were made of all school children, 6 to 14 years of age, in the study area prior to the treatment of the premises in May and later in August and October. Thick and thin blood smears were examined for parasites, and spleen enlargement was recorded by Schüffner's method. During this period spleen rates varied from 43 to 39 per cent, while parasite rates dropped from 21 to 8 per cent.

Castel Volturno, 1945

A study of residual effects of DDT at Castel Volturno in 1945 was conducted by Malaria Control Units, MTOUSA, with the Malaria Control Demonstration Unit retaining responsibility only for the parasite and spleen surveys. A short résumé of a report on this study by Aitken is given below.

The 1944 test area was enlarged to comprise a coastal strip approximately 5 miles wide, extending from the Mondragone hills south to the village of Qualiano, thence following the hills in a southwesterly direction to Mt. Cuma. The zone thus defined included approximately 95 square miles (Fig. 1). Approximately 85 milligrams of DDT were applied per square foot.

Routine captures were made weekly from December 22, 1944, through September 1945 in selected treated premises over a somewhat larger surface than was covered by captures in 1944. No anopheles were captured in December and January in houses sprayed in August, while hibernating mosquitoes in moderate numbers were found in untreated houses.

In April 1945 captures were inaugurated in untreated premises in the Bonifica di Sessa, a thinly populated section south of the Garigliano River and in the town of Minturno, where the surrounding terrain was flooded. Because of the swarms of anopheles present, inspections were made semimonthly and counts were based on estimates when there were presumably more than 1000 mosquitoes on the examined surface. The following record of captures per square yard in treated and untreated sections for the months of April through September speaks for itself:

Area	April	May	June	July	August	September
Treated	0.001	0.003	0.05	0.13	0.04	0.06
Untreated	9.87	41.84[a]	167.04[a]	118.50[a]	185.54[a]	185.54[a]

[a]Based on estimates of over 1000 mosquitoes.

In the area treated in 1944, spleen and parasite surveys were again made in January, May, and August 1945. Although the spleen rates in the test area did not fall significantly during the period of observation, they did not rise, and the rates in the untreated Sessa area were definitely at a higher level. On the other hand, parasite rates in the treated zone dropped significantly from 21 per cent to 1.4 per cent during the interval, while the Sessa rate rose from 18 per cent in May to 41 per cent in August, when transmission was at its height.

The 1945 studies in Castel Volturno indicated that a single preseason application of 85 milligrams per square foot of DDT in kerosene to walls and ceilings in rooms of all buildings on all premises will greatly reduce the density of anopheles in their habitual resting places for the entire breeding season. While spleen rates remained high during the period of observation, parasite rates dropped sharply at a time when both spleen and parasite rates in the untreated area were rising.

TIBER DELTA, 1945

Plan and Sponsorship of the Project

During the summer of 1944 the Malaria Control Demonstration Unit also collaborated in an Allied project in the Tiber Delta by applying a 5 per cent DDT solution in kerosene to the interiors of buildings occupied by troops in Ostia Lido and to all farm buildings in the Isola Sacra formed by two branches of the Tiber River at its mouth. The efficacy of DDT in reducing anopheles density was further demonstrated here.

The 1945 investigation was designed to determine the effect of a single heavy application of a DDT spray in all human habitations and animal shelters in the early spring. The advantages of the Tiber Delta as a site for this study were easy accessibility from Rome, the variety of agricultural development, the high malaria potential, the protection afforded against infiltration of anopheles from outside, together with the willingness of both civil and military authorities to surrender to the Malaria Control Demonstration Unit all responsibility for control of anopheles in the Delta during the 1945 season.

Plans were submitted to, and approved by Brig. G. Parkinson, Chief of the Public Health Sub-Commission of the Allied Commission for Italy, and Col. W. S. Stone, Chief of the Preventive Medicine Section, Office of the Theater Surgeon, MTOUSA. The Rome Area Allied Command Malaria Control Group under the command of Col. T. D. Inch (British) was kept informed of all details of the project.

Excellent cooperation was received from the 10th Malaria Field Unit (Capt. Johnson, British) and Malaria Control Unit No. 133 (Capt. Mood, American), which were responsible for protecting Allied forces in the Rome area. The Italian Hygiene and Health Department for the Commune of Rome, through Prof. Cramarossa, Public Health Officer, collaborated by suspending all antimalaria activity in the test area during the season and by contributing to the project the services of employees usually engaged in such work. Finally, belief in the ultimate success of the project led Prof. Missiroli, of the Istituto Superiore di Sanità, to forego all antimalaria measures in Maccarese, where he had carried on control work for many years and where in 1944 he had made a careful test of the effect of suppressive atabrine treatment.

Test Area

The Tiber Delta, as here designated, is an irregularly shaped district of some 216 square kilometers (120 square miles) bordering the Tyrrhenian Sea about 20 kilometers (12.4 miles) southwest of Rome. It extends from Palo on the north 37.5 kilometers (23.3 miles) to Tor Paterno on the south, with a maximum width of about 18 kilometers (11.2 miles) at the point where the river zigzags across the plain. The terrain is flat, averaging 2 to 3 meters above the level of the sea, and contains some depressions extending below sea level.

The political districts included in the test area were Acilia, Ostia Antica and Ostia Lido, Ponte Galera, Fiumicino, Maccarese, and Palidoro, all belonging to the Commune of Rome. For administrative purposes the test area was subdivided into four sections as shown in Fig. 4; Acilia (E), Ostia (D), Fiumicino (C), and Maccarese (B).

For the conclusive studies planned for 1945 it was important that the test area be so large that infiltration of anopheles at the periphery would not destroy the effect of treatment at the center, and that the district be protected from invasion from without. The Tyrrhenian Sea provides a barrier on the south and west. To the north low rolling hills form a divide, which for about 3˙kilometers is dry and free of permanent water courses. The north-northeast boundary is protected by the Roman hills to a point about 1½ kilometers north of Ponte Galera. Several streams descend from these hills, but during the summer of 1945 these were dry. East of the test area and north of the Tiber, buildings were sprayed at the request of the British 10th Malaria Field Unit, while the area south of the Tiber was similarly treated by the American Malaria Control Unit No. 133. Thus the possibility of infiltration of anopheles from contiguous areas was reduced to a minimum. The periphery to the south was sparsely populated, and no evidence of infiltration there was recorded during the season.

In recent times prior to 1889, the Tiber Delta was virtually uninhabited. When in flood the river overflowed into the wide marshes called "Stagno di Maccarese" and "Stagno della Pagliete." Even the docks of the ancient Porto di Traiano, situated at some distance from the sea, were frequently inundated. The sparse population of shepherds lived in the medieval castles of Ostia Antica, Fusano, Porziano, Maccarese, and Palidoro and on

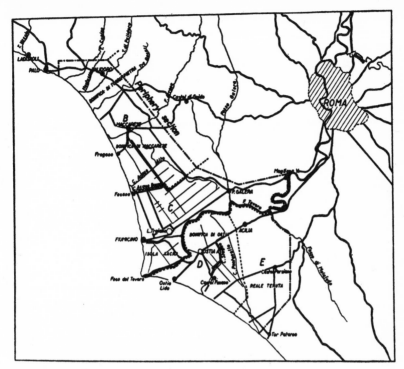

Figure 4. Tiber Delta and coastal plain test area.

occasional farms. Brush and forest covered the remainder of the district. A small fishing village, Fiumicino, was situated near the mouth of the navigable canal of the Tiber.

Reclamation of the Delta was begun by the Italian Government between 1885 and 1890, but it was not until after World War I that extensive agricultural drainage and colonization were seriously undertaken. Thus, within a few years, brush, forest, and swamps were replaced by farms which supported large herds of cattle, extensive vineyards, and market gardens. Modern villages made their appearance. Excellent highways now connect every farm with its market center. Much of the Delta is irrigated as well as drained. The southern and southwestern portion, however, has never been reclaimed. Known as the "Tenuta di Castel Porziano," it is maintained as a royal hunting reserve for the conservation of wild life.

From reliable Italian sources it has been learned that the Germans gave orders that the Maccarese pumping station should stop working on October 9, 1943, but that the pump which lifted water from the Tiber to the distributing canals of the irrigation system should continue to operate, thus causing extensive flooding of the Maccarese plain. On October 19 the drainage pumps on the Isola Sacra ceased to function, by German order, while the tide gates on the outlet canal were permanently opened. Two of the pumps at Ostia Antica were destroyed and the main effluent canal to the sea was blocked in three places. As the coastal area of the Delta is at or slightly below sea level, these steps led to extensive flooding during the rainy season of 1943–1944.

Malaria in the Delta

Data on malaria morbidity are available for this area since 1927 at the Hygiene and Health Department of the Commune of Rome. A case is recorded as primary if the patient has not formerly been treated by the health unit, and as secondary if he is listed in the records as having had prior attacks. Presumably the diagnosis is based on the finding of parasites in a blood smear.

In 1936 malaria morbidity in the units of Fiumicino, Ostia Antica, and Ponte Galera was less than 1 per cent while that in the units of Acilia, Maccarese, and Palidoro was between 4 and 5 per cent. In Fiumicino and Ostia Antica the rates pursued a parallel course, rising to a minor peak in 1939 and then sharply to a major peak in 1944 following the inundation caused by the destruction of the drainage equipment. In Acilia and Ponte Galera there were increases in 1939 and 1944 separated by a period of lower incidence in 1940–1943. The increase in morbidity in 1939 has been attributed to the introduction of nonimmune laborers for the construction of a large hydroplane base on the plain of Magliana. This work was discontinued when Italy entered the war. These areas, located on higher ground were not seriously affected by the inundation of 1943–1944.

Morbidity rates in the Maccarese and Palidoro units pursued similar courses. Incidence in Palidoro dropped continuously from 1936 through 1942 and then rose, while in Maccarese there was a transient rise in 1939 and 1940, a drop to a minimum in 1941 followed by a sharp rise in 1942. Although the Maccarese area suffered extensively from the inundation in 1943–1944, a program of suppressive treatment with atabrine was instituted by Prof. Missiroli in the summer of 1944. Palidoro was not affected by the inundation, but maintenance of its drainage system lapsed. Atabrine was administered here also in 1944.

In May 1945 a survey of 2268 school children in the coastal plain was made by the same group that conducted the surveys in Castel Volturno in 1944 and 1945 to obtain spleen and parasite indices of malaria infection. The rates vary considerably. The proportion of children with enlarged spleens ranged from 12 per cent in Maccarese to 67 per cent in Lingua D'Oca, while the spleen rate for all children was 18 per cent. Parasite rates were lower, ranging from 1 per cent in several towns to 26 per cent in Porto Vecchio, with an average for the total group of 4 per cent.

The Anopheles Vector

Anopheles labranchiae is the most dangerous of the Italian malaria vectors. Missiroli has shown that after the inundation of the Delta area in 1943–1944 the percentage of labranchiae among anopheles caught at three stations rose from 45, 29, and 48 to 96, 100, and 97, respectively. When breeding freely it is found in enormous numbers resting on walls and ceilings of buildings occupied either by man or animals. The choice of resting place of this species renders it particularly vulnerable to the residual effect of DDT.

The records of weekly captures of adult anopheles in 10 stations by the unit of Ostia Antica were obtained from the Hygiene and Health Department of the Commune of Rome, and monthly averages were computed from the data for 1939–1942. It should be noted that these densities pertain to years when there was active control of anopheles breeding through cleaning of ditches and the application of Paris green. For comparison with the earlier densities, captures were made from June through November 1945 following treatment in the area south of the Tiber. (A reduction of about 99 per cent was observed.)

Organization and Equipment of Field Personnel

A chief inspector was assigned to each of the four sections to be responsible for all equipment allocated to his section, to supervise the work, and to keep records of the amount of insecticide issued and applied and of the number of buildings and rooms treated. The date of treatment was permanently stencilled on each group of buildings when the spraying was completed.

Each spraying gang consisted of a foreman and seven laborers traveling in a truck, the driver of which was also a member of the squad. The foreman carried a map of the district and was expected to keep careful records of the premises sprayed.

Raincoats, gloves, goggles, and helmets were provided for each workman. Soap for daily baths was issued weekly together with laundry soap for washing the work garments. The use of gloves was discontinued immediately, and the goggles were discarded soon afterward, since they quickly became covered with a film of kerosene that interfered with vision. The men preferred their own hats or caps to the helmets. At no time during the spraying operations or later were there any complaints of ill effects of DDT, although some cases of dermatitis occurred which usually disappeared after a few days. These were attributed to the effect of kerosene rather than to that of DDT.

The insecticide was applied with a standard farm-type knapsack continuous sprayer, except that the usual nozzle plate giving a cone-shaped spray was replaced by a disc that furnished a flat, fan-shaped spray. The standard delivery arm of 24 inches was too short for most of the work to be done. Two of these could be joined for spraying the lower part of the walls, but longer arms were devised for spraying the upper portions of high walls and ceilings, by inserting a lightweight pipe of 5/16-inch diameter through bamboo poles 2, 3, 4, or 5 meters long to give the required length. Detachable couplings were fitted to the pistol end of each pole so that changes from one length to another could be made quickly. A short piece of curved pipe was inserted in these long poles, giving the nozzle a 30-degree angle to facilitate the proper application of the insecticide.

A detailed map of the test area (scale, 1:12,500), prepared from Italian Government maps, was an essential item of equipment. This map showed rivers, drainage and irrigation canals, pumping stations, highways, bridges, and the location of every group of buildings. While the map was in preparation all premises were visited and the number and location of buildings were verified.

Preparation and Application of the Insecticide

It was found that the kerosene available would readily dissolve considerably more than 5 per cent by weight of DDT, and since a heavy dose was desired, it was decided to use 6.5 per cent by weight in the solution. The insecticide was prepared at headquarters in Rome. After filtration. 205 liters of kerosene was poured into a clean 55-gallon drum into which 11.4 kilograms (25 pounds) of 100 per cent DDT had previously been dumped. The drum was then placed on a platform in the sun and agitated by rolling it frequently back and forth for a period of at least 3 days. In this manner 283 drums of solution were prepared containing 3209 kilograms (7075 pounds) of DDT and 58,015 liters of kerosene. The solution was filtered when transferred to the sprayers since even fine particles in the liquid easily clogged the small orifice of the nozzle. Of the 283 drums of insecticide prepared, the contents of 275 were used in the initial spraying of buildings in the area.

Since an objective of the Tiber Delta study was to obtain information on the maximum effect of an application of DDT under Italian conditions, it was decided to use a dose of 200 milligrams of DDT per square foot of surface. The modern section of the town of Acilia had 226 identical two-family houses which served as a training base for field personnel. Each worker was trained to use approximately 11.5 liters of insecticide to cover the 275 square meters of surface to be sprayed in the interior of each of these houses.

The knapsack sprayer was operated by one man when a short delivery arm could be used, but when a longer arm was required two men were needed. The hose connecting the reservoir with the pole was lengthened to

2½ meters for two-man operation. Where large buildings with high ceilings or unceiled rooms were encountered, one group of operators, using sprayers with long delivery arms, treated the ceilings, another group equipped with sprayers having shorter arms treated the walls just below the ceilings, while a third group (or often a single workman) sprayed the lower part of the walls to within 1½ meters above the floor. The practice of not spraying the floor was adopted because of the impression that labranchiae did not rest low on the walls. It was, however, sometimes found resting in this zone during the summer.

The upper floors of houses were treated first. Everything in position against walls, with the exception of oil paintings, was sprayed—mirrors, wall hangings, pictures, window draperies, bed covering, clothing, and so on. Wardrobes were not sprayed inside. No special effort was made to spray behind pictures or furniture placed close to the walls or behind goods so placed in storerooms. Careful attention was always given to spraying electric-light fixtures, ropes, wires, or other hanging objects on which insects might rest. The housewife was advised to cover foodstuffs. Stables and outbuildings were sprayed without removal of animals.

Summary of Spraying Activities

Structures sprayed in addition to dwellings included all those which might serve as sources of blood meals to anopheles. In all, 5869 buildings were sprayed requiring 1620 man-days, a ratio of 3.6 buildings per man-day. There were 49,951 rooms of various types treated, a ratio of 30.8 per man-day.

Data pertaining to urban as distinct from rural portions of each section have been studied. The area treated covered 286 square kilometers or 110 square miles and housed 35,293 persons according to prewar census figures. From these data, ratios of persons per room and grams of DDT issued per room and per person have been computed for each subdivision of the area. These ratios vary within wide limits according to the type and size of building and to the number and kind of livestock sheltered. For the area as a whole there was less than one person per room (0.71); 63 grams of DDT was issued per room sprayed and 89 grams per person.

Postspraying Capture of Anopheles, Larvae and Adults

As soon as a section had been completely sprayed its personnel was reorganized and routine inspections for larvae and adult anopheles were inaugurated. The section was divided into small zones, each of which could be covered once a week by the inspector on a bicycle. Two men were assigned to each zone, one to look for larvae, the other for adults:

The procedure for adult captures in the Tiber Delta was unlike that in Castel Volturno in that inspections were made in all buildings on nearly all the premises in the rural areas, so the counts should represent a large proportion of the anopheles present. The search for adult anopheles was continued on a reduced scale until February 20, 1946. Sections E (Acilia) and D (Ostia) south of the Tiber were combined for inspection purposes.

Larvae were captured at selected sites and the number taken in 20 dips with a net dipper was considered the count for the station.

Weekly captures of adults rarely exceeded one anopheles per premises and were frequently less than one in 10 premises. Density in Fiumicino (C) rose abruptly to a peak of 2.1 per premises during the week ending June 24 and then dropped, while a similar rise—not so precipitous—occurred in the Acilia–Ostia sections (E and D). Something like a delayed seasonal rise occurred in each section in September. Although density dropped to zero in Fiumicino during the week ending October 28, a minor rise at this time was observed in anopheles captured in the other sections.

All mosquitoes found were captured, and record was made of the number of anophelines and of culicines taken. Only 2978 culicines were captured in the 28 weeks between May 14 and November 25, during which 10,544 inspections of premises were made. This gives an average of only 0.28 per premises inspected. While captures of adults attained a level of one per premises only once during the season in the treated sections, those in the peripheral stations ranged from approximately 4.5 to 25.

Captures of larvae in the treated area attained a level of two per station the week ending July 1, dropped thereafter over a period of 7 weeks, rose to a level of over one per station in August and September, and then dropped sharply.

When adult anopheline density in the section of Fiumicino rose to two per premises the week ending June 24, the terrain and buildings at the site of the heaviest capture near Lago di Traiano were searched and a new pigsty, built after the other buildings had been sprayed, was found with some 300 mosquitoes resting on the walls and roof. Once sprayed it was never again found infested. Anopheles were also found in a large stable which had obviously not been properly sprayed. After treatment only one anopheles was subsequently found. Two pigsties on the Isola Sacra within 300 meters of Lago di Traiano were also found positive and had to be resprayed.

The only known specific effort to control anopheles breeding in the test area during 1945 was made by the estate manager who raised the level of Lago di Traiano and cleared the margins. Nevertheless, larvae were found fairly frequently throughout the season in the canal joining the lake and the sea, and the probable source of the adults was eventually discovered. The ruined storehouses of the old Roman port near the lake had not been sprayed, because searches during the hibernation season of 1944–1945 led to the assumption that labranchiae did not rest there. A careful search of these ruins in the summer of 1945, however, revealed adult anopheles resting on the walls of the dimly lighted chambers. These mosquitoes might well have completed their life cycles without recourse to human blood meals, since livestock grazed at night in the vicinity. There were no human habitations within the direct line of flight between these storehouses and the canal. In the Acilia–Ostia section anopheles were found breeding late in the season in the Tiber River itself.

Maccarese was the last section to be sprayed; and the work there was not completed until June 15, after the breeding season was well advanced, which may account for the higher initial mosquito density. There were also 80 hectares (195 acres) of rice in this section, where larvae were found occasionally until the water was shut off in September. The premises harboring adult anophelines were located in the vicinity of one or another of these plantations, and their number decreased when the fields became dry.

Postspraying Incidence of Malaria

The trend of annual malaria morbidity rates in the six sanitary units for which data were obtained from the Health Department of the Commune of Rome for the years 1936–1945 has been studied.* A sharp rise in incidence occurred in 1944 which was most conspicuous in the units of Ostia Antica and Fiumicino. In 1945 the rates dropped in four of the six units but they continued to rise in Maccarese and Palidoro.

The monthly distribution of malaria cases in all six units, including Ostia Lido, for the years 1944 and 1945 is shown in Figure 10. Late in 1943 many of the civilians in the Delta were evacuated by the Germans, consequently, in the early months of 1944 only a few scattered cases were reported. With the arrival of the Allies people returned to their homes, and an explosive outbreak of malaria occurred which reached a peak of 1242 registered cases in August. The subsequent rapid decline may have been accelerated by measures taken to protect the Allied troops.

An unusual monthly distribution of malaria cases may be noted in 1945. There was an abrupt rise in incidence in January that continued to a peak of 587 cases in March, which was 2½ months before normal seasonal transmisson could have affected the picture. Fewer cases were reported in April, and the number continued to fall during succeeding months of the year. The customary summer peak in August failed to appear. The reasons for

* Sanitary units, Acilia, Ostia Antica, and Fiumicino, were within the treated area; about 60 per cent of the population in the Ponte Galera unit and 70 per cent of that in the Palidoro unit resided in the test area, while four or five premises belonging to the Maccarese unit were situated outside the treated section.

this are believed to have been (1) the appearance of late onsets and winter and spring relapses among persons infected in 1944, and (2) the absence of adult anopheles in 1945 in sufficient numbers to cause the usual summer rise in the number of new infections.

Every effort was made by inspectors and competent staff members to discover instances of recent infection. One new malaria infection was verified in a 3-month-old infant at Fregene, whose mother was reported to have had a relapse at the time of delivery. A thorough search of the neighborhood revealed a few anopheles in a small pigsty which had not been sprayed.

The following statement which summarizes the results of the application of DDT in the Tiber Delta in 1945 is by Prof. A. Missiroli, who has studied malaria in this area for many years: "Not one case of primary malaria has been verified in the Delta of the Tiber, and Ostia has achieved a healthiness the like of which has not been seen there for some 2000 years, that is, since the invasion of Italy by malaria."

As another illustration of the effective use of house spraying with DDT,

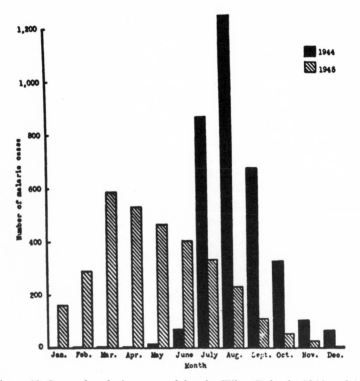

Figure 10. Cases of malaria reported for the Tiber Delta in 1944 and 1945 by month.

Fig. 11 is given. Professor Missiroli undertook to check the epidemic at Fondi, located between Castel Volturno and the Tiber Delta test areas, during the second half of June 1945. A sharp break in the number of new infections was noted 20 days later. Immediate and perfect antilarval work could not have achieved such quick results.

Residual Effect of DDT

When the Tiber Delta project was planned, it was hoped that a single application of insecticide would suffice to keep anopheles density below the level required for transmission of malaria for a full season. Field searches in the Acilia–Ostia sections in February 1946 failed to reveal mosquitoes in treated buildings. The intensive search at this time, however, led to the discovery of labranchiae in many unexpected places, such as empty silos never occupied by animals, open storage sheds, woodpiles near animal shelters, hollow logs, and bundles of cut bamboo. No labranchiae had been found resting under bridges or in culverts during the hot summer months of 1945 but they were discovered in such places in the late fall immediately preceding the period of hibernation.

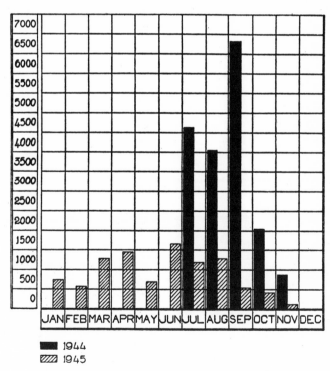

■ 1944
▨ 1945

Figure 11. Cases of malaria reported for Fondi. (*After A. Missiroli.*)

Work of Previous Investigators

At Castel Volturno and in the Delta of the Tiber it was observed that the failure to spray a pigsty or other building might be reflected in the number of anopheles caught in premises at some distance and that the spraying of such neglected shelters would result in the disappearance of anopheles from these other premises. Furthermore, Prof. Missiroli found in 1945 that the spraying of farm buildings and those at the periphery of such towns as Fondi was sufficient to halt the rise of malaria within the towns.

In 1935 Park Ross reported the results of 3 years of control of malaria in Zululand, Natal Province, South Africa, through the weekly spraying of native huts with pyrethrum. Russell and Knipe, following some preliminary work by Covell et al., undertook experiments in India to determine the efficacy of spray insecticides in the control of malaria in areas where *A. culicifacies* is the principal vector. Their results were impressive.

Other Advantages of DDT Application in the Tiber Delta

In the light of the results obtained by other workers, it is believed that a greater reduction was achieved in anopheles density in the Delta than was needed to prevent transmission of malaria. When malaria control is the only consideration a more limited program may be planned at less cost. There were, however, definite advantages achieved by the Delta program in the destruction of all insects inside the premises. Freedom from houseflies, and sandflies, bedbugs, cockroaches, and fleas makes a big impression on people in treated areas and creates a public demand for respraying the following year and for the extension of spraying to neighboring areas. One may conjecture that eventually anopheles control may become a part of a routine program for the elimination of all household insect pests, requiring no special budget and no highly trained staff. The most urgent study now remaining is the determination of what malarious areas exist, if any, where residual DDT alone will not prevent transmission.

Acknowledgments

In addition to the collaboration received from persons whose names have been mentioned, it is a pleasure to record that important contributions were made by the following to the studies described: Col. P. F. Russell, director, Malaria Section, Allied Control Commission in Italy, 1944; Lt. Col. Justin Andrews, malariologist, MTOUSA, 1944; Lt. Col. Richard M. Young and Capt. R. A. Elliot, 12th General Hospital, U.S. Army; Capt. L. M. Klashman and Sgt. C. R. Collins, 137th Malaria Control Detail; Capt. R. A. Fisher, Lt. A. W. Ziegler, and Sgt. C. S. Black, 15th Medical Laboratory; Lt. John S. Wehrle and Sgt. Guy D'Aleo, 2675th Regiment, Allied

Commission; Professoressa Lidia La Face and Sig. Francesco Neri, Istituto Superiore di Sanità, Rome; Drs. Francesco Kongo and Luigo Aloy of the Typhus Control Section of the Allied Control Commission; and Drs. H. W. Kumm and F. S. Markham of the Rockefeller Foundation Health Commission.

Summary and Conclusions

In 1944 and 1945 a 5 per cent DDT–kerosene spray was applied to the walls and ceilings of all buildings in specified areas of the Bonifica di Castel Volturno on the Italian coast just north of Naples. Results in 1944 were so promising that in 1945 a more extensive project was launched in an area of approximately 120 square miles in the Tiber Delta, where a 6.5 per cent solution of DDT in kerosene was applied once at a rate of approximately 200 milligrams per square foot to the interiors of all human habitations and animal shelters between February 27 and June 15. The objective was to determine the residual effect of the spray upon anopheline density in the absence of other control measures.

The organization of the field staff, the preparation of the insecticide and the equipment and methods employed in its application are described.

Routine searches for *Anopheles labranchiae* adults and larvae in Castel Volturno and in the Tiber Delta indicated that density had been greatly reduced. A year after treatment no anopheles were found in previously sprayed buildings examined in the Delta.

In Castel Volturno a significant reduction in the parasite rate of school children occurred during the 16-month period of observation. While malaria morbidity in the Delta in 1945 was higher than in prewar years, its distribution by months showed a rapid rise to a peak in March and a continuous drop thereafter, indicating that most, if not all, of the cases reported came from infections of the previous year. The usual summer rise in incidence failed to appear.

Selection 40 | Nationwide Malaria-Eradication
Projects in the Americas.
V. General Principles of the
Eradication Programs in the
Western Hemisphere*

This 1950 Symposium of the National Malaria Society on "Nationwide Malaria Eradication Projects in the Americas" is a highly significant landmark in the history of tropical medicine. For the first time since 1901, when Gorgas working in Havana demonstrated conclusively that yellow fever and malaria could be controlled by antimosquito measures, the malariologist can legitimately join the yellow fever worker in talking of disease eradication. The advantage is now with the malariologist, who can dry up the sources of human infection, and needs not fear reinfection from animal reservoirs.

The eradication of malaria from rural areas of the tropics may be expected to have more profound effects on these regions than did the elimination of yellow fever from cities and ports several decades ago.

The four papers presented here today describe truly nationwide eradication projects based on a single method: the spraying of human habitations with residual DDT. These projects cover well over half the malarious regions of the Americas, areas infested by such widely varying mosquito vectors as *Anopheles quadrimaculatus, A. darlingi, A. albitarsis,* and *A. cruzii.*

The concept of eradication† implies that the roots of infection are so destroyed that the disease will not reappear, in the absence of reintroduction, even though control measures be discontinued. The worker who is satisfied with disease reduction may well lessen his efforts when the point is

---

* Dr. Soper was the Director, Pan American Sanitary Bureau, and Regional Director for the Americas of the World Health Organization.

This paper was originally published *(70)* in the *Journal of the National Malaria Society 10:* 183–194, 1951.

† It is interesting to note that the word "eradicate" was applied to disease before the work of Pasteur, and long before Finlay, Manson, Ross, Reed, and Gorgas. An *American Dictionary of the English Language* (Noah Webster, 1861) defines "eradicate" thus: "(1) To pull up the roots, or by the roots. Hence to destroy anything that grows; to extirpate; to destroy the roots, so that the plant will not be reproduced; as, to eradicate weeds. (2) To destroy thoroughly; to extirpate; as to

reached at which the cost of eliminating the few remaining infections may be much greater than the cost of preventing other important diseases. The worker looking for eradication must press on to the finish, accepting the fact that the greatest cost per case prevented is incurred just before the final success of the project.

Likewise the worker who leaves the seeds of infection in his own district need take no interest in the reduction of the disease in other areas, nor fear its reintroduction from dirty areas. Eradication, on the other hand, is, and must be, an expanding program, since it is most successful when the clean area is largest. The eradicationist must be an internationalist ready to collaborate with other countries in the simultaneous elimination of common dangers and common enemies.

Disease eradication has been the goal of health workers for many years. We have learned today that Frederick Hoffmann proposed the eradication of malaria in the United States in 1915, just about the time Gorgas was embarking on a program for the eradication of yellow fever from the Americas under the auspices of The Rockefeller Foundation, which was also developing campaigns in many countries for the eradication of hookworm disease. However, at that time available methods proved inadequate for the eradication of malaria in the United States. Likewise, epidemiological factors, then unknown, made elimination of yellow fever impossible, and although the incidence of hookworm disease was reduced greatly, nowhere was the worm eradicated.

Under these circumstances, it is not surprising that The Rockefeller Foundation was unwilling to have the term "eradication" used in the anti–*Anopheles gambiae* project in Brazil in 1938, even though it had been shown in the meantime that the *Aëdes aegypti* mosquito could be eradicated from the principal cities and even from entire states of Brazil. Only after the elimination of gambiae from Brazil did the word "eradicate" become respectable once more and acceptable in good public health circles. Even then the term used was "species eradication," since the word "eradication" itself had been so misused. The dramatic results of the eradication of gambiae in Brazil made it possible to emphasize the importance of the work which was being done in the eradication of aegypti, and in 1940 the Serviço de Febre Amarela of Brazil was reorganized with the declared purpose of eradicating aegypti from the whole of the national territory. This project

---

eradicate errors, or false principles, or vice, or disease." That this reference to disease was to the eradication of disease from a single person rather than from the community is suggested by the classification, at that time, of certain drugs as eradicatives. Definition: "Eradicative, *n*. A medicine that effects a radical cure." And in 1861 very few specific drugs were known, of which quinine was one of the most important.

has made steady progress during the past decade and is now on the eve of completion. Brazil has learned, as all who work with eradication must, that eradication, to be successful, must become an ever-expanding program. In order to protect herself, Brazil proposed to the Directing Council of the Pan American Sanitary Organization in 1947 that a coordinated program for the eradication of aegypti from the Western Hemisphere should be undertaken under the auspices of the Pan American Sanitary Bureau. This proposal was approved, and now almost all of the political units of the Americas are actively participating in this project.

In the meantime, *Anopheles sergenti* has been eradicated from the Oases of Kharga and Dakhla in Egypt, and favorable progress has been reported in campaigns for the eradication of the vectors of malaria in Sardinia and Cyprus. And so the word "eradicate" has come to have once more its original meaning: "to destroy the roots, so that the plant will not be reproduced." In evaluating species eradication, the final test for local eradication is the failure of the species to reappear, in the absence of reintroduction, after all control measures have been discontinued.

The eradication of malaria may be considered as involving first and foremost, the blocking of all transmission by mosquitoes, and second, the spontaneous or therapeutic cure of infective cases in man. When this state has been reached, reappearance of the disease would depend on the introduction of infected humans or of the mosquito vector.

Theoretically, malaria can be eradicated in a closed population, that is, in an area receiving no immigrants, by preventing man–mosquito–man transmission until such time as all infected persons become permanently noninfective. Since the man–mosquito–man transmission of malaria is a complex process influenced by each element, man, mosquito, and parasite, the eradicationist can operate on any one, or cumulatively on all three components.

The prevention of transmission may be obtained by

A. Attack on the parasite
    1. In man, by therapy of the acute attack or by drug suppression
    2. In the mosquito, by agents of interception, effective only against adults which come to attack man
B. Attack on the insect vector
    1. Control of immature stages
       a. Making conditions unfavorable for breeding
       b. Antilarval measures
    2. Antiadult procedures
       a. Prevention of contact, screening, and so on
       b. Spraying, direct and/or residual

During the first three decades after the role of the mosquito in the transmission of malaria became known, little atempt was made to attack specifically the infected or potentially infected adult mosquito. Ironically enough this has come to be recognized as the weakest link in the chain of infection.

In the eradication programs in the United States, Venezuela, British Guiana, and Brazil, the essential factor is the attack on the parasite *in the mosquito* rather than *in man,* which is accomplished by striking at the adult mosquito rather than the larva. The intensity of the attack varies according to the domiciliary habits of the vector species.

Although Le Prince, working in Panama, had used hand captures of anopheles mosquitoes in sleeping quarters as a malaria control measure, and Chagas and James had called attention to the importance of the house as the site of transmission, no one used or advocated attack on the infected mosquito until Park Ross introduced weekly pyrethrum spraying of native quarters for the control of gambiae-transmitted malaria in Natal, South Africa, almost 20 years ago. Russell confirmed the value of this method for *A. culicifacies*-infested regions in India, even though this species is not highly domestic. Knowledge of these and other similar results was essential and basic to the early trial of DDT as a residual spray for preventing transmission of malaria in various parts of the world. Russell, Andrews, and Kumm, all of whom are taking part in this symposium, had some relation to the field trials in Italy at Castel Volturno in 1944 and in the Tiber Delta in 1945. The test in the Tiber Delta was especially important since malaria in this area had been thoroughly studied and controlled by ditching and Paris greening by Hackett and Missiroli for many years previously. Following the 1945 demonstration of the value of DDT residual spray Missiroli publicly (January 1946) announced that drainage and filling was no longer important for the control of malaria in Italy and that, with adequate supplies of DDT, malaria in Italy would disappear as a public health problem within 5 years. This prophecy has been fulfilled.

Since weekly spraying with pyrethrum had given such good results under varied conditions and with vectors which were not highly domestic, it was logical to believe that residual DDT would prevent transmission of malaria by most of the anopheline vectors. Thus by 1946 it was recognized that the most urgent task facing the malariologists of the world was to determine if and where areas existed in which residual DDT would not prevent transmission. From today's reports and others at hand it is apparent that the great bulk of the malaria of the Americas is easily suppressed through residual domiciliary spraying. These results are apparently almost equally good against highly domestic species such as darlingi, in which local species eradication has been achieved by residual spraying, and against species such as *A. albimanus,* of which only a fraction of the adults in an area enter houses. The effect of residual DDT, then, is essentially on the potentially or actually infected adult mosquito, when it visits human habitations.

The reports submitted today merit detailed study and careful consideration by all who are concerned with malaria as a problem in the Americas. For the first time there exists a single efficient and economical method of attack on malaria which can be standardized and applied with confidence to almost all malarious areas of the Americas.

In the United States, beginning in the middle 1930s, long before the advent of DDT, there has been a steady decrease in malaria throughout the endemic regions in uncontrolled as well as in controlled areas. Some workers have attributed this decline to the widespread employment of insecticidal sprays for household use. The U.S. program for the eradication of malaria, which does not contemplate the complete elimination of quadrimaculatus, is the logical one to pursue, considering the difficulty of destroying this species and the enormous area it inhabits. However, after eradication of malaria is achieved, its continued absence will depend on the number and distribution of infective immigrants and the extent to which official agencies or individual families continue to use household insecticides.

The situation in the United States is favorable to the eradication of the disease because

1. Anopheline mosquitoes are generally more susceptible to insecticides than are flies and other noxious insects.

2. The people, once accustomed to homes without insects, will take community and individual measures against these insects.

3. The development of malaria eradication projects in other countries lessens the danger of importation of new cases.

4. The development and use of improved drugs of low cost for suppression and radical cure of malaria will cause a diminution of the disease.

But even so, the United States and every other country, as it becomes free of malaria, can be shown to have a direct stake in the malaria eradication projects of other nations.

This symposium is extremely fortunate in having reports in person from the directors of the malaria studies and control projects in both Venezuela and British Guiana, where careful research has been done for many years (Venezuela since 1936, British Guiana since 1933) before the advent of DDT, and where this agent was introduced early before it became generally available in other parts of the world.

Venezuela lies in a transitional faunal zone in which various vectors of malaria are found, the two most important being albimanus and darlingi, which differ widely in domesticity.

Transmission of malaria by each of these vectors had been found subject to control by weekly spraying with pyrethrum before DDT came on the scene. The early results with residual DDT reported from Venezuela were most important, since they indicated that this measure would be applicable over enormous areas in South and Central America and the West Indies in which one or the other of the two anopheles mentioned above are the principal vectors of malaria.

The malariologists in Venezuela take great care in preparing specifications for the insecticides purchased by them and follow up with routine chemical and other tests on the materials received. The development of satisfactory high-percentage DDT-wettable powders is in large part due to this service, which has set new standards for the marketing of insecticides to the benefit of all purchasers. The fact that workers in Venezuela have always known what they were working with has facilitated the determination of standards for field work under Venezuelan conditions.

With the results of the first 2 years of extensive use of residual DDT at hand, the health authorities of Venezuela realized that a technique for the eradication of malaria was now available, and that with malaria control measures now brought entirely within the domicile, it would be advantageous to have a single service responsible for the control of all diseases transmitted to man by arthropods. At the end of 1947, the malaria service became responsible for the eradication of aegypti from Venezuela. The importance of having a single service responsible for the control of all diseases depending on various types of infestation of human habitations was emphasized in 1949, when it became evident that the prolonged use of residual DDT was bringing about an increase of *Rhodnius prolixus,* an important vector of Chagas' disease (American trypanosomiasis). The malariologist cannot be satisfied with the eradication of malaria but must be ready to work toward freeing human habitations of arthropods of all kinds. Once malaria disappears, interest in household pests, other than mosquitoes, may well be the key to continued work needed to keep malaria out.

One cannot doubt that malaria eradication is imminent in Venezuela, when one learns that persons engaged in smuggling are identified as such by blood examination, as they become infected with malaria before entering Venezuela. So little malaria now occurs that the Malaria Service is willing to consider all cases as new infections unless proved otherwise. The observation that very few malaria relapses occur after the first two years of spraying is very important for an understanding of the epidemiology of the disease and is in accord with the blood survey figures in the gambiae-infested area of Brazil, where the parasite index dropped from 65.5 per cent to 0.9 per cent in 2 years (1939–1941).

The radical changes reported in the vital statistics of Venezuela and British Guiana are most significant and are in keeping with those occurring in malarious regions all over the world following the introduction of residual insecticides. The increasing populations of previously malarious areas are a challenge which must be met by better health services, better schools, better transportation, and especially by improved agricultural methods.

British Guiana has been an ideal setting for the demonstration of the dramatic results which follow when malaria transmission suddenly ceases in a formerly highly endemic area. Because the two principal crops in British Guiana (rice and sugar cane) are irrigated, drainage as an antilarval measure is impossible, and the use of larvicides is impracticable, but conditions are ideal for residual spraying, since the bulk of the population is concentrated in a small area and comparatively few of the houses are of mud and wattle construction. Darlingi is the only important vector of malaria in British Guiana and is so highly domestic there that species eradication has been accomplished, no darlingi having been found in the sprayed areas for 3 years. This experience in British Guiana raises the question whether darlingi is equally domestic throughout its entire range or is highly domestic in British Guiana and semisylvatic in the Amazon Valley and elsewhere in its extensive range in South America. The fixity of habit of a given species is of great practical importance. Aegypti is susceptible to eradication in the Americas largely because it has never become adapted to the forests of the New World, although in its native home in Africa, it is widely dispersed in forests. Are these diverse behaviors in America and Africa due to differences in characteristics of the forests or to discrete differences in the physiology of the mosquito? Tests should be made of the adaptability of the aegypti of African towns to life in the African forest, and of the aegypti of the forests to life in the towns, to determine whether urban eradication of aegypti is feasible in Africa as it is in the New World.

In discussing the attempted eradication of *Anopheles labranchiae* from Sardinia, it has been suggested that it is much more difficult to eradicate an indigenous species than an imported one. This raises the question of where a species is indigenous. Is darlingi indigenous in Venezuela and British Guiana where its local eradication by residual DDT has been observed, or is it a recent importation existing under marginal conditions? The apparent eradication of darlingi from a stretch of the valley of the Rio Doce in Brazil during several years following the intensive use of Paris green as a larvicide may be significant or not. Are the few remaining labranchiae in Sardinia direct descendants of the labranchiae of thousands of years ago before adaptation to life with man occurred and, therefore, incapable of building up the heavy infestation responsible for the previous highly malarious state of the island? Only time and further observation will clarify these points.

In British Guiana, we have an island of eradication established on the mainland of South America, a situation analogous to that which existed in Brazil when aegypti began to disappear from city after city along the coast. The experience with the reinvasion of British Guiana by darlingi in 1941 after a prolonged drought is most encouraging, since this reinvasion was gradual and might have been easily controlled by residual spraying of an adequate barrier area, just as the spread of gambiae in Northeast Brazil was halted in 1939 by a barrier zone of larviciding with Paris green. Although British Guiana plans permanent spraying of only one fourth to one third of the houses to form a barrier zone and to spray these only every 18 months, the mathematics of the situation make it imperative to get as large a zone as possible cleared, since only thus can the cost of the peripheral barrier be reduced to a minimum. It is obviously to the interest of British Guiana to have darlingi eradicated from Dutch Guiana, Venezuela, and North Brazil, so that no barrier zone would be needed. This problem in coordination of national health programs can best be solved by official international organizations such as the Pan American Sanitary Bureau or the World Health Organization.

The remarkable results obtained in British Guiana with rather long intervals between applications of DDT emphasize the disadvantages of mud-and-wattle type of habitations in the tropics. DDT residual spray is less effective in this sort of construction, which is not common in British Guiana. Future studies on suitable housing for the tropics should include investigation of the liability of various kinds of house construction to insect infestation and adaptation to insecticidal action.

An important additional result of the use of residual DDT in British Guiana has been the final eradication of aegypti from the coastal plain, where antilarval measures had been applied since 1939. The yellow fever mosquito is even more vulnerable to DDT residual spray than are the anopheles mosquitoes.

Brazil, the largest of the American republics, has a malaria problem involving all its states and territories. The National Malaria Service has been given greatly increased funds in recent years and has undertaken the gigantic task of eradicating malaria from this vast tropical and subtropical empire. The National Malaria Service works largely through agreements with and contributions from local governments and has come to have the responsibility for malaria control in all of Brazil, except the single powerful state of São Paulo.

Although the control of malaria is highly centralized, evidence of decentralization is already apparent. Malaria control zones have been established in certain areas containing 1000 to 1600 houses and are put in charge of a well-trained local resident who is responsible for the routine spraying of all houses in his zone at regular intervals. The local worker furnishes his own transportation and receives only his salary and the equipment and insecticide required. His work is checked occasionally by the Malaria Service.

Brazil has many types of malaria problems, all of which are apparently soluble with residual DDT. But Brazil also has other important arthropod-borne diseases, including yellow fever, plague, Chagas' disease, and dysentery. Eventually the orientation and follow-up of the general house disinfestation programs now carried out by several decentralized administrative services should rest in the hands of a single central service.

As each country approaches eradication of any disease or of any disease vector in its own territory, it immediately acquires an active interest in measures for similar eradication projects in those countries with which it has direct or indirect contact, and through which it might be reinfected or reinfested.

It is important then to consider the malaria-eradication programs in the United States, Venezuela, Brazil, and British Guiana, in connection with similar projects in other parts of the Americas. Fortunately for this discussion Dr. Carlos Alvarado, Regional Adviser on Malaria to the Pan American Sanitary Bureau, recently completed a survey of antimalarial activities in the Americas which was summarized in the 4th Report to the XIIIth Pan American Sanitary Conference on the campaign against malaria in the American Continent (September 1950). This report is most encouraging, as it indicates that other nations of the Americas are either now or should soon be in the same favorable position as the United States, Venezuela, Brazil, and British Guiana.

The eradication of malaria in Argentina involves two quite distinct problems:

1. Control of *A. pseudopunctipennis,* the sole vector in the northwestern endemic zone, covering parts of seven provinces with an area of 120,000 square kilometers, 225,000 houses, and a population of 1,250,000.

2. Control of *A. darlingi* and *A. albitarsis,* the vectors in the northeastern epidemic zone bordering on Brazil and Paraguay, with an area of 150,000 square kilometers and 500,000 inhabitants.

From the economic point of view, endemic malaria in Argentina has been much more important than epidemic malaria. For many years control measures have been concentrated largely in the zone infested by pseudopunctipennis; the data which follow refer to this zone except as stated otherwise.

In 1947, when the decision was taken to depend entirely on residual DDT, public burial with appropriate funeral rites was held for ditching and larvicidal equipment and materials to impress on the employees of the malaria service and on the public that a new era in the control of malaria had come. In less than 4 years Argentina has practically eliminated the problem of endemic malaria, and the Division of Malaria and Endemic Diseases has become the Department of Health for Northern Argentina.

Although the Argentine law relating to malaria (Law 5195 modified by Law 13266, September 1948, and Decree 9624) does not use the word "eradication," such is obviously the objective. In the endemic zone of Argentina it is obligatory

1. To spray all houses with residual insecticide at regular intervals.

2. To report all suspected malaria cases within 24 hours.

3. To submit blood smears for confirmation.

4. To dispense antimalarial drugs only on the prescription of a physician.

Argentina is handling malaria as a pestilential disease which should not exist in the endemic zone and is taking the responsibility of investigating each case which occurs. The restriction on the sale of antimalarial drugs is used to get information on the incidence of the disease and is quite in contrast to the distribution by the government of large amounts of such drugs in previous years (in 1946, 256,823 treatments).

A solution of DDT in kerosene is generally used, because this solvent is available locally. Only the walls of the sleeping quarters are sprayed, resulting in considerable economy of labor and material. From August 1949 to May 1950, 171,000 (76 per cent) of the houses in the endemic zone were sprayed. The remaining houses were so situated in the center of towns and cities that spraying was not needed. Reported cases of malaria dropped from 129,248 in 1945 to 5324 in 1949. (In the same period reported cases in the United States dropped from 62,763 to 4241.) In 1945, blood examination of 50,866 patients gave 24,161 (47.5 per cent) positives, but in 1949 examination of 9154 patients gave only 568 (6.2 per cent) positives. Only 232 new cases were found in the endemic zone in 1949. A survey of 14,581 school children in 1945 with 10.9 per cent positive bloods is to be compared with a similar survey of 50,652 children in 1949 with only 0.1 per cent of the slides positive. The percentage reduction among preschool children under 5 years of age was even more pronounced (in 1945, 7325 examined; 8.9 per cent positive; in 1949, 9008 examined, 0.05 per cent positive).

In the epidemic zone, where the incidence of malaria may vary greatly from year to year, only 10 per cent of the population was protected by residual DDT in 1949, and 15 per cent in 1950, as compared with 100 per cent of the population in the endemic zone. The plan for 1951 calls for full protection of the epidemic zone, even though 1949 conditions were excellent, with only 152 cases of malaria reported, and a blood parasite index in school children of only 0.1 per cent.

In discussing the eradication of malaria from the Americas, Uruguay and Chile can be eliminated entirely, since Uruguay has no malaria and Chile reported the complete eradication of its only vector, pseudopunctipennis, in 1948.

Ecuador (Law of 2 December 1948) declared the "eradication of malaria to be an urgent national problem" and established the national malaria service under its National Institute of Health. This service has concentrated its efforts on the use of residual DDT. The Government of Ecuador increased the malaria budget from 400,000 sucres in 1948 to 6,220,000 sucres in 1950, or over 1500 per cent. It is estimated that 68 per cent of the houses in the endemic zone have been sprayed once or twice in 1950, and the future program calls for complete coverage of the dangerous area.

Costa Rica, El Salvador, Guatemala, Honduras, British Honduras, and Nicaragua joined in a simultaneous campaign during 1950–1951 against household insects, largely oriented toward the eradication of malaria, under the technical advice of the PASB/WHO, with supplies furnished from a fund of $½ million made available by UNICEF.

Panama had a well-organized service for residual spraying, covering much of the exposed population of the republic when jungle yellow fever was discovered there in January 1949. The additional funds made available for antiaegypti measures were used by the Malaria Service for spraying such towns as were still infested with this mosquito, thereby increasing the coverage against malaria. Although definite figures are not available, malaria has become very uncommon in Panama; unfortunately, following a recent change of government, the rumor has circulated that a return to drainage and antilarval measures is planned.

In Paraguay the PASB/WHO and UNICEF have agreed to collaborate with the government in transforming the aegypti eradication service into a National Malaria Service in 1951.

French Guiana reports having sprayed all the houses in that colony with the consequent suppression of malaria transmission and the eradication of aegypti.

There is not time and space to discuss the situation in each of the remaining countries in detail. Haiti, Nicaragua, and Costa Rica are the only countries which do not have special services for malaria control, and in Honduras and Colombia the Malaria Service is part of the service maintained by the Institute of Inter-American Affairs. In Bolivia, Peru, Colombia, and Mexico, DDT as a residual spray has given the same good results as elsewhere in the Americas, and plans are being made for extension of its use in these countries. Cuba has made a beginning with DDT during the past year, and plans have been made for antimalaria programs in the Dominican Republic and Haiti. In 1950 only in Mexico, Jamaica, and Colombia are more people protected from malaria by engineering projects than by residual insecticide, and in many countries the only control measure used is residual house spraying with DDT.

In the third Pan American Report on Malaria to the XIIth Pan American Sanitary Conference (Caracas, 1947) it was foretold that the introduction of DDT would result in a great reduction in other methods of malaria control, while vast areas of the American tropics which had been untouched by any effective antimalaria measures would begin to receive the benefits of this most practical measure of control. This predicition has been more than borne out by the facts reported here today. It has been amply demonstrated, for the Americas at least, that periodic spraying with DDT will suppress the transmission of malaria within human habitations. Where extradomiciliary transmission of malaria does occur, it must be due in great part to the infection of mosquitoes from gametocyte carriers which were originally infected in habitations. As house transmission of malaria disappears, outside transmission should disappear rapidly also.

Considering that it is only 5 years since DDT became available, and that approximately 75 per cent of the habitations in the malarious regions of the Americas are in countries with nationwide programs for the eradication of malaria, it is not too much to anticipate that the rest of the job can be done during the next 5 years, if full advantage is taken of the services of the international organizations responsible for coordination of health activities in the Americas.

Selection 41 | The Epidemiology of a
Disappearing Disease: Malaria*

The honor of the invitation to deliver the 24th Charles Franklin Craig Lecture is greatly enhanced for me by the presence of Dr. Lewis W. Hackett, my first chief, as our presiding officer. It is significant that the invitation to speak on malaria eradication comes so soon after the masterly 22nd Charles Franklin Craig Lecture on "Malaria Eradication—Growth of the Concept and Its Application" by Dr. Louis L. Williams, Jr., just 2 years ago. This reflects the interest of the American Society of Tropical Medicine and Hygiene in what has come to be the greatest public health effort of all times and the recognition by your leaders that the development of the program for the worldwide eradication of malaria is so rapid that this Society must have frequent reports, if it is to discharge properly the responsibilities assumed in 1951, when the American Society of Tropical Medicine and the National Malaria Society were fused to become the American Society of Tropical Medicine and Hygiene. This Society must be the voice of the tropical public health workers of the United States in all matters related to malaria. The responsibility of this Society is indeed great, since the economic resources for supplies and equipment and for the technical and administrative training of national staffs essential to eradication programs simply are not available in many of the most malarious areas of the world. The continued and increasing support of the U.S. Government through multilateral and bilateral agencies is indispensable. The responsibility of this Society as a source of informed professional opinion will increase as the world program continues to develop and as obvious successes in many areas lead to a false sense of optimism with a natural tendency to relax and reduce the all-out effort before the goal is reached.

The unusual procedure of inviting a Charles Franklin Craig lecturer to speak on a specific subject followed, and may have been suggested by the remarks made a few months ago for the Washington Tropical Diseases Association after a trip to Asia with Dr. Robert Briggs Watson of The Rockefeller Foundation. Our trip to Asia was to observe at first hand eradi-

* The essentials of this paper were given under the title "Some 1959 Impressions of World-Wide Malaria Eradication," as the 24th Annual Charles Franklin Craig Lecture before the American Society of Tropical Medicine and Hygiene, Indianapolis, Indiana, October 28, 1959. Dr. Soper was Director Emeritus of the Pan American Sanitary Bureau.

This article was originally published (97) in the *American Journal of Tropical Medicine and Hygiene 9*: 357–366, 1960. (About 3 pages of the original text have been omitted; they dealt with the development of the *Aëdes aegypti*-eradication program in Brazil.)

cation programs which, after early dramatic declines in malaria incidence, had failed to reach eradication on the anticipated schedule. We visited Taiwan, the Philippines, Ceylon and Mysore State, India, before attending the Third Asian Malaria Conference (March 1959) in New Delhi, where personal contact was established with many malaria workers from Southeast Asia and the Western Pacific. Later I visited the eradication program in Thailand alone. These countries were carefully selected as those which had solved the bulk of their malaria problem but were facing the problem of final extirpation of the infection.

The impressions from this all-too-rapid visit may be summarized as follows:

1. In each of the countries visited the introduction of residual insecticides was followed by a rapid decrease in malaria, almost to eradication, in large heavily populated areas during the first 2 years of overall coverage.

2. No serious technical difficulties were encountered in any of the areas visited; anopheles resistance to DDT was not a problem, nor was extradomiciliary transmission of malaria proved.

3. The administrative difficulty of getting full coverage with residual insecticide of all human habitations in all the malarious areas, and the epidemiological difficulty of identifying areas where transmission continues, both contributed to the failure to eradicate malaria rapidly.

There has been a failure to develop proper supervision and checking of spraying operations and to adapt the techniques suitable for heavily populated, easily accessible populations to fringe populations, to nomadic populations, and to scattered populations living in hilly and forested areas. Particularly has there been a failure in certain instances to recognize the necessity for spraying temporary shelters used by rural populations in connection with seasonal crops. There has been a tendency to be satisfied with the general reduction of malaria, especially during the early years of the program, rather than to evaluate information from local communities to pinpoint places where malaria transmission continues. This blurring of the immediate objective of the eradication program—the interruption of malaria transmission in each local community for the period required for spontaneous clearing of the infection in the human population—has led to costly delays, since partial eradication is always expensive.

In none of the countries visited had high blood parasite indices persisted in the heavily populated, easily accessible areas, following the interruption of transmission. Nowhere was the charge of falsity made against the premise on which the eradication program is based. When properly used DDT had caused transmission to cease and malaria had disappeared rapidly.

The visits to the Asiatic eradication programs were entirely too short to do little more than gather general impressions from reading available reports, discussing details with program leaders, and in some instances observing field operations. Surprisingly, each of the programs with minor variations seemed to fit the same pattern as outlined above. The analysis of the pattern indicates that the difficulties of malaria eradication are in general those of any eradication program and may be classed as (1) administrative difficulties encountered in executing 100 per cent of the necessary program, and (2) epidemiologic difficulties in identifying the places where the program has failed in its immediate objective and permitted transmission to continue. These difficulties seem to plague the health officer whenever he shifts from the concept of communicable disease control to eradication. The public health administrator responsible for the control of communicable diseases, that is, reduction to the point where each disease is no longer a problem of public health importance in his community, tends to lose interest in the individual disease at the point where the eradicationist often encounters his greatest difficulty. This attitude is supported by international quarantine experience, which shows that the threat of international movement of the infectious agents of communicable diseases is correlated with the epidemiological visibility of such diseases. Also, the geographical area for which the public health officer is responsible is generally small and the threat of peripheral reinfection great, so it matters little that the seeds of infection remain in his area. For the eradicationist, continuing unrecognized transmission below the threshold of visibility constitutes the greatest threat to victory in the battle for complete elimination of the sources of infection.

The communicable disease control officer can take satisfaction from the absence of reported cases and of public clamor, but the eradicationist can be happy only when he has proved that transmission has ceased.

To emphasize the need for special study of the manner in which a communicable disease continues near or below the threshold of visibility and of the measures for its final suppression, I proposed some years ago the term, "The Epidemiology of a Disappearing Disease." I was gratified to receive an immediate cash award from Dr. L. L. Williams, Jr., who recognized the value of the term for this concept in malaria eradication. Dr. Louis I. Dublin has since used the term "The Epidemiology of Retreating Tuberculosis" and Dr. Luis Vargas the term "The Epidemiology of Evanescent Malaria."

Malaria eradication in various countries today seems to be following the pattern of endemic yellow fever eradication in Brazil from 1919 to 1934; in the face of an energetic frontal attack malaria disappears, recedes, evanesces, but remains to flare up and ridicule the eradicationist so soon as the attack is abandoned and eradication put to the critical test of the complete suppression of preventive measures. All too often the eradicationist is finding that the insecticidal work in some of his areas has been poorly administered . . . and that his epidemiological investigation has not shown him the silent malaria transmission that was continuing in his "jungle" areas. Without entering into details of anopheles resistance to insecticide and of plasmodial resistance to drugs, it can be said that the technical problems in malaria eradication would be much more easily solved were it possible to recognize every new infection at the time it occurs so that the failure to block transmission in each small delimited area, whether due to technical or administrative failure, could be denounced and corrected. The malariologist does not have any economical method of recognizing each new infection and may well have to settle for the identification of the places where transmission is occurring.

Epidemiological evaluation as a check on the completeness of the interruption of transmission by early insecticidal spraying is hardly less significant than similar information in the terminal stages of the program when surveillance is taking over. Proper evaluation during the attack phase of eradication is essential to the decision to abandon spraying and begin surveillance; precipitate unjustified action can force a highly expensive reorganization whereas continued spraying when no longer required is equally wasteful. The malariologist must decide on the method of evaluation best adapted to his area: (1) routine systematic collection of blood smears from fever cases by local resident representatives, (2) routine collection of blood smears from fever cases by house visits of service employees at frequent intervals, and (3) mass or sampling surveys of all or of certain groups of the population without regard to history of fever.

COMMENTS ON MALARIA ERADICATION IN CERTAIN COUNTRIES
Philippine Islands

In the Philippines after some 4 years of widespread coverage with insecticidal sprays in areas with over 8 million people, field surveys were made (1957–1958) and interpreted to mean that no transmission had occurred during a 2-year period among some 5 million people living in previously malarious areas. Spraying was suppressed in 1958 in these areas. Surveillance was organized on the basis of house-to-house visits every 3 weeks with the examination of blood smears from all fever cases found and of persons reporting fever during the previous 3 weeks. The analysis of the findings at the end of 10 months led to the reorganization of spraying operations throughout much of the area where they had been suppressed. Most of the recrudescence of transmission found was attributed to the introduction of the infection in the "eradication" areas from the sprayed areas where transmission had never been interrupted. Under Philippine conditions, it is apparent that it is not safe to discontinue spraying in one area until the areas from which it can be reinfected have also been cleared of infection.

Ceylon

Ceylon was one of the first countries in Asia to benefit from the introduction of DDT which has been widely used since the malaria epidemic of 1946–1947. The government decided early in 1949 to attempt the complete eradication of malaria from the island and by 1954 considerable areas where transmission could not be found were removed from the spraying program. In many areas *Anopheles culicifacies* could no longer be found. During 1955 the search for fever cases in dispensaries was relied on to show where transmission was occurring; many of these dispensaries were themselves outside the area of transmission. The search for fever cases in dispensaries and the follow-up of these cases to identify the areas where transmission was occurring so that treatment and insecticide could be applied proved ineffective, and in 1956–1957 there was a considerable reinvasion of the "eradicated" area by malaria. In 1958 the spraying program was reorganized and today there is an intensified search for fever cases throughout the island and greater insistence on finding and spraying temporary shelters in the forest clearings. The success of the present program will depend on the seeking out and spraying of all human habitations rather than on finding every infected person and treating him and his contacts.

Taiwan (Nationalist China)

Taiwan is another country in which DDT was introduced fairly early and from which excellent results have always been obtained. Here, although malaria disappeared in a large part of the heavily populated part of the island, the incidence of the disease did not continue to zero, as had been hoped for. An investigation of the situation in 1958 showed that transmission had ceased in the heavily populated agricultural parts of the island, but that in the hilly, mountainous areas with scattered habitations of difficult access, transmission continued. Investigation showed that some of these areas had been poorly sprayed and some had been missed entirely in the general campaign on the island. Reorganization and intensification of the search for infective cases and of the spraying of isolated habitations have led to a month-by-month reduction in the number of cases found since September 1958, and it now appears that practically all the transmission on Taiwan has been blocked and it can be anticipated that this country will become the first of the Asiatic countries to be able to declare the eradication of malaria.

Thailand

In Thailand the application of DDT has resulted in a rapid reduction of malaria and in the practical eradication of *Anopheles minimus* in much of the area covered by the spraying operations. Suppression of spraying has been possible in certain areas without the recurrence of malaria transmission. Impressive settlement of previously uninhabited areas has occurred. The program has, however, developed slowly with initial plans for protecting only the 13 or 14 million people living in the most malarious areas; it is, however, believed that another 9 million of the population live in areas exposed to risk. There is evidence that difficulties similar to those encountered in preventing transmission among peripheral fringe populations in other countries exist in Thailand and will become apparent with the expansion of the program to the forested areas. In summary, the program in Thailand is not sufficiently advanced to permit an appraisal of the problems to be encountered in the terminal stages of eradication.

India

The decision to undertake the eradication of malaria in India marked the inclusion of the largest single malarious population in the world in the eradication program. Although it was initially anticipated that antimalaria measures would be applied in areas populated by some 225 million persons, it is now admitted that measures must be taken throughout areas inhabited by another 170 million people where malaria is relatively a minor problem. Although there are some reports of anopheline resistance to dieldrin, DDT seems to be giving excellent results. The program now being developed to complete the spraying of the homes of some 390 million people during 1960 represents a tremendous effort in financing and in administration. No serious technical difficulties are anticipated; the very size of the effort and the necessity of coordinating the programs of state services and of covering rural, nomadic, and itinerant populations would seem to be the chief obstacles in India.

My remarks on malaria to this point have been devoted to the disappearance of malaria from parts of Asia. The term worldwide malaria eradication implies nothing less than the disappearance of all forms of human plasmodia. This disappearance must be not only from the Americas, from Asia and the Pacific, but also from the USSR, Communist China, Outer Mongolia, North Korea, North Vietnam, East Germany, and Africa. Some workers have tended to discount the possibility of malaria eradication in Asia since little was known of what was being done in those countries not members of the United Nations. In general, it would seem that the communist countries, with a governmental interest in the productivity of their populations and with relatively tight controls over their peoples, may be expected to eradicate malaria as fast as or even faster than the free world, especially since most of these countries are not tropical.

In the USSR a deliberate attempt to eradicate malaria dates from 1952 following an observed reduction in malaria incidence of almost 80 per cent in 2 years. In the USSR, in addition to the spraying of homes with insecticide, all cases are given free treatment, are registered, and supervised for a 2-year period. Malaria cases reported since 1950 by years are 1950, 781,000; 1951, 351,000; 1952, 183,000; 1953, 116,000; 1954, 73,000; 1955, 36,000; 1956, 13,015; 1957, 5095; 1958, 2504.

To quote:
The malaria rate in the Soviet Union has been brought to such a low level that the country is on the threshold of complete eradication of this infection . . . the presence of the high rate of malaria in other countries of the world, especially in the countries adjacent to ours, is of real concern to us. Introduction of malaria . . . is at present gaining importance and increasing significance in the final period of local eradication of malaria . . . The USSR shares this outlook as to the possibility and necessity for eradicating malaria throughout the world.

The participation of the USSR in solving the malaria eradication problem in the world has not been limited solely to the framework of WHO. In 1955, The USSR Ministry of Public Health, at the request of the Government of the Democratic Republic of Vietnam sent a group of Soviet malaria specialists to North Vietnam, where they worked for about three years . . . In 1956, a group of malaria specialists was sent to the Chinese People's Republic for the basic purpose of assisting in training local personnel. As a result of five months work . . . a considerable number of Chinese specialists were trained.

The optimism and firm intent of the USSR malaria workers are apparent in the declaration that "the absence of new local cases for the absolute majority of regions in the country must be attained in the second half semester of 1959, and for the Azerbaidzhan SSR and Yukutsk of the ASSR not later than 1960."

Incomplete reports for 1958 showed 107 cases of malaria imported into the USSR, of which no less than 101 came from China. With regard to China I can do no better than quote from Dr. Williams' paper:

Nothing specific can be said at this time of anti-malaria activities in Communist China but those familiar with her malarious areas perceive no technical difficulties standing in the way. Transportation difficulties are obvious in the various southwest provinces where terrain is rugged. However, roads are not entirely impassable and the local mosquito is notoriously susceptible to DDT.

In Africa, malaria eradication has been planned and is being attempted in a number of the more temperate countries, but there has been a certain reluctance to undertake eradication under present conditions in Africa south of the Sahara and north of Southern Rhodesia. The low economic level, the high rate of transmission, the shortage of trained personnel, and the difficulty of communications in many parts of this region, when taken together, make the problem a formidable one. In spite of reported difficulties and local failures in the past, recent developments suggest there are no sound technical factors which will preclude success of any serious attempt to eradicate malaria when the time comes. A warning should be sounded against any attempt to eradicate malaria on a too-limited basis in tropical Africa since reinfection from the periphery may be expected to be a more serious problem there than in other parts of the world. The creation of national independent governments throughout Africa may well create a demand for international participation in eradication programs for that continent much earlier than would have been the case had previous political conditions been maintained.

In the Americas, practically all the malarious countries are engaged in the eradication effort. Serious difficulties with anopheline resistance to insecticides have been encountered in El Salvador and in Nicaragua and to lesser extent in other countries. Extradomiciliary transmission seems to be a factor delaying eradication in certain areas of Venezuela, Costa Rica, and possibly other countries. The great reaches of the Amazon Valley present a difficult problem in logistics; an attempt is being made to solve this problem with medicated table salt . . . I believe it is not too much to anticipate that just as improvement in administration and in methods for rendering yellow fever and its vector visible resulted in a definite change in the situation for the better at that time, so may we anticipate that the next few years will see tremendous advances in the intensification and improvement of efforts for the eradication of malaria throughout the world. In India where the greatest reservoir of malaria infection has existed, one sees the development of a truly national effort and a national determination to eradicate malaria forever. One cannot fail to be impressed.

There are times when one can take heart from the perspective gained by attempting to look forward from a previous point in the calendar. May I quote for your consideration from a forward looking address of 15 years ago, the Presidential Address of 1945 for the National Malaria Society, one of the parent bodies of this Society:

We are frequently reminded of the possibility of eradicating malaria in the United States, now that it is at a low ebb. I feel this is an untenable concept as we do not yet know in sufficient detail just where and under what conditions the disease occurs, or will occur in its last natural habitat. Possibly malaria will be eliminated but I much prefer to entertain the hope that we will build malaria out in our future developments and that we will attempt to "reduce" rather than "eliminate" it in its existing natural setting . . . it is unwise . . . to put malaria control operations into practice unless the disease is causing a measurable economic loss and unless the cost is in a measure commensurate with the economic ability of the people to pay.

But even as the President of the National Malaria Society was speaking, the die had been cast, and the budget item approved for the extended Malaria Control Program which was to become in 1947 the National Malaria Eradication Program. And indeed in 1950 and 1951 the National Malaria Society took steps for its own dissolution, as no longer necessary.

The action of the XIIIth Pan American Sanitary Conference in 1950 in recommending national programs for the eradication of malaria throughout the Americas was apparently ahead of its time and little stir was created until after the action of the XIVth Pan American Sanitary Conference in 1954. The decision of Mexico to undertake a national malaria eradication program led to support of this program by UNICEF and the action of the Joint UNICEF/WHO Health Policy Committee approving malaria eradication for joint effort of the two organizations. This was followed almost immediately by the action of the Eighth World Health Assembly declaring for a worldwide malaria eradication program. The action and reaction of the 1954-1959 period have been explosive in character in comparison with the slow speed at which international activities usually develop.

In 1957 the Pan American Health Organization received generous contributions to its Malaria Eradication Special Account from the governments of the Dominican Republic, the United States, and Venezuela. In the same year the WHO received a sizable contribution from the United States, and the International Cooperation Administration began to participate officially in malaria eradication with funds earmarked for the purpose by the U.S. Congress. The ICA is participating in malaria eradication in some two dozen countries, including India which has the world's largest population residing in malarious areas.

The governments of nations throughout the world have been most enthusiastic in girding themselves for the task of financing the internal costs of eradication; the difficulties have been related to trained professional staff and international funds to cover materials which must be imported.

The program for the eradication of malaria in the world has implications far beyond the economic, social, health, and cultural effects of this disease. Once the pattern has been set for international collaboration on a worldwide basis in the eradication of a single disease, it is obvious that the road is open for similar action on other human, animal, and plant diseases, and insect and plant pests. On October 22, 1959, the Secretary of Agriculture announced the eradication of vesicular exanthema of swine in the United States. Vesicular exanthema had been present for some 20 years in California in a known but local focus of infection, which suddenly and unexpectedly had an opportunity to spread, apparently on dining cars on interstate railway trains some 7 or 8 years ago. At its peak, 43 states were known to be infected and embargoes were placed on the importation of United States pork products by 10 countries; Canada, the United Kingdom, Colombia, Venezuela, Austria, Belgium, Sweden, Barbados, Jamaica, and British Guiana. California is now free of the infection at the price of having infected the other 42 states and at the price of a 7-year campaign waged by the Department of Agriculture in collaboration with the state governments. In making this announcement Secretary Benson did not announce a program of cooperation with the 10 clean countries which embargoed pork from the United States to help rid the rest of the world of vesicular exanthema, but might well have done so had malaria eradication been completed.

Recent success in the dramatic eradication of the screwworm from its eastern range of distribution in Florida and Georgia leads one to the question: If Florida has no screwworm can Texas be far behind? Eradication of the screwworm in Florida was possible because of the isolation of the eastern focus from other countries by the Gulf of Mexico and the Atlantic Ocean. Texas is not in a similarly favorable position and eradication there would put the United States in a defensive position, vís-à-vís the infested areas of Mexico. As Mexico proceeds in its program for the eradication of the *Aëdes aegypti* mosquito, the urban vector of yellow fever from its territory, it faces a similar problem along the border with the United States and in its contacts with gulf ports. Well may the representatives of agriculture and of health of the two countries hold a combined meeting and arrange broad collaboration in the solution of both problems.

It may be well to close this Charles Franklin Craig Lecture by quoting the words of the Secretary of Health, Education, and Welfare, when on October 20, 1959, he presented at the annual meeting of the American Public Health Association, contributions of $2 and $3 million dollars, respectively, to the Malaria Eradication Special Accounts of the Pan American and World Health Organizations:

> The cause to which this money will be applied is a triumphant one. Never until very recent times has man dared to talk of "eradication." In all war against disease we have moved from helplessness to treatment and thence to prevention and control. As we move toward the eradication of a disease from the face of the earth we stand on the threshold of total victory for man over one of his oldest and deadliest enemies.

But total victory over malaria can come only as there is total coverage of infected populations and as malaria is not permitted to become a disappearing disease before it has been eradicated.

The Relation of Malaria
Eradication to the General
Health Service*

Malaria eradication has a single objective, the elimination of the last
trace of malaria infection in the region; the General Health Service must
cover the important public health problems in the local community. The
most critical period in malaria eradication often comes after the disease is
no longer recognized as a public health problem. The reason for the General Health Service failure to eradicate eradicable diseases is obvious.

At the WHO-PAHO-UNICEF-AID-USPHS Malaria Eradication Coordination Meeting in December 1962, WHO presented the following concept:

There are two important elements in a country for the accomplishment of malaria eradication:

1. A well-organized Malaria Eradication Service with qualified scientific and
administrative staff; and

2. A public health service capable of carrying out a satisfactory case-finding
program and surveillance during the consolidation and maintenance phases.

In countries with well advanced malaria eradication programs, that do not have
the public health infrastructure, it is essential that the public health service be
extended as rapidly as possible to all of the malarious areas of the country.

This concept is the negation of the premise on which disease eradication
has been sponsored by The Rockefeller Foundation, the Pan American
Health Organization, and by the World Health Organization itself. This
premise is that an effective service, dedicated to a single objective, can be
created with relatively untrained workers, each responsible for a routine
operation, for the solution of special disease problems.

It is no exaggeration to state that no country in the Americas, where malaria eradication has been initiated since eradication became a Pan American objective, has had the desired public health infrastructure. Nor has
the speaker seen such infrastructure covering the malaria area in any one
of several countries visited in South East Asia and in the Western Pacific,
where WHO-sponsored malaria eradication campaigns have been developed since 1955.

Experience in programs for the development of rural health services

* Dr. Soper was a Special Consultant, Office of International Health, Public
Health Service.

This summary was originally published (*110*) in the *Proceedings* of the Seventh
International Congresses on Tropical Medicine and Malaria, Rio de Janeiro, September 1–11, 1963, Vol. 5, pp. 196–197, 1964.

over many years and in various countries does not support the thesis that an effective rural health service can be created in a developing country before its more accessible urban areas have been serviced. Nor does experience in campaigns for the eradication of hookworm disease, yellow fever, *Aëdes aegypti, Anopheles gambiae* (Brazil and Egypt), smallpox, yaws, and malaria, support the statement, occurring repeatedly in recent years in WHO documentation on campaigns against other diseases, as well as malaria, that a special disease eradication effort cannot be successful in the absence of a general health service.

The relation between malaria eradication and the General Health Service should be determined by

1. What the General Health Service can do to further malaria eradication within the limits of its routine operation.

2. What malaria eradication can do to prepare the way for the expansion and consolidation of the General Health Service.

The final responsibility for gaining and maintaining freedom from malaria infection should not be delegated to the General Health Service except under very favorable conditions and in limited areas, not obviously subject to reinfection.

The malaria eradicationist, in demanding a preexisting rural health infrastructure, is burdening himself with the labor and expense of its creation and is saddling tropical populations with unnecessary additional years of malaria!

Part XII | Disease Eradication: Yaws, Tuberculosis, Smallpox

Selection 43 | Yaws Eradication in the
Americas: Development of the
Haitian Method*

A great demonstration in public health administration has been in the
making in Haiti since 1950. The field: the eradication technique as applied
to yaws. The administrative staff: the Health Department of Haiti, with
international support. The beneficiaries: the rural people of Haiti and,
indirectly, the millions of people in the world who still suffer from this
disfiguring and crippling disease and those who might get it. For the yaws-
eradication program has served to orient the attack on this disease by the
health departments of many nations.

Yaws is a disease of the tropics, favored by high humidity and heavy
rainfall. Poverty, ignorance, overcrowding, and lack of the facilities for
personal cleanliness all contribute to its spread.

Yaws is a nonvenereal disease caused by a treponema so closely resembling that of syphilis that the two cannot be distinguished under the micro-
scope. Unless treated, yaws may progress through a variety of eruptions and
ulcers, and in advanced stages may eat through the flesh, causing loss of a
finger, a toe, or the nose, leaving ugly scars. Painful lesions on the palms of
the hands and the soles of the feet may incapacitate victims, often preventing them from working or even from walking. The disease causes great
economic loss in addition to human suffering.

Today yaws in the Americas is largely a rural disease, campaigns based
on prolonged treatment with salvarsan having been concentrated for the
past quarter of a century largely in towns and larger villages. The introduction of penicillin, which, in single doses, cures a large proportion of
cases and renders the remaining cases noninfective for others, has facilitated
treatment of entire populations.

Five years ago yaws was the most important health problem in Haiti,
where nearly 1 million cases were estimated for the population of somewhat
over 3 million.

In 1949 the Government of Haiti requested the collaboration of the Pan
American Sanitary Bureau in planning a program for the complete, final
solution to the yaws problem. Previous control campaigns had served to
reduce the number of cases temporarily, but such campaigns had been fol-

* Dr. Soper was the Director, Pan American Sanitary Bureau, and Regional
Director for the Americas of the World Health Organization.

This article was originally published (85) in 1956 by the Office of Public Information of the P.A.S.B. (One figure has been omitted.)

lowed by a recrudescence of the disease. Now Haiti insisted on eradication. The concept of the program for the eradication of yaws in Haiti was essentially similar to that developed in Brazil in the eradication of the yellow fever mosquito, *Aëdes aegypti,* and later applied in Brazil and in Egypt to the eradication of *Anopheles gambiae,* malaria's most dangerous carrier.

The Bureau outlined a plan for the government for the eradication of yaws with the technical collaboration of the Bureau and with material and supplies of UNICEF. Some months later the World Health Organization came to participate in this plan under a general agreement with UNICEF and another with the Pan American Sanitary Organization. Thus it was that the Haitian method of yaws eradication was developed through the collaboration of the government, the Pan American Sanitary Bureau, the World Health Organization and the United Nations Childrens Fund. The PASB/WHO contributed technicians who advised on the organization of the campaign; UNICEF supplied needed equipment, penicillin, and vehicles; the government supplied headquarters and personnel. Teams of workers were recruited locally and intensively trained prior to the launching of the campaign in July 1950.

The eradication of yaws, in the public health sense, may be accepted as accomplished when all transmission from ill to healthy persons ceases, that is, when new infections no longer occur. The importance of eradication as a concept for the solution of the yaws problem can be appreciated only in the light of preexisting practice. Until only a few years ago the control of yaws was limited essentially to the dispensary or hospital treatment of individual cases. This was extremely costly and failed to reach the great mass of cases in infected rural areas.

Haiti has demonstrated that the technique used in its campaign can effectually eradicate yaws in a short period of time at a low per capita cost. The approach has been on a total population, rather than on an individual basis, with, as nearly as possible, simultaneous single injections of penicillin to every infected person in each district. Since infected persons cannot be recognized during the incubation period, all contacts have been treated. In Haiti all persons resident in infected areas have been classified as contacts. Fortunately, the mass treatment of the rural population has been both more rapid and less expensive than any selective procedure could have been.

During the initial training and organizational stage of the eradication campaign in Haiti, the initially planned house-to-house method required for complete coverage of the rural population could not be used. The first year's experience with temporary field clinics showed that treatment centers fail to give adequate population coverage for an eradication program. Some cases do not reach these centers because they cannot walk, while others lack the initiative to seek treatment away from home.

From October 1951 until the end of 1954, house-to-house and family-to-family coverage were the basis of the campaign, which was conducted along a solid front, continually broadening and extending until it embraced all the infected areas. Posttreatment surveys showed that the house-to-house campaign had reached over 95 per cent of the population and that very few infectious cases had been missed. As a matter of fact, such surveys have generally failed to reveal infection rates of more than 0.5 per cent.

With the reduction in yaws to a very low level, intensive mass methods have been abandoned for a countrywide program based on the search for infected individuals, with concentrated treatment of population groups where infection persists. Haiti has been divided into areas, with a trained inspector assigned to each area, under appropriate supervision, to maintain a constant search for cases among the inhabitants of his area.

In 5 years yaws has been virtually eliminated from Haiti and complete eradication shown to be feasible. Haiti has shown that there is no excuse, with the present low cost of penicillin, for the continued existence of yaws anywhere [the cost has been only 30 cents (U.S.) per person treated—20 cents to government and 10 cents to PASB, WHO, and UNICEF].

The day is not far distant when the presence of yaws will be recognized as a public disgrace, seriously reflecting on the technical standing of local and national health services.

The economic benefits to the Haitian economy resulting from the eradication of yaws, a disease that attacked a large percentage of the rural population of this predominantly agricultural country, handicapping and incapacitating many, are incalculable.

In the final analysis, the only safeguard against the reintroduction of yaws into Haiti, once it no longer exists there, is its eradication from other countries.

Fortunately, the striking success of the Haiti program has stimulated the demand for similar eradication campaigns elsewhere, campaigns which are essential for the continued freedom of Haiti itself from reinfection.

Encouraged by the success of the campaigns in Haiti, the health administrations of Brazil and a number of the Caribbean islands have requested the collaboration of PASB/WHO and UNICEF in the eradication of yaws. Plans for several of these eradication campaigns are now in preparation. The eventual objective of the Bureau is, of course, the eradication of yaws from all the Americas.

Statistics on the incidence of yaws elsewhere in the Americas are either lacking or incomplete. The incidence of yaws was higher in Haiti than in other parts of the Americas, but the disease is a serious problem in several other countries and other islands of the Caribbean, particularly Jamaica and the Lesser Antilles. Yaws extends also to the mainland in British and French Guiana and in Surinam, throughout sections of Venezuela, of western Colombia, of Ecuador and Peru, from the slopes of the Andes to the Pacific, and in some scattered rural areas east of the Andes. Treatment campaigns in the contiguous infected areas of Ecuador and Colombia have for some years been coordinated under the auspices of the Institute of Inter-American Affairs, U.S. International Cooperation Administration. In Bolivia high infection rates of up to 50 per cent are reported to have been greatly reduced by treatment during the past 5 or 6 years. A few localities of Central America are known to be infected.

Yaws is found in many parts of Brazil. It is a minor problem in the south, but a serious one throughout the north, northeast, and eastern states, where, in certain areas, it is not uncommon to find up to 15 per cent of the population affected. Available reports indicate from 350,000 to 500,000 cases in the known infected areas in the states of Pará, Maranhão, Ceará, Rio Grande do Norte, Paraíba, Pernambuco, Alagôas, Bahia, Espírito Santo, Minas Gerais, and Rio de Janeiro. Although control measures have been in force for some years, the area of its distribution in Brazil seems to be on the increase, owing, in part, to the recent migrations from the drought-stricken Northeast to other parts of the country.

Although much remains to be done, public health history will surely register the fact that the eradication of yaws in the Americas began with the decision of the Government of Haiti in 1949 to request the Bureau to prepare a plan for the final solution of its problem.

The success of the yaws campaign in Haiti has served to stimulate interest in other health programs in the Republic, whose government is one of the first to accept the challenge of the XIVth Pan American Sanitary Conference to transform malaria control projects into a continental malaria eradication program.

Selection 44 | Problems To Be Solved if the
Eradication of Tuberculosis Is
To Be Realized*

It was only 6 years ago, at Kansas City, that the American Public Health
Association, for the first time, passed a resolution in support of the concept
of eradication in the prevention of communicable diseases. In the 6 years
that have elapsed since the first acceptance of eradication we have advanced
such a tremendous distance that it is now possible to discuss the eradication
of such a difficult problem as tuberculosis. Our discussion is related to the
eradication of what has been and is, probably, the most widespread of
human ills, the most chronic and persistent of infections, with the longest
period of infectivity of any disease, and the disease whose prevention most
clearly depended, until recently, on the improvement of social and economic conditions. The very fact that this session is held will force public
health workers everywhere to consider the possibilities of eradicating not
only tuberculosis, but surely a host of the lesser ills of mankind.

Although I am innocent of direct participation in tuberculosis prevention, I have had long association with eradication projects dating back some
40 years. Not all of these projects have been successful, but I have no regrets
over having promoted and participated in them; rather, I have felt remorse
for not having undertaken and executed some of them much earlier and
before decisive action was forced by destructive epidemics.

In preparing for our discussion I reread and thrilled anew to Carroll
Palmer's paper, "Tuberculosis: A Decade in Retrospect and in Prospect"
prepared at the time of the tenth anniversary of the WHO in 1958. I quote:

> The new challenge for tuberculosis control during the next decade is, therefore,
> to determine what can and should be done in the increasing number of countries
> in which the disease can no longer be regarded as a major public health problem
> . . . In countries where great progress has already been made, tuberculosis work in
> the future will certainly differ from what it has been in the past. Not the least of

* This paper was presented by invitation before a Joint Session of the National
Tuberculosis Association, Tuberculosis Division of the Public Health Service, and
the Epidemiology, Health Officers, Laboratory, Maternal and Child Health, Public
Health Education, and Public Health Nursing Sections of the American Public
Health Association at the Eighty-Ninth Annual Meeting in Detroit, Michigan,
November 16, 1961. When he prepared and read this paper, Dr. Soper was the
Director, Pakistan-SEATO Cholera Research Laboratory, Dacca, East Pakistan.

This article was originally published (*105*) in the *American Journal of Public
Health 52:* 734–745, 1962.

the differences will be a change in objective from control to eradication. At long last, it is not only possible, but, I believe, obligatory to set the goal at eradication and not at some intermediate stage connoted by the term "control". . . .

We are here to discuss how in a specific country, the United States, in which "great progress has already been made, tuberculosis work in the future [should] differ from what it has been in the past." If Palmer in 1958 believed it to be obligatory to set the goal at eradication, surely, we in 1961, with 3 years of additional testing of the tools we have for the job, do not, in conscience, have any choice in the matter. Palmer recognized the supreme importance of the struggle to zero. He said,

Although reductions in mortality, morbidity and infection rates may appear most dramatic in areas in which the present rates are still high, of fundamental importance to tuberculosis workers throughout the world will be the smaller reductions in low prevalence areas, because such reductions will reflect the development of successful methods for pinpointing and eradicating the last remaining sources of infection.

As Palmer clearly foresaw, the outcome of the war to free the human race of tuberculosis depends now on the development of successful mopping-up methods, once the incidence of the disease is at a very low level; tools and techniques are already available for the campaigns for the reduction of mass infection, even in the most heavily infected populations.

I have thrilled also to the challenge issued, later in the same year (1958), by James Perkins for a "firmly concentrated program of eradication of tuberculosis from the whole face of the earth!" Perkins defined "eradication of tuberculosis" as the "ultimate goal of having no human being on this earth react significantly to a skin test with a proper dosage of a standardized tuberculin; in other words, total bacteriologic eradication. . . ."

This apparently overly bold and brash challenge loses these characteristics to one who has seen miracles in his lifetime and is familiar with the present program for the eradication of malaria on a global scale.

The important papers of Palmer and Perkins were followed by the truly remarkable Arden House Conference on Tuberculosis the next year (November 29 to December 2, 1959). The Arden House Report signalizes the transformation of tuberculosis from a social and economic to a public health, medical, and administrative problem and recommends its direct therapeutic solution.

Problems To Be Solved

Experience with other eradication projects suggests that there are many and various problems to be solved in the eradication of such a widespread chronic infection as tuberculosis—psychological, technical, administrative, educational, and financial in nature. The previous measure of these problems is difficult but the solution of entire groups of them may depend on decisions on a few basic points.

Among these points, if the ready eradication of tuberculosis is to be realized, I would put the following:

1. Definition of eradication as an absolute goal; acceptance by the national and state health authorities and by interested voluntary agencies of eradication, thus defined, as a feasible and urgent objective.

2. Acceptance of tuberculosis as no longer essentially a social and economic but rather a public health and medical administrative problem; establishing the responsibility of the community to the infected individual; but also establishing the responsibility of the infected individual to uninfected persons.

3. Provision for a national coordination authority to stimulate through the state health services eradication programs in each of the 3152 counties in the country, backed by technical, epidemiologic, educational, administrative, and finanical support where needed; preparation of a national plan for TB eradication, preferably coordinated with similar national plans for Canada and Mexico.

4. Training of professional staff in the eradication concept of disease prevention; standardization and simplification of procedures to facilitate the training of nonprofessional staff in the routine identification, registration, supervision, and surveillance of infected persons and their intimate contacts.

ACCEPTANCE OF ERADICATION OF TUBERCULOSIS AS A FEASIBLE AND URGENT OBJECTIVE

Although the decision to accept the absolute definition of eradication as the objective of the tuberculosis program is inevitable, it is important that this decision be ratified as soon as possible by all services and agencies participating in tuberculosis prevention.

The acceptance of the concept of eradication in place of control (reduction) forces a radical psychological and administrative change in attitude toward the existence of low-incidence tuberculosis in the community. This change is based on the fundamentally different objectives of control and of eradication.

The objective of control is to reduce the incidence of a given disease to a low level and to maintain this low level forever.

The objective of eradication is completely to eliminate the possibility of the occurrence of a given disease, even in the absence of all preventive measures. This definition, modified by the phrase "unless reintroduction occurs," applies also to local area, state, national, and regional eradication.

In control, one may glory in the percentage reduction of disease incidence, whereas in eradication any reduction short of the absolute leaves one preoccupied with the seeds of infection that remain.

In control, one may measure progress from the high point on the curve of incidence downward, or, that is, what has been done; in eradication one measures always from the base line of the chart upwards, or, that is, what remains to be done.

In control, one tends to lose interest in a disease at the point where, in eradication, many times, the greatest difficulties are encountered.

In control, one may plan on a small local scale, for limited areas; in eradication, one must plan for a program of sufficient scope to minimize, from the beginning, the threat of reinfection from the periphery; in eradication there is no stopping point, no rest period. Eradication must continuously expand at the periphery until all points from which reinfection may occur have been cleared.

In control, one must count the cost as part of continuing unending annual budgets; in eradication, one may capitalize future savings over an indefinite period against the peak costs of the years required for eradication. "Virtual eradication" never merits the full premium of the effort expended; as long as some tuberculosis remains the threat of recrudescence exists and the cost of the control effort must continue. Truly may it be said, "To toil ye have the right, but not to the fruits thereof."

In control, one may disregard the rights of the minority, of those living in sparsely settled areas of difficult access, and take advantage of population distribution to give a low per capita cost and an overall low rate of incidence.

Eradication cannot sacrifice the minority under the blanket classification —"no longer of public health importance." Eradication cannot be made available to part of the people; protection of all the population becomes the only acceptable professional public health standard.

In control, some cases and a few deaths are permissible; in eradication, "any is too many." (Note the singularity of the verb!)

When the public health officer ceases to glory in the partial reduction of disease incidence (control) and accepts the philosophy that in taking credit for any reduction, he accepts responsibility for the residuum, a long step has been taken toward eradication. When the public comes to know that a given communicable disease is completely preventable, another considerable advance has been made.

The proper definition of eradication and the only one which clearly distinguishes it from control goes back to the translation of its Greek roots, "out by the roots." Eradication has no meaning except as an absolute, without modifying phrases or limiting adjectives. For administrative convenience one may speak of area, state, national, continental, and regional eradication programs as steps in global eradication but never of "partial eradication," "virtual eradication," or "eradication as a public health problem!"

The acceptance of eradication as thus defined, as the objective of the Tuberculosis Prevention Program, has the advantage of giving a definite end point against which all progress is measured.

The acceptance of eradication as the objective leads inevitably to careful epidemiological studies as the end point is approached, when basic facts, not previously known, may be more readily uncovered. Thus acceptance of the challenge of eradication leads to the discovery of facts which are needed to bring about eradication. In eradication, one learns what the final difficulties are going to be and their solution through study, while eradicating.

The mathematician knows that geometric regression based on a continued vital index of less than 1 may be as destructive for a species as geometric progression based on an index greater than 1 is favorable to its perpetuation. But the regression curve in many instances cannot be blindly projected down to the zero. Actual experience does not indicate that the factors which effect the gross reduction of an infection will be necessarily effective at the lowest levels of infection. The reduction of *Aëdes aegypti* breeding in the key centers of yellow fever infection in the Americas resulted repeatedly in the practically complete disappearance of yellow fever from the statistics of the continent. Eventually, the chasing and suppression of reported outbreaks was superseded by the routine systematic collection of postmortem material from fever cases over large areas of South America. This so-called viscerotomy revealed two entirely different and unrecognized mechanisms not affected by the antiaegypti campaign by which yellow fever maintained itself during its silent nonepidemic periods: silent endemic rural yellow fever transmitted by *A. aegypti* in a semiarid region and jungle yellow fever among the forest animals.

The phenomena of the hidden focus of infection, of the unrecognized method of transmission, and of the relative increased importance of confusing observations may be very real problems as incidence falls. They have led to the terms "the epidemiology of a disappearing disease," "the epidemiology of a retreating disease," and "the epidemiology of an evanescent disease." They have been and promise to be an important consideration in the eradication of malaria from the world. That this epidemiology of a disappearing disease concept is important is borne out by experience with brucellosis. Biberstein et al. (1961) state:

The brucellosis eradication program in many parts of the country has reached such an advanced stage that certain problems inherent in dealing with the vestiges of a once widespread infection are coming more and more into prominence.

It is a truism that the last residue of infection in a population behaves more erratically in regard to ordinary diagnostic reactions than does a group where no check has ever been applied to the infection previously. This has been the experience in all situations where an infectious disease has been brought under control, as in the cases of bovine tuberculosis and human syphilis and the problem of false tests has assumed proportions it never had when the infections were widespread.

In tuberculosis eradication, it is obvious that as the number of persons infected with the tubercle bacillus declines, the specificity of the tuberculin test will fall, percentually, since nonspecific reactions will chiefly be found.

It is possible that the epidemiology of a disappearing disease differs from the usually recognized epidemiology of that disease only because there are somewhat varied mechanisms of transmission or maintenance of the infection of varying importance when there is no attempt at control. Countermeasures are obviously directed against the most common mechanism, and these measures may be relatively inefficient against less common and unusual mechanisms. These, in turn, may not be sufficiently important to come under scrutiny in a control program because the disease ceases to be a public health problem before they become apparent. One cannot know then whether the long-term downward trend would have continued to regress to zero had tuberculosis continued subject only to the previous pressures; nor can one affirm or deny that the present regression curve will proceed smoothly to zero and not flatten out due to resistance to therapy, to the inability to discover certain foci of transmission, or to other factors. It is only as the pressure drive of eradication is exerted accompanied by careful epidemiological studies that we shall know the answer. The fact that there are already some areas in which all transmission has been blocked suggests that the present tools are sufficiently sharp to preclude any important flattening of the curve on the downward drive.

Acceptance of Eradication as Public Health Administration Problem with Reciprocal Community and Individual Responsibility

The public health worker and the public long have been conditioned to the acceptance of tuberculosis as a chronic disease, that one did or did not have, that one did or did not die of, and that depended on social and economic factors for its solution. To visualize the importance of getting a proper image of tuberculosis before the public, it is only necessary to imagine the reaction were 12,000 people to perish in the United States in 1961 from another febrile hemorrhagic disease, yellow fever. Every one knows that yellow fever is preventable, but not everyone knows that no one has to get tuberculosis.

It is important, if eradication of tuberculosis is to be readily realized, that the public health worker and the public reclassify tuberculosis in the terms of the State Board of Health of New York State in 1899 as a danger-ous, infectious, and communicable disease. To this classification must be added "preventable," "easily preventable," or "completely preventable."

The public health worker has been grouped with the public in this state-ment because the public cannot be expected to go ahead of the public health worker. Striking examples of the present attitude of the public health worker toward tuberculosis are to be found in the reports of two committees appointed by the Public Health Service following the Arden House Conference, the one on Goals and Standards, the other on Case Detection Evaluation. The recommendations of these reports may be rea-sonable in the light of past performance and present capacity of tubercu-losis control services but are not compatible with responsibilities inherent in the present situation.

Tuberculosis has become a public health administrative problem through the development of adequate means to identify infected and in-fectious persons and, for the first time in the long history of tuberculosis prevention, knowledge of and experience with efficient chemotherapeutic drugs. These drugs are both curative and prophylactic; also, although treat-ment is prolonged, most cases become noninfectious during treatment. Treatment is cheap, simple, is taken by mouth, does not require close medical supervision, and may be taken at home and during continued employment. Physical isolation in sanatoriums is now being replaced by chemical isolation under normal living conditions. The prevention of trans-mission is possible without disrupting the lives of infected and infectious individuals. Surely the community through its public health service has a responsibility to prevent the transmission of tuberculosis.

Chemotherapy has become a public health measure not only through the cure of open cases and rendering such cases noninfectious during the neces-sarily prolonged period of treatment, but also by the prevention of infec-tion of contacts of infectious cases. The community cannot discharge its responsibility to its people unless active cases are found and are placed under treatment for the necessary period. It is important, then, in the pub-lic interest, that infected individuals, infectious cases, and their intimate contacts be identified, and, where indicated, be given curative or prophy-lactic therapy. The community should be responsible for making available to all residents, including transients, diagnostic and therapeutic services, either directly or through local hospitals and practicing physicians, under the supervision of the health authority. The community should also, where needed, offer the benefit of social service and rehabilitation to victims of tuberculosis and their families. In synthesis, the community must in its own self-interest make the diagnosis, care, and supervision of persons infected with tuberculosis as attractive as possible.

But the community cannot discharge its responsibility without the acceptance by each citizen of his individual and family responsibility regarding tuberculosis and its transmission.

Ways and means must be found to make the individual responsible for not transmitting tuberculosis infection to any other individual. The discharge of this responsibility will, necessarily, involve periodic testing for infection and infectivity and acceptance of supervised treatment where indicated.

Having accepted the classification of tuberculosis as a dangerous, infectious, communicable, and preventable disease, it is obvious that the untreated open case of tuberculosis is a menace to the community and should merit the same type of interest of public health authorities as does the typhoid carrier. The community is justified in taking such measures as may be required to prevent the dissemination of the infection.

Given the importance of tuberculosis eradication would it not be justified to require that each individual determine periodically whether he is or is not infected with tuberculosis and if infected register for supervision by the health authorities? If Minnesota can tuberculin test all cattle every 2 years in its programs for the eradication of bovine tuberculosis, can one refuse to consider whether Minnesota's calves are worthy of greater consideration than are its children?

As one of the rapidly disappearing hookworm disease workers of a past generation, I would suggest testing the efficiency of the routine sputum-culture test as an early step in high-risk groups rather than as the last step in the identification of open cases of tuberculosis. The distribution of sputum containers could be made to the family, to the school, to the factory or other places of congregation, without the necessity of contacting each individual. The collection of specimens might even be facilitated by sending and receiving containers by post. In the hookworm campaigns of another era containers were distributed and collected for the examination of material coming from the other end of the alimentary canal, which for obvious reasons should be more difficult than the collection of sputum samples. The hookworm campaign was a mass operation and as such the examination of samples received was a routine one carried out by men trained specifically to identify hookworm and other nematode eggs. It should not be difficult to organize the mass sputum-culture examination as a strictly routine procedure involving a minimum of highly trained professional staff. Surely, it will be easier than viscerotomy, the routine systematic collection of postmortem liver tissue for the diagnosis of unsuspected yellow fever cases, already referred to. Just as viscerotomy indicated when transmission of yellow fever was occurring at the time it occurred, so can the sputum-culture test indicate where and when transmission of infection is probably occurring.

The sputum-culture test, if successful as a routine measure, will free the tuberculosis effort of a great deal of intermediate work now performed in sifting out infectious cases from among tuberculin reactors and those with suspect chest films. Used routinely, it will let the infectious case declare itself almost automatically.

NATIONAL COORDINATION AUTHORITY: NATIONAL PLAN FOR ERADICATION

Once eradication of tuberculosis is accepted as a policy, tuberculosis becomes a truly national problem. Experience with eradication programs in other countries has emphasized the importance of central national operation or coordination. In the United States, as has been previously commented, the political structure is not, under normal peacetime conditions, conducive to the organization of effective eradication programs.

The need for a satisfactory mechanism for national planning and coordination of eradication efforts is not limited to the field of tuberculosis but is common to the eradication of a number of presently eradicable diseases and insect vectors. The solution of this problem is of sufficient importance that it should be given full consideration and study before action is taken. There should be consultation of those having experience in the Malaria Control for War Areas, in the Department of Agriculture programs for the eradication of bovine tuberculosis, brucellosis, and the screwworm, and with those who may be interested in the eradication of poliomyelitis, tuberculosis, typhoid fever, syphilis, and *A. aegypti,* to mention only some of the obvious conditions crying out for eradication. The solution will be found through some mechanism taking full advantage of the strength of our city, county, and state health services, and of the unique ability of voluntary agencies in stimulating public interest and marshaling support for health programs. It is to be regretted that the MCWA, with its experience in coordinating the National Malaria Eradication Program and with its relatively large resources in personnel and financing, became the Communicable Disease Center and not the Communicable Disease Eradication Center.

The time has come for the development of a strong coordinating center for eradication efforts devoted to national eradication programs where such are indicated; the U.S. Congress is already conditioned to the approval of budgets for eradication programs in the agriculture and health fields. Special budgets were provided beginning in 1947 for the National Malaria Eradication Program in the United States, and since 1957, the Mutual Security Act has carried provision for many millions of dollars earmarked for malaria-eradication programs in other countries.

Tuberculosis was a local problem until eradication became possible. It is now a national problem and should be planned for on a national basis.

The federal government should be responsible for the overall national plan of eradication and for the coordination of the activities of the various states. Each state in turn must assume the responsibility for the participation of all its cities and counties to give complete national coverage.

It has already been suggested that the community make diagnosis and treatment available and attractive to infected persons and that the individual be made legally responsible for knowing that he and his dependents are not infectious cases of tuberculosis. Accepting tuberculosis as a national problem, is it unreasonable to consider placing this responsibility on the same basis as that of the individual for knowing that he is subject to income and Social Security tax assessments and for taking the initiative of reporting his obligation and making payment? To get effective and agreeable cooperation in maintaining up-to-date reporting and registration of tuberculosis, and to facilitate maintaining infectious cases and their contacts under treatment, might not the U.S. Government establish a system of crediting a certain amount against income tax or Social Security payments to each individual submitting annual certificates of freedom from infectiousness of himself and dependents and a somewhat larger credit for individuals with certification of having undergone an approved period of treatment for himself or members of his family during the year? Such credits would be more than self-compensatory in identifying and getting infectious cases under treatment, in making supervision welcome, and in getting continuing registration of infected persons moving from one area to another. The credits to be established could certainly be less than the cost of searching out individual infectious cases. Such a system adopted by the federal government would be effective in getting uniform provisions for all states and much more rapid and effective in application than measures adopted by each individual state.

As the incidence of tuberculosis in the United States declines, the relative importance of infection introduced from other countries will increase. It would be highly advantageous to plan the eradication program here in conjunction with coordinated plans in Canada and in Mexico. These three countries together have a large land mass easily protected against reinfection by overland immigration; this block could exert a tremendous influence in developing tuberculosis eradication in the Western Hemisphere.

TRAINING OF PROFESSIONAL STAFF IN ERADICATION CONCEPT: SIMPLIFICATION AND STANDARDIZATION OF PROCEDURES FOR ROUTINE HANDLING BY NONPROFESSIONAL STAFF

It is highly important that professional staff entering in eradication programs should be given special training in the concept of eradication and in the differences in administrative approach required for eradication from that satisfactory for control. The basic differences in control and eradication have been discussed at length and these differences are reflected in the administrative techniques acceptable in each case.

There is also a real need for indoctrination of nonprofessional workers in the concept of eradication. They should understand the objective of the program and the reasons for the careful meticulous administration and the disagreeable degree of supervision of all details of an eradication operation; they should know that the big payoff comes only with absolute zero and not with "virtual eradication."

It is obvious that, given the scarcity of professional workers in the public health field, particularly in the field of tuberculosis, any considerable expansion of the present activities must depend very largely on the possibility of using nonprofessional staff wherever possible. Each step of every procedure for identifying, diagnosing, treating, supervising, and registering infected and infectious cases and their contacts should be analyzed and broken down into those elements which require individual judgment of professional staff and those which can be executed by nonprofessional staff under supervision.

In public health administration, once procedure has been simplified and standardized, it is surprising how often it will be found that what the professional can do, he can teach the nonprofessional to do as well or even better, provided it is a routine operation not requiring judgment beyond the training of the individual.

Discussion

The decline of tuberculosis during the past decade and a half surpasses anything one could have imagined at the beginning of this period, and this with a minimal adaptation of preventive measures to the possibilities of the new era of chemotherapeutic cure and prevention of tuberculosis. It has been a period of plunging tuberculosis death rates, of an oversupply of hospital beds for tuberculosis cases, and a rapidly falling infection rate in children and young adults. Significantly, over half of the infectious cases now being found are among elderly, previously infected persons over 45 years of age. This means that tuberculosis has been forced, just to maintain its declining position, to fall back on its capital reserves of infection deposited decades ago in the cohorts of a passing generation.

The full impact of therapy on tuberculosis has not yet been felt and much of the discussion here may seem naive a few years from now. In 1955, after an unforgettable visit to the crowded slums and to the crowded habitations and refugee quarters in Hongkong, I was surprised to find Dr. Moody, the chief of the Hongkong Tuberculosis Program, optimistic over the situation. He had found that, without increases of finance, of staff, or of hospital facilities, the number of patients certified as arrested during the year had risen sixfold in just a few years—from 500 to 3000. Today, we know that available chemotherapy is curative in early cases, is strongly prophylactic in contacts, renders most cases under treatment noninfectious, is cheap, and may be administered orally, under minimal supervision, with a wide margin of safety, at home and during continued employment. Self-medication and medication of family contacts with only occasional supervision is feasible. There are already areas in the United States in which the first stage of eradication has been accomplished—the interruption of transmission to the younger generation. In addition to all this, the program for the eradication of bovine tuberculosis has brought that infection to such a low point that almost no human infections are now occurring. The only serious difficulty of chemotherapy of tuberculosis is the necessity of continued medication over a long period of time. Reading the above statements, one cannot but ask what we are waiting for, what more must we have, what sign do we still require before assuming the responsibility for the eradication of tuberculosis? One does not have to see the end to start; but one must start if one is to see the end.

The existence of areas in the United States where transmission has been stopped has been mentioned above. These "eradicated" areas are tremendously important; they demonstrate that transmission can be prevented and set eradication as an attainable goal. From now on the public health authorities of areas with evidence of continuing transmission must be definitely on the defensive. What man has done, man can do!

The eradicated areas are important also for their power for growth. The power of growth of eradicated areas was first observed in the development of the program for the eradication of the aegypti mosquito and has been facetiously referred to as Soper's law of eradication growth. Eradication of aegypti was first observed in a number of Brazilian port cities; to protect these from reinfestation it was essential to eradicate aegypti, first in the suburbs, then farther and farther afield until eventually pressure built up for the eradication of aegypti in the Western Hemisphere. The islands of tuberculosis eradication should be the cherished seedbeds from which the peripheral spread of eradication is to occur. In 1958 Perkins asked, "Why is it unrealistic, then, to believe that we can enlarge the perimeter of each of these small areas where tuberculosis has been eradicated, until their borders touch, and they coalesce into an ever-expanding tuberculosis free sea, which finally engulfs the last residual island strong-holds of infection?" This is surely the process through which eradication will occur in many states but from a practical standpoint the considerable number of counties in the United States without organized health programs and the lack of coordination of the state programs seriously hamper such a development.

In discussing the "Problems to Be Solved if the Eradication of Tuberculosis Is to Be Realized," I have assumed that we are primarily responsible for the health of the present generation and that the early eradication of tuberculosis is too important to be limited to the speed of execution possible with presently available resources. Tuberculosis eradication should not compete with infant diarrhea, cancer, coronary thrombosis, and other health problems for the given amount of money within existing budgets. Tuberculosis should be lifted from consideration as a disease of declining importance and held up to the focus of public attention as a still dangerous infection which can be blotted out. Eradication of tuberculosis if presented in a bold, decisive way by public health leaders, themselves convinced that eradication is feasible and worthwhile, should easily get the administrative authority and the funds for a coordinated national attack.

In a world of increasing population, a world in which intimacy and rapidity of contact between nations and regions and continents favor the maintenance of known infections and the entry and propagation in man of new disease agents, the eradication concept of communicable-disease prevention has much greater importance than it had a generation ago.

The international acceptance of the eradication concept has outstripped its acceptance by the public health workers of the United States. It has, as a matter of fact, developed certain international political implications. In January 1958 the President of the United States challenged the USSR to cooperate in programs of disease eradication, citing particularly malaria. In June of the same year, the USSR at the World Health Assembly at Minneapolis sponsored a program for the global eradication of smallpox. In 1959, I was told in Accra that the USSR was preaching in Ghana that only under the communist form of government could malaria be readily eradicated from that country.

One of the problems facing health authorities of the American nations at the first Pan American Sanitary Conference in 1902 was the fact that quarantine in some countries was a locally administered activity with the health authorities of individual ports establishing the regulations for quarantine and their application. As local functions, these were not subject to diplomatic negotiation. The United States, as an interested shipping nation, was proposing the nationalization of this function. An analogous situation exists in the United States today with regard to communicable disease and vector eradication. Once disease and vector eradication programs become international in character, the United States assumes certain obligations which cannot be readily discharged, since the prevention of communicable disease in the United States is a state, rather than a national, function. It is essential that the United States as a member of the Pan American and the World Health Organizations develop some mechanism through which the federal government can discharge its international responsibilities in present and future eradication programs. With such a mechanism, the United States could anticipate taking leadership in the eradication of tuberculosis.

In undertaking the eradication of tuberculosis, we are not serving only ourselves. In the failure of the United States to join in the eradication of the aegypti mosquito, it has done a great disservice to other countries which have been reinfested from ships from American ports. Worse, the United States has set the example of nonparticipation in the first official continental eradication effort, merely because yellow fever did not seem to pose an immediate threat to our shores. It is most important to establish the precedent that, once a regional program of eradication has been determined, all nations participate whether directly threatened or not. With our high social and economic level, we may be able to afford the luxury of maintaining tuberculosis permanently; such is not the case in many other countries in which the eradication of tuberculosis could itself become a very important factor in social and economic development.

The insistence on the development of a national eradication coordinating authority and on a national plan should not deter the state, county, and city health services from continuing and extending their present eradication programs. In the final analysis it is these local services which must eradicate tuberculosis and the experience gained and the demonstrations made by them must serve as the basis for the development of the national plan of tuberculosis eradication.

The objective of eradication is eradication and not virtual eradication, and intermediate goals can best be expressed in the number and size of areas and populations in which the complete elimination of transmission of tuberculosis is to be accomplished in a given period of time.

The goal, immediate, intermediate, and final, for the tuberculosis eradication program should be the blocking of all transmission of infection from one person to another. Let us concentrate on this objective, even though we limit it initially to certain areas or population groups, however small.

SUMMARY

Any proposal to eradicate tuberculosis in the United States, other than by slow and uncertain attrition, should be based on

1. Definition of eradication as an absolute; acceptance by the national and state health authorities and by interested voluntary agencies of eradication, thus defined, as a feasible and urgent objective.

2. Acceptance of tuberculosis as no longer essentially a social and economic but, rather, public health and medical administrative problem; establishing the responsibility of the community to the infected individual; but also establishing the responsibility of the infected individual to uninfected persons.

3. Provision for a national coordination authority to stimulate through the state health services eradication programs in each of the 3152 counties in the country, backed by technical, epidemiologic, educational, administrative, and financial support where needed; preparation of a national plan for eradication, preferably coordinated with similar national plans of Canada and Mexico. (This national coordination authority should not be an ad hoc unit devoted to the eradication of tuberculosis but, rather, a permanent agency to coordinate eradication programs for the ever-increasing number of eradicable diseases and disease vectors.)

4. Training of professional staff in the eradication concept of disease prevention; standardization and simplification of procedures to facilitate the training of nonprofessional staff in the routine identification, registration, supervision, and surveillance of infected persons and their intimate contacts.

Selection 45 | Smallpox — World Changes and Implications for Eradication*

The subject under discussion this evening is not smallpox, but smallpox eradication—not local eradication, not national eradication, but eradication as an absolute. We are not here to discuss an alert against smallpox, the defense against smallpox, but the united offensive action of mankind against this disease to bring about its final conquest.

My task as discussant is to relate the papers we have heard to the global eradication of smallpox. Before turning to these papers, I would point out that Thomas Jefferson, 160 years ago, said that "future nations will know by history only that the loathsome smallpox has existed." If the eradication of smallpox were possible 160 years ago, why do we still have this loathsome disease with us? The question we are discussing this evening is what changes favor success in the next decade which were not operative in the previous century and a half of failure?

DISTRICT OF COLUMBIA EPISODE

Dr. Grant's paper on "Smallpox in Washington, D.C." (unpublished) is interesting as an exercise in diagnosis. It is equally interesting as an exercise in emergency epidemiology and high-pressure public health administration. But the importance of this paper to us is its clear demonstration of the failure of the U.S. expenditure of $15 to 20 million annually to protect this country against the threat of smallpox. That the case was actually chickenpox is beside the point. Everyone concerned admitted the threat and the possibility of its being smallpox. This threat establishes once more the fact that quarantine and vaccination certificates are no match for smallpox and jet air travel! (Please note that I said "quarantine and vacci-nation certifiicates" and not quarantine and vaccination.)

The District of Columbia episode emphasizes the stake that all mankind has in smallpox wherever it is; the corollary is that all should be willing to contribute to carry the attack to the remaining endemic regions until there is no more smallpox.

* This paper is based on comments made before the Epidemiology Section of the American Public Health Association at the Ninety-Third Annual Meeting in Chicago, Illinois, October 20, 1965. Dr. Soper was a Special Consultant, Office of International Health, Public Health Service.

This article was originally published (*116*) in the *American Journal of Public Health 56:* 1652–1656, 1966.

International Smallpox Eradication

Dr. Cockburn's paper on "Progress in International Smallpox Eradication" gives the present situation as seen by the World Health Organization. For the benefit of those who do not have a clear map of the world in mind, I shall summarize by broad areas what Dr. Cockburn has told us, noting both what has been done and what remains to be done.

Beginning with the Western Hemisphere, all of North America, Mexico, Central America, and the West Indies have been free of smallpox for over a decade.

In the rest of the world, during the calendar year 1964 no smallpox cases, either imported or local, were reported for all of Europe, all of the USSR, Africa north of the Sahara, and much of the Middle East. Likewise no cases were reported in the entire Western Pacific Region of the WHO, from Korea to New Zealand. USSR sources report that smallpox is nonexistent in China.

Serious eradication efforts are under way in practically all the infected countries of Asia with the exception of Indonesia. In addition to completing the task in these countries, the bulk of the work to be done is in Indonesia, Africa south of the Sahara, and Brazil.

The present favorable situation has come after comparatively little work by the Pan American and World Health Organizations, UNICEF, and the Agency for International Development. The Pan American Health Organization has spent on smallpox from 1948 to 1964 only some $600,000. The World Health Organization has had no significant special organization, or large-scale expenditure, on this problem.

The improvement over the past can be considered only a temporary gain unless the campaign is waged to completion. Within a few years much immunity will be lost and newborn populations will create a new widespread endemicity. While noting that time is of the essence, we note the progress already made clearly demonstrates the feasibility of the global eradication of smallpox. With so much done, all is possible.

We must agree with Dr. Cockburn that in some areas smallpox is not a high-priority public health problem, that outside pressure and assistance are needed, and that countries now free of the disease can best guarantee their continued freedom through such assistance.

The Indian Program

The third paper, "A Critical Examination of the Indian Smallpox Eradication Program," by Dr. Gelfand, is unduly pessimistic. The Indian program, such as it is, and the program in Pakistan, must be credited in large part with the failure of smallpox to spread from Asia to Europe in 1964–

1965. These two countries together constitute one of the greatest masses of infectious smallpox in the world.

The Indian program for the eradication of smallpox was not lightly undertaken, but was preceded by several years of cautious planning and preparation during which the clearly stated objective was the eradication of smallpox. As smallpox continues to occur, we can expect that the defects in the program, such as they are, will be corrected and the campaign carried on to its conclusion.

In eradication programs, when work is inefficient and supervision negligent, the disease itself waits in the background to reveal the true situation. With its dense population concentrated in hundreds of thousands of villages, India represents a most difficult problem. The percentage of vaccination required to terminate smallpox there may well be much higher than in the Americas. Everything possible should be done by the World Health Organization and its member states now free of smallpox to aid in bringing the Indian program to a satisfactory conclusion.

The very scope of the Indian program, with 14,000 persons working with hundreds of millions of doses of vaccine supplied by the USSR, represents a distinct change in the world favoring smallpox eradication. It must be remembered that in the United States itself smallpox persisted until the problem could be taken care of without the organization of a special national campaign. One of the changes favoring the eradication of smallpox in the world today is the recognition by developing countries that they do not have to continue to suffer from certain major eradicable diseases until such time as they are able to develop the finances and staffing for universal general public health programs.

Dr. Gelfand will, in following the eradication program in India during the coming years, find that it, like other serious eradication efforts, has a built-in standard of excellence—zero incidence; this standard is lacking in disease-control programs. In time, the disease being eradicated forces correction of defective administration.

Eradication is never easy and is often slow; inevitably some parts of India will be cleared of smallpox before others; these cleared areas will demand clearance of areas from which reinfection comes. Peripheral pressure from eradicated areas to infected districts works internally within a country as well as internationally.

Changes Favoring Eradication

I would classify the world changes favoring smallpox eradication as (1) improved tools, or improved weapons; (2) international agencies; and (3) altered attitudes.

Among improved tools, better methods of preservation and application of vaccine are most important to success in tropical zones. The first to be mentioned would be electrical refrigeration. In 1943, Dr. James P. Leake wrote: "The electric refrigerator is perhaps the chief cause of the remarkable decline in the number of smallpox cases which the United States has experienced in recent years."

The next important tool is the freeze-dried heat-resistant vaccine. This development makes it unnecessary for developing countries to await the widespread use of electrical refrigeration before eradicating smallpox. This important tool was largely neglected during two decades after its first demonstration. The rehabilitation of this technic can be traced directly to the introduction of smallpox in New York City in 1947. This outbreak called attention to the failure of the Pan American Sanitary Bureau, operating under the Pan American Sanitary Code, to prevent the intercountry spread of smallpox. As director of the Bureau and having no funds with which to call an expert committee on smallpox prevention, I did the next best—or should I say the best—thing; I called in Dr. Leake, a lifelong student of smallpox, retired from the U.S. Public Health Service. In discussing procedures and difficulties of smallpox eradication in the tropics, Dr. Leake spoke of the previous use of freeze-dried vaccine by both The Netherlands and France in their colonial territories. In spite of their success with the freeze-dried vaccine, its use had never reached the Western Hemisphere.

I approached the Surgeon General of the U.S. Public Health Service, who forthwith asked the National Institutes of Health to look into the matter. The National Institutes of Health, in turn, farmed the project out to the Michigan State Laboratory at Lansing, and by the end of 1949, 50,000 doses of freeze-dried vaccine were ready for testing. The field tests, carried out in Peru, showed great superiority of the freeze-dried vaccine over the glycerinated product. Childern vaccinated on one arm with freeze-dried vaccine and on the other with the glycerinated product, each of which had been exposed to room temperature for 30 days, had 94 per cent of takes on one arm and 35 per cent on the other. With this new tool available, the Pan American Sanitary Conference, in 1950, voted a resolution calling for the eradication of smallpox throughout the Western Hemisphere. The campaign for the eradication of smallpox in the Western Hemisphere began with the installation of freeze-dried equipment and the training of technicians in its manufacture in a number of Latin American countries. The results have been most gratifying.

The last paper, "Integration of Jet Injection into a National Smallpox Campaign," (unpublished) read by Dr. Morris, tells how the jet injector reduced the cost of vaccination during field tests in Brazil with increased speed and diminished consumption of vaccine. In spite of the difficulties in servicing and maintaining such mechanical equipment in the field, and in spite of the difficulties of concentrating people for vaccination, the jet injector does hold promise of greatly facilitating the completion of global eradication of smallpox.

The international health agencies—the Pan American Health Organization, the World Health Organization, UNICEF, and the (U.S.) Agency for International Development—each has an important part to play in the eradication of smallpox.

The Pan American Health Organization and the World Health Organization are especially responsible for the coordination of the activities of neighboring countries, the pooling of technical and financial resources, communications at the technical level between workers in different countries, and finally the incrimination and stimulation possible in international meetings. These are all important factors in the organization of regional and global eradication programs; today the situation is entirely different from the days when health workers of neighboring countries communicated with each other only through diplomatic channels.

A most important world change favoring smallpox eradication and the eradication of other diseases is the altered attitude of the technical workers of many nations.

This session, devoted to the global eradication of smallpox, epitomizes this altered attitude. Two decades ago it would have been impossible to hold such a meeting as this in the American Public Health Association. Today there is acceptance of the eradication concept as applicable to certain communicable diseases. It is recognized that certain communicable diseases must be attacked at their sources, that offensive action must be taken against remaining seedbeds of infection. Today we recognize a community of interest of all nations in what happens anywhere; national interest and responsibility do not stop at the frontier. There is a recognition of the responsibility of a nation to its neighbors; we have seen in recent years the response of the United States to pressure brought by neighboring countries for the eradication of the urban vector of yellow fever.

CONCLUSION

I would point to three important steps in developing the global smallpox eradication effort:

1. The rehabilitation of freeze-dried vaccine and the Pan American Health Organization's program for the eradication of smallpox (1950).

2. The USSR proposal for global smallpox eradication and its approval by the World Health Assembly (1958).

3. The U.S. pledge of support for a special drive to complete the eradication of smallpox within the next decade and the World Health Assembly's simultaneous declaration that the eradication of smallpox is one of the main objectives of the World Health Organization (May 1965).

Our generation has no excuse to offer future generations if we continue to permit half of the human race to suffer from smallpox while we attempt to defend ourselves with costly and inefficient quarantine and vaccination certificates.

The selling has been done; the tools are available; support has been assured; the program is already well advanced. The only question is whether our national and the international administrative agencies can measure up to the challenge.

Bibliography
of the Papers of Fred L. Soper

1. N. C. Davis, F. L. Soper, and W. L. Rocha. Field study of hookworm infection. *Bull. Int. Health Board 4:* 155–168, 1924. (Unpublished house organ.)
2. Notas sobre la distribución geográfica de la uncinaria en el Paraguay. *Rev. Soc. Cient. (Paraguay) 1:* 81–82, 1924.
3. Treatment of hookworm disease with a combination of carbon tetrachloride and oil of chenopodium. Comparison of results of simultaneous and delayed administration of magnesium sulphate. *Amer. J. Hyg. 4:* 699–709, 1924.
4. G. E. Coghill and F. L. Soper. The development of the pronephros in relation to the behavior pattern in *Amblystoma. Anat. Rec. 30:* 321–325, 1925.
5. Factors which should determine the selection of an anthelmintic in a geographical area. *Amer. J. Hyg. 5:* 408–453, 1925. Spanish translation: Factores que deben determinar la elección de un antihelmíntico en un área geográfico. *Rev. Soc. Cient. (Paraguay) 2:* 17–66, 1925. (Includes 28 tables not published in the English version.)
6. A simple punch card system for cross-tabulations, adapted to the study of hookworm survey data. *Bull. Int. Health Board 5:* 158–166, 1925. (Unpublished house organ.)
7. Comparison of Stoll and Lane egg-count methods for the estimation of hookworm infestation. *Amer. J. Hyg. 6 (Suppl.):* 62–102, 1926.
8. Tetrachlorethylene (C_2Cl_4) in the treatment of hookworm disease. *Amer. J. Trop. Med. 6:* 451–454, 1926.
9. The report of a nearly pure *Ancylostoma duodenale* infestation in native South American Indians and a discussion of its ethnological significance. *Amer. J. Hyg. 7:* 174–184, 1927.
10. The relative egg-laying function of *Necator americanus* and *Ancylostoma duodenale. Amer. J. Hyg. 7:* 542–560, 1927. Spanish translation: La relación entre el desove del *Necator americanus* y el del *Ancylostoma duodenale.* Sociedad Argentina de Patologia Regional del Norte, Tercera Reunión, Tucuman, Julio 7, 8 y 10 de 1927. Buenos Aires, Imprenta de la Universidad, 16 pp., 1927.
11. Notas sobre a distribuição do *Necator americanus* e o *Ancylostoma duodenale* no Continente Americano; a importancia de uma determinação ulterior. *Bol. Ofic. Sanit. Panamer. 7:* 283–288, 1928.
12. Serviços de febre amarella no Sector Norte do Brasil, de 1 de Janeiro a 31 de Agosto de 1930. *Rev. Hyg. Saude Pub. (Rio) 5:* 1–7, 1931.
13. (With M. Frobisher, Jr., J. A. Kerr, and N. C. Davis.) Studies of the distribution of immunity to yellow fever in Brazil. I. Postepidemic survey of Magé, Rio de Janeiro, by complement-fixation and monkey-protection tests. *J. Prev. Med. 6:* 341–377, 1932.
14. (With Alvaro de Andrade.) Studies of the distribution of immunity to yellow fever in Brazil. II. The disproportion between immunity distribution as re-

vealed by complement-fixation and mouse-protection tests and history of yellow fever attack at Cambucy, Rio de Janeiro. *Amer. J. Hyg. 18:* 588–617, 1933.

15. (With H. Penna, E. Cardoso, J. Serafim, Jr., M. Frobisher, Jr., and J. Pinheiro.) Yellow fever without *Aëdes aegypti.* Study of a rural epidemic in the Valle do Chanaan, Espírito Santo, Brazil, 1932. *Amer. J. Hyg. 18:* 555–587, 1933.

16. (With José Serafim, Jr.) Note on the breeding of *Aëdes (Taeniorhynchus) fluviatilis,* Lutz, in artificial water deposits. *Amer. J. Trop. Med. 13:* 589–590, 1933.

17. Algumas notas a respeito da epidemiologia da febre amarela no Brasil. *Rev. Hyg. Saude Pub. (Rio) 7:* 343–388, 1933. English translation: Some notes on the epidemiology of yellow fever in Brasil. *Rev. Hyg. Saude Pub. (Rio) 8:* 37–61, 73–94, 1934.

18. (With E. R. Rickard and P. J. Crawford.) The routine postmortem removal of liver tissue from rapidly fatal fever cases for the discovery of silent yellow fever foci. *Amer. J. Hyg. 19:* 549–566, 1934.

19. Fiebre amarilla. (Observaciones sobre el problema de la fiebre amarilla en América del Sur.) IXa Conferencia Sanitaria Panamericana, Buenos Aires, Nov. 12–22, 1934. *Actas,* Washington, Pan American Sanitary Bureau, pp. 96–118, 1935. Also published with the title: El problema de la fiebre amarilla en América. *Bol. Ofic. Sanit. Panamer. 14:* 204–213, 1935. Published again in Peru: Las nuevas ideas sobre la fiebre amarilla y sobre la existencia de focos amarilógenos en América. *Reforma Med. (Lima) 20:* 849–857, 1934.

20. Paludismo. (Observaciones sobre la presencia en el continente americano del *Anopheles gambiae.*) IXa Conferencia Sanitaria Panamericana, Buenos Aires, November 12–22, 1934. *Actas,* Washington, Pan American Sanitary Bureau, pp. 226–227. (*Correction:* For Dr. Chagas read Dr. Shannon, and for Argelia read Natal, Brazil.)

21. Fiebre amarilla rural, fiebre amarilla de la selva, como problema nuevo de sanidad en Colombia. *Rev. Hig. (Bogota) 4:* 47–84, 1935. English translation: Rural and jungle yellow fever: a new public health problem in Colombia. Bogota, Editorial Minerva, S.A., 42 pp., 1935.

22. Febre amarella silvestre: novo aspecto epidemiologico da doença. *Rev. Hyg. Saude Pub. (Rio) 10:* 31–70, 1936. English translation: Jungle yellow fever: a new epidemiological entity in South America. *Rev. Hyg. Saude Pub. (Rio) 10:* 107–144, 1936.

23. Recent extensions of knowledge of yellow fever. *Quart. Bull. Health Org. League Nations 5:* 19–68, 1936.

24. The newer epidemiology of yellow fever. *Amer. J. Public Health 27:* 1–14, 1937. Portuguese translation: see paper 26.

25. The geographical distribution of immunity to yellow fever in man in South America. *Amer. J. Trop. Med. 17:* 457–511, 1937. Portuguese translation: Distribuição geográfica na América do Sul da imunidade amarílica no homem. *Rev. Hyg. Saude Pub. (Rio) 12:* 173–228, 1938.

26. Epidemiologia da febre amarella. *Folha Med. (Rio) 18:* 423–430, 1937. (Portuguese translation of paper 24.)

27. Present day methods for the study and control of yellow fever. *Amer. J. Trop. Med. 17:* 655–676, 1937.

28. Vacinação contra a febre amarela no Brasil, de 1930 a 1937. *Arq. Hig. (Rio) 7:* 379–390, 1937.

29. (With H. H. Smith.) Yellow fever vaccination with cultivated virus and immune and hyperimmune serum. *Amer. J. Trop. Med. 18:* 111–134, 1938.

30. (With Henry Beeuwkes, N. C. Davis, and J. A. Kerr.) Transitory immunity to yellow fever in the offspring of immune human and monkey mothers. *Amer. J. Hyg. 27:* 351–363, 1938.

31. Situation de la fièvre jaune au Brésil. *Bull. Office Int. Hyg. Pub. (Paris) 30:* 1205–1208, 1938. English translation: The yellow fever situation in Brazil. Laval (France), Barnéoud, 4 pp., 1938. Spanish translation: La situación de la fiebre amarilla en el Brasil. *Bol. Ofic. Sanit. Panamer. 17:* 510–512, 1938.

32. Yellow fever: the present situation (October, 1938) with special reference to South America. *Trans. Roy. Soc. Trop. Med. Hyg. 32:* 297–332, 1938.

33. (With H. H. Smith.) Vaccination with virus 17D in the control of jungle yellow fever in Brazil. Third International Congresses on Tropical Medicine and Malaria, Amsterdam, Sept. 24–Oct. 1, 1938. *Transactions,* Vol. 1, pp. 295–313, 1938.

34. Progresos en el estudio y control de la fiebre amarilla en Sur América alcanzados entre la IXa y la Xa Conferencias Sanitarias Panamericanas (1934–1938). Xa Conferencia Sanitaria Panamericana, Bogota, Sept. 4–14, 1938. *Actas,* Washington, Pan American Sanitary Bureau, pp. 44–61, 1938. Portuguese translation: Progressos realizados nos estudos e combate da febre amarela entre a IXa e a Xa Conferencias Sanitarias Panamericanas, 1934–1938. *Arq. Hig. (Rio) 9:* 65–86, 1939.

35. El problema del mosquito *Anopheles gambiae* como vector de paludismo. Xa Conferencia Sanitaria Panamericana, Bogota, Sept. 4–14, 1938. *Actas,* Washington, Pan American Sanitary Bureau, pp. 347–349.

36. Summary of activities of the Yellow Fever Service of Ministry of Education of Brazil. *Brazilian Medical Contributions,* Rio de Janeiro, Imprensa Nacional, 17 pp., 1939.

37. (With H. H. Smith and Henrique Penna.) Yellow fever vaccination: field results as measured by the mouse protection test and epidemiological observations. (Abstract and Discussion.) Third International Congress of Microbiology, New York, Sept. 2–9, 1939. *Proceedings,* pp. 351–353, 1939.

38. Yellow fever. In: G. M. Piersol, ed., *The Cyclopedia of Medicine, Surgery and Specialities.* Philadelphia, F. A. Davis Co., Vol. 15, pp. 1086–1108, 1940. Reprinted in 1946 and 1948. Portuguese translation: Febre amarela. *O Hospital (Rio) 22:* 141–171, 1942.

39. Book review: *Carlos Finlay and Yellow Fever* by Carlos E. Finlay. *J. Parasit. 27:* 367–368, 1941.

40. Address (in Portuguese) at the meeting of the Academia Nacional de Medicina (Brazil) celebrating the 25th anniversary of The Rockefeller Foundation in Brazil, held on Nov. 13, 1941. *Bol. Acad. Nac. Med. (Rio) 113:* 45–54, 1941.

41. The pharmacopeia and the physician: treatment of yellow fever. *J. Amer.*

Med. Assn. 118: 374–378, 1942. Correction, *119:* 1212. Spanish translation: La farmacopea y el médico: tratamiento de la fiebre amarilla. *Bol. Ofic. Sanit. Panamer. 21:* 647–656, 1942.

42. (With D. B. Wilson.) Species eradication: a practical goal of species reduction in the control of mosquito-borne disease. *J. Nat. Malaria Soc. 1:* 5–24, 1942. Portuguese translation: Erradicação da espécie, em vez da sua redução, como fim práctico no combate a doenças transmitidas por mosquitos. *Bol. Hig. Saude Pub. (Rio) 1:* 26–46, 1943.

43. Febre amarela panamericana, 1938 a 1942. XIth Pan American Sanitary Conference, Rio de Janeiro, Sept. 7–18, 1942. *Atas* da XIa Conferencia Sanitaria Panamericana, Rio de Janeiro, Government of Brazil, pp. 379–394, 1942. Reprinted in: *Bol. Ofic. Sanit. Panamer. 21:* 1207–1222, 1942.

44. (Observações sobre a campanha contra o mosquito gambiae.) *Atas* da XIa Conferencia Sanitaria Panamericana, Rio de Janeiro, Government of Brazil, pp. 874–875, 1942.

45. (With D. B. Wilson.) Anopheles gambiae in Brazil, 1930 to 1940. New York, The Rockefeller Foundation, 262 pp., 1943.

46. (With D. B. Wilson.) Campanha contra o "Anopheles gambiae" no Brasil, 1939–1942. Rio de Janeiro, Ministério da Educação e Saúde, Serviço de Documentação, 150 pp., 1945. *(Note:* The Portuguese version describes the terminal period of the eradication campaign, giving more details of surveys and statistical data; it omits the detailed description of *Anopheles gambiae* and the discussion of operational procedures used in the campaign.)

47. (With D. B. Wilson, Servulo Lima, and Waldemar Sá Antunes.) The Organization of Permanent Nation-Wide Anti-*Aëdes aegypti* Measures in Brazil. New York, The Rockefeller Foundation, 137 pp., 1943.

48. Yellow fever. In: Z. T. Bercovitz, ed., *Clinical Tropical Medicine.* New York, P. B. Hoeber, Chap. 32, pp. 391–420, 1944.

49. (With W. A. Davis, F. S. Markham, L. A. Riehl, and Paul Buck.) Louse powder studies in North Africa (1943). *Arch. Inst. Pasteur Algerie 23:* 183–223, 1945.

50. La febbre gialla come attuale probleme sanitario. *Rendic. Ist. Sup. Sanit. (Roma) 9:* 529–542, 1946.

51. (With F. W. Knipe, G. Casini, L. A. Riehl, and A. Rubino.) Reduction of anopheles density effected by the preseason spraying of building interiors with DDT in kerosene, at Castel Volturno, Italy, in 1944–1945 and in the Tiber Delta in 1945. *Amer. J. Trop. Med. 27:* 177–200, 1947.

52. (With W. A. Davis, F. S. Markham, and L. A. Riehl.) Typhus fever in Italy, 1943–1945, and and its control with louse powder. *Amer. J. Hyg. 45:* 305–334, 1947.

53. Editorial: Continental eradication of *Aëdes aegypti. Bol. Ofic. Sanit. Panamer. 26:* 898–899, 1947. Spanish translation: Erradicación continental del *Aëdes aegypti. Bol. Ofic. Sanit. Panamer. 26:* 899–901, 1947.

54. (With F. S. Markham, W. A. Davis, and L. A. Riehl.) Notes on experience with powders in the control of typhus in Italy, 1943 to 1945. Primera Reunión Interamericana del Tifo, Mexico, D.F., Oct. 7–13, 1945. *Memorias,* pp. 441–450, 1947.

55. Jungle yellow fever. In: T. G. Hull, ed., *Diseases Transmitted from Animals to Man.* Springfield, Ill., Charles C Thomas, 3d ed., pp. 432–453, 1947. Revised in 1955, 4th ed., pp. 606–625.

56. La fiebre amarilla. *Medico (Buenos Aires) 20:* 253–256, 1948.

57. The pioneer international health organization. *Record (Washington) 4:* 39–44, 1948 (special edition). Reprinted in: *Bol. Ofic. Sanit. Panamer. 27:* 912–916, 1948.

58. Actividades de salubridad internacional en las Américas. *Bol. Ofic. Sanit. Panamer. 27:* 798–805, 1948.

59. Informe sobre el programa de la Oficina Sanitaria Panamericana. *Bol. Ofic. Sanit. Panamer. 27:* 977–997, 1948.

60. (Remarks espousing early regional organizations of the World Health Organization at the First World Health Assembly.) *Official Records of the W.H.O., No. 13,* pp. 69, 70, 117, 253, 254, 255, 258, 259, 271, 272, 274, 1948.

61. Address of the Chairman at the Special Exercises commemorating the demonstration by Walter Reed of mosquito transmission of yellow fever. Fourth International Congresses on Tropical Medicine and Malaria, Washington, D.C., May 10–18, 1948. *Proceedings,* Vol. 1, pp. 40–44, 1948.

62. Species sanitation as applied to the eradication of (a) an invading or (b) an indigenous species. Fourth International Congresses on Tropical Medicine and Malaria, Washington, D.C. May 10–18, 1948. *Proceedings,* Vol. 1, pp. 850–857. Spanish translation: Saneamiento de especies aplicado a la erradicación de (a) una especie invasora o (b) indígena. *Bol. Ofic. Sanit. Panamer. 27:* 603–610, 1948.

63. Foreword. In: G. Giglioli, *Malaria, Filariasis and Yellow Fever in British Guiana.* Georgetown, British Guiana, Mosquito Control Service, Medical Department, 1 p., 1948.

64. Yellow fever. In: *Nelson Loose-Leaf Medicine.* New York, Thomas Nelson & Sons, Vol. II, pp. 87–102, 1948.

65. Species sanitation and species eradication for control of mosquito-borne diseases. In: M. F. Boyd, ed., *Malariology.* Philadelphia, W. B. Saunders, Vol. 2, pp. 1167–1174, 1949.

66. Salubridad internacional. *Bol. Ofic. Sanit. Panamer. 29:* 163–164, 1950.

67. Control de las infecciones oculares en el continente. *Bol. Ofic. Sanit. Panamer. 30:* 457–470, 1951.

68. Introductory remarks of the Director of the Pan American Sanitary Bureau to the IVth Meeting of the Directing Council, Pan American Sanitary Organization, Ciudad Trujillo, Dominican Republic, Sept. 25–30, 1950. Mimeographed Document CD4/7 (Add. 1), pp. 1–7, 1950. (In both English and Spanish.)

69. Notes on the Progress of the Pan American Health Organization, 1947–1950 (translated from the Spanish), XIIIa Conferencia Sanitaria Panamericana, Ciudad Trujillo, Dominican Republic, Oct. 1–10, 1950. *Actas,* Washington, Pan American Sanitary Bureau (Publication No. 261), Vol. 1, pp. 37–44, 1952. Other remarks: pp. 67–68. English version of pp. 37–44: Mimeographed document CSP13/6 (Annex I), pp. 1–9, Sept. 29, 1950.

70. Nation-wide malaria eradication projects in the Americas. V. General princi-

ples of the eradication programs in the Western Hemisphere. *J. Nat. Malaria Soc. 10:* 183–194, 1951.

71. International health. 3. Some aspects of WHO's program in the Americas. *Amer. J. Public Health 41:* 1464–1468, 1951.

72. Yellow fever in the Caribbean. *Bol. Ofic. Sanit. Panamer. 32:* 197–204, 1952.

73. The elephant never forgets. *Amer. J. Trop. Med. Hyg. 1:* 361–368, 1952.

74. Discussion of M.A.C. Dowling's paper: Control of malaria in Mauritius— Eradication of *Anopheles funestus* and *Aëdes aegypti. Trans. Roy. Soc. Trop. Med. Hyg. 47:* 191–193, 1953.

75. Director's General Review, in the Annual Report for 1952 of the Director, Pan American Sanitary Bureau and Regional Office for the Americas of the World Health Organization. Washington, P.A.S.B., Document CD7/3 (Engl.), pp. 3–10, Oct. 1953.

76. *Aëdes aegypti*-transmitted yellow fever as a factor in the international spread of yellow fever. In: African Seminar on Yellow Fever, Kampala, Uganda, Sept. 7–12, 1953. Brazzaville, WHO Regional Office for Africa. Document MH/CT/ 2.54, pp. 104–109, 1954. (Mimeographed, unpublished.)

77. Director's General Review, in the Annual Report for 1953 of the Director, Pan American Sanitary Bureau and Regional Office for the Americas of the World Health Organization. Washington, P.A.S.B., Document CSP14/4 (Engl.), pp. 3–13, July 1954.

77a. International health organization. *J. Amer. Med. Assn. 156:* 1145–1146, 1954. Spanish translation: Organización sanitaria internacional. *Bol. Ofic. Sanit. Panamer. 37:* 503–507, 1954.

78. Address (Inaugural Session). XIVth Pan American Sanitary Conference, Santiago, Chile, Oct. 7–22, 1954. *Proceedings,* Washington, Pan American Sanitary Bureau, Official Document No. 14, English edition, pp. 32–34, 1954. Other remarks: pp. 201, 265–266, 346–347, 351–352. Spanish translation: Official Document No. 14, Spanish edition, pp. 33–34, 212–213, 280–281, 364–366, 370–371, respectively.

79. La erradicación de la malaria en el Hemisferio Occidental. *Bol. Ofic. Sanit. Panamer. 38:* 231–236, 1955.

80. Yellow Fever Conference, Washington, D.C., Dec. 21–22, 1954. Remarks of the Chairman on: Review of the yellow fever menace, pp. 573–582; The question of the yellow fever threat to Asia, pp. 559–603; *Aëdes aegypti* eradication in the Americas, pp. 609–614; and Concluding remarks, pp. 653–654. *Amer. J. Trop. Med. Hyg. 4:* 571–661, 1955. Spanish translation published simultaneously: Conferencia de Fiebre Amarilla. Observaciones del Presidente sobre: Recapitulación histórica del problema de la fiebre amarilla, pp. 2–9; La posibilidad de invasión del continente asiático por la fiebre amarilla, pp. 25–28; Erradicación del *Aëdes aegypti* en las Américas, pp. 34–39; y Observaciones finales, pp. 73–75. *Bol. Ofic. Sanit. Panamer. 39:* 1–82, 1955.

81. *Aëdes aegypti* and malaria eradication programs in Latin America. In: Twenty-Third Annual Conference of the California Mosquito Control Association and the Eleventh Annual Meeting of the American Mosquito Control Association, Los Angeles, Jan. 24–27, 1955. *Proceedings and Papers,* pp. 20–22, 1955.

82. Yellow fever control. *Phila. Med. 51:* 380–381, 409–413, 1955.
83. The unfinished business with yellow fever. In: *Yellow Fever: A Symposium in Commemoration of Carlos Juan Finlay.* Philadelphia, Jefferson Medical College, Sept. 22–23, 1955, pp. 79–88, 1955.
84. Introductory Section—Eight-Year Summary, in the Annual Report for 1954 of the Director, Pan American Sanitary Bureau and Regional Office for the Americas of the World Health Organization. Washington, P.A.S.B., Official Documents No. 11, pp. 1–21, 1955.
85. *Yaws: Its eradication in the Americas.* Washington, Pan American Sanitary Bureau, Office of Public Information, 5 pp., 1956.
86. El concepto de erradicación de las enfermedades transmisibles. *Bol. Ofic. Sanit. Panamer. 42:* 1–5, 1957.
87. La colaboración internacional en el desarrollo y mejoramiento de los servicios de alimentos y drogas en las Américas. *Bol. Ofic. Sanit. Panamer. 44:* 187–190, 1958.
88. International health in the Americas: ten significant years. *J. Lancet 78:* 223–225, 1958. Spanish translation: La salud internacional en las Américas. Diez años trascendentales. *Informaciones de la OPS 2:* 1–4, 1958. (P.A.S.B. house organ.)
89. More about malaria eradication. *Mosquito News 18:* 53–58, 1958.
90. The 1957 status of yellow fever in the Americas. *Mosquito News 18:* 203–216, 1958.
91. International Health in the Americas, 1954–1957: Director's Review. In: 1954–1957 Quadrennial Report and 1957 Annual Report of the Director, Pan American Sanitary Bureau and Regional Director for the Americas of the World Health Organization. Washington, Pan American Sanitary Bureau, Official Documents No. 25, pp. 1–20, 1958.
92. Address (Inaugural Session). XVth Pan American Sanitary Conference, San Juan, Puerto Rico, Sept. 23–Oct. 3, 1958. *Proceedings,* Washington, Pan American Sanitary Bureau, Official Document No. 27, English edition, pp. 52–53, 1958. Status of *Aëdes aegypti* eradication in the Americas, pp. 105–108; Status of Malaria eradication in the Americas, pp. 137–138; (Remarks after being designated Director Emeritus), pp. 212–215. Spanish translations, as published in the Spanish edition of Official Document No. 27: pp. 52–54, 108–111, 142–143, 223–226, respectively.
93. Some international aspects of virus diseases. *Minnesota Med. 42:* 88–91, 1959.
94. Address as Retiring Director at Oath of Office Ceremonies for Dr. Abraham Horwitz, Washington, Jan. 15, 1959. *PAHO Quart. 3:* 18–20, 1959. Excerpts in *Public Health Rep. 74:* 274–275, 1959.
95. Introduction of DDT to Italy, 1943–1945. *Riv. Parassit. 20:* 403–409, 1959.
96. Discussions. In: International Conference on Live Poliovirus Vaccines, 1st, Washington, D.C., June 22–26, 1959. Washington, Pan American Sanitary Bureau, Scientific Publication No. 44, pp. 301, 637, 647, 684–685, 1959.
97. The epidemiology of a disappearing disease: malaria. *Amer. J. Trop. Med. Hyg. 9:* 357–366, 1960.
98. Eradication versus control in communicable disease prevention. *J. Amer. Vet.*

Med. Assn. 137: 234–238, 1960. Spanish translation: La erradicación y el control en la prevención de enfermedades transmisibles. *Bol. Ofic. Sanit. Panamer. 49:* 121–131, 1960.

99. (Address on receiving the Order of Boyacá.) Eleventh Meeting, Directing Council of the Pan American Health Organization, Washington, Sept. 21–30, 1960. Washington, Pan American Sanitary Bureau, Official Document No. 32, English edition, p. 114. Spanish original in Official Document No. 32, Spanish edition, pp. 124–125, 1960.

100. (Discussion.) In: Symposium on Pesticides, Brazzaville, Republic of the Congo, Nov. 9–13, 1959. Geneva, World Health Organization, Doc. MHO/PA/40.60, pp. 144–145, 160, 192–193, 1960. (Mimeographed, unpublished.)

101. (Discussion.) In: Second International Conference on Live Poliovirus Vaccines, Washington, D.C., June 6–10, 1960. Washington, Pan American Sanitary Bureau, Scientific Publication No. 50, pp. 598–599, 1960.

102. Epidemiology (summary). In: SEATO Conference on Cholera, Dacca, East Pakistan, Dec. 5–8, 1960. *Public Health Rep. 76:* 330–331, 1961.

103. International Cooperation Administration Expert Panel on Malaria (Chairman: F. L. Soper). Report and recommendations on malaria: a summary. *Amer. J. Trop. Med. Hyg. 10:* 451–502, 1961. Spanish translation: El paludismo: métodos para su erradicación. Mexico City, Agencia para el Desarrollo Internacional, p. 126, 1963.

104. Public health on an international basis. Conference of State and Provincial Health Authorities of North America, 75th annual meeting, Detroit, Nov. 11, 1961. *Proceedings,* pp. 26–32, 1961.

105. Problems to be solved if the eradication of tuberculosis is to be realized. *Amer. J. Public Health 52:* 734–745, 1962. Spanish translation: Problemas por resolver para lograr la erradicación de la tuberculosis. *Bol. Ofic. Sanit. Panamer. 52:* 378–390, 1962.

106. The elimination of urban yellow fever in the Americas through the eradication of *Aëdes aegypti. Amer. J. Public Health 53:* 7–16, 1963.

107. Book review: *A Textbook of Malaria Eradication* by Emilio Pampana. *Amer. J. Trop. Med. Hyg. 12:* 936–939, 1963.

108. An island of eradication—the college campus. *J. Amer. Coll. Health Assn. 12:* 153–169, 1963.

109. Aegypti and gambiae: eradication of African invaders in the Americas. In: 50th Annual Meeting of the New Jersey Mosquito Extermination Association and the 19th Annual Meeting of the American Mosquito Control Association, Atlantic City, New Jersey, March 12–15, 1963. *Proceedings,* pp. 152–160. Spanish translation: Erradicación en las Américas de los invasores africanos *Aëdes aegypti* y *Anopheles gambiae. Bol. Ofic. Sanit. Panamer. 55:* 259–266, 1963.

110. The relation of malaria eradication to the general health service (summary). In: Seventh International Congresses on Tropical Medicine and Malaria, Rio de Janeiro, Sept. 1–11, 1963. *Proceedings,* Vol. 5, pp. 196–197, 1964.

111. Gorgas Memorial Laboratory. *Trop. Med. Hyg. News 14:* 14–18, 1965.

112. Rehabilitation of the eradication concept in prevention of communicable diseases. *Public Health Rep. 80:* 855–869, 1965.

113. The 1964 status of *Aëdes aegypti* eradication and yellow fever in the Americas. *Amer. J. Trop. Med. Hyg. 14:* 887–891, 1965.

114. What price tuberculosis? *Clin. Proc. Child. Hosp. District of Columbia 21:* 293–295, 1965.

115. Book review: *Papeles de Finlay* by César Rodríguez Expósito. *Bull. Hist. Med. 40:* 490, 1966.

116. Smallpox—world changes and implications for eradication. *Amer. J. Public Health 56:* 1652–1656, 1966.

117. Paris green in the eradication of *Anopheles gambiae:* Brazil, 1940; Egypt, 1945. *Mosquito News 26:* 470–476, 1966.

118. The eradication of *Aëdes aegypti:* a world problem. Ninth International Congress for Microbiology, Moscow, USSR, July 24–30, 1966. *Proceedings Symposia.* Oxford, Pergamon Press, pp. 599–605, 1966.

119. Sedgwick Memorial Medal for 1966: response by Dr. Soper. *Amer. J. Public Health 57:* 164–165, 1967. Spanish translation: Palabras de aceptación. *Bol. Ofic. Sanit. Panamer. 62:* 177–178, 1967.

120. Book review: *World Eradication of Infectious Diseases* by E. Harold Hinman. *Amer. J. Trop. Med. Hyg. 16:* 381–384, 1967.

121. *Aëdes aegypti* and yellow fever. *Bull. WHO 36:* 521–527, 1967. Spanish translation, with summaries in Portuguese and French: *Bol. Ofic. Sanit. Panamer. 64:* 187–196, 1968.

122. Acceptance Speech—Leon Bernard Foundation Medal and Prize. Geneva, World Health Organization, Official Records No. 161, Part II, pp. 123–125, 1967.

123. Dynamics of *Aëdes aegypti* distribution and density: seasonal fluctuations in the Americas. *Bull. WHO 36:* 536–538, 1967.

The publications listed in the Bibliography have been placed on file with the National Library of Medicine, Bethesda, Maryland.

Addendum

In his position of Director of the Pan American Sanitary Bureau and Regional Director for the Americas of the World Health Organization, Dr. Soper attended all the World Health Assemblies that took place during his tenure of office. The World Health Organization is the Secretariat of the World Health Assembly.

The published proceedings of six of the Assemblies contain summaries of the remarks that Dr. Soper made. These summaries are not verbatim reports and have been omitted from the Bibliography. They are cited below:

A. Summary of statements regarding the International Sanitary Regulations. Fourth World Health Assembly, Geneva, Switzerland, May 1951. Geneva, World Health Organization Official Records No. 37, pp. 246–247, 292, 295, 297, 1952.

B. Summary of statements regarding the Annual Report of the Director-General (of W.H.O.) for 1953. Seventh World Health Assembly, Geneva, May 1954. Geneva, W.H.O. Official Records No. 55, pp. 194, 196, 1954.

C. Summary of statements regarding the Annual Report of the Director-General (of W.H.O.) for 1954. Eighth World Health Assembly, Mexico, D.F., May 1955. Geneva, W.H.O. Official Records No. 63, pp. 169–170, 1955.

D. Summary of statements regarding the Annual Report of the Director-General (of W.H.O.) for 1955. Ninth World Health Assembly, Geneva, May 1956. Geneva, W.H.O. Official Records No. 71, pp. 179–180, 1956.

E. Summary of statements regarding the Annual Report of the Director-General (of W.H.O.) for 1956. Tenth World Health Assembly, Geneva, May 1957. Geneva, W.H.O. Official Records No. 79, pp. 220–222, 226–228, 1957.

F. Summary of statements regarding the Annual Report of the Director-General (of W.H.O.) for 1957. Eleventh World Health Assembly, Minneapolis, Minnesota, May–June 1958. Geneva, W.H.O. Official Records No. 87, pp. 172–176, 179–180, 1958.

Index

545